PRIMARY CARE
Tools for Clinicians

PRIMARY CARE
Tools for Clinicians

A Compendium of Forms, Questionnaires, and Rating Scales
for Everyday Practice

LORRAINE LORETZ, DPM, MSN, FNP

Family Nurse Practitioner
UMassMemorial – Marlborough Hospital
Marlborough, Massachusetts

Formerly:
Podiatric Physician
Davis, California

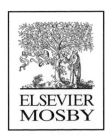

ELSEVIER
MOSBY

11830 Westline Industrial Drive
St.Louis, Missouri 63146

NOTICE

International Standard Book Number 0-323-01983-8

Executive Publisher: *Robin Carter*
Developmental Editor: *Deanna Davis*
Publishing Services Manager: *Catherine Albright Jackson*
Senior Project Manager: *Celeste Clingan*
Designer: *Amy Buxton*

Printed in the USA

Last digit is the print number: 9   8   7   6   5   4   3   2   1

Preface

When I entered primary care practice as a nurse practitioner, I was overwhelmed with the volume of information necessary for documentation of patient encounters. During my years as a specialist in podiatric medicine and surgery, I had developed a concise number of documentation forms, easily organized and pertaining to one specific area. In contrast, the breadth of primary care encounters was astounding. Well-child visits, preoperative 'clearances', sports physicals, well-woman 'check-ups', disability exams, not to mention routine office visits and physicals, were all completed in the course of a day's work. Each of these encounters required different pieces of information to be clearly documented in order to satisfy the needs of the practice, the insurance industry, and governmental agencies. How was I to be sure of gathering and documenting all of the information essential to current standards of care and required by supervisory administrative bodies?

Another area of practice which left me frazzled was the inability to access practice tools. In my professional graduate education, I had been introduced to hundreds of useful rating scales, standardized questionnaires, charts and measures on a variety of topics. Most of these were now buried deeply in my class notes that were filed away at home by subject. If only all of these practical tools could be gathered in one place for immediate access at my place of employment. Thus the seed for *Primary Care Tools for Clinicians* was planted.

The concept of combining documentation forms and published rating scales, measures and charts into one text is unique, yet makes sense. Both groups of tools are used to document patient findings. Forms, questionnaires, and logs record information gathered by the clinician in a logical and organized fashion. Rating scales and measures use responses to questions that have been scientifically tested for accuracy to calculate a score that assists in diagnosis and treatment planning. Charts are used to compare patient findings to a norm or standard. By placing a wide variety of these instruments in one text, the reader has a choice of tools for documentation in everyday practice.

This text is divided into two parts. Part One compiles documentation forms and questionnaires into seven chapter headings encompassing areas of adult evaluations, logs and records, pediatric evaluations, sports medicine, mental health, nutrition and specialized evaluations. Because clinicians have individual preferences for documentation style, many of these forms are customizable by the reader by using interactive versions of the files provided on CD-ROM. Part Two contains nine chapters of quantifiable measures within the subject headings of pediatrics and development, mental health, geriatrics, general health status, pain assessment, wound evaluation, nutrition, specialty tools, and social/spiritual assessment. Intended to be used as a reference volume without recommending one tool over another, this book is designed to promote awareness of the types of measures that have been developed from many health-related areas that are of interest to primary care practitioners.

Throughout this text the terms 'clinician' and 'primary care provider' are used to represent all professional primary care providers. These include medical doctors, doctors of osteopathy, nurse practitioners, physician assistants, clinical nurse specialists, and other health care professionals who provide primary care services. It is my hope that this text will be of value to the clinician and health professional student who seek to improve patient data collection, and will serve as a resource for primary care documentation needs.

Reader Comments

If you would like to express your opinions about *Primary Care Tools for Clinicians*, you may e-mail your comments to tools4clinicians@yahoo.com. The author and publisher of this text welcome suggestions for additions, changes, or other topic areas to include in future editions.

Lorraine Loretz, DPM, MSN, FNP

Acknowledgments

I am indebted to the many people who made this text possible. My heartfelt gratitude goes to Robin Carter, Executive Publisher at Elsevier, for believing in this project and for the opportunity to bring my dream of this volume from concept to reality. Editorial thanks also goes to Deanna Davis and Barbara Cicalese for their help with keeping me on track, to Marie Thomas for accomplishing the daunting task of obtaining permissions to reproduce the tools, to the Elsevier production team, headed by Celeste Clingan, for creating the look and style for this text, and multimedia team with Ken Wendling and Tyson Sturgeon for producing the CD-ROM. Copyright permission was requested to reproduce tools included in this text, and I am grateful to the scale developers and distributors for their consent. The staff at the Lamar Soutter Library at the University of Massachusetts Medical School in Worcester, Massachusetts, assisted me in locating elusive reference materials; I am thankful for their help.

Constructive criticism and review of book material by colleagues were essential for completion of this compendium. Without the thoughtful input and suggestions from innumerable people, compilation of the wide breadth of materials contained in this text would not have been possible. I would like to acknowledge the following persons for tool recommendations, formatting suggestions, review of documentation forms, testing of customizable forms, and professional dialogue: Pamela Alix-Bloznalis, MD; Eileen Aubuchon, NP; Christine Betzold, NP; Lois Brenneman, NP; Eric Cardin, PT; Jean Casello, MD; Andy Craig NP; Marilyn Edmunds, PhD, NP; Sylvia Escott-Stump, RD; Linda Greenspan, DO; Kristal Imperio, NP; Sonia Lawson, OT; L. Kathleen Mahan, RD; Priscilla Merrill, NP; Karima Miller NP; David Mittman, PA; Ira Monka, DO; Leonard Moss, DO; Connie Paczkowski, NP; Ellen Pateman, RN; Lori Martin Plank NP; Judy Pollacheck, PhD, NP; Melinda L. Poso, NP; Lori Quinn, PT; Chris Robertozzi, DPM; Judi Shea-Vaillancourt, NP ; Yvonne Shelton, MD; Lynn Speed, NP; Tracey Stesner, Gail Stuart, PhD, RN, Karen Wetherbee NP; Frank Winn, PA; and Debbie Woods NP. Additionally, the encouragement and support from my many colleagues and friends was invaluable and convinced me of the need for this text.

Lastly I would like to thank my family, Michael, Rebecca, and Eric Leach, for tolerating the late nights and the stress that came with this project; their patience is very much appreciated.

Contributor

Eric Cardin, MS, PT
Fitness Forum
Raynham, Massachusetts

Chapter 11: *Health Status Measures*

Contents

Italicized page numbers refer to page locations of the reprinted tool.

PART TWO

MEASUREMENT TOOLS AND RATING SCALES

8   Developmental and Pediatric Tools, 195

9 Behavioral and Psychiatric Instruments, 237

PRIMARY CARE
Tools for Clinicians

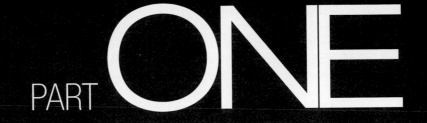

PART ONE

Documentation Forms, Logs, and Questionnaires

Introduction to Chapters One through Seven

Many thousands of forms are developed by individuals, clinics, hospitals, private and public institutions, and educators. Health care professionals are notorious for having independent opinions regarding documentation; often, the first change implemented in a new practice is the redesign of medical record forms. Rarely do two clinicians within one office agree on the precise method of documentation. Concerns about reimbursement, third-party audits, standards of care, patient privacy, and the need to efficiently communicate medical findings serve to complicate the often anguishing search for the ideal documentation device.

Because of the tremendous effort required for the development of medical record documentation systems, the clinician often continues with an older and familiar but ineffective system. Practice commitments may preclude the time it takes to research and develop improvements in record-keeping. Resources for current standardized clinical guidelines, performance measurement data, and insurance reimbursement requirements are widely scattered in handbooks, newsletters, journals, and cyberspace and may be buried within agency publications. The busy clinician may choose to purchase printed forms or invest in an electronic medical record system; but preprinted forms may have deficiencies, and expensive electronic medical records require a steep learning curve. Neither system may provide the flexibility in documentation design that a clinician desires, nor does either system usually address specialized medical topics.

The goal of this portion of the text is to provide the user with a range of concise documentation forms covering a variety of primary care areas. Newly created forms and logs incorporating current clinical standards have been designed to allow customization of forms by the reader. Previously published specialty forms and questionnaires are gathered here for providers to use as needed. Because guidelines for clinical practice are updated regularly, resources for access to this information are cited in this Introduction. Lastly, resources for the reader to seek further information on clinical topics and sources for additional forms and tools are provided within each chapter.

Contents of Part One

The purpose of this section is to provide forms, logs, and questionnaires to be used for medical information collection and documentation. A form may be used in three ways: as direct documentation that becomes part of a legal, paper-based medical record; as a collection tool, used to gather data that are later dictated or entered into an electronic record; and as a training tool that assists the health care professional student in organizing thought processes for gathering pertinent medical data in a standardized fashion.

Documentation forms printed in Part One and included on the CD-ROM have been designed to include the standard components of the history and physical examination for each patient subgroup. The history and physical examination forms are intended to document a baseline record of patient information. Logs and records provide the reader with the tools necessary to incorporate health maintenance and disease prevention into daily practice by tracking health care information such as vaccinations, prescription medications, and results of laboratory tests and other studies. Previously published questionnaires provide the clinician with more focused information in specific clinical areas.

When they are not copyright-protected, forms may be personalized with letterhead and photocopied for office use. However, each user should carefully examine the form to ensure that it meets all patient documentation needs for the practice. With the use of the enclosed CD-ROM, many forms may be altered to meet the needs of the practice by following instructions included on the CD-ROM. Customization can include the addition of practice-identifying information in the upper right corner of the form, or this space may be used for patient addressograph data. Clinicians may choose to add or delete cue boxes, increase or decrease space allowed for undirected narrative notes, add or delete lines for note space, and modify medical terminology. Forms are composed with the standard SOAP (Subjective, Objective, Assessment, Plan) format; however, clinicians may choose to alter or expand the format to incorporate a different model, such as SOOOAAP (Subjective, Objective, Opinion, Options, Advice, Agreed Plan).[1]

Use of these forms in a paper-based medical record system offers several advantages. The forms are inexpensive, may be easily customized to meet the needs of the clinician, and require little training to use. Paper systems are not prone to mechanical failure, are completely portable, and provide a means for simple data entry. Drawbacks to the paper-based record include increased requirements for personnel to maintain, organize, and file the charts; likelihood of misplacement of records; and unavailability at multiple clinical sites. Issues of legibility, inconsistencies in the ways that different providers record data, and difficulty in tracking health maintenance behaviors are also disadvantages to a paper-based system.

Electronic medical records systems have become technologically advanced and offer many advantages over handwritten documentation. It is not the focus of this text to debate the advantages and disadvantages of electronic medical record systems in comparison with paper. Although forms in this text have been designed for use in a paper-based system, the clinician can also use the forms for gathering information, which can later be incorporated into an electronic record.

Box **1**   What this text does:
• Provides a variety of history and physical documentation forms from which to choose or adapt for individual practice purposes • Provides documentation logs and records for health maintenance management • Summarizes the content of the forms and tools within subject chapters • Cites current guidelines for standards of primary care practice and incorporates these standards into documentation forms

---

Box **2**   What this text does not do:
• Instruct the reader in how to implement the forms within his or her practice management structure • Teach techniques for gathering histories or performing examinations • Recommend one form over another • Provide patient health counseling information

The Medical Record

A medical record is a confidential document kept for each patient by a health care professional, group, or organization. In addition to patient demographic information, it contains the patient's medical history and documentation of each encounter, which includes symptoms, examination findings, assessment, and treatment provided. Copies of results of laboratory tests and other studies, records of prescribed medications, and professional correspondence are also included. The medical record is used to monitor patient care, support billing claims, and assess patterns of medical service delivery. With permission, it can be shared with or transferred to other professionals who are involved in the patient's care. The structured record also facilitates coding, compliance monitoring, and auditing procedures. The medical record can be submitted as evidence in a court case and, as such, is considered to be part of the legal record. It may also be used to substantiate disability or other insurance claims. Because the medical record may be used for these diverse purposes, it is important for the provider to include as much pertinent information as possible in the database.

In light of its uses, the following criteria are of utmost importance in maintaining a medical record:

- At a minimum, the patient's name, medical record number, and date of encounter should appear on every page.
- Late entries must be clearly and accurately noted as such.
- All entries must be legibly recorded.
- All statements, observations, procedures, recommendations, actions, and outcomes must be accurately and completely reported.
- Notes should contain sufficient detail to clearly demonstrate why the course of treatment was chosen.
- The medical record must clearly indicate who entered the data.
- The record should be organized in a fashion that facilitates retrieval of patient data by clinicians, staff, auditors, and researchers with permitted access.

Health Care Quality and Performance Measurement

Medical records are reviewed by health care organizations to conduct performance measurements in order to promote health care quality improvement, to monitor use of medical services, and to demonstrate accountability to the public. The clinician needs to be aware of standards set by various agencies and the performance tracking measures that are conducted by private health care organizations. By following guidelines set by these agencies, the clinician can create a medical record that incorporates documentation of recommended preventive practice measures and meets the requirements of private health care organizations for reimbursement.

Health care quality is tracked by government agencies, private nonprofit organizations, and private health care organizations. The generalized goal for all agencies is improvement of health care quality for everyone. Underlying objectives include reimbursement issues and malpractice risk reduction. Many public and private groups set health care standards and track performance. The organizations described here are prominent in their activities.

Government agencies include the U.S. Department of Health and Human Services' Office of Disease Prevention and Health Promotion (ODPHP),[2] which launched the PPIP (Put Prevention Into Practice) program in 1994 to improve implementation of the recommendations of the U.S. Preventive Services Task Force (USPSTF). The USPSTF is an independent panel of experts in primary care and prevention that systematically reviews the evidence of effectiveness and develops recommendations for clinical preventive services. The USPSTF produced the *Guide to Clinical Preventive Services* (second edition), which provides recommendations on preventive interventions: screening tests, counseling, immunizations, and chemoprophylactic regimens for more than 80 conditions.[3] The most recent edition of the *Guide to Clinical Preventive Services* updates some recommendations from the second edition and evaluates additional new topics.[4] Recommendations from the Task Force are being released incrementally, as they become available.

PIPP is a program designed to increase the appropriate use of clinical preventive services—such as screening tests, immunizations, and counseling—according to USPSTF recommendations.[5] In 1998 management of the PIPP project was transferred to the U.S. Department of Health and Human Services' Agency for Healthcare Research and Quality (AHRQ) and is now part of AHRQ's integrated program in clinical disease prevention services.[6] AHRQ, in partnership with the American Medical Association and the American Association of Health Plans, also sponsors the National Guideline Clearinghouse, a public resource for evidence-based clinical practice guidelines.[7]

The U.S. Department of Health and Human Services agency Centers for Medicare & Medicaid Services produces the *Documentation Guidelines for Evaluation and Management Services*.[8] These medical record documentation guidelines explain appropriate use of the evaluation and management codes related to Medicare comprehensive multisystem examination and single-system examination. Compliance with these guidelines for documentation is critical for receiving reimbursement for Medicare services.

Independent nonprofit organizations include the National Committee for Quality Assurance, which evaluates and reports on the quality of managed care plans with the Health Plan Employer Data and Information Set (HEDIS) and through a comprehensive member satisfaction survey.[9] HEDIS is a tool used to measure performance of many significant public health issues by managed health care plans and includes a standardized survey of consumers' experiences that evaluates plan performance in areas such as customer service, access to care, and claims.[10] Foundation for Accountability is another not-for-profit national organization that conducts research and disseminates information to consumers with the goal of encouraging them to help shape the system and hold it accountable for quality.[11] The Joint Commission on Accreditation of Healthcare Organizations (JCAHO) is an independent, not-for-profit organization that evaluates and accredits nearly 17,000 health care organizations and programs in the United States.[12] Since 1951, the JCAHO has developed professionally based standards and evaluated the compliance of health care organizations against these benchmarks. Integration of performance measurement data into the accreditation process was accomplished through the implementation of the ORYX initiative in 1997.[13] Identification and use of standardized, or core, performance measures is a primary component of the ORYX initiative.

The reader who is interested in examining the various health care performance measures can access the individual websites cited in Resources and References. The reference text by Carolyn Buppert[14] gives an excellent summary and comparison of performance measures, as well as extensive guidelines for managing medical data to meet auditing standards, and is highly recommended for all practicing clinicians.

Support for Use of Forms

Scientific studies that compare the use of a documentation form or template with use of a narrative note can be found throughout the literature. Significant advantages of using a form include more consistent and detailed information transfer,[15] higher gross billing and greater physician satisfaction,[16] higher rates of completion of specific clinical details and clinical staff acceptance for use of the form,[17] and more complete documentation as compared with handwritten charts.[18] Formatted charts have been found to improve the documentation process and to allow more time for patient-physician interaction.[19] Additionally, a structured encounter form was found to be very effective in improving documentation of almost all aspects of well-child care.[20] Structured questionnaires also provided more and better information, and their use improved clinical response to risk factors.[21]

Delivery of preventive health care services has been improved through effective office systems for documentation and tracking,[22] and use of checklists has been shown to facilitate identification of health problems among adolescent girls.[23] Summary reports indicate that structured encounter forms have been effective in improving documentation of well-child care and well-adult care,[24] and case-finding and screening instruments can dramatically

Box **3**	Advantages in the use of documentation forms

- Improves organized documentation of data collected during the office visit
- Allows more time for the patient visit by reducing documentation time
- Increases clinician satisfaction with the documentation process
- Allows for consistency in documentation among clinicians in group practice
- Provides cues for the medical evaluation that may assist the clinician during busy or stressful times
- Collects data systematically, which makes leaving important facts out less likely
- Facilitates communication between clinicians regarding an individual patient's care
- Improves legibility, which facilitates review of records by other persons
- Allows more effective and efficient searching for patient data
- Allows ease in documentation of negative findings, which may be overlooked in handwritten documentation because of time constraints, providing protection from litigation
- Reduces errors associated with transcription when form is completed at the time of patient visit
- Reduces malpractice and audit risks by consistently and comprehensively recording patient encounters
- Increases gross billing by minimizing downcoding caused by inadequate documentation
- Facilitates third-party payer review for quality assurance and coding issues
- Is relatively inexpensive and requires minimal training

Box **4**	Disadvantages in the use of documentation forms

- Requires cooperation among staff members for consistent implementation of forms
- Necessitates acceptance and cooperation by all clinicians in a group practice
- May be redundant if narrative, dictated, or computerized documentation is also used
- May encourage clinician dependence on cues contained in the form rather than critical thinking and engagement of the patient in conversation
- May limit documentation to the form components (i.e., not all information discussed or gathered may be recorded)

improve the practitioner's efficiency and increase the productivity of clinicians in finding new and treatable problems in older patients.[25]

In summary, use of forms or templates helps to guide and improve the accuracy of patient evaluation documentation. Systematic presentation, ease of use, and convenience reduce the burden of documentation and allow the clinician more time to focus on his or her relationship with the patient.

Drawbacks in Use of Forms

Records in which paper forms are used require cooperation among staff and clinicians for completion of patient data entries or a redistribution of responsibilities among office staff. Inadequate staffing, frequent staff turnover, or unwillingness of staff or clinicians to comply with form systems will undermine attempts to institute consistent form completion.

Use of a form for data collection or documentation may lead to attention being focused only on the points listed on the form, which may result in the clinician missing nuances in the patient history or examination findings. A patient evaluation without dependence on forms may allow the clinician an opportunity to fully investigate and engage with the patient, without the distraction of a form. This undirected method of patient assessment, with resultant detailed narrative documentation, is ideally suited for the student or inexperienced clinician, so that he or she may gain more speed and confidence in interviewing, examination, and documentation skills. Because of time constraints, the experienced clinician may choose to document findings on a template form after conducting an undirected patient interview.

Content Disclaimer

With the exception of questionnaires, the forms contained in this chapter are not meant for patient use. They are a means for the clinician to record information essential for documentation in the medical record. Although the forms contain cues for history-taking and physical examination components, sole reliance on the cues contained within the forms is inappropriate. Optimal clinical skills include knowledge of investigative questions; sensitivity to the autonomy of the patient; and awareness of the patient's perceptions, beliefs, expectations, and goals. Proficiency in performing the physical examination, knowledge of appropriate diagnostic and treatment options, and provision of educational information cannot be implied by completion of a form.

Forms included in this book are not meant to be a substitute for competent didactic and practical knowledge, nor can use of these forms substitute for insufficient primary care skills. It is assumed that the reader and user of these forms has adequate knowledge of the complete history-taking process and is competent in performing all aspects of the physical examination. If the reader is unfamiliar with any of the components of the forms, he or she may refer to one of the sources listed in Resources and References at the end of each chapter for more information. It is also presumed that the reader understands the terminology and standard medical abbreviations contained in the forms. If terminology is unfamiliar to the reader, referral to Appendix B or one of the listed references is recommended for clarification before the form is used in practice. The forms included in this text provide no guidance for diagnosis and treatment protocols. The user should be capable of making an effective differential diagnosis and formulating a treatment plan before he or she uses these forms.

Content of the forms contained in this text is based on current published guidelines for health care of infants, children, adolescents, and adults. However, the information included in these forms does not indicate an exclusive course of action, nor does it represent a standard of medical care. Because standards in the field may change rapidly, information may need to be updated according to release of new data or recommendations. The reader is advised to consult other sources to confirm information contained within this text and to update information as necessary. The author and publisher do not assume responsibility for omissions or inaccuracies in materials in this text or for any consequences resulting from the use of information from this text.

Website link citations are independently run sites outside of the publisher's domain. The author and publisher are not responsible for the privacy practices, activities, or content of such independent sites. Inclusion of website citations does not indicate endorsement of any claims or recommendations made by said websites. Website information and link addresses may change frequently; although website information is accurate at press time, the reader is advised to conduct a general online search for the reference information if the website link becomes invalid.

Resources and References

1. Teichman PG: Documentation tips for reducing malpractice risk, *Fam Pract Manag* 7:29-33, 2000.
2. Office of Disease Prevention and Health Promotion, United States Department of Health and Human Services, Washington, DC. Created by Congress in 1976, the Office of Disease Prevention and Health Promotion (ODPHP) plays a vital role in developing and coordinating a wide range of national disease prevention and health promotion strategies. Links to current projects, resources, infrastructure policies and publications are included at this website. Website: http://www.odphp.osophs.dhhs.gov/
3. Agency for Healthcare Research and Quality: U.S. Preventive Services Task Force (USPSTF), 1996. *Reviews and recommendations: guide to clinical preventive services*, ed 2. Provides the latest available recommendations on preventive interventions: screening tests, counseling, immunizations, and chemoprophylactic regimens for more than 80 conditions. Includes periodic health examination and age-specific charts. Website: http://www.ahrq.gov/clinic/cpsix.htm
4. Agency for Healthcare Research and Quality: U.S. Preventive Services Task Force (USPSTF), 2004. *Reviews and recommendations: guide to clinical preventive services*, ed 3. Updates some recommendations from the second edition and evaluates additional new topics. Recommendations from the Task Force are being released incrementally, as they become available. Website: http://www.ahcpr.gov/clinic/cps3dix.htm
5. Agency for Healthcare Research and Quality (AHRQ): *Put Prevention into Practice (PPIP)*. A program to increase the appropriate use of clinical preventive services, such as screening tests, immunizations, and counseling, based on U.S. Preventive Services Task Force recommendations. Website: http://www.ahrq.gov/clinic/ppipix.htm
6. Agency for Healthcare Research and Quality (AHRQ): A division of the United States Department of Health and Human Services, the AHRQ offers extensive information and publications on clinical practice guidelines, clinical preventive services, information quality guidelines, grants, research findings, quality assessment, public health preparedness, and other health care issues. Website: http://www.ahcpr.gov/
7. Agency for Healthcare Research and Quality (AHRQ): National Guideline Clearinghouse (NGC). The NGC is a comprehensive database of evidence-based clinical practice guidelines and related documents produced by the Agency for Healthcare Research and Quality (AHRQ), U.S. Department of Health and Human Services, in partnership with the American Medical Association (AMA) and the American Association of Health Plans–Health Insurance Association of America (AAHP-HIAA). The NGC mission is to provide physicians, nurses, and other health professionals, health care providers, health plans, integrated delivery systems, purchasers, and others an accessible mechanism for obtaining objective, detailed information on clinical practice guidelines and to further their dissemination, implementation and use. Website: http://www.guideline.gov
8. Centers for Medicare & Medicaid Services: *Documentation guidelines for evaluation and management services*. Baltimore: 1997, Centers for Medicare & Medicaid Services. Available at http://www.cms.hhs.gov/medlearn/emdoc.asp
9. National Committee for Quality Assurance (NCQA): NCQA is a private, nonprofit organization dedicated to improving health care quality everywhere. NCQA is active in quality oversight and improvement initiatives at all levels of the health care system. NCQA is best known for its work in assessing and reporting on the quality of the nation's managed care plans through accreditation and performance measurement programs. Website: http://www.ncqa.org
10. National Committee for Quality Assurance (NCQA): Health Plan Employer Data and Information Set (HEDIS). Sponsored, supported, and maintained by the NCQA, HEDIS is a set of standardized performance measures designed to ensure that purchasers and consumers have the information they need to reliably compare the performance of managed health care plans. The performance measures in HEDIS are related to many significant public health issues such as cancer, heart disease, smoking, asthma, and diabetes. Website: http://www.ncqa.org/programs/hedis/index.htm
11. Foundation for Accountability (FAACT): FAACT is a national organization improving health care for Americans by advocating for an accountable and accessible system in which consumers are partners in their care and help shape the delivery of care. Consumer and provider resources include quality measures, presentations, and news updates on health care delivery issues. Web site: http://www.facct.org
12. Joint Commission on Accreditation of Healthcare Organizations (JCAHO): An independent, not-for-profit organization, the JCAHO evaluates and accredits more than 16,000 health care organizations and programs in the United States. Information for providers and the general public includes information on facility accreditation, disease-specific care certification, performance measurement, news updates, and public policy initiatives. Website: http://www.jcaho.org
13. Joint Commission on Accreditation of Healthcare Organizations (JCAHO): Facts about ORYX. The ORYX initiative integrates outcomes and other performance measurement data into the accreditation process to increase the value of accreditation. Data collected on standardized, or core, performance measures are identified and used by the JCAHO to assist in on-site survey evaluation activities. Website: http://www.jcaho.org/accredited+organizations/hospitals/ oryx/oryx+facts.htm
14. Buppert C: *The primary care provider's guide to compensation and quality: how to get paid and not get sued*, Boston, 2003, Jones and Bartlett Publishers.

15. Reid WA et al: Effect of using templates on the information included in histopathology reports on specimens of uterine cervix taken by loop excision of the transformation zone, *J Clin Pathol* 52:825-828, 1999.

16. Marill KA et al: Prospective, randomized trial of template-assisted versus undirected written recording of physician records in the emergency department, *Ann Emerg Med* 33:500-509, 1999.

17. Wallace SA et al: Use of a pro forma for head injuries in the accident and emergency department—the way forward, *J Accid Emerg Med* 11:33-42, 1994.

18. Cole AB, Counselman FL: Comparison of transcribed and handwritten emergency department charts in the evaluation of chest pain, Ann Emerg Med 25:445-450, 1995.

19. Humphreys T et al: Preformatted charts improve documentation in the emergency department, *Ann Emerg Med* 21:534-540, 1992.

20. Madlon-Kay DJ: Use of a structured encounter form to improve well-child care documentation, *Arch Fam Med* 7:480-483, 1998.

21. Lilford RJ et al: Effect of using protocols on medical care: randomised trial of three methods of taking an antenatal history, *BMJ* 305:1181-1184, 1992.

22. Bordley WC: Improving preventive service delivery through office systems, *Pediatrics* 108:E41, 2001.

23. Wilf-Miron R: Using a health concerns checklist as a bridge from reason for encounter to diagnosis of girls attending an adolescent health service, *Pediatrics* 106:1065-1069, 2000.

24. Standridge JB: Putting prevention into practice, *Clin Fam Pract* 2:485, 2000.

25. Yoshikawa TT, Cobbs EL, Brummel-Smith K: *Practical ambulatory geriatrics,* St. Louis, 1998, Mosby.

CHAPTER 1

Adult History and Physical Examination Forms

Chapter Contents

ICON KEY: ▤ Tool Printed   ⊘ Tool on CD ROM   ∞ Customizable Tool   **i** Information and Resources Provided for Further Acquisition

Content of Forms

The adult history and physical forms presented in this chapter were composed with reference to standard physical assessment textbooks. The traditional essential baseline components included in an adult history and physical examination are the history of present illness (HPI) or chief complaint (CC), past medical history (PMH), past surgical history (PSH), family history (FH), social history (SH), current medications, known allergies, a review of systems (ROS), physical examination, assessment, and plan (Box 1-1). Primary prevention by incorporation of health maintenance screening and recommendations into the periodic physical examination has become the standard of care in the past decade.

Description of Forms

Comprehensive Adult History and Physical Form   ⊘ ▤ ∞

This four-page form includes a complete health history and full physical examination form, suitable for primary care practices. Included on this form are the essential components of a medical history record, as outlined above.

Text block areas, most with detailed, cued documentation, are included for the following:

History:
    History of Present Illness
    Past Medical History
    Past Surgical History/Trauma/Hospitalization
    Medications
    Allergies
    Reproductive History
    Social History
    Family History
    Health Maintenance History
    Immunizations
    Safety Record
    Review of Systems
Physical Examination:
    Vital Signs
    Visual Acuity
    Systems Exam
    Labs/Studies
Assessment and Plan
    Periodic Health Screening Plan
    Immunizations

Box **1-1**   Adult History and Physical Essential Components

HISTORY OF PRESENT ILLNESS/CHIEF COMPLAINT
- System analysis of presenting complaint including review of system(s) affected
- Symptom characteristics such as onset, location, duration, quality, quantity, timing, setting, exacerbating and alleviating factors, associated manifestations, prior treatment
- Impact of illness on patient's usual lifestyle

PAST MEDICAL HISTORY
- General health
- Past major adult illnesses including current chronic illnesses and conditions
- Past and present psychiatric illnesses
- Nonsurgical hospitalizations
- Childhood illnesses and immunization status
- Transfusions
- Health maintenance history

PAST SURGICAL HISTORY
- Surgeries
- Accidents and injuries with resulting disabilities

FAMILY HISTORY
- Age and health or age and cause of death of parents, siblings, grandparents, children, other relatives
- Family occurrence of major diseases, hereditary disorders, psychiatric problems

SOCIAL HISTORY
- Personal and family status
- Residence conditions and cohabitants, pets
- Occupational history and education
- Hobbies and interests
- Travel
- Exposure to toxic substances, radiation, wild or domestic animals
- Caffeine use
- Tobacco and alcohol use, past and present
- Recreational drug use, intravenous drug abuse
- Diet, sleep, and exercise habits
- Sexual history
- Cultural and religious influences
- Stress and coping patterns, social support systems, financial status

MEDICATIONS
- Current and recently prescribed medications
- Nonprescription and home remedies
- Vitamin and supplement use
- Prosthetic devices: limbs, braces, corrective lenses, dentures, hearing aids

ALLERGIES
- Medications
- Environmental allergens, latex
- Foods
- Intravenous contrast material

REVIEW OF SYSTEMS
- Detailed questions for each body system to include general constitutional, dermatologic, HEENT (head, ears, eyes, nose and, throat), breast, respiratory, cardiovascular, peripheral vascular, gastrointestinal, genitourinary, endocrine, hematologic, immunologic, musculoskeletal, neurologic, and psychiatric reviews

PHYSICAL EXAMINATION
- Objective findings on physical examination with use of inspection, auscultation, percussion, and palpation processes
- Laboratory testing, radiographs, and other special procedures
- Use of validated and reliable screening tools

ASSESSMENT
- Problem list
- Assessment or differential diagnosis for each problem
- Anticipated potential problems

PLAN
- Diagnostic tests or studies to be performed
- Treatment plan including prescription and nonprescription medications, physical therapy, assistive devices, home remedies, behavioral changes, and referrals for specialist or home services
- Health maintenance review
- Patient education
- Follow-up plan for reevaluation

Health Counseling

Lab tests and other studies ordered

The form contains a combination of narrative documentation space, check-off boxes and tables, and lines for short answers/explanations of findings. The reader may use this form as printed or modify the form to best suit individual practice by following instructions in Appendix A.

Adult History and Physical Form— Female and Male

These two-page forms contain the essential components of the comprehensive history and physical examination; however, there are fewer check-off box cues and less space for narrative documentation of specifics. The health care professional may supplement this form with a dictated or handwritten note if the exam findings warrant more documentation.

Adult History and Physical Form— Female and Male Short Forms

These one-page forms contain an abbreviated version of the Adult History and Physical forms. There is minimal space for narrative documentation of specifics. These forms are intended for use with the patient who has a previously completed Comprehensive Adult History and Physical, which is documented in the medical record.

It is recommended that the health care professional supplement this form with a dictated or handwritten note.

Well-Woman History and Physical Form

This two-page form contains an expanded Female Reproductive History with cues and spaces for recording data. Space for recording of Past Medical History, Social History, and Family History is reduced. The physical exam is modified to focus on gynecologic examination. Labs and Health Counseling specify needs particular to women and include standard health maintenance, safety, and immunization cues. This form is recommended for documentation of the periodic gynecologic exam.

Comprehensive Older Adult History and Physical Form

This four-page form contains the essential components of the history and physical examination with changes relevant to the needs of the geriatric patient. Reproductive and Family Histories are consolidated and Social History is extensively expanded to reflect the concerns of the older adult. The Review of Systems and Physical Exam are modified to cue the user to symptoms and findings that occur more frequently in the older adult patient. The Plan includes health screenings, immunizations, and health counseling sections. Additional lab and procedure check-off boxes and indicators for risk factors and referral services that pertain to the elderly are also included.

Office Visit Form

This form provides an alternative to the narrative progress record. Space is provided for narrative History of Present Illness and updates for Medications, Allergies, and Past Medical History. Check-off boxes for review of systems and focal exam areas, with notation space for length of visit facilitate quick review by office personnel for coding accuracy. Narrative space is provided for exam findings, Assessment and Plan. Check-off boxes for commonly ordered labs, studies and follow-up visit complete the form.

Medication History

A thorough medication history may provide important information related to ineffective management of chronic conditions, new symptoms, masking of subclinical diagnoses, and risks for drug-drug and drug-food interactions. This two-page form allows documentation of current medical diagnoses, allergies, and family history of allergies. Questions on occupation, hobbies, travel, immunizations, diet, substance use, sources of medications, access issues, and drug storage safety are listed. Tables are available to document current and past prescription medication use, as well as over-the-counter medication use for common symptoms. Information may be obtained by patient interview, keeping in mind that the average person may not be familiar with generic and brand names of drugs or medical terminology. Suggestion of trade name over-the-counter medications and use of open-ended questions are recommended to best communicate with the level of understanding appropriate for the patient. For more thorough coverage of herbal products and supplements, please see the Herbal and Supplement History Form in Chapter 6.

Resources and References

Online Resources

Agency for Healthcare Research and Quality (AHRQ): *Put Prevention into Practice (PPIP).*
A program to increase the appropriate use of clinical preventive services, such as screening tests, immunizations, and counseling, based on U.S. Preventive Services Task Force recommendations. Web site: http://www.ahrq.gov/clinic/ppipix.htm

Agency for Healthcare Research and Quality: U.S. Preventive Services Task Force (USPSTF): *Reviews and recommendations: guide to clinical preventive services,* 2nd ed. 1996.
Provides the latest available recommendations on preventive interventions: screening tests, counseling, immunizations, and chemoprophylactic regimens for more than 80 conditions. Includes periodic health examination and age-specific charts. Web site: http://www.ahrq.gov/clinic/cpsix.htm

Agency for Healthcare Research and Quality: U.S. Preventive Services Task Force (USPSTF): *Reviews and recommendations: guide to clinical preventive services,* 3rd ed. 2000-2004.
Updates some recommendations from the second edition and evaluates additional new topics. Recommendations from the Task Force are being released incrementally, as they become available. Web site: http://www.ahcpr.gov/clinic/cps3dix.htm

Centers for Disease Control and Prevention (CDC) National Immunization Program. Complete, current information on immunizations. Web site: http://www.cdc.gov/nip

Centers for Disease Control and Prevention (CDC) National Immunization Program—Recommended Adult Immunization Schedule, United States, 2002-2003 and Recommended Immunizations for Adults with Medical Conditions, United States, 2002-2003. Web site: http://www.cdc.gov/nip/recs/adult-schedule.pdf

References and Suggested Readings

Barkauskas VH, Baumann LC, Darling-Fisher CS: *Health and physical assessment,* ed 3, St Louis, 2002, Mosby.
Bickley LS, Szilagyi PG, Stackhouse JG: *Bates' guide to physical examination and history taking,* ed 8, Philadelphia, 2002, Lippincott.
Burke M, Laramie JA: *Primary care of the older adult—a multidisciplinary approach,* St Louis, 2000, Mosby.
Carlson KJ et al: *Primary care of women,* ed 2, St Louis, 2002, Mosby.
Coffield AB: Priorities among recommended clinical preventive services, *Am J Prev Med* 21:1-9, 2001.
Dains JE, Baumann LC, Scheibel P: *Advanced health assessment and clinical diagnosis in primary care,* ed 2, St Louis, 2003, Mosby.
Epstein O et al: *Clinical examination,* ed 3, St Louis, 2003, Mosby.
Fields SD: History-taking in the elderly: obtaining useful information, *Geriatrics* 46(8):26-35, 1991.
Fields SD: Special considerations in the physical exam of older patients, *Geriatrics* 46(8):39-44, 1991.
Goldberg TH, Chavin SI: Preventive medicine and screening in older adults, *J Am Geriatr Soc* 45:344-354, 1997.
Jarvis C: *Physical examination and health assessment,* ed 3, Philadelphia. 2000, WB Saunders.

Rubenstein LZ: Comprehensive geriatric assessment. In Abrams WB, Beers MH, Berkow R, editors: *Merck manual of geriatrics*, Whitehouse Station, NJ, 1995, Merck Research Laboratories.

Seidel HM et al: Mosby's guide to physical examination, ed 5, St Louis, 2003, Mosby.

Swartz MH: *Textbook of physical diagnosis*, ed 4, Philadelphia, 2002, WB Saunders.

Wilson SF, Giddens JF: *Health assessment for nursing practice*, ed 2, St Louis, 2001, Mosby.

Yoshikawa TT, Cobbs EL, Brummel-Smith K: *Practical ambulatory geriatrics*, St Louis, 1998, Mosby.

Youngkin E, Davis MS: *Women's health: a primary care clinical guide*, ed 2, Stamford, CT, 1998, Prentice Hall.

Comprehensive Adult History and Physical

Date of Visit: _____

Patient Name: _____

Medical Record #: _____

Address: _____

Telephone: (home)_____ (business) _____ Informant/Relationship: _____

Date of Birth: _____ Age: _____ Gender: Male Female   Language _____ Interpreter present: ☐ Yes ☐ No

Provider: _____ Reliability: ☐ Adequate ☐ Inadequate

History of Present Illness

Past Medical History

☐ HTN	☐ Asthma/COPD	☐ Seizure Disorder	☐ Breast Disease
☐ DM	☐ GERD	☐ Renal Disease	☐ Anemia
☐ CVD/CAD	☐ Hepatitis	☐ Thyroid Disorder	☐ Transfusions
☐ CVA	☐ Osteoporosis	☐ Bleeding Disorder	☐ Psychiatric
☐ CA	☐ Arthritis	☐ Infectious Disease	☐ Childhood Illnesses

Other/Details of Above:

Past Surgical History/Trauma/Hospitalization

☐ T & A: Other/Details:

☐ Appendectomy:

☐ Cholecystectomy:

☐ Hernia repair:

☐ Hysterectomy:

☐ Laparotomy:

☐ Cesarean section:

☐ Biopsy: _____ ☐ ORIF: _____

Medications

☐ OTC

☐ Vitamins

☐ Supplements/Herbals

Allergies

☐ Drugs

☐ Environment

☐ Foods ☐ Latex

☐ IV Contrast

Reproductive History

Menstrual: _____ Age at menarche _____ LMP _____

Interval _____ Duration _____ Flow _____

☐ Reg ☐ Irreg ☐ Cramping ☐ Intermenstrual Bleeding ☐ PMS

Obstetrical: G _____ T _____ P _____ A _____ L _____

Complications: _____

Menopause: Age _____ Abnl Bleeding: _____

Symptoms: _____

Hormones: ☐ ERT ☐ HRT ☐ topical _____

Contraceptives: _____

Sexual Activity:

☐ same sex   ☐ opposite sex   ☐ abstinent

☐ single partner ☐ multiple partners ☐ >4 lifetime partners

STD hx:_____

Concerns:

Comprehensive Adult History and Physical - 2

Patient Name: _____

Date of Birth: _____ Date of Exam: _____

Social History

Marital Status: ☐ Single ☐ Married ☐ Domestic Partner
☐ Divorced ☐ Widowed

Cohabitants: _____

Children: _____

Education: _____

Occupation: _____

Interests/Activities: _____

Exercise: ☐ Aerobic ☐ Weights _____

Diet: ☐ Balanced ☐ Calcium _____

Sleep/Rest: _____ **Caffeine:** ☐ No ☐ Yes cups/day _____

Tobacco: ☐ No ☐ Yes PPD _____ # Years _____ Quit Year _____

Smoking in home: ☐ Yes ☐ No _____

ETOH: ☐ Yes ☐ No ☐ Daily ☐ Weekly ☐ Monthly # drinks _____

Recreational Drugs: _____

Support Systems/Coping Skills: ☐ Adequate ☐ Inadequate

Family History

☐ **Family History Unknown**

Father: _____

Mother: _____

Siblings: _____

_____

MGF: _____

MGM: _____

PGF: _____

PGM: _____

Other: _____

_____

Cultural/Religious Influences: _____

Health Maintenance History

Exam	Last Date	Results	N/A	Refused	Exam	Last Date	Results	N/A	Refused
Pap test					Dental				
Mammogram					Vision				
SBE/TSE					Hearing				
Stool guaiac					Lipid Profile				
Flex sig/Colonoscopy					FBS				
CXR					PSA				
ECG					PPD				

Immunizations (dates):

Td		MMR/titers		Hep B		Polio
Varicella vaccine/chickenpox			Influenza		Pneumovax	

Safety:

☐ Seatbelt Use ☐ Cycling Helmet ☐ Sunscreen ☐ Occupational
☐ Smoke Detectors ☐ Housing ☐ Dom. Violence ☐ Firearms

Review of Systems (Check box at left if all systems negative.)

Comments/Details:

☐ **General:** ☐ fever ☐ chills ☐ night sweats ☐ fatigue ☐ unexplained weight loss ☐ weight gain

☐ **Skin:** ☐ pruritus ☐ rash ☐ hair loss ☐ worrisome lesion ☐ pigment change ☐ moles ☐ sweating ☐ dry skin ☐ nail change

☐ **HEENT:** ☐ headache ☐ dizziness ☐ earache ☐ hearing loss ☐ tinnitus ☐ vision change ☐ eye pain/sensitivity ☐ excessive tearing ☐ eyeglasses/contact use ☐ glaucoma ☐ rhinorrhea ☐ nasal congestion ☐ postnasal drip ☐ sinus pain ☐ nosebleeds ☐ hay fever ☐ sore throat ☐ mouth sores ☐ hoarseness ☐ toothache ☐ bleeding gums ☐ dentures

☐ **Breast:** ☐ pain ☐ lumps ☐ discharge ☐ history of breast disease ☐ implants

☐ **Pulmonary:** ☐ cough ☐ sputum ☐ hemoptysis ☐ SOB ☐ pain with respiration ☐ wheezing ☐ cyanosis

☐ **CV:** ☐ chest pain ☐ palpitations ☐ DOE ☐ orthopnea ☐ PND ☐ diaphoresis ☐ syncope ☐ heart murmur ☐ leg edema

☐ **PVD:** ☐ claudication ☐ varicose veins ☐ phlebitis ☐ coldness of hands/feet ☐ leg ulcers

☐ **GI:** ☐ dysphagia ☐ heartburn ☐ change in appetite ☐ food intol ☐ nausea ☐ vomiting ☐ hematemesis ☐ abdominal pain ☐ bloating ☐ flatulence ☐ diarrhea ☐ constipation ☐ melena ☐ jaundice ☐ dark urine ☐ BRBPR ☐ change in BM ☐ hemorrhoids ☐ hernia

☐ **GU:** ☐ dysuria ☐ urgency ☐ frequency ☐ hematuria ☐ nocturia ☐ polyuria ☐ suprapubic pain ☐ flank pain ☐ incontinence ☐ lesions ♂ ☐ hesitancy ☐ dribbling ☐ decreased force stream ☐ testicular pain ☐ testicular mass/swelling ☐ penile discharge ☐ erectile dysfunction ♀ ☐ vaginal itch ☐ abnl vaginal discharge ☐ vaginal dryness ☐ dyspareunia ☐ sexual dysfunction ☐ abnl vaginal bleeding

☐ **Endocrine:** ☐ polyuria ☐ polydipsia ☐ polyphagia ☐ heat/cold intol ☐ tremor ☐ lump in throat ☐ unexplained wt change ☐ hair changes

☐ **Heme:** ☐ anemia ☐ easy bruising ☐ swollen glands ☐ bleeding of skin/mucous membranes ☐ freq infections ☐ allergies ☐ delayed healing

☐ **MSK:** ☐ joint pain (location _____) ☐ stiffness ☐ restriction of motion ☐ swelling ☐ erythema ☐ bony deformity ☐ myalgia ☐ muscle cramps ☐ weakness ☐ antalgic gait ☐ back pain

☐ **Neuro:** ☐ focal weakness ☐ paralysis ☐ numbness ☐ tremor ☐ seizure ☐ syncope ☐ gait disturbance ☐ memory loss ☐ aphasia

☐ **Psych:** ☐ anxiety ☐ panic attacks ☐ depression ☐ mood changes ☐ irritability ☐ nervousness ☐ decreased libido ☐ eating disorder ☐ sleep disturbance ☐ suicidal thoughts ☐ impaired judgment ☐ hallucinations ☐ confusion

Comprehensive Adult History and Physical - 3

Patient Name: _____

Date of Birth: _____ Date of Exam: _____

Physical Exam

N = Normal A = Abnormal (Check appropriate box)	N	A
1. General Appearance: age • LOC • nutrition • development • mobility • affect • speech • hygiene		
2. Skin: hydration • color • texture • hair • nails • lesions		
3. Head: shape • size • symmetry • scalp • TMJ • lesions		
4. Eyes: lids • conjunctiva • sclera		
Extraocular Muscles		
Visual fields		
Pupils: size, reaction to light and accommodation		
Fundi		
5. Ears: pinna • canals • TMs • hearing		
6. Nose: patency • nares • sinuses • nasal mucosa • septum • turbinates		
7. Mouth: lips • gums • teeth • mucosa • palate • tongue		
8. Throat: pharynx • tonsils • uvula		
9. Neck: ROM • symmetry • palpation • thyroid • trachea • carotids • jugular veins • lymph nodes		
10. Breasts: size • symmetry • skin • nipples • palpation • nodes		
11. Chest/Lungs: excursion • palpation • percussion • auscultation		
12. Cardiac: PMI • palpation • rate • rhythm • S1 • S2 • murmurs • gallops • bruits • extra sounds		
13. Abdomen: appearance • bowel sounds • bruits • percussion • palpation • liver • spleen • flank • suprapubic • hernia		
14. Anorectal: perianal		
digital rectal		
stool guaiac		
prostate exam		
15. Female perineum • labia • urethral meatus • introitus		
Genitalia: Internal: vaginal mucosal • cervix		
Bimanual: vagina • cervix • uterus • adnexa		
16. Male Genitalia: penis • scrotum • testes • hernia		
17. Lymph Nodes: cervical • subclavian • axillary • inguinal • other		
18. Musculoskeletal: Back/Spine: ROM • palpation		
Upper Extremity: ROM • strength • palpation		
Lower Extremity: ROM • strength • palpation		
19. Peripheral Upper extremity: pulses • appearance • temp		
Vascular: Lower extremity: pulses • appearance • temp		
20. Neurologic: cranial nerves • motor • sensory • cerebellar • reflexes • gait • mental status		

Vitals

Ht _____ Wt _____ Temp _____ Resp _____ Pulse _____

BP (upright) _____ (supine) _____ Staff Initials _____

Visual Acuity

Right   /   Left   /

Corrective lenses   ☐ Yes   ☐ No

Document Abnormals (by number)/Comments

Lab/Studies

Assessment and Plan

Comprehensive Adult History and Physical - 4

Patient Name: _____

Date of Birth: _____ *Date of Exam:* _____

Assessment and Plan (continued)

Periodic Health Screening Plan

Exam	Performed	Scheduled	N/A	Refused
Breast Exam				
Mammogram				
Pap Test				
Prostate exam				
Testicular exam				
Digital rectal with stool guaiac				
Flexible Sigmoidoscopy/Colonoscopy				
Bone Density				
PPD				

Health Counseling (check if discussed, describe any intervention)

☐ Smoking cessation _____

☐ Alcohol/Drug Use _____

☐ Diet/Weight _____

☐ Vitamins/Calcium _____

☐ Periodic Dental/Vision care _____

☐ Exercise/Sleep _____

☐ Sun exposure _____

☐ Seatbelts/Helmets _____

☐ Stress/Family issues _____

☐ Safety: Weapons/ Domestic Violence _____

☐ BSE/TSE _____

☐ Sexual issues/risks _____

☐ Contraception _____

☐ Living Will/Power of atty/DNR _____

Immunizations

Immunizations current: ☐ Yes ☐ No

Vaccine	Given	Planned	Refused
Td			
Hepatitis B			
Influenza			
Pneumonia			
Other:			

Lab/Studies Ordered

☐ CXR   ☐ Lipids   ☐ Creat/BUN   ☐ HbA$_1$C

☐ ECG   ☐ CBC/diff   ☐ LFTs   ☐ TSH

       ☐ Electrolytes   ☐ FBS   ☐ UA/UC

☐ Other: _____

_____
Provider's Signature   Date

☐ Note dictated/written

Adult History and Physical - Female

Date of Visit: _____

Patient Name: _____

Medical Record #: _____

Address: _____

Telephone: (home)_____ (business)_____   Informant/Relationship: _____

Date of Birth: _____ Age: _____ Gender: Male Female   Language _____ Interpreter present: ☐ Yes ☐ No

Provider: _____   Reliability: ☐ Adequate ☐ Inadequate

History of Present Illness

Past Medical History

Past Surgery, Biopsy, Trauma

1. _____
2. _____
3. _____
4. _____
5. _____

Allergies

☐ NKDA

Medications (R$_x$ and OTC)

Sexual History

Menstrual:

Menarche _____ LMP _____ Regular/Irreg

Interval _____ Duration _____ Flow _____

☐ Cramping ☐ Intermenstrual bleeding ☐ PMS

Obstetrical: G ___ T ___ P ___ A ___ L ___

Complications:

Menopause:

Age ____ Symptoms: _____

Abnl Bleeding: _____ Hormones: _____

Sexual Activity:

Contraceptives: _____

☐ same sex ☐ opposite sex ☐ abstinent

☐ single/multiple partner(s)

☐ >4 lifetime partners

STD hx: _____

Concerns:

Social History

Marital Status: _____ Children: _____

Cohabitants: _____

Education: _____

Occupation: _____

Caffeine: ☐ No ☐ Yes cups/day _____

Tobacco: ☐ No ☐ Yes PPD _____

       # Years _____

Quit year _____ Smoking in home? _____

ETOH: _____

Recreational drugs: _____

Activities: (√ if adequate)

☐ Exercise: aerobic•weights

☐ Diet ☐ Sleep

Hobbies: _____

Support Systems/Coping Skills:

Cultural/Religious Influences:

Family History   ■ Unknown

Father:

Mother:

Siblings:

MGF: MGM:

PGF: PGM:

Other:

Health Maintenance History

Pap test:		Lipid Profile:	
Mammogram SBE:		FBS:	
Stool guaiac:		PPD:	
FOBT/Flex sig/colonoscopy:		Dental:	
CXR:		Vision:	
ECG:		Hearing:	
Other:			

Review of Systems

N=normal A=Abnormal	N	A		N	A
Constitutional			GI		
Skin			GU		
HEENT			Endocrine		
Breast			Heme/Immune		
Pulmonary			MSK		
Cardiovascular			Neuro		
Peripheral Vascular			Psych		
Other Details:					

Safety

Seatbelts: _____ Helmets: _____

Smoke Detectors: ____ Sunscreen: ____

Housing:

Guns: _____ Dom. Violence: _____

Occupational:

Immunizations

Td: _____ MMR/titers: _____

Hep B: _____ Polio: _____

Influenza: _____ Pneumovax: _____

Varicella vaccine/chickenpox: _____

Other:

Adult History and Physical - Female 2

Patient Name: _____

Date of Birth: _____

Physical Exam

Vitals Ht _____ Wt _____ Temp _____ Resp _____ Pulse _____

BP (upright) _____ (supine) _____ Staff Initials _____

Visual Acuity Right / Left / Corrective lenses ☐ Yes ☐ No

N = normal A = abnormal (√ appropriate box)	N	A
1. General Appearance		
2. Skin: hydration • color • texture • hair • nails • lesions		
3. Head: shape • size • symmetry • scalp • TMJ • lesions		
4. Eyes: lids • conjunctiva • sclera • EOM • VF • pupils • fundi		
5. Ears: pinna • canals • TMs • hearing		
6. Nose: nares • sinuses • mucosa • septum • turbinates		
7. Mouth: lips • gums • teeth • mucosa • palate • tongue		
8. Throat: pharynx • tonsils • uvula		
9. Neck: ROM • thyroid • trachea • carotids • jugulars • nodes		
10. Breasts: size • symmetry • skin • nipples • palpation • nodes		
11. Chest/Lungs: excursion • palpation • percussion • auscultation		
12. CV: rate • rhythm • S1 • S2 • murmur • extra sounds		
13. Abd: BS • liver • spleen • flank • suprapubic • hernia		
14. Anorectal: perianal • digital rectal • stool guaiac		
15. Genitalia: perineum • labia • urethral meatus • introitus		
Internal: vaginal mucosal • cervix		
Bimanual: vagina • cervix • uterus • adnexa		
16. Lymph Nodes: cervical • subclavian • axillary • inguinal • other		
17. Musculoskeletal: Back/Spine • UE • LE • ROM • strength		
18. Peripheral Vascular: pulses • appearance • temperature		
19. Neurologic: CNs • motor • sensory • cerebellar • DTRs • mental		
20. Psychiatric: mental status • mood • affect		

Document Abnormals (by number)/Comments:

Lab/Studies:

Assessment and Plan:

Anticipatory Guidance	**√ Topics Discussed**
Smoking cessation	BSE: ☐ doing ☐ declines
Alcohol/Drug use	Seatbelts/Helmets
Diet/Weight	Personal safety/Domestic violence
Vitamins/Calcium	Parenting/Family issues
Periodic Dental care	Adequate sleep
Exercise: aerobic • weights	Stress: home • job
Sun exposure	Sexual issues • safe sex
	Living Will

Periodic Health Screening Plan:

Exam:	Performed	Scheduled	N/A	Refused
Breast exam				
Mammogram				
Pap test				
Digital rectal/ FOBT				
Flex sig/Colonoscopy				
Bone density				

Immunizations: current: ☐ Yes ☐ No

Vaccine:	Given	Planned	Refused
Td			
Hepatitis B			
Influenza			
Pneumonia			
Other:			

Provider's Signature
☐ Note dictated/written

Date

Adult History and Physical - Male

Date of Visit: _____

Patient Name: _____

Medical Record #: _____

Address: _____

Telephone: (home)_____ (business)_____ Informant/Relationship: _____

Date of Birth: _____ Age: _____ Gender: Male Female Language _____ Interpreter present: ☐ Yes ☐ No

Provider: _____ Reliability: ☐ Adequate ☐ Inadequate

History of Present Illness

Past Medical History

Past Surgery, Biopsy, Trauma

1. _____
2. _____
3. _____
4. _____
5. _____

Allergies

☐ NKDA

Medications (R$_x$ and OTC)

Sexual History

Sexual Activity:

Contraceptives: _____

☐ same sex ☐ opposite sex ☐ abstinent

☐ single partners ☐ multiple partners

STD hx: _____

Condoms/Contraceptives: _____

Concerns: ☐ Libido ☐ ED ☐ PE

Social History

Marital Status: _____ Children: _____

Cohabitants:_____

Education: _____

Occupation: _____

Caffeine: ☐ No ☐ Yes cups/day _____

Tobacco: ☐ No ☐ Yes PPD _____

    # Years _____

Quit Year _____ Smoking in Home?_____

ETOH: _____ Recreational Drugs: _____

Activities: (√ if adequate) _____

☐ Exercise: aerobic · weights ☐ Diet ☐ Sleep

Hobbies: _____

Support Systems/Coping Skills:

Cultural/Religious Influences:

Family History   ■ Unknown

Father:

Mother:

Siblings:

MGF: MGM:

PGF: PGM:

Other:

Health Maintenance History

PSA	Lipid Profile:	
Digital rectal:	FBS:	
Stool guaiac:	PPD:	
FOBT/Flex sig/colonoscopy:	Dental:	
CXR:	Vision:	
ECG:	Hearing:	
Other:		

Review of Systems

N=normal A=Abnormal	N	A		N	A
Constitutional			GI		
Skin			GU		
HEENT			Endocrine		
Breast			Heme/Immune		
Pulmonary			MSK		
Cardiovascular			Neuro		
Peripheral Vascular			Psych		

Other Details:

Safety

Seatbelts: Helmets:	
Smoke Detectors: Sunscreen:	
Housing:	
Guns: Dom. Violence:	
Occupational:	

Immunizations

Td: MMR/titers:	
Hep B: Polio:	
Influenza: Pneumovax:	
Varicella vaccine/chickenpox:	
Other:	

Adult History and Physical - Male 2

Patient Name: _____

Date of Birth: _____

Physical Exam

Vitals Ht _____ Wt _____ Temp _____ Resp _____ Pulse _____

BP (upright) _____ (supine) _____ Staff Initials _____

Visual Acuity Right / Left / Corrective lenses ☐ Yes ☐ No

N = normal A = abnormal (√ appropriate box)	N	A
1. General Appearance		
2. Skin: hydration • color • texture • hair • nails • lesions		
3. Head: shape • size • symmetry • scalp • TMJ • lesions		
4. Eyes: lids • conjunctiva • sclera • EOM • VF • pupils • fundi		
5. Ears: pinna • canals • TMs • hearing		
6. Nose: nares • sinuses • mucosa • septum • turbinates		
7. Mouth: lips • gums • teeth • mucosa • palate • tongue		
8. Throat: pharynx • tonsils • uvula		
9. Neck: ROM • thyroid • trachea • carotids • jugulars • nodes		
10. Breasts: size • symmetry • skin • nipples • palpation • nodes		
11. Chest/Lungs: excursion • palpation • percussion • auscultation		
12. CV: rate • rhythm • S1 • S2 • murmur • extra sounds		
13. Abd: BS • liver • spleen • flank • suprapubic • hernia		
14. Anorectal: perianal • digital rectal • prostate • stool guaiac		
15. Male Genitalia: penis • scrotum • testes • hernia		
16. Lymph Nodes: cervical • subclavian • axillary • inguinal • other		
17. Musculoskeletal: Back/Spine • UE • LE • ROM • strength		
18. Peripheral Vascular: pulses • appearance • temperature		
19. Neurologic: CNs • motor • sensory • cerebellar • DTRs • mental		
20. Psychiatric: mental status • mood • affect		

Document Abnormals (by number)/Comments:

Lab/Studies:

Assessment and Plan:

Anticipatory Guidance	√ Topics Discussed
Smoking cessation	TSE: ☐ doing ☐ declines
Alcohol/Drug use	Seatbelts/Helmets
Diet/Weight	Personal safety/Domestic violence
Vitamins/Calcium	Parenting/Family issues
Periodic Dental care	Adequate sleep
Exercise: aerobic • weights	Stress: home • job
Sun exposure	Sexual issues • safe sex
	Living Will

Periodic Health Screening Plan:

Exam:	Performed	Scheduled	N/A	Refused
Prostate exam				
Testicular exam				
Digital rectal/ FOBT				
Flex. sig/Colonoscopy				
Bone density				

Immunizations:	current: ☐ Yes ☐ No		
Vaccine:	**Given**	**Planned**	**Refused**
Td			
Hepatitis B			
Influenza			
Pneumonia			
Other:			

_____

Provider's Signature   Date
☐ Note dictated/written

Adult Female History & Physical - Short Form

Date of Visit: _____

Patient Name: _____

Medical Record #: _____

Address: _____

Telephone: (home)_____ (business) _____   Informant/Relationship: _____

Date of Birth: _____ Age: _____ Gender: Male Female   Language _____ Interpreter present: ☐ Yes ☐ No

Provider: _____   Reliability: ☐ Adequate   ☐ Inadequate

History of Present Illness

Past Medical, Surgical, and Trauma History

☐ Unchanged since: _____

☐ Changed since: _____

Allergies
☐ NKDA

Family History
☐ Unchanged
☐ New

Medications

1. _____
2. _____
3. _____
4. _____
5. _____
6. _____
7. _____
8. _____

Reproductive History:

Menstrual: LMP _____ Regular/Irreg

Interval _____ Duration _____ Flow _____

Obstetrical: P ___ G ___ Complications: ____

Menopause: Age ____ Symptoms: _____

Abnl Bleeding: _____ Hormones: _____

Sexual Activity:

Contraceptives:_____

Concerns:

Social History:

☐ Unchanged ☐ New _____

Activities: (√ if adequate) ☐ Exercise ☐ Diet ☐ Sleep

☐ Caffeine ☐ No ☐ Yes cups/day _____

Tobacco: ☐ No ☐ Yes PPD __ # Years __ Quit year ___

ETOH/Drugs: _____ Smoking in home? _____

Support Systems: _____

Safety: (√ if adequate) ☐ Seatbelts ☐ Helmets ☐ Sunscreen

☐ Smoke Detectors ☐ Housing ☐ Occupational

Guns in home? _____ Domestic violence: _____

Immunizations current: ☐ Yes ☐ No _____

Review of Systems

N=Normal A=Abnormal	N	A
Constitutional		
Skin		
HEENT		
Breast		
Pulmonary		
Cardiovascular		
Peripheral Vascular		
GI		
GU		
Endocrine		
Heme/Immune		
MSK		
Neuro		
Psych		
Other:		

Assessment and Plan

Physical Exam

Vitals:

Height	Weight	☐ Kg ☐ Lb	BMI:	Visual Acuity: Right / Left /
				Corrective lenses ☐ Yes ☐ No

BP	Pulse	☐ Regular ☐ Irregular	Resp Rate	Temperature	Staff Initials

N = Normal A = Abnl →	N	A		N	A		N	A
1. General			8. Throat			15. Genitalia: External		
2. Skin			9. Neck			Internal		
3. Head			10. Breasts			Bimanual		
4. Eyes			11. Chest/Lungs			16. Lymph Nodes		
5. Ears			12. CV			17. Musculoskeletal		
6. Nose			13. Abdomen			18. Peripheral Vascular		
7. Mouth			14. Anorectal guaiac ☐			19. Neurologic		

Document Abnormals (by number)/Comments:

Guidance & Plan (√ if done)

☐ Pap test ☐ Mammogram
☐ Flex sig ☐ colonoscopy
☐ CXR ☐ ECG ☐ Audiogram
☐ Lipid profile ☐ FBS ☐ CBC
☐ PPD ☐ Vaccine:
Smoking cessation
Alcohol/Drug use
Diet • Weight • Exercise • Sleep
Vitamins • Calcium
☐ Dental ☐ Vision
BSE: ☐ doing ☐ declines
Stress: home/job/family/parenting
Sexual issues • safe sex
Living Will • Proxy • DNR

_____

Provider's Signature   Date

☐ Note dictated/written

Adult Male History & Physical - Short Form

Date of Visit: _____

Patient Name: _____

Medical Record #: _____

Address: _____

Telephone: (home)_____ (business) _____   Informant/Relationship: _____

Date of Birth: _____ Age: _____ Gender: Male Female   Language _____ Interpreter present: ☐ Yes ☐ No

Provider: _____   Reliability: ☐ Adequate ☐ Inadequate

History of Present Illness

Past Medical, Surgical, and Trauma History

☐ Unchanged since: _____

☐ Changed since: _____

Allergies

☐ NKDA

Family History

☐ Unchanged
☐ New

Medications

1.
2.
3.
4.
5.
6.
7.
8.

Reproductive History:

Sexual Activity:

Condoms/Contraceptives:

Concerns: ☐ Libido ☐ ED ☐ PE

Social History:

☐ Unchanged ☐ New _____

Activities: (√ if adequate) ☐ Exercise ☐ Diet ☐ Sleep
☐ Caffeine ☐ No ☐ Yes cups/day

Tobacco: ☐ No ☐ Yes PPD __ # Years __ Quit year ___

ETOH/Drugs: _____ Smoking in home? _____

Support Systems: _____

Safety: (√ if adequate) ☐ Seatbelts ☐ Helmets ☐ Sunscreen
☐ Smoke Detectors ☐ Housing ☐ Occupational

Guns in home? _____ Domestic violence: _____

Immunizations current: ☐ Yes ☐ No _____

Review of Systems

N=Normal A=Abnormal	N	A
Constitutional		
Skin		
HEENT		
Breast		
Pulmonary		
Cardiovascular		
Peripheral Vascular		
GI		
GU		
Endocrine		
Heme/Immune		
MSK		
Neuro		
Psych		
Other:		

Assessment and Plan

Physical Exam

Vitals:

Height	Weight	☐ Kg ☐ Lb	BMI:	Visual Acuity: Right / Left /
				Corrective lenses ☐ Yes ☐ No

BP	Pulse	☐ Regular ☐ Irregular	Resp Rate	Temperature	Staff Initials

N = Normal A = Abnl →	N	A		N	A		N	A
1. General			8. Throat			15. Prostate		
2. Skin			9. Neck			16. Genitalia		
3. Head			10. Breasts			17. Lymph Nodes		
4. Eyes			11. Chest/Lungs			18. Musculoskeletal		
5. Ears			12. CV			19. Peripheral Vascular		
6. Nose			13. Abdomen			20. Neurologic		
7. Mouth			14. Anorectal guaiac ☐					

Document Abnormals (by number)/Comments:

Guidance & Plan (√ if done)

☐ Digital rectal ☐ PSA

☐ Flex sig ☐ colonoscopy

☐ CXR ☐ ECG ☐ Audiogram

☐ Lipid profile ☐ FBS ☐ CBC

☐ PPD ☐ Vaccine:

Smoking cessation

Alcohol/Drug use

Diet • Weight • Exercise • Sleep

Vitamins • Calcium

☐ Dental ☐ Vision

TSE: ☐ doing ☐ declines

Stress: home/job/family/parenting

Sexual issues • safe sex

Living Will • Proxy • DNR

Provider's Signature _____ Date _____

☐ Note dictated/written

Well-Woman History & Physical

Date of Visit: _____

Patient Name: _____

Medical Record #: _____

Address: _____

Telephone: (home)_____ (business) _____

Date of Birth: _____ Age: _____ Gender: Male Female   Informant/Relationship: _____

Provider: _____   Language _____ Interpreter present: ☐ Yes ☐ No

Last visit to PCP: _____ Last Completed H & P: _____   Reliability: ☐ Adequate ☐ Inadequate

Reason for Visit

- ☐ Well-check
- ☐ Request for contraception
- ☐ Increased risk for cancer
- ☐ Child-bearing age
- ☐ Menopausal symptoms
- ☐ >3 years since last Pap
- ☐ Breast problem
- ☐ Other:

Past Medical History   data reviewed/updated/unchanged

- ☐ Negative

_____

_____

Surgeries ☐ None _____

Hospitalizations ☐ None _____

Allergies

- ☐ None

Medications/Vit/Ca++:

Immunizations ☐ Td ☐ MMR ☐ Hep B ☐ Varicella ☐ Polio

Social History

Marital Status: _____ Children: _____

Occupation: _____

Exercise: ☐ aerobic ☐ weights _____

Diet: ☐ Balanced _____

Sleep: ☐ Adequate _____

Tobacco: ☐ No ☐ Yes PPD _____

    # Years _____

Caffeine: ☐ No ☐ Yes cups/day _____

ETOH: _____

Street Drugs: _____

Violence:_____

Stress: _____

Reproductive History:

Last pelvic exam:_____ ☐ Never

Last Pap test:_____ ☐ Never

Last mammogram: _____ ☐ Never

SBE: ☐ No ☐ Yes Frequency _____

☐ DES exposure in utero   ☐ last Pap > 7 yrs

Breast:

- ☐ implants ☐ lactating ☐ lumps ☐ pain
- ☐ nipple discharge ☐ no complaints

Breastfed: ☐ No ☐ Yes # months _____

Obstetrical: G ___ T ___ P ___ A ___ L ___

Age at 1st pregnancy: _____ Last pregn: _____

Complications: _____

Infertility hx: ☐ yes ☐ no _____

Urinary History:

- ☐ no complaints ☐ frequent urination
- ☐ nocturia _____ # times ☐ initiation difficulty
- ☐ incontinence: stress/urge/mixed

pads/Depends _____

UTI Hx: _____

Gynecologic History:

Vaginal discharge/odor/itch: ☐ Yes ☐ No

Bleeding with intercourse: ☐ Yes ☐ No

Vaginal infections: ☐ never ☐ <one per year

    ☐ 1-2 per year ☐ >2 per year

Vaginal/Vulval lesion: ☐ Yes ☐ No

Abdominal pain/bloating: ☐ Yes ☐ No

Previous:

- ☐ Abnl vaginal bleeding_____
- ☐ Abnl Pap smear _____
- ☐ PID _____
- ☐ Uterine biopsy _____
- ☐ Uterine growths_____
- ☐ Other gyn:

Menstrual:

Menarche _____ LMP _____ Regular/Irreg

Interval _____ Duration _____ Flow: heavy/mod/light

- ☐ Cramping: none/mild/moderate/severe
- ☐ Intermenstrual Bleeding: Freq _____ # pads _____
- ☐ Mood changes: none/mild/moderate/marked

Menopause:

Age _____ natural/oophorectomy/hysterectomy

Symptoms: ☐ vasomotor ☐ vaginal ☐ urinary

Abnl Bleeding: _____

Hormones: ☐ ERT ☐ HRT ☐ topical ☐ ring

Sexual Activity:

- ☐ same sex ☐ opposite sex ☐ abstinent
- ☐ single/multiple partner(s) ☐ vaginal/oral/anal
- ☐ age at onset <17 ☐ >4 lifetime partners

Sexual Dysfunction:

- ☐ no complaints ☐ loss of interest
- ☐ painful intercourse ☐ poor lubrication
- ☐ no orgasm

Contraceptives:

_____

Condom use:

- ☐ always ☐ sometimes
- ☐ infrequent ☐ never

STD hx:

- ☐ None ☐ Nonspecific ☐ Chlamydia
- ☐ Gonorrhea ☐ Syphilis ☐ Warts
- ☐ HSV ☐ HIV
- ☐ Other:

Family History   ■ Unknown

Breast CA:

GU CA:

Colon CA:

CVD:

DM:

HTN:

Other:

Review of Systems

N=normal A=abnormal	N	A
Constitutional		
Skin		
HEENT		
Breast		
Pulmonary		
Cardiovascular		
Peripheral Vascular		
GI		
Endocrine		
Heme/Immune		
MSK		
Neuro		
Psych		
Other/Details:		

Well-Woman History and Physical 2

Patient Name: _____

Medical Record #: _____

Date of Birth: _____

Physical Exam

Vitals Ht _____ Wt _____ Temp _____ Resp _____ Pulse _____

BP (upright) _____ (supine) _____ Staff Initials _____

Visual Acuity Right / Left / Corrective lenses ☐ Yes ☐ No

N = Normal A = Abnormal D = Deferred (√ appropriate box)	N	A	D	Describe variance
General Appearance				
Skin: hydration • color • texture • hair • nails • lesions				
HEENT				
Neck: ROM • thyroid • trachea • carotids • jugulars • nodes				
Breasts: size • symmetry • skin • nipples • palpation • nodes				
Chest/Lungs: excursion • palpation • percussion • auscultation				
CV: rate • rhythm • S1 • S2 • murmur • extra sounds				
Abd: BS • liver • spleen • flank • suprapubic • hernia				
Genitalia: perineum • labia • urethral meatus • introitus				
Internal: vaginal mucosal • cervix				CMT ☐
Bimanual: vagina • cervix • uterus • adnexa				AV ☐ RV ☐ Mid ☐
Anorectal: perianal • digital rectal • stool guaiac				
Lymph Nodes: cervical • subclavian • axillary • inguinal • other				
Musculoskeletal: Back/Spine • UE • LE • ROM • strength				
Peripheral Vascular: pulses • appearance • temperature				
Neurologic: CNs • motor • sensory • cerebellar • DTRs • mental				

Office Labs/Results: Hb/Hct ☐   urine HCG ☐   UA ☐   RBS ☐

Right   Left
Breasts

Vulva/Anus   Cervix

Lab Preps:

	Done	*Declined*	*N/A*
Pap: TP/slide			
GC			
Chlamydia			
HSV			
FOBT			
Wet Mount			

Result: ☐ Candida ☐ BV ☐ trich ☐ other

Lab/Studies Ordered:

☐ CXR   ☐ Lipids   ☐ Creat/BUN   ☐ HbA$_1$C
☐ ECG   ☐ CBC/diff   ☐ LFTs   ☐ TSH
☐ Flex sig   ☐ Electrolytes   ☐ FBS   ☐ UA/UC
☐ Colonoscopy   ☐ RPR   ☐ Serum HCG
☐ Bone density   ☐ Hormones:
☐ Other:

Immunizations Updated: ☐ Yes ☐ No

Assessment and Plan:

☐ Well Woman

Health Counseling — ✔ Topics discussed

Smoking cessation	BSE
Alcohol/Drug use	Personal safety/Domestic violence
Diet/Weight	Parenting/Family issues
Vitamins/Calcium	Stress: home • job
Exercise: aerobic • weights	STD Risk • safe sex
Adequate sleep	Family Planning
Sun exposure	Emergency Contraception Rx
Seatbelts/Helmets	Menopause
Periodic Dental care	Living Will

Provider's Signature   Date
☐ Note dictated/written

Comprehensive Older Adult History and Physical

Date of Visit: _____

Patient Name: _____

Medical Record #: _____

Address: _____

Telephone: (home)_____ (business)_____

Date of Birth: _____ Age: _____ Gender: Male   Female _____

Provider: _____

Informant/Relationship: _____

Prior Medical Records: ☐ Office   ☐ Hospital _____

Language _____   Interpreter present: ☐ Yes   ☐ No

Reliability: ☐ Adequate   ☐ Inadequate

☐ Hard of hearing   ☐ Confirming history from caregiver

History of Present Illness/Troubling Symptoms

Past Medical History

☐ HTN   ☐ Asthma/COPD   ☐ Seizure Disorder   ☐ Breast Disease

☐ DM   ☐ Pneumonia   ☐ Renal Disease   ☐ Anemia

☐ CVD/CAD   ☐ GERD/PUD   ☐ Thyroid Disorder   ☐ Transfusions

☐ CVA   ☐ Hepatitis   ☐ Bleeding Disorder   ☐ Cataracts

☐ CA   ☐ GBD   ☐ Infectious Disease   ☐ Glaucoma

☐ TB   ☐ Arthritis/Gout   ☐ Psychiatric/ETOH   ☐ Osteoporosis

Other/Details of Above:

Past Surgical History/Trauma/Hospitalization (dates):

☐ T & A: Other/Details:

☐ Appendectomy:

☐ Cholecystectomy:

☐ Hernia repair:

☐ Hysterectomy:

☐ Cesarean section:

☐ Fracture: _____

☐ ORIF: _____

☐ Biopsy: _____

Medications

☐ OTC

☐ Vitamins

☐ Supplements/Herbals

Allergies

☐ Drugs   Other/Details:

☐ Environmental

☐ IV contrast

☐ Latex

☐ Foods

Reproductive History

Obstetrical: G _____ T _____ P _____ A _____ L _____

Complications:_____

Menopause: Age _____   Symptoms _____

Abnl Bleeding: _____

Hormones: ☐ ERT   ☐ HRT   ☐ topical _____

Sexual Activity:

☐ ability present   ☐ interest present   ☐ active

☐ abstinent   ☐ STD risk

Concerns: _____

Family History:

☐ Family History Unknown

_____

_____

_____

_____

Comprehensive Older Adult History and Physical - 2

Patient Name: _____

Medical Record #: _____ *Date of Birth:* _____

Social History

Marital Status: ☐ Single ☐ Married ☐ Domestic Partner
☐ Divorced ☐ Widowed

Cohabitants: _____

Children: _____

Occupation: Current: _____ Prior: _____ Education: _____

Interests/Activities: _____

Exercise: ☐ Aerobic ☐ Weights _____

Diet: ☐ Balanced ☐ Special _____

Supplements: ☐ Calcium ☐ Vitamins ☐ Other _____

Sleep/Rest: # hours_____ # naps _____

Tobacco: ☐ No ☐ Yes PPD ____ # Years ____ Quit Year _____

Smoking in home: ☐ Yes ☐ No _____

ETOH: ☐ No ☐ daily ☐ weekly ☐ monthly # drinks_____

Caffeine: ☐ No ☐ Yes cups/day ____ Substance abuse: _____

Cultural/Religious Influences: _____

Activities of Daily Living (ADL)

check if adequate:

☐ ambulation ☐ stairs ☐ transfers
☐ bathing ☐ toileting ☐ dressing/grooming
☐ bowel function ☐ bladder function ☐ eating/feeding
☐ mouth care ☐ endurance

Issues:

Instrumental Activities of Daily Living (IADL)

check if adequate:

☐ cooking/food prep ☐ cleaning ☐ laundry
☐ telephone use ☐ transportation ☐ financial management
☐ taking medicines ☐ shopping

Access to grocery store/meal service: _____

Issues:

Support Services:

☐ Family ☐ Community ☐ Agency _____ Financial means: ☐ adequate ☐ inadequate

Health Maintenance History

Exam	Last Date	Results	N/A	Refused	Exam	Last Date	Results	N/A	Refused
Pap test					Vision				
Mammogram/SBE					Foot care				
Stool guaiac					Hearing				
Flex sig/Colonoscopy					Lipid Profile				
CXR					FBS				
ECG					PSA				
Dental					PPD				

Immunizations (dates): Td _____ Influenza _____ Pneumovax _____ Other: _____

Safety: ☐ Seatbelt Use ☐ Firearms ☐ Sunscreen ☐ Smoke Detectors ☐ Falls risks **Housing**:_____ # stairs _____

Abuse: ☐ physical ☐ verbal ☐ financial ☐ neglect _____

Transportation: ☐ public ☐ community ☐ private ☐ Driving issues: _____

Appliances: ☐ hearing aid ☐ glasses ☐ reading glasses ☐ contacts ☐ dentures ☐ cane ☐ walker ☐ wheelchair ☐ prosthesis
Condition of appliances:

Review of Systems (Check box at left if all systems negative.)

☐ **General:** ☐ fever ☐ chills ☐ night sweats ☐ fatigue ☐ unexplained weight loss ☐ weight gain ☐ stopped eating or drinking

☐ **Skin:** ☐ pruritus ☐ rash ☐ hair loss ☐ worrisome lesion ☐ pigment change ☐ moles ☐ sweating ☐ dry skin ☐ nail change

☐ **HEENT:** ☐ headache ☐ dizziness ☐ scalp tenderness ☐ earache ☐ hearing loss ☐ tinnitus ☐ blurred vision ☐ loss of peripheral vision
☐ diplopia ☐ decr central vision ☐ difficulty reading ☐ eye pain/sensitivity ☐ glare intolerance ☐ excessive tearing ☐ eyeglasses/contact use
☐ glaucoma ☐ rhinorrhea ☐ nasal congestion ☐ postnasal drip ☐ sinus pain ☐ nosebleeds ☐ hay fever ☐ sore throat
☐ mouth sores ☐ hoarseness ☐ toothache ☐ bleeding gums ☐ difficulty speaking ☐ pain on chewing ☐ dentures/fit _____

☐ **Breast:** ☐ pain ☐ lumps ☐ discharge ☐ history of breast disease ☐ implants

☐ **Pulmonary:** ☐ cough ☐ sputum ☐ hemoptysis ☐ SOB ☐ pain with respiration ☐ wheezing ☐ cyanosis

☐ **CV:** ☐ chest pain ☐ palpitations ☐ DOE ☐ orthopnea ☐ PND ☐ diaphoresis ☐ syncope ☐ heart murmur ☐ leg edema

☐ **PVD:** ☐ claudication ☐ varicose veins ☐ phlebitis ☐ coldness of hands/feet ☐ leg ulcers

☐ **GI:** ☐ dysphagia ☐ heartburn ☐ change in appetite ☐ food intolerance ☐ nausea ☐ vomiting ☐ hematemesis ☐ abdominal pain ☐ bloating
☐ flatulence ☐ diarrhea ☐ constipation ☐ melena ☐ jaundice ☐ dark urine ☐ BRBPR ☐ BM incontinence ☐ hemorrhoids ☐ hernia

☐ **GU:** ☐ dysuria ☐ urgency ☐ frequency ☐ hematuria ☐ nocturia ☐ polyuria ☐ suprapubic pain ☐ flank pain ☐ incontinence ☐ genital lesions
♂ ☐ hesitancy ☐ dribbling ☐ decreased force stream ☐ testicular pain ☐ testicular mass/swelling ☐ penile discharge ☐ erectile dysfunction
♀ ☐ vaginal itch ☐ abnl vaginal discharge ☐ vaginal dryness ☐ dyspareunia ☐ sexual dysfunction ☐ abnl vaginal bleeding

☐ **Endocrine:** ☐ polyuria ☐ polydipsia ☐ polyphagia ☐ heat/cold intol ☐ tremor ☐ lump in throat ☐ unexplained wt change ☐ facial/body hair changes

☐ **Heme/Immune:** ☐ anemia ☐ easy bruising ☐ swollen glands ☐ bleeding of skin/mucous membranes ☐ frequent infections ☐ allergies ☐ delayed healing

☐ **MSK:** ☐ joint pain (location _____) ☐ stiffness ☐ restriction of motion ☐ immobility ☐ swelling ☐ erythema
☐ bony deformity ☐ myalgia ☐ muscle cramps ☐ weakness ☐ antalgic gait ☐ back pain

☐ **Neuro:** ☐ falls ☐ memory loss ☐ tremor ☐ gait disturbance ☐ paralysis ☐ numbness ☐ focal weakness ☐ seizure ☐ syncope ☐ aphasia

☐ **Psych:** ☐ anxiety ☐ confusion: acute/chronic ☐ depression ☐ mood changes ☐ irritability ☐ agitation ☐ apathy ☐ self-neglect ☐ taken to bed
☐ sleep disturbance/insomnia ☐ suicidal thoughts ☐ panic attacks ☐ personality change ☐ impaired judgment ☐ hallucinations ☐ decreased libido

Other/Details of Above:

Comprehensive Older Adult History and Physical - 3

Patient Name: _____

Date of Birth: _____ *Date of Exam:* _____

Physical Exam

N = Normal A = Abnormal (Check appropriate box)	N	A
1. General Appearance: age • LOC • nutrition • development • mobility • affect • speech • hygiene		
2. Skin: hydration • color • texture • hair • nails • feet • lesions		
3. Head: shape • symmetry • scalp • temporal art • TMJ • lesions		
4. Eyes: lids • conjunctiva • sclera		
Extraocular Muscles		
Visual fields		
Pupils: size, reaction to light and accommodation		
Fundi		
5. Ears: pinna • canals • TMs • hearing audioscope ☐		
6. Nose: patency • nares • sinuses • nasal mucosa • septum • turbinates		
7. Mouth: lips • gums • teeth • mucosa • palate • tongue		
8. Throat: pharynx • tonsils • uvula		
9. Neck: ROM • symmetry • palpation • thyroid • trachea • carotids • jugular veins • lymph nodes		
10. Breasts: size • symmetry • skin • nipples • palpation • nodes		
11. Chest/Lungs: excursion • palpation • percussion • auscultation		
12. Cardiac: PMI • palpation • rate • rhythm • S1 • S2 • murmurs • gallops • bruits • extra sounds		
13. Abdomen: appearance • bowel sounds • bruits • percussion • palpation • liver • spleen • flank • suprapubic • hernia		
14. Anorectal: perianal		
digital rectal		
stool guaiac		
prostate exam		
15. *Female Genitalia:* perineum • labia • urethral meatus • introitus		
Internal: vaginal mucosal • cervix		
Bimanual: vagina • cervix • uterus • adnexa • bladder		
16. Male Genitalia: penis • scrotum • testes • hernia		
17. Lymph Nodes: cervical • subclavian • axillary • inguinal • other		
18. *Musculoskeletal:* Back/Spine: ROM • palpation • curvature		
Upper Extremity: ROM • strength • palpation		
Lower Extremity: ROM • strength • palpation		
19. Peripheral Vascular: *Upper extremity:* pulses • appearance • temperature		
Lower extremity: pulses • appearance • temperature • CFT • Ankle-brachial index: _____		
☐ elevation pallor/dependent rubor		
20. Neurologic: cranial nerves • motor • sensory • cerebellar • reflexes • RAM • gait • mental status		

Assessment and Plan

Vitals

Ht _____ Wt _____ Temp _____ Resp _____ Pulse _____

BP (upright) _____ (supine) _____ Staff Initials _____

Visual Acuity

Right   /   Left   /

Corrective lenses ☐ Yes   ☐ No

Document Abnormals (by number)/Comments

Lab/Studies

Screenings:

☐ Mini-mental _____
☐ Depression _____
☐ Other: _____

Comprehensive Older Adult History and Physical - 4

Patient Name: _____

Medical Record #: _____ *Date of Birth:* _____

Assessment and Plan (continued)

Periodic Health Screening Plan

Exam	Performed	Scheduled	N/A	Refused
Breast exam				
Mammogram				
Pap test				
Prostate exam				
Testicular exam				
Digital rectal stool guaiac ☐				
Flexible Sigmoidoscopy/Colonoscopy				
Bone density				
PPD				

Health Counseling: (check if discussed, describe any intervention)

☐ Smoking cessation _____

☐ Alcohol/Drug Use _____

☐ Diet/Weight _____

☐ Vitamins/Calcium _____

☐ Medications/Interactions _____

☐ Periodic Dental/Vision care _____

☐ Podiatric care _____

☐ Exercise/Sleep _____

☐ Sun exposure _____

☐ Injury/Falls Prevention/Seatbelts _____

☐ Stress/Family issues _____

☐ Safety: Weapons/Violence/Abuse _____

☐ Housing _____

☐ Sexual issues/risks _____

☐ Loss/bereavement _____

☐ Living will/Power of atty/DNR _____

☐ End of life care _____

Immunizations

Immunizations current: ☐ Yes ☐ No

Vaccine	Given	Planned	Refused
Td			
Hepatitis B			
Influenza			
Pneumonia			
Other:			

Risk Factors:

☐ over 85   ☐ lives alone/ill spouse

☐ dementia   ☐ recently bereaved

☐ inadequate financial means

Lab/Studies Ordered

☐ ECG   ☐ UA/UC   ☐ FBS   ☐ Iron studies

☐ Spirometry   ☐ CBC/diff   ☐ HbA$_1$C   ☐ Folate

☐ Audiogram   ☐ Electrolytes   ☐ TSH   ☐ Albumin

                 ☐ Creat/BUN   ☐ Lipids   ☐ PSA

☐ CXR: _____

☐ CT/MRI: _____

☐ X-ray: _____

Referrals:

☐ Family contacted   ☐ Home assessment

☐ Long-term care program   ☐ Rehab/PT

☐ Community agency _____

☐ Specialist _____

_____

Provider's Signature   Date

☐ Note dictated/written

Office Visit

Date of Visit: _____

Patient Name: _____

Medical Record #: _____

Date of Birth: _____ Age: _____

Provider: _____ Length of visit: _____

History of Present Illness

PMH, Surgical, and Trauma History

☐ Unchanged since: _____

☐ Change: _____

Allergies

LMP: _____ Pregnant: ☐ Yes ☐ No

Contraceptives: _____

Tobacco: ☐ Yes ☐ No _____

ETOH: ☐ Yes ☐ No _____

Review of Systems (✔ system if done)

N=Normal A=Abnl	N	A		N	A	Findings:
Constitutional			GI			
Skin			GU			
HEENT			Endocrine			
Breast			Heme/Immune			
Pulmonary			MSK			
Cardiovascular			Neuro			
Peripheral Vascular			Psych			

Medications

Physical Exam (✔ system if done)

Vitals Ht _____ Wt _____ Temp _____ Resp _____ BP (upright) _____ (supine) _____ Pulse _____ Staff Initials _____

N = nl A = abnl	N	A		N	A		N	A		N	A
1. General			6. Nose			11. Chest/Lungs			16. Lymph Nodes		
2. Skin			7. Mouth			12. CV			17. Musculoskeletal		
3. Head			8. Throat			13. Abdomen			18. Peripheral Vascular		
4. Eyes			9. Neck			14. Anorectal guaiac ☐			19. Neurologic		
5. Ears			10. Breasts			15. Genitalia			Labs/Studies		

Document Abnormal Findings (by number):

Assessment and Plan

Lab/Studies Ordered

☐ UA/UC   ☐ Pap

☐ RBS/FBS   ☐ Bone density

☐ CBC/diff   ☐ ECG

☐ SMAC 7   ☐ CXR

☐ PT/INR   ☐ Mammogram

☐ Lipids   ☐ US _____

☐ TSH   ☐ CT/MRI _____

☐ PSA   ☐ X-Ray _____

☐ LFTs   ☐ _____

_____

Provider's Signature   Date

Referrals: _____

☐ Return to Office: _____

Medication History

Date of Visit: _____

Patient Name: _____

Medical Record #: _____

Date of Birth: _____ Age: _____

Provider: _____ Length of visit: _____

Current Medical Diagnoses	Allergies

Family History of Allergies:

Occupation: _____ Location _____

Hobbies: _____

Travel: ☐ Domestic ☐ International _____

Immunizations (last 5 yrs) ☐ Td _____

☐ Flu _____ ☐ Pneumonia _____

Diet: ☐ Balanced ☐ Frequency _____

Caffeine: ☐ No ☐ Yes cups/day _____ source _____

Tobacco: ☐ No ☐ Yes PPD _____ # Years ____ Quit Year ____

ETOH: ☐ No ☐ daily ☐ weekly ☐ monthly # drinks _____

Recreational Drugs:

Source of drugs: ☐ local pharmacy ☐ mail order ☐ Internet ☐ samples ☐ foreign (Can/Mex) ☐ Other _____

Cost Issues: ☐ No ☐ Yes _____

Accessibility Issues: ☐ No ☐ Yes _____

Where are drugs kept? _____

Drugs stored in unlabeled containers: ☐ Yes ☐ No _____

Drugs out of reach of small children: ☐ Yes ☐ No _____

Drugs discarded after expiration: ☐ Yes ☐ No _____

Current Medications: Prescription

Name of Drug	Dose	Frequency	Last Taken?	Takes Regularly?	Side Effects	Is Drug Helping?

Prior Prescription Medications: Previous 3 Months, No Longer Taking

Name of Drug	Dose	Frequency	Last Taken?	Side Effects	Reason for Discontinuation

Medication History - 2

Over-the-Counter Medication Use

Symptom	Drug(s) and Dose(s)	Frequency	Last Taken?	Helping Sx?	Side Effects
Pain (HA, muscle, back, tooth)					
Diarrhea					
Constipation					
Heartburn, Nausea					
Cough					
Congestion, Sinus, Colds					
Allergies					
Sleep Aid					
Stimulants (sleep avoidance)					
Weight loss					
Anxiety					
Depression					
Menstrual/Menopause					
Fluid Retention					
Skin (Itching, dryness, psoriasis, tinea)					
Vitamins/Minerals/Salt Substitutes					
Herbals (pills, roots, teas)					
Food Supplements					

Other/Details:

Assessment/Plan:

_____
Provider's Signature   Date

CHAPTER 2

Patient Information Logs and Records

Chapter Contents

ICON KEY: ▤ Tool Printed ✐ Tool on CD-ROM ∞ Customizable Tool **i** Information and Resources Provided for Further Acquisition

Purpose of Logs, Records, and Flow Sheets

In today's practice environment, it has become increasingly important to develop record-keeping practices that enhance expedient access to patient information. Multiple providers within and outside the practice, internal and external medical record auditors, and claims processors all benefit from consistent, legible, and concise patient record summaries. Rapid review of current care and health status promotes efficiency in modern practices, in which patient interaction time is often limited.

In addition, the past decade has seen tremendous growth of studies demonstrating improved patient outcomes through detection procedures and behavioral interventions. Consumer and government agencies have developed guidelines by which to measure the quality of preventive care. (For current guidelines on evidence-based preventive services, the reader may access the second and third editions of the *Guide to Clinical Services* from the Agency for Healthcare Research and Quality: Report of the U.S. Preventive Services Task Force [see Online Resources section].)

Increasingly, health insurance payers encourage preventive screening and have developed quality audit procedures to ensure compliance among their providers. For the purposes of effective delivery and accountability, preventive health services need to be accurately documented and tracked over time. Studies have shown that reminder systems that allow quick review of patient data will increase the delivery of preventive care. Such systems can also

---

- Organizes a summary of patient information
- Allows immediate overview of health status without need to consult progress notes
- Improves provider and staff efficiency by reducing time spent searching for patient information
- Allows more expedient handling of acute-care visits during busy times
- Minimizes the effort needed for adequate documentation
- Facilitates communication among multiple staff providers involved in a patient's care
- Facilitates communication with nonprovider office staff
- Makes leaving important facts out less likely through systematic information collection
- Improves the delivery of preventive health care services
- Meets the requirements of various insurance and government organizations

Box **2-2** Recommendations for Effective Use of Information Logs

- Office staff should be educated as to the importance of implementation of information log documentation and access.
- Instruction on how to use the flow sheets must be provided to office staff and providers.
- Responsibilities for completion of log entries at each patient encounter must be clearly assigned to providers and staff.
- Data need to be consistently and promptly entered.
- Flow sheet entries must be legible.
- Information logs are best kept in a separate section in the front of the medical record, which facilitates immediate retrieval by providers and staff.
- Periodic random chart review for compliance in information log maintenance is recommended.

> **Information must be consistently and promptly entered by all providers to ensure successful use of these forms!!**

ease insurance audits, facilitate coding and billing services, and promote effective communication among staff members regarding an individual patient's care.

A simple, but important, office tool for tracking patient health data and provider interventions is a flow sheet or log in the patient medical record. Data records provide a concise and organized approach to documentation of ongoing health monitoring (Box 2-1). Relevant patient information may be summarized in one place in the chart. Information logs may be designed to correspond with preventive services provided and the health care needs of the patient population. Forms may track an array of patient information including problem lists, medication and vaccine history, prescriptions dispensed, preventive care, and monitoring of common chronic health problems. Compilation of medical data on one page permits an immediate overview of health status and prior interventions. Accurately maintained flow sheets alert the provider to health issues influencing a current visit, guide preventive care services, and assist office staff with coding and billing issues. Opportunities to schedule and deliver preventive care and monitor ongoing health issues are enhanced by easy access to patient data.

Content of Forms

The forms in this chapter offer a range of patient information logs and records. The reader may choose to use the forms most pertinent to his or her practice. The reader may use these forms as printed or modify them to best suit individual practice by following instructions on the CD-ROM. Forms previously published or adapted may be printed, but are not available for modification.

Recommendations for effective use of patient information logs are listed in Box 2-2. When a new patient information log is introduced into a medical record system,

responsibilities for printing the forms, inserting forms into charts, and entering log data must be clearly assigned and monitored.

Adult Health Profile

This form contains demographic information, allergies, code status, and emergency contact information. Personal risk factors, such as smoking, and familial risk factors, such as cardiovascular disease, may be noted in the upper right table. Problem lists for both chronic and acute illnesses are centrally located. An area to document referrals to specialists is also included. It is recommended that this form be placed on the first page or inner cover of the medical record.

Adult Health Care Maintenance Record

This form provides an overview of the preventive care measures and anticipatory guidance provided for individual patients.

Medication Log

Injection Record

Adult Vaccine and PPD Administration Record

Pediatric Vaccine and PPD Administration Record

These forms document medications, injections, and vaccines that are prescribed or administered by the provider.

Medication Refill Log

This form permits documentation of all medication prescriptions and refills. It differs from the medication log in that it documents the quantity and frequency of medication use. The user may choose to highlight narcotic and benzodiazepine prescriptions to better track use of these substances.

Laboratory Results

X-ray and Special Procedure Results

Coagulation Monitoring Log

These forms compile laboratory and procedure orders and results in one location. Properly maintained, these logs dramatically increase efficiency by eliminating a search through pages of prior reports to glean patient lab value history. Log entry may be delegated to a staff member as reports are received by the office, before or after review by the provider.

Vital Signs Flow Sheet

The vital signs flow sheet allows for rapid review of vital signs, past office visits, routine health care, and medications. By scanning the vital signs flow sheet, the provider can get a feel for the patient without reading the progress notes. All scheduled office visits are entered, including no-show and nursing appointments. A brief entry including the diagnosis, medications prescribed, and comments gives the provider a concise review of prior care. Highlighting no-show appointments and narcotic/benzodiazepine prescriptions in different colors allows better tracking of these important issues.

Blood Pressure Log

Diabetes Monitoring Log

Asthma Monitoring Log

These forms organize patient data relevant to hypertension, diabetes, and asthma management. Monitoring laboratory values, medication use, pertinent screenings, and teaching serves to improve overall care of patients with these chronic illnesses.

Telephone Triage Call Record

Telephone triage may be rendered by clinicians or office staff. Telephone protocols are available for a variety of specialties and may be used to assist the triage personnel in prescreening the patient caller. The triage staff must determine the urgency of the patient's problem and advise the patient of the appropriate actions he or she must take to treat the problem. Documentation of patient calls is essential to maintain continuity of patient care and to provide a written record of the encounter for legal protection.

Telephone triage documentation should include the date and time of the call, identifying information for the patient and the caller, the reason for the call, and information regarding the patient's current health status, medications, and allergies. The triage staff should also record their impression, the protocol used (if any), and the suggested advice. Caller response, time of the end of the call, and the name of the professional taking the call provide additional essential details.

The telephone triage call record form reprinted in this chapter contains the essential information outlined above. Additional health status information, a useful mnemonic device (SCHOLAR) to help elicit important patient history, and a listing of activities of daily living (ADL) pertinent to assessment of the patient's complaint are also included. After completion of the triage process, it is recommended that the triage form be placed in the patient's record.

Resources and References

Online Resources

Agency for Healthcare Research and Quality (AHRQ): *Put Prevention into Practice (PPIP).* A program to increase the appropriate use of clinical preventive services, such as screening tests, immunizations, and counseling, based on U.S. Preventive Services Task Force recommendations. Web site: http://www.ahrq.gov/clinic/ppipix.htm.

Agency for Healthcare Research and Quality: U.S. Preventive Services Task Force (USPSTF): *Reviews and recommendations: guide to clinical preventive services,* ed 2, 1996, and ed 3, 2000-2004. An independent panel of experts in primary care and prevention systematically reviews the evidence of effectiveness and develops recommendations for clinical preventive services. Web site: http://www.ahcpr.gov/clinic/uspstfix.htm.

Centers for Disease Control and Prevention (CDC) National Immunization Program: Complete, current information and schedules for immunizations. Web site: http://www.cdc.gov/nip.

Centers for Disease Control and Prevention (CDC) National Immunization Program: Recommendations of the ACIP (Advisory Committee on Immunization Practices): comprehensive and current recommendations on immunizations. Web site: http://www.cdc.gov/nip/publications/acip-list.htm.

References and Suggested Readings

Buppert C: *The primary care provider's guide to compensation and quality: how to get paid and not get sued,* Boston, 2003, Jones and Bartlett Publishers.

Caffee AE, Teichman PG: Improving anticoagulation management at the point of care, *Fam Pract Manag* 9:35-37, 2002. Web site: www.aafp.org/fpm/20020200/35impr.html.

Giovino JM: Reimbursement strategies: coding level-one office visits: a refresher course, *Fam Pract Manag* 7:39-42, 2000. Web site: www.aafp.org/fpm/20000700/39codi.html.

Standridge JB: Putting prevention into practice, *Clin Fam Pract* 2:485, 2000.

Studdiford JS III, et al: The telephone in primary care. *Prim Care* 23(1):83-102, 1996.

Wheeler S: Telephone triage: SAVED by the form, *Nursing* 30:54-55, 2000.

Adult Health Profile

Patient Name: _____

Medical Record #: _____

Address: _____

*Telephone: (home)*_____ *(business)* _____

Date of Birth: _____ *Gender:* ☐ *Male* ☐ *Female*

Allergies: _____

_____

_____

Code Status: _____

Advance Directives on File: ☐ *Yes* ☐ *No*

Emergency Contact: _____

_____

Risk Factors

Risk Factor: Personal or Familial History	Personal	Familial

Problem List: Chronic

Entry Date	Description: Chronic Problem	Date Begun

Problem List: Acute

Entry Date	Description: Acute Problem	Date Begun	Date Ended

Referrals

Specialist	Problem	Date of Referral	Letter Received

Adult Health Maintenance Record

Patient Name: _____

Medical Record #: _____

Telephone: (home)_____ (business) _____

Date of Birth: _____ Gender: ☐ Male ☐ Female

Primary Provider: _____

Examination	Date	Result	Date	Result	Date	Result	Date	Result	Date	Result	Date	Result
Blood Pressure												
Weight (Height:)												
Pap												
Pelvic Exam												
Breast Exam												
Bone Density												
Digital Rectal Exam												
Stool Guaiac												
Flex Sig/Colonoscopy												
Testicular Exam												
Skin Exam												
Foot Exam												
Vision Exam												
Glaucoma Screening												
Dental Care												
Audiogram												
Cholesterol Screen												
CBC												
Blood Glucose (RBG/FBG)												
Thyroid Screen												
PSA												
UA												

Health Counseling

Issues Discussed	Dates ▶										
Smoking Cessation											
Alcohol and Drugs											
Diet and Weight											
Vitamins and Calcium											
Physical Activity											
Dental Care											
Vision Care											
Foot Care											
Sun Exposure											
Safety: Seatbelts, helmets											
Safety: Housing, falls, guns											
Occupational Health											
Stress/Family Issues											
Domestic Violence											
Sexual Issues and Risks											
Contraception											
Self-Exams (BSE, TSE, skin)											
Polypharmacy											
Advance Directives											

Medication Log

Patient Name: _____

Medical Record #: _____

Telephone: (home)_____ (business) _____

Date of Birth: _____ Gender: ☐ Male ☐ Female

Primary Provider: _____

Medication	Dose	Sig	Start	Stop	Medication	Dose	Sig	Start	Stop

Medication Refill Log

Patient Name: _____

Medical Record #: _____

Telephone: (home)_____ (business) _____

Date of Birth: _____ Gender: ☐ Male ☐ Female

Primary Provider: _____

Date	Medication	Dosage	Qty	Sig	Refills	Pharmacy	Prescriber	Caller

Injection Record

Patient Name: _____

Medical Record #: _____

*Telephone: (home)*_____ *(business)* _____

Date of Birth: _____ *Gender:* ☐ *Male* ☐ *Female*

Primary Provider: _____

Date	Medication	Dosage	Lot #	Exp	Inj Site	Reaction	Initials/Provider

Adult Vaccine & PPD Administration Record

Patient Name: _____

Medical Record #: _____

Telephone: (home) _____ *(business)* _____

Date of Birth: _____ *Gender:* ☐ *Male* ☐ *Female*

I have read, or have had explained to me, information about the diseases and the vaccines listed below. I have had a chance to ask questions that were answered to my satisfaction. I believe I understand the benefits and risks of the vaccines listed and ask that the vaccine(s) listed below be given to me or to the person named above (for whom I am authorized to make this request).

VACCINE	Date Given (mm/dd/yr)	Vaccine Manufacturer	Vaccine Lot #	Site Given	Initials of Vaccine Adm*	Signature of Patient or Guardian
Td						
MMR						
Hep B 1						
Hep B 2						
Hep B 3						
Varicella 1						
Varicella 2						
Meningococcal						
Pneumovax						
Influenza						

Immunization History

Vaccine	Year Primary Series Complete	Year of Last Booster	Facility
DTP/DTaP			
Polio			
MMR			
Hep B			
Varicella			

PPD-Mantoux Testing

Date Adm	Initials of Adm*	Date Read	Result	Read By

*Signature of Vaccine Administrator

Use reverse side if more signatures are needed.

Pediatric Vaccine & PPD Administration Record

Patient Name: _____

Medical Record #: _____

Telephone: (home)_____ (business) _____

Date of Birth: _____ Gender: ☐ Male ☐ Female

I have read, or have had explained to me, information about the diseases and the vaccines listed below. I have had a chance to ask questions that were answered to my satisfaction. I believe I understand the benefits and risks of the vaccines listed and ask that the vaccine(s) listed below be given to me or to the person named above (for whom I am authorized to make this request).

VACCINE	Date Given (mm/dd/yr)	Vaccine Manufacturer	Vaccine Lot #	Site Given	Initials of Vaccine Adm*	Signature of Patient or Guardian
DtaP/DT 1						
DtaP/DT 2						
DtaP/DT 3						
DtaP/DT 4						
DtaP/DT 5						
Td						
Hib 1						
Hib 2						
Hib 3						
Hib 4						
IPV 1						
IPV 2						
IPV 3						
IPV 4						
MMR 1						
MMR 2						
Hep B 1						
Hep B 2						
Hep B 3						
PCV 1						
PCV 2						
PCV 3						
PCV 4						
Varicella 1						
Varicella 2						
Meningococcal						
Pneumovax						
Influenza						

*Signature of Vaccine Administrator

PPD				
Date Adm	Initials of Adm*	Date Read	Result	Read By

Use reverse side if more signatures are needed.

Laboratory Results

Patient Name: _____

Medical Record #: _____

Telephone: (home) _____ *(business)* _____

Date of Birth: _____ *Gender:* ☐ *Male* ☐ *Female*

Primary Provider: _____

Test	Date	Result	Informed (initials)	Plan

X-Ray and Special Procedure Results

Patient Name: _____

Medical Record #: _____

*Telephone: (home)*_____ *(business)* _____

Date of Birth: _____ *Gender:* ☐ *Male* ☐ *Female*

Primary Provider: _____

Test	Date	Result	Informed (initials)	Plan

Coagulation Monitoring Log

Patient Name: _____

Medical Record #: _____

Telephone: (home)_____ (business) _____

Date of Birth: _____ Gender: ☐ Male ☐ Female

Primary Provider: _____

Device _____

Date	PT (sec)	INR	Current Coumadin Dose	Action/Comments	Tech/Provider

Blood Pressure Log

Patient Name: _____

Medical Record #: _____

Telephone: (home) _____ *(business)* _____

Date of Birth: _____ *Gender:* ☐ *Male* ☐ *Female*

Primary Provider: _____

Date	BP	Medications	Initials	Date	BP	Medications	Initials

Enter the date below; place a dot on the line closest to systolic pressure; in the *same* column place a dot on the line closest to diastolic pressure.

mm Hg
> 240
230
220
200
190
180
170
160
150
140
130
120
110
100
90
80
70
60
< 60
Date ▶

Vital Signs Flow Sheet

Patient Name: _____

Medical Record #: _____

Telephone: (home)_____ (business) _____

Date of Birth: _____ Gender: ☐ Male ☐ Female

Primary Provider: _____

Height _____ Ideal Weight Range _____

Date	Initials	Weight	BP	Pulse	Resp	Temp	Pain	Diagnosis, plan, meds, notes

Diabetes Monitoring Log

Patient Name: _____

Medical Record #: _____

Telephone: (home) _____ *(business)* _____

Date of Birth: _____ *Gender:* ☐ *Male* ☐ *Female*

Primary Provider: _____

Height _____ *Ideal Weight Range* _____ ☐ *Wears Medic Alert*

Each Visit

Date	Initials	Weight	BP	RBS	Diet & Exercise	Foot exam	Tobacco	Diagnosis, plan, meds, notes

Periodic Screening

Visit Date/Initials →							
Fasting Blood Glucose							
HgA$_1$C (desired <7%)							
Total Cholesterol/HDL/LDL/TG							
Microalbumin/creatinine							
Comprehensive foot exam							
Dilated eye exam							

Teaching

Date/Initials →							
Pathophysiology of Diabetes							
Glucometer use							
Insulin administration/meds							
Nutrition counseling							
Foot care							

Asthma Monitoring Log

Patient Name: _____

Medical Record #: _____

Telephone: (home)_____ (business) _____

Date of Birth: _____ Gender: ☐ Male ☐ Female

Primary Provider: _____

Height _____ Goal PFM Reading _____ ☐ Wears Medic Alert

Each Visit

Date	Initials	Weight	BP	Peak Flow Demo	Tobacco	Allergy Prevention	Diagnosis, plan, meds, notes

Teaching

Date/Initials →								
Pathophysiology of Asthma								
Use of peak flow meter								
Inhaler use and care								
Types and use of medications								
Allergen avoidance								

Emergency Department Visits: _____

Hospitalizations: _____

Referrals: _____

Telephone Triage Call Record

Patient Name: _____

Medical Record #: _____

Telephone: (home) _____ *(business)* _____

Date of Birth: _____ *Age:* _____ *Gender: Male   Female*

Primary Provider: _____

Triage/Advice Form

				4. Scholar
1. Adult?	**Pediatric?**		**Name**	

						4. Scholar
Age DOB M F		Date Time AM PM				Sx
Caller/Relation to Pt.		Hx Prematurity? Y N Wt.				Char.
Temp. Oral Ax Rec. BP		2. Immz Up-to-Date? Y N (N = Needs Appt.)				Course

3. Chief Complaint

Hx of Sx

Onset

Loc.

4. SCHOLAR, ADLs (see right margin)

Ag. Fac.

5. Home Tx Administered?   Y   N

Rel. Fac.

ADL

6. *Last Menstrual Period?* 7. *Pregnant?* Y N	8. *Breast-feeding?* Y N	Intake
9. *Allergies?* Y N	10. *Chronic Illness?* Y N	Liquid
		Solid
	11. *Emotional State?*	Output
12. *Medications?* Y N	13. *Recent Injury?* Y N	Urine
	14. *Recent Illness?* Y N	BM
		Emesis
	15. *Recent Ingestion?* Y N	Sleep

16. Impression:

Activity

Color

17. Protocol Advice/18. Modifications:

19. Mode of Transport:	20. Advised to Be Here within Min. Hr.
21. Appt. Date Time	22. Precautions Stated? Y N
23. Client Agreement to Plan? Y N	
24. RN Sig/Title	25. Time Ended

From Wheeler S: Telephone triage: SAVED by the form, *Nursing* 30:54–55, 2000.

CHAPTER 3

Pediatric History and Physical Examination Forms and Tools

Chapter Contents

TOOL	DESCRIPTION	LOCATION OF TOOLS	FORMAT
Pediatric History and Physical Forms			
Pediatric Initial Health Questionnaire	p. 50	p. 56-57	📋 ✐ ∞
Pediatric Well Visit Forms:			
0 to 1-Month Well-Child Visit	p. 51-52	p. 58-59	📋 ✐ ∞
2-Month Well-Child Visit	p. 51-52	p. 60-61	📋 ✐ ∞
4-Month Well-Child Visit	p. 51-52	p. 62-63	📋 ✐ ∞
6-Month Well-Child Visit	p. 51-52	p. 64-65	📋 ✐ ∞
9-Month Well-Child Visit	p. 51-52	p. 66-67	📋 ✐ ∞
12-Month Well-Child Visit	p. 51-52	p. 68-69	📋 ✐ ∞
15-Month Well-Child Visit	p. 51-52	p. 70-71	📋 ✐ ∞
18-Month Well-Child Visit	p. 51-52	p. 72-73	📋 ✐ ∞
2-Year Well-Child Visit	p. 51-52	p. 74-75	📋 ✐ ∞
3-Year Well-Child Visit	p. 51-52	p. 76-77	📋 ✐ ∞
4-Year Well-Child Visit	p. 51-52	p. 78-79	📋 ✐ ∞
5-Year Well-Child Visit	p. 51-52	p. 80-81	📋 ✐ ∞
6-7 Year Well-Child Visit	p. 51-52	p. 82-83	📋 ✐ ∞
8-10 Year Well-Child Visit	p. 51-52	p. 84-85	📋 ✐ ∞
11-14 Year Well-Child Visit	p. 51-52	p. 86-87	📋 ✐ ∞
15-17 Year Well Visit	p. 51-52	p. 88-89	📋 ✐ ∞
18-20 Year Well Visit	p. 51-52	p. 90-91	📋 ✐ ∞
Pediatric Well Care Summaries:			
Well-Child Visit: Newborn to 4 Months	p. 52	p. 92	📋 ✐ ∞
Well-Child Visit: 6 to 12 Months	p. 52	p. 93	📋 ✐ ∞
Well-Child Visit: 15 Months to 2 Years	p. 52	p. 94	📋 ✐ ∞
Well-Child Visit: 3 to 5 Years	p. 52	p. 95	📋 ✐ ∞
Well-Child Visit: 6 to 11 Years	p. 52	p. 96	📋 ✐ ∞
Well-Adolescent Visit: 12 to 18 Years	p. 52	p. 97	📋 ✐ ∞
Pediatric Screening Forms			
Screening Form for Early Follow-up of Breastfed Infants	p. 52	p. 98	📋 ✐
Breastfeeding Infant Triage Form	p. 52	p. 99	📋 ✐
Periodic Blood Lead Screening Risk Questionnaire	p. 52	p. 100	📋 ✐ ∞
Tuberculosis Risk Questionnaire	p. 52	p. 101	📋 ✐ ∞

Chapter Contents—cont'd

ICON KEY: 📄 Tool Printed ⊘ Tool on CD-ROM ∞ Customizable Tool **i** Information and Resources Provided for Further Acquisition

Introduction and Contents

Preventive pediatric health care focuses on optimal monitoring and care for the developing child, with anticipatory guidance for parents. Pediatric preventive care includes an initial health history, completed at the child's first health visit, and a well-child examination. This initial visit is followed by incremental well visits, at which the child's developmental progress is evaluated. Components in the pediatric initial health history include patient demographics, birth and pregnancy history, family social and health histories, nutrition history, past medical history, immunization status and screening history, medications, allergies, and brief developmental and behavioral histories (Box 3-1).

The pediatric initial and interval well examinations include updating of family and social history, interval history, review of systems, daily activities, behavioral assessment, developmental screening, physical examination, assessment and plan (Box 3-2).

Guidelines and standards have been established by numerous organizations and governmental agencies; several national organizations are listed in Box 3-3, with references cited at the end of this introduction. The forms in this chapter are designed to include the guidelines set by the groups listed in Box 3-3, but have not been endorsed by these groups.

PEDIATRIC HISTORY AND PHYSICAL FORMS

Pediatric Initial Health Questionnaire

This two-page form documents information obtained during an initial pediatric visit. Included on this form are patient demographics, pregnancy and birth history, family social and health histories, nutrition history, brief

---

Box **3-1** **Pediatric Initial Health History Essential Components**

INITIAL HISTORY
- Birth and Pregnancy History
- Family Social History
  - Parental marital status, occupations, siblings
  - Residence age and conditions, cohabitants, pets
  - Cultural and religious influences
  - Financial status, medical insurance
  - Family social support
- Family Health History
  - Age and health or age and cause of death of parents, siblings, grandparents
  - Family occurrence of major diseases, hereditary disorders, psychiatric problems
- Nutrition History
  - Feeding during infancy
  - Food intolerances

PAST MEDICAL HISTORY
- Previous illnesses
- Nonsurgical hospitalizations
- Serious injuries, accidents, or abuse
- Surgeries
- Transfusions

IMMUNIZATION STATUS AND SCREENING HISTORY
- Immunization status
- Vision, hearing, and dental screening
- Previous laboratory screening: TB, lead, SCA, urine, hemoglobin/hematocrit

MEDICATIONS
- Current and recently prescribed medications
- Nonprescription and home remedies
- Vitamin, fluoride, and supplement use
- Prosthetic devices, glasses, orthodontia, corrective shoes

ALLERGIES
- Medications
- Environmental allergens, latex
- Foods, lactose

DEVELOPMENTAL HISTORY
- Growth history
- Developmental milestones

BEHAVIORAL HISTORY
- School and peer issues
- Family and relationship issues

TB, Tuberculosis; SCA, sickle cell anemia.

Box 3-2 Pediatric Well-Visit Essential Components

UPDATE FAMILY AND SOCIAL HISTORY

INTERVAL HISTORY (subsequent to initial well visit)
- Parental concerns
- Injuries, accidents, or abuse
- Surgeries
- Hospitalizations
- Medications
- Allergies

REVIEW OF SYSTEMS
- Detailed questions for each body system to include general constitutional, dermatologic, HEENT, breast, respiratory, cardiovascular, peripheral vascular, gastrointestinal, genitourinary, endocrine, hematologic, immunologic, musculoskeletal, neurologic, and psychiatric reviews as indicated by age

DAILY ACTIVITIES
- Nutrition
- Sleep
- Hygiene
- Dental
- Exercise
- Recreation
- Caregivers
- School
- Safety

BEHAVIORAL ASSESSMENT
- School and peer issues
- Family and relationship issues
- Adolescent risk assessment: substance use, sexual history, safety, relationships, and emotional development

DEVELOPMENTAL SCREENING
- Personal, social, cognitive, self-care development
- Gross and fine motor development
- Language

PHYSICAL EXAMINATION
- Measurements: Head circumference (to age 3 yr), height, and weight monitored for growth rate; vital signs
- Sensory screening: vision and hearing
- Objective findings on physical examination by means of inspection, auscultation, percussion, and palpation processes
- Laboratory testing, radiographs, and other special procedures
- Use of validated and reliable screening tools, if necessary

ASSESSMENT
- Well child status
- Additional problems
- Assessment or differential diagnosis for each problem
- Anticipated potential problems

PLAN
- Diagnostic tests or studies to be performed
- Treatment plan for any problem including prescription and nonprescription medications, physical therapy, assistive devices, home remedies, behavioral changes, and referrals for specialist or home services
- Laboratory screening tests (age-appropriate)
- Immunization update and administration
- Anticipatory guidance
- Patient referrals: dental, smoking cessation, other
- Follow-up plan for reevaluation of any problems
- Schedule next age-appropriate well-child visit

HEENT, Head, ears, eyes, nose, and throat.

Box 3-3 Organizations with Guidelines on Preventive Pediatric Practice

Agency for Healthcare Research and Quality (AHRQ):
   Put Prevention into Practice (PPIP)
   U.S. Preventive Services Task Force
American Academy of Pediatrics Committee on
   Practice and Ambulatory Medicine:
   Recommendations for Preventive Pediatric Practice
National Center for Education in Maternal and Child
   Health at Georgetown University: Bright Futures
   Guidelines
Institute for Clinical Systems Improvement: Preventive
   Services for Children and Adolescents
American Medical Association: Guidelines for
   Adolescent Preventive Services (GAPS)
Centers for Disease Control and Prevention (CDC):
   National Immunization Program
CDC: National Center for Environmental Health:
   Screening Young Children for Lead Poisoning
CDC: Advisory Council for the Elimination of Tuberculosis

developmental and behavioral histories, past medical history, medications, allergies, and immunization and screening history. This form is designed to be completed by the parent or guardian of the child before the appointment for the first well visit and to be reviewed by the provider.

Pediatric Well Visit Forms

The 17 pediatric well-visit forms presented in this chapter were adapted from the age-related documentation forms for pediatric well-care visits created by the Child & Teen Checkup Documentation Template Workgroup consisting of the Minnesota Department of Health and Human Services, physicians, coding/billing representatives, clinic quality improvement staff, and representatives from health plans and public health departments.

   Each two-page form includes the age-appropriate essential components of the pediatric well visit, as outlined previously. Text block areas with cues for documentation, check-off boxes and tables, lines for short answers, and narrative documentation space are included for the following age-appropriate categories:

Patient and Office Identifying Information
Measurements
Vision/Hearing
Child Health History:
    Update on Family/
        Social History
    Parental/Child Concerns
    Interval History
    Review of Systems
    Daily Activities:
        Nutrition   Sleep
        Hygiene   Dental
        Recreation   Exercise
        Caregivers
        Safety
        Environmental Risks
        Community Support
        Behavior Risks

Development:
    Personal/social/cognitive
    Fine motor/adaptive
    Language
    Gross motor
    School/Activities
    Relationships: family/peer
    Emotional
Physical Examination:
    Systems Exam
Assessment
Plan:
    Anticipatory Guidance
    Immunization Plan
    Laboratory Tests/Other
        Studies
    Dental
    Other Referrals

The reader may use these forms as printed or modify them to suit individual practice by following instructions on the CD-ROM.

Seventeen Child & Teen Checkups (C&TC) Provider Documentation forms acknowledgements: Allina Health Systems/Medica Health Plans, Blue Cross and Blue Shield/Blue Plus of Minnesota, Children's Physician Network, HealthPartners, Hennepin County Community Health, Hennepin County Medical Center, Metropolitan Health Plan, Minnesota Department of Health, Minnesota Department of Human Services, UCare, University Affiliated Family Physicians, University of Minnesota, and many other individuals who contributed valuable feedback throughout the development process.

Pediatric Well-Care Summaries

These one-page forms contain space for documentation for three age-interval well visits. There are spaces for measurement and vital signs documentation and small areas for interval history, daily activities, and nutrition. There is minimal space for narrative documentation of specifics. Check-off boxes are provided for major developmental tasks; acknowledgement of vision, hearing, and dental screening; physical examination; anticipatory guidance; and age-appropriate immunizations and laboratory tests. These forms are created for the provider who prefers brief-form documentation, supplemented by a dictated or handwritten note.

PEDIATRIC SCREENING FORMS

Screening Form for Early Follow-up of Breastfed Infants

This one-page questionnaire, developed by The Lactation Program, Rose Medical Center, Denver, Colorado, is designed to detect early breastfeeding problems. It is ideally administered to the breastfeeding mother 4 to 6 days after delivery. If an office visit is not scheduled for this time, the form can be given to the mother at the time of hospital discharge and can be completed at home. Alternatively, triage personnel can assist the mother with completion of the form by phone at the appropriate time interval.

Breastfeeding Infant Triage Form

This one-page triage form designed by Christine Betzold, NP, IBCLC, MSN, targets identification of breastfeeding problems in the newborn and mother dyad. It is recommended that all breastfeeding mothers complete this form during the infant's first week of life; the form provides good documentation of breastfeeding concerns and subsequent advice. The form may be completed in the office or during telephone conversations regarding a breastfeeding problem in a newborn.

Periodic Blood Lead Screening Risk Questionnaire

This brief questionnaire follows guidelines for lead screening set by the Centers for Disease Control and Prevention (CDC) National Center for Environmental Health in 1997 and American Academy of Pediatrics (AAP) Committee on Environmental Health in 1998. Guidelines suggest that all children be assessed for possible lead exposure annually between 6 months and 6 years of age by using community-specific risk assessment questions. In communities where universal blood lead level screening is recommended, the suggested guidelines call for routine blood lead level screening to be done once at age 9 to 12 months, with consideration of a second screening at age 24 months. In communities where targeted screening is recommended, guidelines suggest determining which patients are at risk and screening when necessary. If at any time an item on the questionnaire elicits a "yes" or "not sure" response, further questioning about environmental risk factors for lead poisoning is indicated, and blood lead level screening should be considered. For more information or to determine whether your community is recommended for universal screening, please contact your local health department or the online resources cited for CDC and AAP guidelines.

Tuberculosis Risk Questionnaire

This questionnaire is designed to assess risk of tuberculosis (TB) on the basis of factors identified by The American Thoracic Society and CDC Advisory Council for the Elimination of Tuberculosis. Recommendations by these groups have been adopted as policy by the American Academy of Pediatrics. The policy directives include the following:

1. All children need routine health care evaluations that include assessment of their risk of exposure to TB (Box 3-4).
2. Routine tuberculin skin testing of children with no risk factors residing in low-prevalence communities is not indicated.

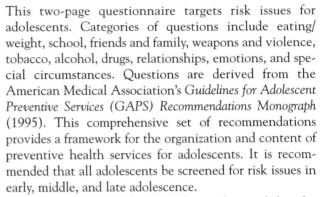

Box 3-4 Children at High Risk for Tuberculosis Exposure

- Close contact with persons known or suspected to have tuberculosis (TB) (i.e., those sharing the same household or other enclosed environments)
- Child with human immunodeficiency virus (HIV)
- Birth or travel within 5 years to endemic TB areas: Africa, Middle East, Asia, Latin America, or Caribbean and/or significant contact with indigenous persons from such countries
- Regular contact with adults at high risk for TB:
  - Homeless person
  - Incarcerated person
  - Illicit drug user
  - HIV-positive patient
- Residents of high-risk congregate settings (e.g., mental institutions, other long-term residential facilities, and shelters for the homeless)
- Some medically underserved, low-income populations
- High-risk racial or ethnic minority populations, as defined locally

From http://www.cdc.gov/mmwr/preview/mmwrhtml/00038873.htm

3. Tuberculin skin testing should generally be performed only in persons who belong to at least one of the high-risk groups identified in Box 3-4.

4. Children who have no risk factors but who reside in high-prevalence regions and children whose histories for risk factors are incomplete or unreliable should be considered for tuberculin (Mantoux) skin testing at 4 to 6 and 11 to 16 years of age. The decision to test should be based on the local epidemiology of tuberculosis in conjunction with advice from regional TB control officials.

5. Family investigation is indicated whenever a tuberculin skin test result of a parent or guardian converts from negative to positive (indicating recent infection).

6. Children with human immunodeficiency virus (HIV) infection or disease should have annual tuberculin skin tests.

The questionnaire included in this chapter is designed to be completed by the parent or guardian of the child before the office visit. Frequency of administration of a TB risk questionnaire after the first completion has not been suggested by pediatric organizations. It is recommended that clinicians consult their local health departments for information on risk groups within their community and follow local recommendations for frequency of risk assessment.

ADOLESCENT RISK ASSESSMENT FORMS

Adolescent Risk Monitoring Log

This form for tracking of adolescent risk assessment contains space for documentation at four age-interval well visits. Risk categories include nutrition, school, safety, substance abuse, sexuality, violence and abuse, and special circumstances. Columns provide space for brief documentation of individual risks and education provided.

Adolescent Questionnaire

This two-page questionnaire targets risk issues for adolescents. Categories of questions include eating/weight, school, friends and family, weapons and violence, tobacco, alcohol, drugs, relationships, emotions, and special circumstances. Questions are derived from the American Medical Association's *Guidelines for Adolescent Preventive Services (GAPS) Recommendations Monograph* (1995). This comprehensive set of recommendations provides a framework for the organization and content of preventive health services for adolescents. It is recommended that all adolescents be screened for risk issues in early, middle, and late adolescence.

Additional comprehensive forms designed by the American Medical Association (AMA) to support the implementation of the *Guidelines for Adolescent Preventive Services* (GAPS) are available for reproduction at http://www.ama-assn.org/ama/pub/category/2280.html.

Younger adolescent, middle/older adolescent, and parent/guardian questionnaires in English and Spanish are included on this site.

Adolescent Psychosocial History Tools

Numerous mnemonic tools exist to cue the clinician on history taking and anticipatory guidance processes. Two of the more common mnemonic tools used in obtaining an adolescent risk history are *HEADSSS* and *SAFETEENS* (Box 3-5).

Box 3-5 Adolescent Psychosocial History Tools

HEADSSS*
H - Home and family
E - Education and school
A - Activities and associates
D - Drugs, alcohol, and tobacco
S - Sexuality and sexual activity
S - Suicide and depression
S - Safety, violence and abuse

SAFETEENS†
S - Sexuality
A - Accident, abuse
F - Firearms, homicide
E - Emotions (suicide, depression)
T - Toxins (tobacco, alcohol, other)
E - Environment (school, home, friends)
E - Exercise
N - Nutrition
S - Shots (immunization status)

*Goldenring JM, Cohen E: Getting into adolescents heads, *Contemp Pediatr* 5:75-90, 1988; with permission.
†Gilchrist VJ: Preventive health care for the adolescent, *Am Fam Physician* 43:869-878, 1991; with permission.

One of these mnemonics may be stamped in the adolescent's chart at each visit or be incorporated into the customized age-appropriate well-visit form. The provider may then cross off the appropriate letter in the mnemonic as each area is discussed.

Resources and References

Online Resources

Agency for Healthcare Research and Quality: *Guide to clinical preventive services,* ed 2. 1996. Report of the U.S. Preventive Services Task Force: Provides the latest available recommendations on preventive interventions: screening tests, counseling, immunizations, and chemoprophylactic regimens for more than 80 conditions. Includes periodic health examination and age-specific charts. Website: http://www.ahrq.gov/clinic/cpsix.htm

Agency for Healthcare Research and Quality: *Guide to clinical preventive services,* ed 3, periodic updates, Rockville, Md, 2003. Website: http://www.ahrq.gov/clinic/gcpspu.htm

American Academy of Pediatrics: Pediatric visit documentation forms are available for purchase on the website: http://www.aap.org/bst/showprod.cfm?&DID=15&CATID=133&ObjectGroup_ID=620

American Academy of Pediatrics Committee on Environmental Health: Screening for elevated blood lead levels, *Pediatrics* 101:1072-1078, 1998. Website: http://www.aappolicy.aappublications.org/cgi/content/full/pediatrics%3b101/6/1072

American Academy of Pediatrics Committee on Practice and Ambulatory Medicine: Recommendations for preventive pediatric health care (RE9939), *Pediatrics* 105:645-646, 2000. Website: http://www.aappolicy.aappublications.org/cgi/content/full/pediatrics%3b105/3/645

American Medical Association (AMA): *Guidelines for Adolescent Preventive Services (GAPS). Recommendations monograph.* A comprehensive set of recommendations that provides a framework for the organization and content of preventive health services for adolescents. Website: http://www.thoracic.org/adobe/statements/latenttb1-27.pdf

American Thoracic Society/Centers for Disease Control and Prevention: Targeted tuberculin testing and treatment of latent tuberculosis infection, *Am J Respir Crit Care Med* 161:S221-S247, 2000. Website: http://www.thoracic.org/adobe/statements/latenttb1-27.pdf

Bright Futures: A national initiative initiated in 1990 and guided by the Health Resources and Services Administration's Maternal and Child Health Bureau, with additional program support from the Health Care Financing Administration's Medicaid Bureau. The panel developed comprehensive health supervision guidelines with the collaboration of four interdisciplinary panels of experts in infant, child, and adolescent health; these guidelines were reviewed by nearly 1000 health professionals, educators, and child health advocates throughout the United States. Bright Futures publishes practical tools and materials with a developmental approach to providing health supervision for children and adolescents from birth through age 21 years. Website: http://www.brightfutures.org/

Centers for Disease Control and Prevention (CDC): Division of Tuberculosis Elimination. 2000. *Core curriculum on tuberculosis: what the clinician should know,* ed 4. Website: http://www.cdc.gov/nchstp/tb/pubs/corecurr/default.htm

Centers for Disease Control and Prevention (CDC) Advisory Council for the Elimination of Tuberculosis: Screening for tuberculosis and tuberculosis infection in high-risk populations. Recommendations of the Advisory Council for the Elimination of Tuberculosis, *MMWR*

Recomm Rep Sep 8; 44(RR-11):19-34, 1995. Website: http://www.cdc.gov/mmwr/preview/mmwrhtml/00038873.htm

Centers for Disease Control and Prevention (CDC) National Center for Environmental Health: *Screening young children for lead poisoning: guidance for state and local public health officials,* November 1997. Website: http://www.cdc.gov/nceh/lead/guide/guide97.htm

Centers for Disease Control and Prevention (CDC) National Immunization Program: Complete, current information on immunizations. Website: http://www.cdc.gov/nip

Centers for Disease Control and Prevention (CDC) National Immunization Program–2003: Childhood & Adolescent Immunization Schedule and Catch-up Schedule. Website: http://www.cdc.gov/nip/recs/child-schedule.htm#catchup

GAPS Implementation Materials: Forms designed by the American Medical Association (AMA) to support the implementation of the *Guidelines for Adolescent Preventive Services* (GAPS) are available for reproduction. Younger adolescent, middle/older adolescent, and parent/guardian questionnaires in English and Spanish are included. Website: http://www.ama-assn.org/ama/pub/category/2280.html

Harriet Lane Links. The Harriet Lane Links (formerly Pediatric Points of Interest) provide an edited collection of pediatric resources (5928 links) on the World Wide Web. Maintained and edited at Johns Hopkins University, this site attempts to catalog, review, and score existing links to pediatric information on the Internet. Website: http://derm.med.jhmi.edu/hll/

Institute for Clinical Systems Improvement: Preventive Services for Children and Adolescents: A comprehensive approach to the provision of preventive services, counseling, education, and disease screening for low-risk, asymptomatic individuals from birth through age 18 years. Website: http://www.icsi.org/knowledge/detail.asp?catID=29&itemID=190

KidsGrowth: Pediatric Practice Management and Child Advocacy: This exceptional online resource provides pediatric health information for clinicians, parents, and adolescents. Among the many resources in the parents' section are growth charts, parenting tips, and an extensive collection of medical handouts appropriate for primary care office use. Website: http://www.kidsgrowth.com

La Leche League, Schaumburg, Illinois: Through a large volunteer network, this organization trains group leaders who bring breastfeeding information and support to families throughout the world. This organization provides communities, individuals, and health care professionals with breastfeeding information, telephone counseling, and extensive breastfeeding literature resources. Website: http://www.lalecheleague.org

Minnesota's Early and Periodic Screening, Diagnosis and Treatment (EPSDT) Program. The Minnesota Department of Health (MDH) provides a comprehensive child health program for children and teens from birth through the age of 20 years who are enrolled in Medical Assistance or MinnesotaCare. Information contained at this site includes comprehensive Child & Teen Checkups (C&TC) Program documentation forms, C&TC Screening Training, FACT Sheets on various C&TC components, Denver II training, and Early Childhood & Family Initiatives. Website: http://www.dhs.state.mn.us/healthcare/ctc/default.htm

Put Prevention Into Practice, May 2000. Agency for Healthcare Research and Quality (AHRQ), Rockville, Md: A program to increase the appropriate use of clinical preventive services, such as screening tests, immunizations, and counseling, based on U.S. Preventive Services Task Force recommendations. Website: http://www.ahrq.gov/clinic/ppipix.htm

TIPP–The Injury Prevention Program: An educational program for parents of infants and children through 12 years of age designed to help prevent common injuries. TIPP includes a policy statement on injury prevention approved by the American Academy of Pediatrics and a package of materials consisting of age-related safety surveys and age-specific, color-coded safety information sheets for use in providing anticipatory guidance to parents and children. Website: http://www.aap.org/family/tippintr.htm

References and Suggested Readings

Eiger MS, Olds SW: *The complete book of breastfeeding*, ed 3, New York, 1999, Workman.

Elster AB: Comparison of recommendations for adolescent clinical preventive services developed by national organizations, *Arch Pediatr Adolesc Med* 152:193-198, 1998.

Elster AB, Kuznets NJ: *AMA guidelines for adolescent preventive services (GAPS): recommendations and rationale*, Chicago, 1994, American Medical Association.

Feldman E: Risks, resilience, prevention: the epidemiology of adolescent health, *Clin Fam Pract* 2:767-790, 2000.

Froehlich H, Ackerson LM, Morozumi PA: Targeted testing of children for tuberculosis: validation of a risk assessment questionnaire, *Pediatrics* 107:E54, 2001.

Goldenring JM, Cohen E: Getting into adolescents' heads, *Contemp Pediatr* 5:75-90, 1988.

Green M, Palfrey J, editors: *Bright Futures: guidelines for health supervision of infants, children, and adolescents*, Arlington, Va, 2000, National Center for Education in Maternal and Child Health.

Joffe A: Why adolescent medicine? *Med Clin North Am* 84:769-85, 2000.

Levenberg PB, Elster AB: *Guidelines for adolescent preventive services (GAPS): clinical evaluation and management handbook*, Chicago, 1995, American Medical Association.

Mohrbacher N, Stock J: *The breastfeeding answer book*, ed 3 revised, Schaumburg, Ill, 2002, La Leche League International.

Neifert MR: Part 2: the management of breastfeeding, *Pediatr Clin North Am* 48:273-297, 2001.

Tenore JL: Preventive services for the adolescent (13-20 years), *Clin Fam Pract* 2:289-311, 2000.

U.S. Preventive Services Task Force: *United States Preventive Service Task Force report*, ed 2, Baltimore, 1996, Williams & Wilkins.

Pediatric Initial Health Questionnaire

Date of Visit: _____

Your Name: _____

Child's Name: _____

Relationship to Child: _____

THIS FORM IS FOR MEDICAL RECORD USE ONLY AND WILL REMAIN CONFIDENTIAL. PLEASE ANSWER EACH QUESTION TO THE BEST OF YOUR ABILITY.

Vital Information

Child's Birth date _____ ❑ Boy ❑ Girl

Birthplace: City/State_____

  Hospital _____ Other _____

Mother's Name _____ Birth date: _____

  Occupation _____ Ht _____ Wt _____

Father's Name _____ Birth date: _____

  Occupation _____ Ht _____ Wt _____

Names of living brothers and sisters   *Birth dates*

_____

_____

_____

_____

Was child adopted? ❑ Yes ❑ No At what age? _____

  If adopted, country of origin _____

Religious Preference _____

Pregnancy

Number of pregnancies before this one: _____

How long was this pregnancy? _____ weeks

How many months pregnant when prenatal care was begun? _____

Were there any of the following illnesses or problems?

❑ Rubella (measles)   ❑ Accident/Injury   ❑ Bleeding

❑ High blood pressure   ❑ Swelling   ❑ Sugar in urine

❑ Excessive weight gain   ❑ Other infections

Explain: _____

Medicines or drugs used during pregnancy:

_____

_____

Smoking while pregnant: ❑ None ❑ Moderate ❑ Heavy

Alcohol while pregnant: ❑ None ❑ <1 per week ❑ >1 per week

Birth

How long was labor? _____ Was labor induced? _____

At delivery (check all that apply):

❑ Breech (feet or bottom first)   ❑ Cesarean section   ❑ VBAC

❑ Breathed and cried immediately   ❑ Resuscitated   ❑ In oxygen

Did baby require:

❑ special nursery   ❑ blood transfusion   ❑ antibiotics   ❑ lights

Did baby have:

❑ breathing problems   ❑ yellow jaundice   ❑ Other _____

At birth:

Weight: _____ Length: _____ Apgar score _____

Discharge weight: _____ Length of hospital stay: _____

Describe any problems: _____

_____

Family Background

Ethnic origin/Race: Mother: _____ Father: _____

❑ Married ❑ Living together ❑ Separated ❑ Divorced ❑ Single

Child lives with:

❑ Both parents ❑ Mother ❑ Father ❑ Guardian

Other members of household: _____

Age of home or apartment: _____ Any pets? _____

Has any parent, brother, or sister died? _____ Who? _____

Cause of death _____ Age _____

Please check the box of your child's blood relatives who have ever had any of the following conditions; circle examples in parentheses or write in name of disease, if known:	Father	Mother	Father's side	Mother's side	Siblings
Headaches (migraine, cluster, tension)					
Eye Disease (blindness, tumor, glaucoma)					
Ear Disease (deafness, infections, defects)					
Allergies (eczema, hay fever, sinus, hives)					
Lung Disease (asthma, cystic fibrosis, bronchitis)					
Tuberculosis					
High Blood Pressure					
High Cholesterol					
Heart Attack (age _____)					
Heart Disease					
Anemia (Sickle Cell, Mediterranean, other)					
Bleeding Disorders (hemophilia)					
Stomach or Duodenal Ulcers					
Liver or Gallbladder Disease (hepatitis)					
Intestinal Disease (colitis, polyps)					
Kidney Disease (nephritis, cysts, stones)					
Diabetes					
Thyroid Problems (goiter, nodules, hyper-, hypo-)					
Bone or Joint Disease (arthritis, osteoporosis)					
Muscle Weakness or Dystrophy					
Seizure Disorder (epilepsy)					
Neurologic Disorder					
Learning Disability					
Mental Retardation (Down Syndrome, other)					
Mental Illness (depression, anxiety, other)					
Alcoholism or Drug Abuse					
Birth Defects (cleft lip, other deformity)					
Obesity					
Cancer: Breast, Cervix, Uterine, or Ovarian					
Lung, Thyroid, Pancreas, or Kidney					
Bladder, Prostate, or Testicular					
Colon, Stomach, or Oral Cavity					
Leukemia, Myeloma, or Lymphoma					
Skin, Brain, or Bone					
Other _____					

Pediatric Initial Health Questionnaire - 2

Nutrition in Infancy

Feeding: Breast ☐ Duration _____ months/weeks

Formula ☐ Type _____

☐ Vitamins ☐ Fluoride ☐ Iron ☐ Uses Pacifier

Problems: ☐ Vomiting ☐ Colic ☐ Diarrhea ☐ Allergies

Solid foods: Age when started _____ Intolerances _____

Growth and Development

At what age did your child:

Sit alone _____ Walk alone _____ Feed self _____

Talk (2-3-word sentences) _____ Dress self _____

Toilet trained: Day _____ Night _____

School-age child: Current grade _____ Days missed this year _____

School Problems: ☐ reading, writing ☐ behavior ☐ special needs

Are there any behavior problems at home? _____

Please describe: _____

_____

_____

Medical History

Please check the diseases that your child has had and give age:

☐ Measles, Rubella _____   ☐ Anemia _____

☐ Mumps _____   ☐ Heart Disease _____

☐ Chickenpox _____   ☐ Allergies/Hay fever _____

☐ Whooping cough _____   ☐ Eczema _____

☐ Scarlet fever _____   ☐ Asthma _____

☐ Rheumatic fever _____   ☐ Pneumonia _____

☐ Convulsions/Seizures _____   ☐ Hepatitis _____

☐ Strep throat _____   ☐ Ear Infection _____

☐ Other illnesses _____

Has your child ever been injured? _____ Age _____

Injury _____

Any fractures? _____ Which bone(s)? _____

Any loss of consciousness or concussion? _____

Any accidental poisoning? _____ Age _____ Substance _____

Has your child ever had surgery? _____ Age _____

Type of operation _____

Has your child ever been hospitalized other than for the above? _____

Describe: _____

Has your child ever had a blood transfusion? _____ Age _____

Does your child take any medications regularly? _____

Please list: _____

_____

_____

Does your child take any of the following:

☐ Vitamins ☐ Fluoride ☐ Food supplements _____

Has your child worn:

☐ Glasses ☐ Contact lenses ☐ Dental braces ☐ Leg braces

☐ Corrective shoes ☐ Orthotics in shoes ☐ Other braces

Does your child have allergies to any of the following?

☐ Penicillin ☐ Sulfa ☐ Other medicines _____

☐ Pollen Foods _____ ☐ Animals _____

Type of allergic reaction to above: _____

Please check if your child has had:

☐ Frequent headaches   ☐ Crossed eyes

☐ Pinkeye   ☐ More than two earaches a year

☐ Trouble hearing   ☐ Frequent nosebleeds

☐ Stuffy nose most of time   ☐ More than 6 colds a year

☐ Chronic cough   ☐ Shortness of breath with exercise

☐ Heart murmur   ☐ Constant or frequent fatigue

☐ Frequent stomachaches   ☐ Frequent diarrhea or constipation

☐ Poor appetite   ☐ Frequent urination or accidents

☐ Bloody, red, or brown urine ☐ Frequent bed-wetting after age 5

☐ Joint pains or swelling   ☐ Dizziness or fainting spells

☐ Inability to get to sleep   ☐ Frequent nightmares or sleepwalking

☐ Excessive thirst   ☐ Excessive weight gain

☐ Signs of sexual development before age 9

Other concerns: _____

_____

_____

Immunizations & Screenings

Please give approximate dates for each immunization, if known:

Series	#1	#2	#3	#4	#5
DtaP/DT					
Tetanus booster					
Polio IPV/OPV					
MMR					
Hib					
Hepatitis B					
Pneumococcal					
Varicella					
Meningococcal					
Influenza					

Please give approximate dates for the following, if done:

Test	No	Yes	Date(s)	Result
Lead blood test				
TB skin test				
Vision exam				
Hearing test				
Hemoglobin blood test				
Urine test				

0 to 1-Month Well-Child Visit

Date of Visit: _____

Medical Record Number: _____

Child's Name: _____

Address: _____

Telephone: _____

Date of Birth: _____ Age: _____ Gender: Male   Female

Provider: _____

Informant: _____

Relationship to child: _____

Interpreter present: ❑ Yes   ❑ No

Language _____

Measurements

Ht _____ _____ % Wt _____ _____ % OFC _____ _____ % Staff

Temp _____ Pulse _____ Resp _____ Initials _____

Birth Data

Ht _____   Wt _____   OFC _____   Gest Age _____ Wks

L&D record on baby's chart?   ❑ Yes   ❑ No

Significant prenatal history on baby's chart?   ❑ Yes   ❑ No

Hepatitis B vaccine given in nursery?   ❑ Yes   ❑ No

Newborn Metabolic Screening

❑ Normal   ❑ Abnormal (specify):

Vision/Hearing

Newborn Hearing Screening

❑ Normal   ❑ Not screened   ❑ Abnormal (specify):

Vision concerns   ❑ No   ❑ Yes (explain)_____

Hearing concerns   ❑ No   ❑ Yes (explain)_____

Child Health History

Family/social history (refer to chart)   ❑ Completed   ❑ Updated

Parental concerns: _____

_____

Recent injury/illness/surgery/hospitalizations:

Allergies: _____

Medications: _____

Review of Systems

	N	AB
HEENT (eye discharge, thrush)		
Skin (rashes)		
CV (color)		
Resp (wheezing)		
GI (projectile vomiting/stools)		
GU (pain/stream/frequency)		
Neuromuscular (moves all extremities equally)		

Remainder of review of systems (unlisted) negative ❑

Daily Activities

Nutrition/Elimination

❑ Breast frequency _____   # feedings/day _____

❑ Formula _____   # feedings/amount _____

❑ Iron/Vitamins   # stools/day _____   # voids/day _____

Sleep (arrangements/patterns) _____

Hygiene (cord/circ care) _____

Caregivers   ❑ Mother   ❑ Father   ❑ Other relative

Caregiver working/in school   ❑ Yes   ❑ No

Who cares for baby during day or other time?   ❑ Parent/other relative

❑ Day care

Stresses for Caregivers _____

Environmental Risks—Check if assessed

❑ Lead risk   ❑ Guns in house/bldg   ❑ TB exposure

❑ Alcohol use in house/bldg ❑ Housing inadequate   ❑ Domestic violence

❑ Smokers in house/bldg   ❑ Drug use in house/bldg   ❑ Other

❑ Identified risks _____

Active community supports/resources:

_____

Mental Health/Behavior Risks:

❑ No concerns

❑ Concerns (explain) _____

Observation of parent/child interaction:

❑ Appropriate

❑ Not appropriate (explain)_____

Other:

Development

Personal/Social/Cognitive	N	AB
• Regards face		
• Smiles responsively		
Fine motor/adaptive		
• Follows to midline		
Language		
• Vocalizes		
• Responds to sound		
• "Ooo/aah"		
Gross motor		
• Lifts head 45°		
Breastfeeding		
• Latch-on/positioning		
• Quality of suck		

❑ Development screening tool, if used:

Name of tool _____

_____

Staff initials _____

❑ By observation/exam/ parent report. No tool used.

0 to 1-Month Well-Child Visit - 2

Child's Name: _____   *Medical Record Number:* _____

Physical Exam

N = normal Ab = abnormal (check appropriate box)	N	AB
1. General appearance:		
2. Skin: color • character • birthmarks • jaundice		
3. Nodes: cervical • axillary • inguinal		
4. Head: shape • AF size • PF size • sutures • scalp		
5. Eyes: tear ducts • EOM • red reflex • corneal light reflex PERL • lids		
6. Vision: follows light, movement		
7. Ears: pinna • canals • TMs		
8. Hearing: responds to loud sound		
9. Nose: patency • nares		
10. Mouth: gums • tongue • frenulum • palate • mucosa • throat		
11. Neck: position • ROM • thyroid		
12. Chest: shape • symmetry • lungs • respiration rate • clavicles		
13. CV: rate • rhythm • S1 • S2 • murmur • femoral pulses		
14. ABD: contour • umbilicus • liver • spleen • masses • anus • bowel sounds		
15. GU: ♀ labia • vaginal mucosa • discharge ♂ circ • penis • testes • hydrocele • hernia		
16. MS: ROM • Ortolani • spine		
17. Neuro: jitteriness • head control • posture • tone • DTRs • clonus • Babinski • Moro • TNR • suck • root • grasp • stepping crossed • extension • positive supporting		

Document Abnormals (by number):

Anticipatory Guidance

✔ *Topics discussed*

Nutrition

No solids	Spitting up/vomiting
Always hold to feed/ Never prop bottle	Encourage continuation of breastfeeding (if appropriate) on demand
No honey before one year	

Safety

Car seat	Supervise sibling and pet interaction
Never leave unattended	Safe crib/sleep on back or side
Support head and neck	No strings
Care with talc	Smoke detectors
Sun protection	No smoking around baby
Hot water temp <125° F	

Parenting

Show affection to baby	Diarrhea care
Interact by responding to cry	Thermometer use
Never punish, jerk, or shake	When to call office
Day care concerns	Bulb syringe for congestion
Fever care	Infection risk reduction
Skin care	

Other:

Laboratory Tests (None routinely required at this age)

Assessment

☐ Child well

☐ Additional Diagnoses (specify):

Plan

Immunizations

Are immunizations on schedule? ☐ Yes ☐ No (Update Record Card)

If not, catch-up plan? _____

Previous reaction? ☐ Yes   ☐ No

Comments: _____

Immunizations ordered/given: ☐ Hepatitis B ☐ PCV

☐ DTaP ☐ IPV ☐ Hib ☐ Other _____

If immunization(s) due but not given, explain:

Additional Plan

Referrals

☐ *Smoking cessation class*

☐ *Breastfeeding class/support group*

☐ *Other:*

☐ *Encouraged smoking cessation*

☐ *Need for financial assistance*

☐ *Social services*

☐ *Requires additional health education*

☐ *Schedule 2-month visit*

Provider Signature

☐ Note dictated

2-Month Well-Child Visit

Date of Visit: _____

Medical Record Number: _____

Child's Name: _____

Address: _____

Telephone: _____

Date of Birth: _____ Age: _____ Gender: Male Female

Provider: _____

Informant: _____

Relationship to child:_____

Interpreter present: ☐ Yes ☐ No

Language _____

Measurements

Ht _____ _____ % Wt _____ _____ % OFC _____ _____ % Staff

Temp _____ Pulse _____ Resp _____ Initials _____

Birth Data

Ht _____ **Wt** _____ **OFC** _____ **Gest Age** _____ **Wks**

L&D record on baby's chart? ☐ Yes ☐ No

Significant prenatal history on baby's chart? ☐ Yes ☐ No

Hepatitis B vaccine given in nursery? ☐ Yes ☐ No

Newborn Metabolic Screening

☐ Normal ☐ Abnormal (specify):

Vision/Hearing

Newborn Hearing Screening

☐ Normal ☐ Not screened ☐ Abnormal (specify):

Vision concerns ☐ No ☐ Yes (explain)_____

Hearing concerns ☐ No ☐ Yes (explain)_____

Child Health History

Family/social history (refer to chart) ☐ Completed ☐ Updated

Parental concerns:_____

Recent injury/illness/surgery/hospitalizations:

Allergies: _____

Medications: _____

Review of Systems

	N	AB
CV (color)		
Resp (wheezing)		
GI (projectile vomiting/stools)		
GU (pain/stream/frequency)		
Skin (rashes)		
Neuromuscular (moves all extremities equally)		

Remainder of review of systems (unlisted) negative ☐

Daily Activities

Nutrition/Elimination

☐ Breast frequency _____ # feedings/day_____

☐ Formula _____ # feedings/amount _____

☐ Iron/Vitamins # stools/day _____ # voids/day _____

Sleep (arrangements/patterns) _____

Hygiene (cord/circ care) _____

Caregivers ☐ Mother ☐ Father ☐ Other relative

Caregiver working/in school ☐ Yes ☐ No

Who cares for baby during day or other time? ☐ Parent/other relative

☐ Day care

Stresses for Caregivers _____

Environmental Risks—Check if assessed

☐ **Lead risk** ☐ Guns in house/bldg ☐ TB exposure

☐ Alcohol use in house/bldg ☐ Housing inadequate ☐ Domestic violence

☐ Smokers in house/bldg ☐ Drug use in house/bldg ☐ Other

☐ **Identified risks** _____

Active community supports/resources:

_____

Mental Health/Behavior Risks:

☐ No concerns

☐ Concerns (explain)_____

Observation of parent/child interaction:

☐ Appropriate

☐ Not appropriate (explain) _____

Other:

Development

Personal/Social/Cognitive	N	AB
• Regards face		
• Smiles responsively		
Fine motor/adaptive		
• Follows to midline		
Language		
• Vocalizes		
• Responds to sound		
• "Ooo/aah"		
Gross motor		
• Lifts head 45°		
Breastfeeding		
• Latch-on		
• Begins to position self		

☐ Developmental screening tool, if used:

Name of tool _____

_____

Staff initials _____

☐ By observation/exam/parent report. No tool used.

2-Month Well-Child Visit - 2

Child's Name: _____   *Medical Record Number:* _____

Physical Exam

N = normal Ab = abnormal (check appropriate box)	N	AB
1. General appearance:		
2. Skin: color • character • birthmarks		
3. Nodes: cervical • axillary • inguinal		
4. Head: shape • AF size • PF size • sutures • scalp		
5. Eyes: tear ducts • EOM • red reflex • corneal light reflex PERL • lids		
6. Vision: follows light, movement		
7. Ears: pinna • canals • TMs		
8. Hearing: responds to loud sound		
9. Nose: patency • nares		
10. Mouth: gums • tongue • frenulum • palate • mucosa • throat		
11. Neck: position • ROM • thyroid		
12. Chest: shape • symmetry • lungs • respiration rate		
13. CV: rate • rhythm • S1 • S2 • murmur • femoral pulses		
14. Abd: contour • umbilicus • liver • spleen • masses • anus • bowel sounds		
15. GU: ♀ labia • vaginal mucosa ♂ circ • penis • testes • hydrocele • hernia		
16. MS: ROM • Ortolani • spine		
17. Neuro: head control • posture • tone • DTRs • clonus • Babinski • Moro • TNR • suck • root • grasp • stepping crossed • positive supporting		

Document Abnormals (by number): _____

Anticipatory Guidance

✔ Topics discussed

Nutrition

No solids	Milk supply maintenance
Always hold to feed/ Never prop bottle	Encourage continuation of breast-feeding (if appropriate) on demand
Spitting up/vomiting	Breastmilk storage
No honey before one year	

Safety

Car seat	Care with talc
Never leave unattended	Sun protection
Support head and neck	Hot water temp <125° F
Supervise sibling and pet interaction	Smoke detectors
Safe crib/sleep on back or side	No smoking around baby
No strings	

Parenting

Show affection to baby	Diarrhea care
Interact by responding to cry	Thermometer use
Never punish, jerk, or shake	When to call office
Day care concerns	Bulb syringe for congestion
Fever care	Infection risk reduction
Skin care	

Other: _____

Laboratory Tests (None routinely required at this age)

Assessment

☐ Child well

☐ Additional Diagnoses (specify):

Plan
Immunizations

Are immunizations on schedule?   ☐ Yes ☐ No (Update Record Card)

If not, catch-up plan? _____

Previous reaction?   ☐ Yes   ☐ No

Comments: _____

Immunizations ordered/given: ☐ Hepatitis B   ☐ PCV

☐ DTaP   ☐ IPV ☐ Hib   ☐ Other _____

If immunization(s) due but not given, explain:

Additional Plan

Referrals

☐ *Smoking cessation class*

☐ *Breastfeeding support group*

☐ *Other:*

☐ *Encouraged smoking cessation*

☐ *Need for financial assistance*

☐ *Social services*

☐ *Requires additional health education*

☐ *Schedule 4-month visit*

Provider Signature

☐ Note dictated

4-Month Well-Child Visit

Date of Visit: _____

Medical Record Number: _____

Child's Name: _____

Address: _____

Telephone: _____

Date of Birth: _____ Age: _____ Gender: Male   Female

Provider: _____

Informant: _____   Interpreter present: ☐ Yes   ☐ No

Relationship to child: _____   Language _____

Measurements

Ht _____ _____ % Wt _____ _____ % OFC _____ _____ % Staff

Temp _____ Pulse _____ Resp _____ Initials ____

Vision/Hearing

Vision concerns   ☐ No   ☐ Yes (explain) _____

Hearing concerns   ☐ No   ☐ Yes (explain) _____

Child Health History

Family/social history (refer to chart)   ☐ Completed   ☐ Updated

Parental concerns: _____

_____

Recent injury/illness/surgery/hospitalizations:

Allergies: _____

Medications: _____

Review of Systems

	N	AB
HEENT (eye discharge, thrush)		
Skin (rashes)		
CV (color)		
Resp (wheezing)		
GI (vomiting/stools)		
GU (pain/stream/frequency)		
Neuromuscular (moves all extremities equally)		

Remainder of review of systems (unlisted) negative ☐

Daily Activities

Nutrition

☐ Breast frequency _____ # feedings/day _____

☐ Formula _____ # feedings/amount _____

☐ Juice (oz/day) _____

☐ Cereal

☐ Iron/Vitamins

Sleep (arrangements/patterns) _____

Hygiene (bathing frequency) _____

Child Health History (continued)

Caregivers   ☐ Mother   ☐ Father   ☐ Other relative

Caregiver working/in school   ☐ Yes   ☐ No

Who cares for baby during day or other time?   ☐ Parent/other relative

☐ Day care

Stresses for Caregivers _____

Environmental Risks—Check if assessed

☐ **Lead risk**   ☐ Guns in house/bldg   ☐ TB exposure

☐ Alcohol use in house/bldg   ☐ Housing inadequate   ☐ Domestic violence

☐ Smokers in house/bldg   ☐ Drug use in house/bldg   ☐ Other

☐ **Identified risks**

Active community supports/resources:

_____

Mental Health/Behavior Risks:

☐ No concerns

☐ Concerns (explain) _____

Observation of parent/child interaction:

☐ Appropriate

☐ Not appropriate (explain) _____

Other:

Development

Personal/Social/Cognitive	N	AB
• Regards own hand		
• Smiles spontaneously		
Fine motor/adaptive		
• Grasps rattle		
• Hands together		
• Follows 180°		
Language		
• Laughs		
• Squeals		
Gross motor		
• Head up 90°		
• Sits—head steady		
• Rolls over		
• Bears weight on legs		
• Chest up—arm support		
Breastfeeding		
• Efficiently nursing		

☐ Developmental screening tool, if used:

Name of tool _____

_____

Staff initials _____

☐ By observation/exam/ parent report. No tool used.

4-Month Well-Child Visit - 2

Child's Name: _____   *Medical Record Number:* _____

Physical Exam

N = normal Ab = abnormal (check appropriate box)	N	AB
1. General appearance:		
2. Skin: color • character • birthmarks		
3. Nodes: cervical • axillary • inguinal		
4. Head: shape • AF size • scalp		
5. Eyes: tear ducts • EOM • red reflex • corneal light reflex PERL • lids		
6. Vision: follows light, movement		
7. Ears: pinna • canals • TMs		
8. Hearing: responds to loud sound		
9. Nose: patency • nares		
10. Mouth: gums • tongue • frenulum • palate • mucosa • throat		
11. Neck: position • ROM • thyroid		
12. Chest: shape • symmetry • lungs • respiration rate		
13. CV: rate • rhythm • S1 • S2 • murmur • femoral pulses		
14. Abd: contour • liver • spleen • masses • anus • bowel sounds		
15. GU: ♀ labia • vaginal mucosa ♂ penis • testes • hydrocele • hernia		
16. MS: ROM • Ortolani • spine		
17. Neuro: head control • posture • tone • DTRs • clonus • Babinski • Moro		

Document Abnormals (by number):

Anticipatory Guidance

✔ *Topics discussed*

Nutrition

No solids	No honey before one year
Always hold to feed/ Never prop bottle	Encourage continuation of breast-feeding (if appropriate) on demand
Spitting up/vomiting	Breastmilk storage

Safety

Car seat	Supervise sibling and pet interaction
Never leave unattended	Safe crib/sleep on back or side
Support head and neck	No strings
Care with talc	Smoke detectors
Sun protection	No smoking around baby
Hot water temp <125° F	No walkers

Parenting

Show affection to baby	Fever care
Interact by talking, singing, playing	When to call office
Never punish, jerk, or shake	Infection risk reduction
Day care concerns	

Other:

Laboratory Tests (None routinely required at this age)

Additional Plan

Assessment

☐ Child well
☐ Additional Diagnoses (specify):

Plan

Immunizations

Are immunizations on schedule? ☐ Yes ☐ No (Update Record Card)

If not, catch-up plan? _____

Previous reaction? ☐ Yes   ☐ No

Comments: _____

Immunizations ordered/given: ☐ Hepatitis B   ☐ PCV

☐ DTaP   ☐ IPV   ☐ Hib   ☐ Other _____

If immunization(s) due but not given, explain:

Referrals
☐ *Smoking cessation class*
☐ *Breastfeeding support group*
☐ *Other:*

☐ *Encouraged smoking cessation*
☐ *Need for financial assistance*
☐ *Social services*
☐ *Requires additional health education*
☐ *Schedule 6-month visit*

Provider Signature
☐ Note dictated

6-Month Well-Child Visit

Date of Visit: _____

Medical Record Number: _____

Child's Name: _____

Address: _____

Telephone: _____

Date of Birth: _____ Age: _____ Gender: Male Female

Provider: _____

Informant: _____

Relationship to child: _____

Interpreter present: ☐ Yes   ☐ No

Language _____

Measurements

Ht _____ _____ % Wt _____ _____ % OFC _____ _____ % Staff

Temp _____ Pulse _____ Resp _____ Initials _____

Vision/Hearing

Vision concerns   ☐ No ☐ Yes (explain)_____

Hearing concerns ☐ No ☐ Yes (explain)_____

Child Health History

Family/social history (refer to chart) ☐ Completed ☐ Updated

Parental concerns:_____

_____

Recent injury/illness/surgery/hospitalizations:

Allergies: _____

Medications: _____

Review of Systems

	N	AB
HEENT (strabismus, ear infections, colds, teething)		
Skin (rashes)		
CV (color)		
Resp (wheezing)		
GI (vomiting/stools)		
GU (pain/stream/frequency)		
Neuromuscular (moves all extremities equally)		

Remainder of review of systems (unlisted) negative ☐

Daily Activities

Nutrition

☐ Breast frequency _____ # feedings/day _____

☐ Formula _____ # feedings/amount_____

☐ Juice (oz/day) _____

☐ Solids

☐ Iron/Vitamins

Sleep (arrangements/patterns) _____

Hygiene (bathing frequency)_____

Child Health History (continued)

Caregivers ☐ Mother ☐ Father ☐ Other relative

Caregiver working/in school ☐ Yes ☐ No

Who cares for baby during day or other time? ☐ Parent/other relative

☐ Day care

Stresses for Caregivers _____

Environmental Risks—Check if assessed

☐ Lead risk   ☐ Guns in house/bldg   ☐ TB exposure

☐ Alcohol use in house/bldg ☐ Housing inadequate ☐ Domestic violence

☐ Smokers in house/bldg ☐ Drug use in house/bldg ☐ Other

☐ **Identified risks**

Active community supports/resources:

_____

Mental Health/Behavior Risks:

☐ No concerns

☐ Concerns (explain)_____

Observation of parent/child interaction:

☐ Appropriate

☐ Not appropriate (explain) _____

Other:

Development

Personal/Social/Cognitive	N	AB
• Feeds self		
• Works for toy		
Fine motor/adaptive		
• Regards raisin		
• Reaches		
Language		
• Turns to voice		
• Imitates speech sounds		
Gross motor		
• Pulls to sit—no head lag		
• Rolls over		
• Chest up—arm support		
• Bears weight on legs		
Breastfeeding		
• Nurses sitting up		
• Signs of weaning		

☐ Developmental screening tool, if used:

Name of tool _____

Staff initials _____

☐ By observation/exam/ parent report. No tool used.

6-Month Well-Child Visit - 2

Child's Name: _____   Medical Record Number: _____

Physical Exam

N = normal Ab = abnormal (check appropriate box)	N	AB
1. General appearance:		
2. Skin: color • character • birthmarks		
3. Nodes: cervical • axillary • inguinal		
4. Head: shape • AF size • scalp		
5. Eyes: tear ducts • EOM • red reflex • corneal light reflex PERL • strabismus • lids		
6. Vision: follows light, movement		
7. Ears: pinna • canals • TMs		
8. Hearing: responds to loud sound		
9. Nose: patency • nares		
10. Mouth: gums • tongue • frenulum • teeth • mucosa • throat		
11. Neck: position • ROM • thyroid		
12. Chest: shape • symmetry • lungs • respiration rate		
13. CV: rate • rhythm • S1 • S2 • murmur • femoral pulses		
14. Abd: contour • liver • spleen • masses • anus • bowel sounds		
15. GU: ♀ labia • vaginal mucosa ♂ penis • testes • hydrocele • hernia		
16. MS: ROM • Ortolani • spine		
17. Neuro: head control • posture • tone • DTRs • clonus • Babinski • Moro		

Document Abnormals (by number):

Anticipatory Guidance

✔ *Topics discussed*

Nutrition

Fluoride if using well water (after tested)	Finger food
Breast/formula for one year	Choking prevention
Always hold to feed/Never prop bottle	Discourage excess sweets
Introduce cup	Gradual solids introduction

Safety

Car seat	Lower crib mattress
Never leave unattended	Sun protection
Hot water temp <125° F	Poison control number
Smoke detectors	Electrical cords/drapery pulls
No smoking around baby	Plastic bags/balloons
No walkers	Toys with small parts
Poisonous plants	Stair gates

Parenting

Interact by talking, singing, playing	Use of OTC meds
Never punish, jerk, or shake	Teething
Day care concerns	Thumbsucking normal
Stranger/separation anxiety	Infection risk reduction
Sibling and pet interaction	

Other:

Laboratory Tests (None routinely required at this age)

Additional Plan

Assessment

☐ Child well
☐ Additional Diagnoses (specify):

Plan
Immunizations

Are immunizations on schedule? ☐ Yes ☐ No (Update Record Card)

If not, catch-up plan? _____
Previous reaction? ☐ Yes   ☐ No

Comments: _____
Immunizations ordered/given: ☐ Hepatitis B ☐ PCV
☐ DTaP   ☐ IPV ☐ Hib   ☐ Other _____
If immunization(s) due but not given, explain:

Referrals
☐ *Smoking cessation class*
☐ *Other:*

☐ *Encouraged smoking cessation*
☐ *Need for financial assistance*
☐ *Social services*
☐ *Requires additional health education*
☐ *Schedule 9-month visit*

Provider Signature
☐ Note dictated

9-Month Well-Child Visit

Date of Visit: _____

Medical Record Number: _____

Child's Name: _____

Address: _____

Telephone: _____

Date of Birth: _____ Age: _____ Gender: Male Female

Provider: _____

Informant: _____

Relationship to child: _____

Interpreter present: ☐ Yes ☐ No

Language _____

Measurements

Ht _____ _____ % Wt _____ _____ % OFC _____ _____ % Staff

Temp _____ Pulse _____ Resp _____ Initials _____

Vision/Hearing

Vision concerns ☐ No ☐ Yes (explain) _____

Hearing concerns ☐ No ☐ Yes (explain) _____

Child Health History

Family/social history (refer to chart) ☐ Completed ☐ Updated

Parental concerns: _____

_____

Recent injury/illness/surgery/hospitalizations:

Allergies: _____

Medications: _____

Review of Systems

	N	AB
HEENT (strabismus, ear infections, colds, teething)		
Skin (rashes)		
CV (color)		
Resp (wheezing)		
GI (vomiting/stools)		
GU (pain/stream/frequency)		
Neuromuscular (moves all extremities equally)		

Remainder of review of systems (unlisted) negative ☐

Daily Activities

Nutrition

☐ Breast frequency _____ # feedings/day _____

☐ Formula _____ # feedings/amount _____

☐ Juice (oz/day) _____

☐ Solids

☐ Iron/Vitamins

Sleep (arrangements/patterns) _____

Hygiene (bathing frequency) _____

Child Health History (continued)

Caregivers ☐ Mother ☐ Father ☐ Other relative

Caregiver working/in school ☐ Yes ☐ No

Who cares for baby during day or other time? ☐ Parent/other relative
  ☐ Day care

Stresses for Caregivers _____

Environmental Risks—Check if assessed

☐ Lead risk ☐ Guns in house/bldg ☐ TB exposure

☐ Alcohol use in house/bldg ☐ Housing inadequate ☐ Domestic violence

☐ Smokers in house/bldg ☐ Drug use in house/bldg ☐ Other

☐ **Identified risks**

Active community supports/resources: _____

_____

Mental Health/Behavior Risks:

☐ No concerns

☐ Concerns (explain) _____

Observation of parent/child interaction:

☐ Appropriate

☐ Not appropriate (explain) _____

Other:

Development

Personal/Social/Cognitive	N	AB
• Feeds self		
• Works for toy		
• Waves bye-bye		
Fine motor/adaptive		
• Passes cube		
• Rakes raisin		
• Takes 2 cubes		
• Thumb—finger grasp		
Language		
• Imitates speech sounds		
• Dada/Mama nonspecific		
• Single syllables		
• Jabbers		
Gross motor		
• Stands holding on		
• Sits/no support		
• Pulls to sit/no head log		
• Pulls to stand		
Breastfeeding		
• Comfort nurses		

☐ Developmental screening tool, if used:

Name of tool _____

_____

Staff initials _____

☐ By observation/exam/ parent report. No tool used.

9-Month Well-Child Visit - 2

Child's Name: _____

Medical Record Number: _____

Physical Exam

N = normal Ab = abnormal (check appropriate box)	N	AB
1. **General appearance:**		
2. **Skin:** color • character • birthmarks		
3. **Nodes:** cervical • axillary • inguinal		
4. **Head:** shape • AF size • scalp		
5. **Eyes:** tear ducts • EOM • red reflex • corneal light reflex PERL • strabismus • lids		
6. **Vision:** follows light, movement		
7. **Ears:** pinna • canals • TMs		
8. **Hearing:** localization of sound		
9. **Nose:** patency • nares		
10. **Mouth:** gums • mucosa • teeth • throat		
11. **Neck:** position • ROM • thyroid		
12. **Chest:** shape • symmetry • lungs • respiration rate		
13. **CV:** rate • rhythm • S1 • S2 • murmur • femoral pulses		
14. **Abd:** contour • liver • spleen • masses • anus • bowel sounds		
15. **GU:** ♀ labia • vaginal mucosa ♂ penis • testes • hydrocele • hernia		
16. **MS:** ROM • hips • spine		
17. **Neuro:** posture • tone • DTRs • clonus • Babinski		

Document Abnormals (by number):

Anticipatory Guidance

✔ *Topics discussed*

Nutrition

Fluoride if using well water (after tested)	Highchair safety
Breast/formula for one year	Self-feeding with spoon/messy OK
Begin weaning to cup	Discourage excess sweets

Safety

Car seat	Hot water temp <125° F
Never leave unattended	Smoke detectors
Sun protection	No smoking around baby
No walkers	Stair gates
Poisonous plants	Window guards
Poison control number	Lock up medications/cleaning products
Plastic bags/balloons	Socket plugs
Toys with small parts/sharps	Eliminate lead risks

Parenting

Interact by talking, singing, playing	Use of OTC meds
Never punish, jerk, or shake	Teething
Day care concerns	Thumbsucking normal
Stranger/separation anxiety	Teach "no" and use of distraction
Infection risk reduction	

Other:

Laboratory Tests (None routinely required at this age)

☐ **Hemoglobin** (once between 9 & 15 mo)

Assessment

☐ Child well
☐ Additional Diagnoses (specify):

Additional Plan

Referrals
☐ *Smoking cessation class*
☐ *Other:*

☐ *Encouraged smoking cessation*
☐ *Need for financial assistance*
☐ *Social services*
☐ *Requires additional health education*
☐ *Schedule 12-month visit*

Plan
Immunizations

Are immunizations on schedule? ☐ Yes ☐ No (Update Record Card)
If not, catch-up plan? _____
Previous reaction? ☐ Yes ☐ No

Comments: _____
Immunizations ordered/given: ☐ Hepatitis B ☐ PCV
☐ DTaP ☐ IPV ☐ Hib ☐ Other _____
If immunization(s) due but not given, explain:

Provider Signature
☐ Note dictated

12-Month Well-Child Visit

Date of Visit: _____

Medical Record Number: _____

Child's Name: _____

Address: _____

Telephone: _____

Date of Birth: _____ Age: ____ Gender: Male Female

Provider: _____

Informant: _____   Interpreter present: ☐ Yes   ☐ No

Relationship to child: _____   Language _____

Measurements

Ht _____ _____ % Wt _____ _____ % OFC _____ _____ % Staff

Temp _____ Pulse _____ Resp _____ Initials ____

Vision/Hearing

Vision concerns   ☐ No ☐ Yes (explain) _____

Hearing concerns ☐ No ☐ Yes (explain) _____

Child Health History

Family/social history (refer to chart)   ☐ Completed   ☐ Updated

Parental concerns: _____

_____

Recent injury/illness/surgery/hospitalizations:

Allergies: _____

Medications: _____

Review of Systems

	N	AB
HEENT (strabismus, ear infections, colds, teething)		
Skin (rashes)		
CV (color)		
Resp (wheezing)		
GI (vomiting/stools)		
GU (pain/stream/frequency)		
Neuromuscular (moves all extremities equally)		

Remainder of review of systems (unlisted) negative ☐

Daily Activities

Nutrition

☐ Breast frequency _____ # feedings/day _____

☐ Whole milk/amount _____

☐ Juice (oz/day) _____

☐ Solids

☐ Iron/Vitamins/Fluoride

Sleep (arrangements/patterns) _____

Hygiene (bathing frequency) _____

Dental (brushing) _____

Child Health History (continued)

Caregivers   ☐ Mother   ☐ Father   ☐ Other relative

Caregiver working/in school   ☐ Yes   ☐ No

Who cares for baby during day or other time?   ☐ Parent/other relative
                                                ☐ Day care

Stresses for Caregivers _____

Environmental Risks—Check if assessed

☐ Lead risk   ☐ Guns in house/bldg   ☐ TB exposure

☐ Alcohol use in house/bldg ☐ Housing inadequate   ☐ Domestic violence

☐ Smokers in house/bldg ☐ Drug use in house/bldg   ☐ Other

☐ **Identified risks**

Active community supports/resources: _____

_____

Mental Health/Behavior Risks:

☐ No concerns

☐ Concerns (explain) _____

_____

Observation of parent/child interaction:

☐ Appropriate

☐ Not appropriate (explain) _____

Other:

Development

Personal/Social/Cognitive	N	AB
• Plays pat-a-cake		
• Indicates wants		
Fine motor/adaptive		
• Bangs 2 cubes		
Language		
• Dada/Mama nonspecific		
• Combines syllables		
• Jabbers		
Gross motor		
• Pulls to stand		
• Stands 2 seconds		
Breastfeeding		
• Uses words for nursing		

☐ Developmental screening tool, if used:

Name of tool _____

_____

Staff initials _____

☐ By observation/exam/parent report. No tool used.

12-Month Well-Child Visit - 2

Child's Name: _____   Medical Record Number: _____

Physical Exam

N = normal Ab = abnormal (check appropriate box)	N	AB
1. General appearance:		
2. Skin: color • character • birthmarks		
3. Nodes: cervical • axillary • inguinal		
4. Head: shape • AF size • scalp • hair		
5. Eyes: EOM • red reflex • corneal light reflex • PERL • strabismus • lids		
6. Vision: follows objects		
7. Ears: pinna • canals • TMs		
8. Hearing: localization of sound		
9. Nose: patency • nares		
10. Mouth: gums • mucosa • teeth • throat		
11. Neck: position • ROM • thyroid		
12. Chest: shape • symmetry • lungs • respiration rate		
13. CV: rate • rhythm • S1 • S2 • murmur • femoral pulses		
14. Abd: contour • liver • spleen • masses • anus • bowel sounds		
15. GU: ♀ labia • vaginal mucosa ♂ penis • testes • hydrocele • hernia		
16. MS: ROM • hips • spine		
17. Neuro: posture • tone • DTRs • clonus • Babinski		

Document Abnormals (by number):

Anticipatory Guidance

✔ *Topics discussed*

Nutrition

Table food	Iron, calcium sources
Wean off bottle	Avoid food conflicts
Vary diet	Age-related decrease in appetite
Choking prevention—no popcorn, nuts, gum, raisins, etc.	
Toddler nursing/manners/setting limits	

Safety

Car seat	Sun protection
Never leave unattended, especially in water, near stove, fan, machinery, in car	Hot water temp <125° F
	Eliminate lead risks
	Toys with small parts/sharps
Smoke detectors	Stair gates
No smoking around baby	Window guards
No walkers	Lock up medications/cleaning products
Poisonous plants	
Poison control number	Socket plugs
Plastic bags/balloons	Rescue of choking baby

Parenting

Interact by talking, singing, playing	Safe child care
Autonomy/dependency needs	Use of OTC meds/minor illness care
Consistent scheduling	Teeth brushing
Tantrums	Thumbsucking normal
Never punish, jerk, or shake	Infection risk reduction
	Read books

Other:

Assessment

☐ Child well
☐ Additional Diagnoses (specify):

Laboratory Tests

☐ *Blood lead*
☐ *Hemoglobin* (once between 9 and 15 mo)

Additional Plan

Plan

Immunizations

Are immunizations on schedule? ☐ Yes ☐ No (Update Record Card)

*If not, catch-up plan?*_____

Previous reaction?   ☐ Yes   ☐ No

Comments: _____

Immunizations ordered/given: ☐ Hepatitis B ☐ PCV

☐ DTaP   ☐ IPV ☐ Hib   ☐ Other _____

If immunization(s) due but not given, explain:

☐ Has had chickenpox infection
☐ Other _____

| **Referrals** |
| ☐ *Smoking cessation class* |
| ☐ *Other:* |

☐ *Encouraged smoking cessation*
☐ *Need for financial assistance/Social services*
☐ *Requires additional health education*
☐ *Schedule 15-month visit*

Provider Signature
☐ Note dictated

15-Month Well-Child Visit

Date of Visit: _____

Medical Record Number: _____

Child's Name: _____

Address: _____

Telephone: _____

Date of Birth: _____ Age: _____ Gender: Male Female

Provider: _____

Informant: _____

Relationship to child: _____

Interpreter present: ☐ Yes   ☐ No

Language _____

Measurements

Ht _____ _____ % Wt _____ _____ % OFC _____ _____ % Staff

Temp _____ Pulse _____ Resp _____ Initials _____

Vision/Hearing

Vision concerns   ☐ No   ☐ Yes (explain)_____

Hearing concerns   ☐ No   ☐ Yes (explain)_____

Child Health History

Family/social history (refer to chart)   ☐ Completed   ☐ Updated

Parental concerns:_____

_____

Recent injury/illness/surgery/hospitalizations:

Allergies: _____

Medications: _____

Review of Systems

	N	AB
HEENT (strabismus, ear infections, colds, teething)		
Skin (rashes)		
CV (color)		
Resp (wheezing)		
GI (vomiting/stools)		
GU (pain/stream/frequency)		
Neuromuscular (moves all extremities equally)		

Remainder of review of systems (unlisted) negative ☐

Daily Activities

Nutrition

☐ Breast frequency _____ # feedings/day _____

☐ Whole milk/amount _____

☐ Juice (oz/day) _____

☐ Solids

☐ Iron/Vitamins/Fluoride

Sleep (arrangements/patterns) _____

Hygiene (bathing frequency)_____

Dental (brushing) _____

Child Health History (continued)

Caregivers   ☐ Mother   ☐ Father   ☐ Other relative

Caregiver working/in school   ☐ Yes   ☐ No

Who cares for baby during day or other time?   ☐ Parent/other relative

☐ Day care

Stresses for Caregivers _____

Environmental Risks—*Check if assessed*

☐ Lead risk   ☐ Guns in house/bldg   ☐ TB exposure

☐ Alcohol use in house/bldg   ☐ Housing inadequate   ☐ Domestic violence

☐ Smokers in house/bldg   ☐ Drug use in house/bldg   ☐ Other

☐ Identified risks _____

Active community supports/resources:

_____

Mental Health/Behavior Risks:

☐ No concerns

☐ Concerns (explain)_____

Observation of parent/child interaction:

☐ Appropriate

☐ Not appropriate (explain) _____

Other:

Development

Personal/Social/Cognitive	N	AB
• Waves bye-bye		
• Drinks from cup		
• Imitates activities		
• Plays ball with examiner		
Fine motor/adaptive		
• Scribbles		
• Puts block in cup		
Language		
• Has 2-6 words		
• Dada/Mama specific		
Gross motor		
• Walks well		
• Stoops and recovers		
• Stands alone		
• Walks backwards		

☐ Developmental screening tool, if used:

Name of tool _____

_____

Staff initials _____

☐ By observation/exam/ parent report. No tool used.

15-Month Well-Child Visit - 2

Child's Name: _____   Medical Record Number: _____

Physical Exam

N = normal Ab = abnormal (check appropriate box)	N	AB
1. *General appearance:*		
2. *Skin:* color • character • birthmarks		
3. *Nodes:* cervical • axillary • inguinal		
4. *Head:* shape • AF size • scalp • hair		
5. *Eyes:* EOM • red reflex • corneal light reflex • PERL • strabismus • lids		
6. *Vision:* follows objects		
7. *Ears:* pinna • canals • TMs		
8. *Hearing:* localization of sound		
9. *Nose:* patency • nares		
10. *Mouth:* gums • mucosa • teeth • throat		
11. *Neck:* position • ROM • thyroid		
12. *Chest:* shape • symmetry • lungs • respiration rate		
13. *CV:* rate • rhythm • S1 • S2 • murmur • femoral pulses		
14. *Abd:* contour • liver • spleen • masses • anus • bowel sounds		
15. *GU:* ♀ labia • vaginal mucosa ♂ penis • testes • hydrocele • hernia		
16. *MS:* ROM • hips • spine		
17. *Neuro:* posture • tone • DTRs • clonus • Babinski		

Document Abnormals (by number):

Assessment

☐ Child well

☐ Additional Diagnoses (specify):

Plan

Immunizations

Are immunizations on schedule? ☐ Yes ☐ No (Update Record Card)

If not, catch-up plan? _____

Previous reaction? ☐ Yes   ☐ No

Comments: _____

Immunizations ordered/given: ☐ Hepatitis B   ☐ PCV
☐ DTaP   ☐ IPV   ☐ Hib   ☐ MMR   ☐ Varicella

If immunization(s) due but not given, explain:

☐ Has had chickenpox infection

☐ Other _____

Anticipatory Guidance

☑ *Topics discussed*

Nutrition

Balanced diet/nutritious snacks	Iron, calcium sources
Self-feeding/drinking from cup	Avoid food conflicts
No bottles	Family mealtime
Choking prevention—no popcorn, nuts, gum, raisins, etc.	
Toddler nursing/manners/setting limits	

Safety

Car seat	Sun protection
Never leave unattended, especially in water, near stove, fan, machinery, in car	Hot water temp <125° F
	Toys with small parts/sharps
Smoke detectors	Stair gates
No smoking around baby	Window guards
No walkers	Lock up medications/cleaning products
Poisonous plants	
Poison control number	Socket plugs
Plastic bags/balloons	Rescue of choking baby
Eliminate lead risks	

Parenting

Interact by talking, singing, playing	Role model healthy habits
Autonomy/dependency needs	Media violence
Consistent scheduling	Safe child care
Tantrums	Use of OTC meds/minor illness care
Hitting/biting/aggressive behavior	
Never punish, jerk, or shake	Teeth brushing
Read books	Infection risk reduction

Other:

Laboratory Tests

☐ **Blood lead if not tested at 12 months**

☐ **Hemoglobin** *(once between 9 & 15 mo)*

Additional Plan

Referrals
☐ **Smoking cessation class**
☐ **Other:**

☐ **Encouraged smoking cessation**

☐ **Need for financial assistance/Social services**

☐ **Requires additional health education**

☐ **Schedule 18-month visit**

_____

Provider Signature

☐ Note dictated

18-Month Well-Child Visit

Date of Visit: _____

Medical Record Number: _____

Child's Name: _____

Address: _____

Telephone: _____

Date of Birth: _____ Age: _____ Gender: Male Female

Provider: _____

Informant: _____

Relationship to child: _____

Interpreter present: ☐ Yes ☐ No

Language _____

Measurements

Ht _____ _____ % Wt _____ _____ % OFC _____ _____ % Staff

Temp _____ Pulse _____ Resp _____ Initials _____

Vision/Hearing

Vision concerns ☐ No ☐ Yes (explain)_____

Hearing concerns ☐ No ☐ Yes (explain)_____

Child Health History

Family/social history (refer to chart) ☐ Completed ☐ Updated

Parental concerns:_____

_____

Recent injury/illness/surgery/hospitalizations:

_____

Allergies: _____

Medications: _____

Review of Systems

	N	AB
HEENT (strabismus, ear infections, colds, teething)		
Skin (rashes)		
CV (color)		
Resp (wheezing)		
GI (vomiting/stools)		
GU (pain on voiding/ urinary stream)		
Neuromuscular (moves all extremities equally)		

Remainder of review of systems (unlisted) negative ☐

Daily Activities

Nutrition
☐ Breast frequency _____ # feedings/day _____
☐ Whole milk/amount _____
☐ Juice (oz/day) _____
☐ Solids
☐ Iron/Vitamins/Fluoride

Sleep (arrangements/patterns) _____

Hygiene (bathing frequency)_____

Dental (brushing) _____

Child Health History (continued)

Caregivers ☐ Mother ☐ Father ☐ Other relative

Caregiver working/in school ☐ Yes ☐ No

Who cares for baby during day or other time? ☐ Parent/other relative ☐ Day care

Stresses for Caregivers _____

Environmental Risks—Check if assessed

☐ Lead risk   ☐ Guns in house/bldg   ☐ TB exposure

☐ Alcohol use in house/bldg ☐ Housing inadequate ☐ Domestic violence

☐ Smokers in house/bldg ☐ Drug use in house/bldg ☐ Other

☐ Identified risks _____

Active community supports/resources:

_____

Mental Health/Behavior Risks:

☐ No concerns

☐ Concerns (explain)_____

Observation of parent/child interaction:

☐ Appropriate

☐ Not appropriate (explain) _____

Other:

Development

Personal/Social/Cognitive	N	AB
• Removes garment		
• Uses spoon and cup		
• Shows affection, kisses		
• Imitates activities		
Language		
• Says 6-20 words		
• Listens to story		
• Uses two-word phrases		
• Points to some body parts		
Gross motor		
• Throws ball		
• Walks backwards		
• Runs		
Fine motor/adaptive		
• Makes tower of 3 cubes		
• Scribbles		
• Pulls a toy along ground		

☐ Developmental screening tool, if used:

Name of tool _____

_____

Staff initials _____

☐ By observation/exam/ parent report. No tool used.

18-Month Well-Child Visit - 2

Child's Name: _____   Medical Record Number: _____

Physical Exam

N = normal Ab = abnormal (check appropriate box)	N	AB
1. General appearance:		
2. Skin: color • character • birthmarks		
3. Nodes: cervical • axillary • inguinal		
4. Head: shape • AF size • scalp • hair		
5. Eyes: EOM • red reflex • corneal light reflex • PERL • strabismus • lids		
6. Vision: follows objects		
7. Ears: pinna • canals • TMs		
8. Hearing: localization of sound		
9. Nose: patency • nares		
10. Mouth: gums • mucosa • teeth • throat		
11. Neck: position • ROM • thyroid		
12. Chest: shape • symmetry • lungs • respiration rate		
13. CV: rate • rhythm • S1 • S2 • murmur • femoral pulses		
14. Abd: contour • liver • spleen • masses • anus • bowel sounds		
15. GU: ♀ labia • vaginal mucosa ♂ penis • testes • hydrocele • hernia		
16. MS: ROM • hips • spine		
17. Neuro: posture • tone • DTRs • clonus • Babinski		

Document Abnormals (by number):

Assessment

❑ Child well
❑ Additional Diagnoses (specify):

Plan
Immunizations

Are immunizations on schedule? ❑ Yes ❑ No (Update Record Card)
*If not, catch-up plan?*_____
Previous reaction? ❑ Yes   ❑ No

Comments: _____
Immunizations ordered/given: ❑ Hepatitis B ❑ PCV
❑ DTaP   ❑ IPV   ❑ Hib   ❑ MMR
❑ Varicella
If immunization(s) due but not given, explain:
❑ Has had chickenpox infection
❑ Other _____

Anticipatory Guidance

✔ *Topics discussed*

Healthy Habits

Car seat/air bags	Self-feeding, drinking from cup
Smoke detectors/childproof home	Family meals/healthy meals & snacks
Close supervision	First aid/poison control
Smoke-free environment	Choke foods
Eliminate lead risks	Toddler nursing

Social Competence

Limit but enforce rules consistently	Help with fears/strategies for nightmares
Curiosity about genitalia	
Acceptable alternative behaviors	Toilet training
Self-care, self-expression, choices	Hitting, biting, aggressive behavior
Reassure once negative behavior stops	

Family Relationships

Affection	Sharing toys
Sibling relationships	Help child express joy, anger
Listen, respect, interest in activities	Family playtime/short family outings
Role model healthy habits	Infection risk reduction
	Read books

Other:

Laboratory Tests

❑ *Blood lead if not tested at 12 months*

Additional Plan

Referrals
❑ *Smoking cessation class*
❑ *Other:*

❑ *Encouraged smoking cessation*
❑ *Need for financial assistance/Social services*
❑ *Requires additional health education*
❑ *Schedule 2-year visit*

Provider Signature
❑ Note dictated

2-Year Well-Child Visit

Date of Visit: _____

Medical Record Number: _____

Child's Name: _____

Address: _____

Telephone: _____

Date of Birth: _____ Age: _____ Gender: Male Female

Provider: _____

Informant: _____   Interpreter present: ☐ Yes   ☐ No

Relationship to child: _____   Language _____

Measurements

Ht _____ _____ % Wt _____ _____ % OFC _____ _____ % Staff

Temp _____ Pulse _____ Resp _____ Initials _____

Vision/Hearing

Vision concerns   ☐ No   ☐ Yes (explain) _____

Hearing concerns   ☐ No   ☐ Yes (explain) _____

Child Health History

Family/social history (refer to chart)   ☐ Completed   ☐ Updated

Parental concerns: _____

_____

Recent injury/illness/surgery/hospitalizations:

Allergies: _____

Medications: _____

Review of Systems

	N	AB
HEENT (strabismus, ear infections, frequent URIs)		
Skin (rashes)		
CV (color)		
Resp (wheezing)		
GI (vomiting/stools)		
GU (pain on voiding/urinary stream)		
Neuromuscular (coordination, gait, balance)		

Remainder of review of systems (unlisted) negative ☐

Daily Activities

Nutrition: (variety/misses meals/wt concern) _____

Milk: (whole, 2%, 1%, skim, breast) _____

Sleep: bedtime _____ awakes _____ naps _____

Dental: (brushing) _____

Exercise: _____

Recreation/TV: _____

Preschool/Childcare: _____

Child Health History (continued)

Environmental Risks—Check if assessed

☐ **Lead risk**   ☐ Guns in house/bldg   ☐ TB exposure

☐ Alcohol use in house/bldg   ☐ Housing inadequate   ☐ Domestic violence

☐ Smokers in house/bldg   ☐ Drug use in house/bldg   ☐ Other

☐ **Identified risks** _____

Active community supports/resources:

_____

Mental Health/Behavior Risks:

☐ No concerns

☐ Concerns (explain) _____

Observation of parent/child interaction:

☐ Appropriate

☐ Not appropriate (explain) _____

Other:

Development

Personal/Social/Cognitive	N	AB
• Removes garment		
• Uses spoon/fork		
• Brushes teeth with help		
Language		
• Uses at least 6-20 words		
• Points to 2 pictures		
• Follows 2-step commands		
• Uses two-word phrases		
Gross motor		
• Kicks ball forward		
• Walks up steps		
• Runs		
• Jumps up		
Fine motor/adaptive		
• Makes tower of 6 cubes		
• Holds cup securely		

☐ Developmental screening tool, if used:

Name of tool _____

_____

Staff initials _____

☐ By observation/exam/ parent report. No tool used.

2-Year Well-Child Visit - 2

Child's Name: _____   *Medical Record Number:* _____

Physical Exam

N = normal Ab = abnormal (check appropriate box)	N	AB
1. General appearance:		
2. Skin: color • character • birthmarks		
3. Nodes: cervical • axillary • inguinal		
4. Head: shape • hair		
5. Eyes: EOM • red reflex • corneal light reflex • PERL • cross cover accommodation • lids		
6. Ears: pinna • canals • TMs		
7. Nose: patency • nares • turbinates		
8. Mouth: mucosa • tonsils • teeth • throat		
9. Neck: ROM • thyroid		
10. Chest: shape • symmetry • lungs • respiration rate		
11. CV: rate • rhythm • S1 • S2 • murmur • femoral pulses		
12. Abd: contour • liver • spleen • masses • anus • bowel sounds		
13. GU: ♀ labia • vaginal mucosa • urethra ♂ penis • testes • hernia		
14. MS: ROM • gait • spine		
15. Neuro: DTRs • clonus • motor strength • sensory • Babinski		

Document Abnormals (by number):

Anticipatory Guidance

✔ *Topics discussed*

Healthy Habits

Car seat/air bags	Family meals/healthy meals & snacks
Smoke detectors/childproof home	First aid/poison control
Close supervision	Curiosity about sex, use correct terms
Smoke-free environment	Infection risk reduction
Eliminate lead risks	Toddler nursing

Social Competence

Individual attention	Help with fears/strategies for nightmares
Praise, talking, interactive reading	
Socialization	Toilet training
Choices, limits, time out	Exploration, physical activity
	Community programs/preschool

Family Relationships

Affection	Preparation for new baby
Sibling relationships	Help child express joy, anger
Listen, respect, interest in activities	Play with child
Role model healthy habits	Read books

Other:

Laboratory Tests

☐ *Blood lead*

Additional Plan

Assessment

☐ Child well
☐ Additional Diagnoses (specify):

Plan
Immunizations

Are immunizations on schedule? ☐ Yes ☐ No (Update Record Card)
If not, catch-up plan? _____
Previous reaction? ☐ Yes ☐ No

Comments: _____
Immunizations ordered/given: ☐ Hepatitis B ☐ DTaP ☐ IPV ☐ Hib ☐ MMR ☐ Varicella
If immunization(s) due but not given, explain:
☐ Has had chickenpox infection
☐ Other _____

Referrals
☐ *Smoking cessation class*
☐ *Other:*

☐ *Encouraged smoking cessation*
☐ *Need for financial assistance/Social services*
☐ *Requires additional health education*
☐ *Verbal referral for preventive dental visit*
☐ *Schedule 3-year preventive visit*

Provider Signature
☐ Note dictated

3-Year Well-Child Visit

Date of Visit: _____

Medical Record Number: _____

Child's Name: _____

Address: _____

Telephone: _____

Date of Birth: _____ Age: _____ Gender: Male Female

Provider: _____

Informant: _____   Interpreter present: ☐ Yes   ☐ No

Relationship to child:_____   Language _____

Measurements

Ht _____ _____ % Wt _____ _____ % OFC _____ _____ % Staff

Temp _____ Pulse _____ Resp _____ Initials _____

Vision/Hearing

Hearing (if able)								Vision
Right Ear				Left Ear				Glasses ☐ Yes ☐ No
500	1000	2000	4000	500	1000	2000	4000	Right eye /
								Left eye /

☐ Normal ☐ Abnormal ☐ Question validity/retest   ☐ Normal
Comments: Staff Initials _____   ☐ Refer to eye clinic
                                                  ☐ Question validity/ retest

Vision concerns   ☐ No   ☐ Yes (explain) _____

Hearing concerns   ☐ No   ☐ Yes (explain) _____

Child Health History

Family/social history (refer to chart)   ☐ Completed   ☐ Updated

Parental concerns:_____

_____

Recent injury/illness/surgery/hospitalizations:

_____

Allergies: _____

Medications: _____

Review of Systems

	N	AB
HEENT		
Skin (rashes)		
CV (activity level)		
Resp (wheezing)		
GI (vomiting/stools)		
GU (pain on voiding/urinary stream)		
Neuromuscular (coordination, gait, balance)		

Remainder of review of systems (unlisted) negative ☐

Daily Activities

Nutrition: (variety/misses meals/wt concern)

Milk: (whole, 2%, 1%, skim, breast) _____

Sleep: bedtime _____ awakes _____ naps _____

Child Health History (continued)

Dental: (brushing) _____

Exercise: _____

Recreation/TV: _____

Preschool/Childcare: _____

Environmental Risks—Check if assessed

☐ Lead risk   ☐ Guns in house/bldg   ☐ TB exposure

☐ Alcohol use in house/bldg   ☐ Housing inadequate   ☐ Domestic violence

☐ Smokers in house/bldg   ☐ Drug use in house/bldg ☐ Other

☐ Identified risks

Active community supports/resources:

_____

Mental Health/Behavior Risks:

☐ No concerns

☐ Concerns (explain)_____

Observation of parent/child interaction:

☐ Appropriate

☐ Not appropriate (explain)_____

Other:

Development

Personal/Social/Cognitive	N	AB
• Knows name, age, & sex		
• Washes and dries hands		
• Brushes teeth with help		
• Puts on T-shirt		
Language		
• Names 4 pictures		
• Points to 6 body parts		
• Speech more than ½ understandable		
Gross motor		
• Throws ball overhand		
• Jumps up		
• Balances on each foot 1 second		
Fine motor/adaptive		
• Makes tower of 8 cubes		
• Imitates vertical line		
• Copies circle, cross		

☐ Developmental screening tool, if used:

Name of tool _____

_____

Staff initials _____

☐ By observation/exam/ parent report. No tool used.

3-Year Well-Child Visit - 2

Child's Name: _____   *Medical Record Number:* _____

Physical Exam

N = normal Ab = abnormal (check appropriate box)	N	AB
1. General appearance:		
2. Skin: color • character • birthmarks		
3. Nodes: cervical • axillary • inguinal		
4. Head: shape • hair		
5. Eyes: EOM • red reflex • corneal light reflex • PERL • cross cover accommodation • fundi • lids		
6. Ears: pinna • canals • TMs		
7. Nose: patency • nares • turbinates		
8. Mouth: mucosa • tonsils • teeth • throat		
9. Neck: ROM • thyroid		
10. Chest: shape • symmetry • lungs • respiration rate		
11. CV: rate • rhythm • S1 • S2 • murmur • femoral pulses		
12. Abd: contour • liver • spleen • masses • anus • bowel sounds		
13. GU: ♀ labia • vaginal mucosa • urethra ♂ penis • testes • hernia		
14. MS: ROM • hips • spine		
15. Neuro: DTRs • clonus • motor strength • sensory		

Document Abnormals (by number):

Assessment

☐ Child well
☐ Additional Diagnoses (specify):

Plan
Immunizations

Are immunizations on schedule? ☐ Yes ☐ No (Update Record Card)

If not, catch-up plan? _____
Previous reaction? ☐ Yes ☐ No

Comments: _____
Immunizations ordered/given: ☐ Hepatitis B ☐ DTaP ☐ IPV
☐ Hib   ☐ MMR   ☐ Varicella
If immunization(s) due but not given, explain:
☐ Has had chickenpox infection
☐ Other _____

Anticipatory Guidance

✔ *Topics discussed*

Healthy Habits

Limit TV	Sucking habits
Safety: matches/poisons/guns	Family meals/healthy meals & snacks
Safety: water/playground/stranger	Adequate sleep/physical activity
Safety: car seat	Curiosity about sex
Infection risk reduction	Eliminate lead risks

Social Competence

Individual attention	Choices, limits, time out
Praise, talking, interactive reading	Help with fears
Socialization	

Family Relationships

Affection	Role model healthy habits
Sibling relationships	Preparation for new baby
Listen, respect, interest in activities	

Other:

Laboratory Tests

☐ **Blood lead** *(if never tested)*
☐ **UA** *(optional)*
☐ **Other** _____

Dental

☐ **Verbal referral for preventive dental visit/resource information given**

Additional Plan

Referrals
☐ **Smoking cessation class**
☐ **Other:**

☐ **Encouraged smoking cessation**
☐ **Need for financial assistance/Social services**
☐ **Requires additional health education**
☐ **Schedule 4-year preventive visit**

Provider Signature _____
☐ Note dictated

4-Year Well-Child Visit

Date of Visit: _____

Medical Record Number: _____

Child's Name: _____

Address: _____

Telephone: _____

Date of Birth: _____ Age: ____ Gender: Male Female

Provider: _____

Informant: _____   Interpreter present: ❑ Yes ❑ No

Relationship to child: _____   Language _____

Measurements

Ht _____ _____ % Wt _____ _____ % OFC _____ _____ % Staff

Temp _____ Pulse _____ Resp _____ Initials _____

Vision/Hearing

Hearing (if able)								Vision
Right Ear				Left Ear				Glasses ❑ Yes ❑ No
500	1000	2000	4000	500	1000	2000	4000	Right eye /
								Left eye /

❑ Normal ❑ Abnormal ❑ Question validity/retest   ❑ Normal
Comments: Staff Initials _____   ❑ Refer to eye clinic
                                              ❑ Question validity/retest

Vision concerns   ❑ No   ❑ Yes (explain) _____

Hearing concerns   ❑ No   ❑ Yes (explain) _____

Child Health History

Family/social history (refer to chart)   ❑ Completed   ❑ Updated

Parental concerns: _____

_____

Recent injury/illness/surgery/hospitalizations: _____

Allergies: _____

Medications: _____

Review of Systems

	N	AB
HEENT		
Skin (rashes)		
CV (activity level)		
Resp (wheezing)		
GI (vomiting/stools)		
GU (pain on voiding/urinary stream)		
Neuromuscular (headaches, limb pain)		

Remainder of review of systems (unlisted) negative ❑

Daily Activities

Nutrition: (variety/misses meals/wt concern)

Milk: (whole, 2%, 1%, skim, breast) _____

Sleep: bedtime _____ awakes _____ naps _____

Child Health History (continued)

Dental: (brushing) _____

Exercise: _____

Recreation/Hobbies/TV: _____

Preschool/Childcare: _____

Environmental Risks—*Check if assessed*

❑ **Lead risk**   ❑ Guns in house/bldg   ❑ TB exposure

❑ Alcohol use in house/bldg ❑ Housing inadequate   ❑ Domestic violence

❑ Smokers in house/bldg   ❑ Drug use in house/bldg ❑ Other

❑ **Identified risks** _____

Active community supports/resources:

_____

Mental Health/Behavior Risks:

❑ No concerns

❑ Concerns (explain) _____

Observation of parent/child interaction:

❑ Appropriate

❑ Not appropriate (explain) _____

Other:

Development

Personal/Social/Cognitive	N	AB
• Puts on T-shirt		
• Names friend		
• Gives first and last name		
Language		
• Names 1-2 colors		
• Counts 1 block		
• Knows 3 adjectives (cold, hungry, tired)		
• Speech all understandable		
Gross motor		
• Balances on each foot 3 seconds		
• Hops on one foot		
• Broad jump		
Fine motor/adaptive		
• Builds 10-block tower		
• Thumb wiggle		
• Copies 0		

❑ Developmental screening tool, if used:

Name of tool _____

_____

Staff initials _____

❑ By observation/exam/parent report. No tool used.

4-Year Well-Child Visit - 2

Child's Name: _____   *Medical Record Number:* _____

Physical Exam

N = normal Ab = abnormal (check appropriate box)	N	AB
1. General appearance:		
2. Skin: color • character • birthmarks		
3. Nodes: cervical • axillary • inguinal		
4. Head: shape • hair		
5. Eyes: EOM • red reflex • corneal light reflex • PERL • cross cover accommodation • fundi • lids		
6. Ears: pinna • canals • TMs		
7. Nose: patency • nares • turbinates		
8. Mouth: mucosa • tonsils • teeth • throat		
9. Neck: ROM • thyroid		
10. Chest: shape • symmetry • lungs • respiration rate		
11. CV: rate • rhythm • S1 • S2 • murmur • femoral pulses		
12. Abd: contour • liver • spleen • masses • anus • bowel sounds		
13. GU: ♀ labia • vaginal mucosa • urethra ♂ penis • testes • hernia		
14. MS: ROM • gait • spine		
15. Neuro: DTRs • clonus • motor strength • sensory		

Document Abnormals (by number):

Assessment

☐ Child well

☐ Additional Diagnoses (specify):

Plan

Immunizations

Are immunizations on schedule?   ☐ Yes ☐ No (Update Record Card)

If not, catch-up plan? _____

Previous reaction?   ☐ Yes   ☐ No

Comments: _____

Immunizations ordered/given: ☐ Hepatitis B   ☐ DTaP   ☐ IPV
☐ Hib   ☐ MMR   ☐ Varicella

If immunization(s) due but not given, explain:

☐ Has had chickenpox infection

☐ Other _____

Anticipatory Guidance

☑ *Topics discussed*

Healthy Habits

Limit TV	Sucking habits
Safety: matches/poisons/guns	Family meals/healthy meals & snacks
Safety: water/playground/stranger	Adequate sleep/physical activity
Safety: car seat/seat belt/bike helmet	Curiosity about sex
	Eliminate lead risks
Infection risk reduction	

Social Competence

Limits/Time out	School enrollment: preschool, Sunday school
Praise, encourage	
Assertiveness, not aggression	Interactive talking/reading

Family Relationships

Affection	Listen, respect, interest in activities
Sibling relationships	Role model healthy habits

Other:

Laboratory Tests

☐ **Blood lead** *(if never tested)*

☐ **UA** *(optional)*

☐ **Other** _____

Dental

☐ **Verbal referral for preventive dental visit/resource information given**

Additional Plan

Referrals

☐ **Smoking cessation class**

☐ **Other:**

☐ **Encouraged smoking cessation**

☐ **Need for financial assistance/Social services**

☐ **Requires additional health education**

☐ **Schedule 5-year preventive visit**

Provider Signature

☐ Note dictated

5-Year Well-Child Visit

Date of Visit: _____

Medical Record Number: _____

Child's Name: _____

Address: _____

Telephone: _____

Date of Birth: _____ Age: ____ Gender: Male Female

Provider: _____

Informant: _____

Relationship to child: _____

Interpreter present: ❑ Yes   ❑ No

Language _____

Measurements

Ht _____ _____ % Wt _____ _____ % BP _____ Staff

Temp _____ Pulse _____ Resp _____ Initials ____

Vision/Hearing

Hearing								Vision
Right Ear				**Left Ear**				Glasses ❑ Yes ❑ No
500	1000	2000	4000	500	1000	2000	4000	Right eye /
								Left eye /

❑ Normal ❑ Abnormal ❑ Question validity/retest
Comments: Staff Initials _____

Vision:
❑ Normal
❑ Refer to eye clinic
❑ Question validity/retest

Vision concerns   ❑ No   ❑ Yes (explain) _____

Hearing concerns   ❑ No   ❑ Yes (explain) _____

Child Health History

Family/social history (refer to chart) ❑ Completed ❑ Updated

Parental concerns: _____

_____

Recent injury/illness/surgery/hospitalizations: _____

Allergies: _____

Medications: _____

Review of Systems

	N	AB
HEENT		
Skin (rashes)		
CV (activity level)		
Resp (wheezing)		
GI (vomiting/stools)		
GU (pain on voiding/stream/bedwetting)		
Neuromuscular (headaches, limb pain)		

Remainder of review of systems (unlisted) negative ❑

Daily Activities

Nutrition: (variety/misses meals/wt concern) _____

Milk: (whole, 2%, 1%, skim) _____

Sleep: bedtime _____ awakes _____

Child Health History (continued)

Dental: (brushing) _____

Exercise: _____

Recreation/Hobbies/TV: _____

Environmental Risks—Check if assessed

❑ Lead risk   ❑ Guns in house/bldg   ❑ TB exposure

❑ Alcohol use in house/bldg ❑ Housing inadequate   ❑ Domestic violence

❑ Smokers in house/bldg   ❑ Drug use in house/bldg   ❑ Other

❑ Identified risks _____

Active community supports/resources:

_____

Mental Health/Behavior Risks:

❑ No concerns

❑ Concerns (explain) _____

Observation of parent/child interaction:

❑ Appropriate

❑ Not appropriate (explain) _____

Other:

Development

Personal/Social/Cognitive	N	AB
• Dresses without help		
• Plays make believe		
• Plays board games		
Language		
• Names 4 colors		
• Counts 5 blocks		
• Understands 4 prepositions		
• Able to define 5 words		
• Speech all understandable		
Gross motor		
• Balances each foot 5 sec		
• Heel-to-toe walk		
Fine motor/adaptive		
• Copies square demonstrated		
• Copies +		
• Recognizes some letters		
• Draws a person with 6 parts		

❑ Developmental screening tool, if used:

Name of tool _____

_____

Staff initials _____

❑ By observation/exam/parent report. No tool used.

5-Year Well-Child Visit - 2

Child's Name: _____   *Medical Record Number:* _____

Physical Exam

N = normal Ab = abnormal (check appropriate box)	N	AB
1. General appearance:		
2. Skin: color • character • birthmarks		
3. Nodes: cervical • axillary • inguinal		
4. Head: shape • hair		
5. Eyes: EOM • red reflex • corneal light reflex • PERL • cross cover accommodation • fundi • lids		
6. Ears: pinna • canals • TMs		
7. Nose: patency • nares • turbinates		
8. Mouth: mucosa • tonsils • teeth • throat		
9. Neck: ROM • thyroid		
10. Chest: shape • symmetry • lungs • respiration rate		
11. CV: rate • rhythm • S1 • S2 • murmur • femoral pulses		
12. Abd: contour • liver • spleen • masses • anus • bowel sounds		
13. GU: ♀ labia • vaginal mucosa • urethra ♂ penis • testes • hernia		
14. MS: ROM • gait • spine		
15. Neuro: DTRs • clonus • motor strength • sensory		

Document Abnormals (by number):

Assessment

☐ Child well

☐ Additional Diagnoses (specify):

Plan

Immunizations

Are immunizations on schedule? ☐ Yes ☐ No (Update Record Card)

If not, catch-up plan? _____

Previous reaction? ☐ Yes   ☐ No

Comments: _____

Immunizations ordered/given: ☐ Hepatitis B   ☐ DTaP   ☐ IPV
☐ Hib   ☐ MMR   ☐ Varicella

If immunization(s) due but not given, explain:

☐ Has had chickenpox infection

☐ Other _____

Anticipatory Guidance

✔ **Topics discussed**

Healthy Habits

Limit TV	Food choices (friuts, vegetables, grains)
Safety: matches/poisons/guns	Safe after-school environment
Safety: water/playground/stranger	Adequate sleep/physical activity
Safety: car seat/seat belt/ bike helmet	Curiosity about sex
	Infection risk reduction
Dental sealants	Eliminate lead risk

Social Competence

School readiness	Family rules, respect, right from wrong
Praise, encourage	
Knows address and phone number	Anger control/conflict resolution

Family Relationships

Affection	Know child's friends/families
Sibling relationships	Ethical role model

Other:

Laboratory Tests

☐ **Blood lead** *(if never tested)*   ☐ **UA** *(optional)*

☐ **Other**

Dental

☐ **Verbal referral for preventive dental visit**

Additional Plan

Referrals
☐ **Smoking cessation class**
☐ **Other:**

☐ **Encouraged smoking cessation**

☐ **Need for financial assistance/Social services**

☐ **Requires additional health education**

☐ **Dental resource information given**

☐ **Schedule 6-year preventive visit**

Provider Signature

☐ Note dictated

82

6 to 7-Year Well-Child Visit

Date of Visit: _____

Medical Record Number: _____

Child's Name: _____

Address: _____

Telephone: _____

Date of Birth: _____ Age: ____ Gender: Male Female

Provider: _____

Informant: _____

Relationship to child: _____

Interpreter present: ☐ Yes ☐ No

Language _____

Measurements

Ht _____ _____ % Wt _____ _____ % BP _____ Staff

Temp _____ Pulse _____ Resp _____ Initials _____

Vision/Hearing

Hearing								Vision
Right Ear				Left Ear				Glasses ☐ Yes ☐ No
500	1000	2000	4000	500	1000	2000	4000	Right eye /
								Left eye /

☐ Normal ☐ Abnormal ☐ Question validity/retest

Comments: Staff Initials _____

☐ Normal
☐ Refer to eye clinic
☐ Question validity/retest

Vision concerns ☐ No ☐ Yes (explain) _____

Hearing concerns ☐ No ☐ Yes (explain) _____

Child Health History

Family/social history (refer to chart) ☐ Completed ☐ Updated

Parental concerns: _____

_____

Recent injury/illness/surgery/hospitalizations:

Allergies: _____

Medications: _____

Review of Systems

	N	AB
HEENT		
Skin (rashes)		
CV (dizziness, chest pain)		
Resp (wheezing)		
GI (vomiting/stools)		
GU (pain/stream/bedwetting)		
Neuromuscular (headaches)		

Remainder of review of systems (unlisted) negative ☐

Child Health History (continued)
Daily Activities

Nutrition: (variety/misses meals/wt concern)_____

Milk: (whole, 2%, 1%, skim) _____

Sleep: bedtime _____ awakens _____

Dental: (brushing) _____

Exercise: _____

Recreation/Hobbies/TV: _____

Childcare: _____

Environmental Risks—Check if assessed

☐ Lead risk ☐ Guns in house/bldg ☐ TB exposure
☐ Alcohol use in house/bldg ☐ Housing inadequate ☐ Domestic violence
☐ Smokers in house/bldg ☐ Drug use in house/bldg ☐ Other
☐ Identified risks _____

Active community supports/resources:

_____

Mental Health/Behavior Risks:
☐ No concerns
☐ Concerns (explain)_____

Observation of parent/child interaction:
☐ Appropriate
☐ Not appropriate (explain) _____

Other:

Development

	N	AB	Comments:
School performance (reading/math at grade level)			Grades:
Ability to complete age-appropriate tasks			
Ability to form/maintain peer relationships			
Emotional stability			
Family relationships			
Team activities (social competence)			
Communication			

Copyright © 2005 by Mosby, Inc. All rights reserved.

6 to 7-Year Well-Child Visit - 2

Child's Name: _____   Medical Record Number: _____

Physical Exam

N = normal Ab = abnormal (check appropriate box)	N	AB
1. General appearance:		
2. Skin: color • character • birthmarks • rashes		
3. Nodes: cervical • axillary • inguinal		
4. Head: shape • scalp • hair		
5. Eyes: EOM • red reflex • corneal light reflex • PERL • lids • fundi		
6. Ears: pinna • canals • TMs		
7. Nose: patency • nares		
8. Mouth: mucosa • pharynx • tonsils • teeth • throat		
9. Neck: ROM • thyroid		
10. Chest: shape • symmetry • lungs • respiration rate		
11. CV: rate • rhythm • S1 • S2 • murmur • femoral pulses		
12. Abd: contour • liver • spleen • masses • anus • bowel sounds		
13. GU: ♀ labia • vaginal mucosa ♂ penis • testes • hernia		
14. MS: ROM • gait • feet		
15. Neuro: tone • DTRs • coordination • motor strength		

Document Abnormals (by number):

Assessment

☐ Child well

☐ Additional Diagnoses (specify):

Plan

Immunizations

Are immunizations on schedule?   ☐ Yes ☐ No (Update Record Card)

If not, catch-up plan? _____

Previous reaction?   ☐ Yes   ☐ No

Comments: _____

Immunizations ordered/given: ☐ Hepatitis B   ☐ DTaP/Td
☐ IPV   ☐ MMR   ☐ Varicella

If immunization(s) due but not given, explain:

☐ Has had chickenpox infection

☐ Other _____

Anticipatory Guidance

✔ Topics discussed

Healthy Habits

Limit TV	Adequate sleep/physical activity
Safety: matches/poisons/guns	Safe after-school environment
Safety: seat belts/bike helmet	Questions about sex/education at home
Food choices (fruits, vegetables, grains)	Infection risk reduction

Social Competence

Reading	Personal space
Self-discipline/limits & consequences	Chores/family rules/ family activities
Anger control/conflict resolution	

Family Relationships

Affection	Know child's friends/families
Sibling relationships	Ethical role model

Other:

Laboratory Tests

☐ Blood lead (up to 6 years if never tested)

☐ Other

Dental

☐ Verbal referral for preventive dental visit

Additional Plan

Referrals

☐ Smoking cessation class

☐ Other:

☐ Encouraged smoking cessation

☐ Need for financial assistance/Social services

☐ Requires additional health education

☐ Dental resource information given

☐ Schedule 8-year preventive visit

Provider Signature

☐ Note dictated

8 to 10-Year Well-Child Visit

Date of Visit: _____

Medical Record Number: _____

Child's Name: _____

Address: _____

Telephone: _____

Date of Birth: _____ Age: _____ Gender: Male Female

Provider: _____

Informant: _____

Relationship to child: _____

Interpreter present: ☐ Yes ☐ No

Language _____

Measurements

Ht _____ _____ % Wt _____ _____ % BP _____ Staff

Temp _____ Pulse _____ Resp _____ Initials _____

Vision/Hearing

Hearing								Vision
Right Ear				**Left Ear**				Glasses ☐ Yes ☐ No
500	1000	2000	4000	500	1000	2000	4000	Right eye /
								Left eye /

☐ Normal ☐ Abnormal ☐ Question validity/retest

Comments: Staff Initials _____

☐ Normal
☐ Refer to eye clinic
☐ Question validity/retest

Vision concerns ☐ No ☐ Yes (explain) _____

Hearing concerns ☐ No ☐ Yes (explain) _____

Child Health History

Family/social history (refer to chart) ☐ Completed ☐ Updated

Parental concerns: _____

_____

Recent injury/illness/surgery/hospitalizations:

_____

Allergies: _____

Medications: _____

Review of Systems

	N	AB
HEENT		
Skin (rashes)		
CV (dizziness, chest pain)		
Resp (wheezing)		
GI (vomiting/stools)		
GU (pain/stream)		
Neuromuscular (headaches)		

Remainder of review of systems (unlisted) negative ☐

Child Health History (continued)
Daily Activities

Nutrition: (variety/misses meals/wt concern) _____

Milk: (whole, 2%, 1%, skim) _____

Sleep: bedtime _____ awakes _____

Dental: _____

Exercise: _____

Recreation/Hobbies/TV: _____

Childcare: _____

Tobacco/Alcohol/Drugs: _____

Menstrual Hx (female):

    Menarche _____ LMP _____

Environmental Risks—Check if assessed

☐ Guns in house/bldg ☐ TB exposure ☐ Alcohol use in house/bldg

☐ Housing inadequate ☐ Domestic violence ☐ Smokers in house/bldg

☐ Drug use in house/bldg ☐ Other:

☐ Identified risks _____

Active community supports/resources:

_____

Mental Health/Behavior Risks:

☐ No concerns

☐ Concerns (explain) _____

Observation of parent/child interaction:

☐ Appropriate

☐ Not appropriate (explain) _____

Other:

Development

	N	AB	Comments:
School performance (reading/math at grade level)			Grades:
Ability to complete age-appropriate tasks			
Ability to form/maintain peer relationships			
Emotional stability			
Family relationships			
Team activities (social competence)			

8 to 10-Year Well-Child Visit - 2

Child's Name: _____   *Medical Record Number:* _____

Physical Exam

N = normal Ab = abnormal (check appropriate box)	N	AB
1. General appearance:		
2. Skin: color • character • rashes • acne		
3. Nodes: cervical • axillary • inguinal		
4. Head: scalp • hair		
5. Eyes: EOM • red reflex • corneal light reflex • PERL • lids		
6. Ears: pinna • canals • TMs		
7. Nose: patency • nares		
8. Mouth: gums • mucosa • teeth/caries • throat		
9. Neck: ROM • thyroid		
10. Chest: shape • symmetry • lungs • respiration rate		
11. CV: rate • rhythm • S1 • S2 • murmur • femoral pulses		
12. Abd: liver • spleen • masses • anus • bowel sounds		
13. GU: ♀ labia • vaginal mucosa ♂ penis • testes • hernia		
14. MS: ROM • spine • gait		
15. Neuro: posture • DTRs • coordination		

Document Abnormals (by number):

Anticipatory Guidance

✔ *Topics discussed*

Healthy Habits

Drugs, alcohol, tobacco		Healthy food choices/family meals
Seat belts, bike helmets		Dental
Safety: water, sports		Puberty, sexual development, education
Safety: home alone, stranger		Limit TV, video games
Adequate sleep/physical activity		Infection risk reduction
Personal hygiene		

Social Competence

Reading, hobbies		Positive interactions with adults
Family activities/rules		Personal space
Talents		Anger/conflict resolution
Community/school programs		

Family Relationships

Know child's friends/families		Role model
Reasonable expectations		

Other:

Laboratory Tests (None routinely required at this age)

Dental

❏ *Verbal referral for preventive dental visit*

Assessment

❏ Child well

❏ Additional Diagnoses (specify):

Additional Plan

Plan

Immunizations

Are immunizations on schedule? ❏ Yes ❏ No (Update Record Card)

If not, catch-up plan? _____

Previous reaction? ❏ Yes ❏ No

Comments: _____

Immunizations ordered/given: ❏ Hepatitis B ❏ Td ❏ IPV
❏ MMR ❏ Varicella

If immunization(s) due but not given, explain:

❏ Has had chickenpox infection

❏ Other _____

Referrals

❏ *Smoking cessation class*

❏ *Other:*

❏ *Encouraged smoking cessation*

❏ *Need for financial assistance/Social services*

❏ *Requires additional health education*

❏ *Dental resource information given*

❏ *Schedule next visit in 1 to 2-years*

Provider Signature

❏ Note dictated

11 to 14-Year Well-Child Visit

Date of Visit: _____

Medical Record Number: _____

Child's Name: _____

Address: _____

Telephone: _____

Date of Birth: _____ Age: ____ Gender: Male Female

Provider: _____

Informant: _____

Relationship to child: _____

Interpreter present: ☐ Yes   ☐ No

Language _____

Measurements

Ht _____ _____ % Wt _____ _____ % BP _____ Staff _____

Temp _____ Pulse _____ Resp _____ Initials _____

Vision/Hearing

Hearing								Vision
Right Ear				Left Ear				
500	1000	2000	4000	500	1000	2000	4000	Glasses ☐ Yes ☐ No
								Right eye /
								Left eye /

☐ Normal ☐ Abnormal ☐ Question validity/retest
Comments: Staff Initials _____

Vision:
☐ Normal
☐ Refer to eye clinic
☐ Question validity/retest

Vision concerns   ☐ No   ☐ Yes (explain) _____

Hearing concerns   ☐ No   ☐ Yes (explain) _____

Health History

Family/social history (refer to chart) ☐ Completed ☐ Updated

Adolescent/parental concerns: _____

_____

Recent injury/illness/surgery/hospitalizations:

_____

Allergies: _____

Medications: _____

Review of Systems

	N	AB
HEENT		
Skin (rashes/acne)		
CV (dizziness, chest pain)		
Resp (wheezing)		
GI (vomiting/stools)		
GU (pain/stream)		
Neuromuscular (headaches)		

Remainder of review of systems (unlisted) negative ☐

Daily Activities

Nutrition: (variety/misses meals/wt concern) _____

Milk: (whole, 2%, 1%, skim) _____

Sleep: bedtime _____ awakes _____

Health History (continued)

Dental: _____

Exercise: _____

Recreation/Hobbies/TV: _____

Tobacco/Alcohol/Drugs: _____

Menstrual Hx (female):

  Menarche _____ LMP _____ Regularity _____

Sexual History (activity, partners, birth control, STDs, pregnancy):

_____

Practices self-breast/testicular exam?:   ☐ Yes   ☐ No

Environmental Risks—Check if assessed

☐ Guns in house/bldg   ☐ TB exposure   ☐ Alcohol use in house/bldg

☐ Housing inadequate   ☐ Violence/rape   ☐ Smokers in house/bldg

☐ Drug use in house/bldg   ☐ Other:

☐ Identified risks _____

Active community supports/resources:

_____

Mental Health/Behavior Risks:

☐ No concerns

☐ Concerns (explain) _____

Observation of parent/child interaction:

☐ Appropriate

☐ Not appropriate (explain) _____

Other: _____

☐ Adolescent risk assessment tool (if used)

Development

	N	AB	Comments:
School performance (reading/math at grade level)			Grades:
Ability to complete age-appropriate tasks			
Ability to form/maintain peer relationships			
Emotional stability			
Family relationships			
Team activities (social competence)			
Communication			
Dating/sexual activity			

11 to 14-Year Well-Child Visit - 2

Child's Name: _____   Medical Record Number: _____

Physical Exam

N = normal Ab = abnormal (check appropriate box)	N	AB
1. General appearance:		
2. Skin: rash • acne		
3. Nodes: cervical • axillary • inguinal		
4. Head: scalp • hair		
5. Eyes: EOM • red reflex • corneal light reflex • PERL • lids		
6. Ears: pinna • canals • TMs		
7. Nose: patency • nares		
8. Mouth: gums • teeth/caries • occlusion • throat		
9. Neck: ROM • thyroid		
10. Chest: lungs • respiration rate		
♀ Female: Breasts • Tanner Stage:		
♂ Male: Gynecomastia		
11. CV: rate • rhythm • S1 • S2 • murmur • femoral pulses		
12. Abd: liver • spleen • masses • anus • bowel sounds		
13. GU: ♀ labia • vaginal mucosa		
♂ penis • testes • hernia		
Tanner Stage: _____		
Pelvic: EG _____ Vag _____ BUS _____ CX _____ Uterus _____ Adnexa _____		
14. MS: ROM • spine • gait		
15. Neuro: DTRs • coordination • sensory • motor		

Document Abnormals (by number):

Anticipatory Guidance

✔ Topics discussed

Healthy Habits

Adequate sleep/exercise	Family meals
Athletic conditioning, fluids	Weight management/food choices
Weight training, changes	Sexual feelings
Weapons	How to say no, abstinence
Seat belts, bike helmets	Alcohol/Drugs/Tobacco use
Stress, nervousness, sadness	Infection risk reduction

Social Competence

Family time	Social activities/groups/sports
Peer pressure/Peer refusal	Respect parents' limits/consequences

Responsibility

Respect others	Rules, chores, responsibility
Ethical role model	Religious, cultural, volunteer activities

School Achievement

Attendance, homework	Future plans, college, career

Other:

Laboratory Tests

☐ Hgb/Hct (once in adolescence for menstruating females) _____

☐ Urinalysis (once in adolescence) _____

Dental

☐ Verbal referral for preventive dental visit

Additional Plan

Assessment

☐ Child well

☐ Additional Diagnoses (specify):

Plan

Immunizations

Are immunizations on schedule?   ☐ Yes ☐ No (Update Record Card)

If not, catch-up plan? _____

Previous reaction?   ☐ Yes   ☐ No

Comments: _____

Immunizations ordered/given: ☐ Hepatitis B   ☐ Td   ☐ IPV
☐ MMR   ☐ Varicella

If immunization(s) due but not given, explain:

☐ Has had chickenpox infection

☐ Other _____

Referrals

☐ Smoking cessation class

☐ Other:

☐ Encouraged smoking cessation

☐ Need for financial assistance/Social services

☐ Requires additional health education

☐ Dental resource information given

☐ Schedule visit in 1 to 2 years

Provider Signature

☐ Note dictated

15 to 17-Year Well Visit

Date of Visit: _____

Medical Record Number: _____

Child's Name: _____

Address: _____

Telephone: _____

Date of Birth: _____ Age: _____ Gender: Male Female

Provider: _____

Informant: _____

Relationship to child: _____

Interpreter present: ☐ Yes ☐ No

Language _____

Measurements

Ht _____ _____ % Wt _____ _____ % BP _____ Staff

Temp _____ Pulse _____ Resp _____ Initials _____

Vision/Hearing

Hearing								Vision
Right Ear				**Left Ear**				Glasses ☐ Yes ☐ No
500	1000	2000	4000	500	1000	2000	4000	Right eye /
								Left eye /

☐ Normal ☐ Abnormal ☐ Question validity/retest

Comments: Staff Initials _____

Vision:
☐ Normal
☐ Refer to eye clinic
☐ Question validity/ retest

Vision concerns ☐ No ☐ Yes (explain) _____

Hearing concerns ☐ No ☐ Yes (explain) _____

Health History

Family/social history (refer to chart) ☐ Completed ☐ Updated

Adolescent/parental concerns: _____

_____

Recent injury/illness/surgery/hospitalizations:

_____

Allergies: _____

Medications: _____

Review of Systems

	N	AB
HEENT		
Skin (rashes/acne)		
CV (dizziness, chest pain)		
Resp (wheezing)		
GI (vomiting/stools)		
GU (pain/stream)		
Neuromuscular (headaches)		

Remainder of review of systems (unlisted) negative ☐

Daily Activities

Nutrition: (variety/misses meals/wt concern) _____

Milk: (whole, 2%, 1%, skim) _____

Sleep: bedtime _____ awakes _____

Health History (continued)

Dental: _____

Exercise: _____

Recreation/Hobbies/TV: _____

Tobacco/Alcohol/Drugs/Driving: _____

Menstrual Hx (female):

Menarche _____ LMP _____ Regularity _____

Sexual History (activity, partners, birth control, STDs, pregnancy):

_____

Practices self-breast/testicular exam?: ☐ Yes ☐ No

Environmental Risks—Check if assessed

☐ Guns in house/bldg ☐ TB exposure ☐ Alcohol use in house/bldg

☐ Housing inadequate ☐ Violence/rape ☐ Smokers in house/bldg

☐ Drug use in house/bldg ☐ Other:

☐ **Identified risks** _____

Active community supports/resources:

_____

Mental Health/Behavior Risks:

☐ No concerns

☐ Concerns (explain) _____

Observation of parent/child interaction:

☐ Appropriate

☐ Not appropriate (explain) _____

Other: _____

☐ Adolescent risk assessment tool (if used)

Development

	N	AB	Comments:
School (employment) performance/attendance:			
Future plans, college, career			
Family relationships			
Ability to form/maintain peer relationships			
Dating/sexual activity			
Activities or sports involvement			
Emotional stability			

15 to 17-Year Well Visit - 2

Child's Name: _____ *Medical Record Number:* _____

Physical Exam

N = normal Ab = abnormal (check appropriate box)	N	AB
1. General appearance:		
2. Skin: rash • acne		
3. Nodes: cervical • axillary • inguinal		
4. Head: scalp • hair		
5. Eyes: EOM • red reflex • corneal light reflex • PERL • lids		
6. Ears: pinna • canals • TMs		
7. Nose: patency • nares		
8. Mouth: gums • teeth/caries • occlusion • throat		
9. Neck: ROM • thyroid		
10. Chest: lungs • respiration rate		
♀ **Female:** Breasts • Tanner Stage:		
♂ **Male:** Gynecomastia		
11. CV: rate • rhythm • S1 • S2 • murmur • femoral pulses		
12. Abd: liver • spleen • masses • anus • bowel sounds		
13. GU: ♀ labia • vaginal mucosa		
♂ penis • testes • hernia		
Tanner Stage: _____		
Pelvic: EG _____ Vag _____ BUS _____ CX _____ Uterus _____ Adnexa _____		
14. MS: ROM • spine • gait		
15. Neuro: DTRs • coordination • sensory • motor		

Document Abnormals (by number):

Assessment

☐ Adolescent well

☐ Additional Diagnoses (specify):

Plan
Immunizations

Are immunizations on schedule? ☐ Yes ☐ No (Update Record Card)

If not, catch-up plan? _____

Previous reaction? ☐ Yes ☐ No

Comments: _____

Immunizations ordered/given: ☐ Hepatitis B ☐ Td ☐ IPV ☐ MMR ☐ Varicella ☐ Meningococcal

If immunization(s) due but not given, explain:

☐ Has had chickenpox infection

☐ Other _____

Anticipatory Guidance

☑ *Topics discussed*

Healthy Habits

Self-protection	Adequate sleep/exercise
Weight management/food choices	Athletic conditioning, weight training
Sexual feelings	Handle anger/conflict resolution
How to say no, abstinence	Weapons
Birth control, STDs, safer sex	Seat belts, bike helmets
Alcohol/Drugs/Tobacco use	Stress, nervousness, sadness
Infection risk reduction	

Social Competence

Family time	Social activities/groups/sports
Peer pressure/peer refusal	Respect parents' limits/consequences

Responsibility

Respect others	Rules, chores, responsibility
Ethical role model	Religious, cultural, volunteer activities

School Achievement

Attendance, homework	Frustrations, dropping out
Future plans, college, career	

Other:

Laboratory Tests

☐ **Hgb/Hct** (once in adolescence for menstruating females) _____

☐ **Urinalysis** (once in adolescence) _____

☐ **Other** (STD, Pap, TB, Cholesterol if at risk) _____

Dental

☐ **Verbal referral for preventive dental visit**

Additional Plan

Referrals
☐ **Smoking cessation class**
☐ **Other:**

☐ **Encouraged smoking cessation**
☐ **Need for financial assistance/Social services**
☐ **Requires additional health education**
☐ **Dental resource information given**
☐ **Schedule visit in 1 to 2 years**

Provider Signature
☐ Note dictated

18 to 20-Year Well Visit

Date of Visit: _____

Medical Record Number: _____

Child's Name: _____

Address: _____

Telephone: _____

Date of Birth: _____ Age: _____ Gender: Male Female

Provider: _____

Informant: _____

Relationship to child: _____

Interpreter present: ☐ Yes ☐ No

Language _____

Measurements

Ht _____ _____ % Wt _____ _____ % BP _____ Staff

Temp _____ Pulse _____ Resp _____ Initials _____

Vision/Hearing

Hearing								Vision
Right Ear				Left Ear				Glasses ☐ Yes ☐ No
500	1000	2000	4000	500	1000	2000	4000	Right eye /

☐ Normal ☐ Abnormal ☐ Question validity/retest

Comments: Staff Initials _____

Vision: Left eye /
☐ Normal
☐ Refer to eye clinic
☐ Question validity/retest

Vision concerns ☐ No ☐ Yes (explain) _____

Hearing concerns ☐ No ☐ Yes (explain) _____

Health History

Family/social history (refer to chart) ☐ Completed ☐ Updated

Adolescent/parental concerns: _____

Recent injury/illness/surgery/hospitalizations:

Allergies: _____

Medications: _____

Review of Systems

	N	AB
HEENT		
Skin (rashes/acne)		
CV (dizziness, chest pain)		
Resp (wheezing)		
GI (vomiting/stools)		
GU (pain/stream)		
Neuromuscular (headaches)		

Remainder of review of systems (unlisted) negative ☐

Daily Activities

Nutrition: (variety/misses meals/wt concern) _____

Milk: (whole, 2%, 1%, skim) _____

Sleep: bedtime _____ awakes _____

Health History (continued)

Dental: _____

Exercise: _____

Recreation/Hobbies/TV: _____

Tobacco/Alcohol/Drugs/Driving: _____

Menstrual Hx (female):

Menarche _____ LMP _____ Regularity _____

Sexual History (activity, partners, birth control, STDs, pregnancy):

Practices self-breast/testicular exam?: ☐ Yes ☐ No

Environmental Risks—Check if assessed

☐ Guns in house/bldg ☐ TB exposure ☐ Alcohol use in house/bldg
☐ Housing inadequate ☐ Violence/rape ☐ Smokers in house/bldg
☐ Drug use in house/bldg ☐ Other:
☐ Identified risks _____

Active community supports/resources:

Mental Health/Behavior Risks:
☐ No concerns
☐ Concerns (explain) _____

Observation of parent/child interaction:
☐ Appropriate
☐ Not appropriate (explain) _____

Other: _____

☐ Adolescent risk assessment tool (if used)

Development

	N	AB	Comments:
School (employment) performance/attendance:			
Future plans, college, career			
Family relationships			
Ability to form/maintain peer relationships			
Dating/sexual activity			
Activities or sports involvement			
Emotional stability			

18 to 20-Year Well Visit - 2

Child's Name: _____   *Medical Record Number:* _____

Physical Exam

N = normal Ab = abnormal (check appropriate box)	N	AB
1. General appearance:		
2. Skin: rash • acne		
3. Nodes: cervical • axillary • inguinal		
4. Head: scalp • hair		
5. Eyes: EOM • red reflex • corneal light reflex • PERL • lids		
6. Ears: pinna • canals • TMs		
7. Nose: patency • nares		
8. Mouth: gums • teeth/caries • occlusion • throat		
9. Neck: ROM • thyroid		
10. Chest: lungs • respiration rate		
♀ **Female:** Breasts • Tanner Stage:		
11. CV: rate • rhythm • S1 • S2 • murmur • femoral pulses		
12. Abd: liver • spleen • masses • anus • bowel sounds		
13. GU: ♀ labia • vaginal mucosa		
♂ penis • testes • hernia		
Tanner Stage: _____		
Pelvic: EG _____ Vag _____		
DUS _____ CX _____		
Uterus _____ Adnexa _____		
14. MS: ROM • spine • gait		
15. Neuro: DTRs • coordination • sensory • motor		

Document Abnormals (by number):

Assessment

☐ Adolescent well
☐ Additional Diagnoses (specify):

Plan
Immunizations

Are immunizations on schedule? ☐ Yes ☐ No (Update Record Card)

If not, catch-up plan? _____

Previous reaction? ☐ Yes ☐ No

Comments: _____

Immunizations ordered/given: ☐ Hepatitis B ☐ Td ☐ IPV
☐ MMR ☐ Varicella ☐ Meningococcal

If immunization(s) due but not given, explain:
☐ Has had chickenpox infection
☐ Other _____

Anticipatory Guidance

✔ **Topics discussed**

Healthy Habits

Self-protection	Adequate sleep/exercise
Weight management/food choices	Athletic conditioning, weight training
Sexual feelings	Handle anger/conflict resolution
How to say no, abstinence	Gay/lesbian issues
Birth control, STDs, safer sex	Seat belts, bike helmets, weapons
Alcohol/Drugs/Tobacco use	Stress, nervousness, sadness
Infection risk reduction	

Social Competence

Peer pressure/peer refusal	Family, sibling, peer relationship
Social activities/groups/sports	

Responsibility

Respect others	Chores, responsibility
Ethical role model	Religious, cultural, volunteer activities
Health care consumer	

School Achievement

Talents, new skills	Future plans, college, career

Other:

Laboratory Tests

☐ **Hgb/Hct** (once in adolescence for menstruating females) _____
☐ **Urinalysis** (once in adolescence) _____
☐ **Other** (STD, Pap, TB, Cholesterol if at risk) _____

Dental

☐ **Verbal referral for preventive dental visit**

Additional Plan

Referrals
☐ **Smoking cessation class**
☐ **Other:**

☐ **Encouraged smoking cessation**
☐ **Need for financial assistance/Social services**
☐ **Requires additional health education**
☐ **Dental resource information given**
☐ **Schedule visit in 1 to 2 years**

Provider Signature
☐ Note dictated

Well-Child Visit: Newborn to 4 Months

Name: _____ Birth Date: _____

2 weeks

Date _____ Age _____
Length _____ Wt _____ HC _____
Temp _____ Pulse _____ Resp _____
Birth wt _____ D/C wt _____

Recent Problems:

Nutrition:
- ☐ Breast: Freq _____ min/feeding _____
- ☐ Formula: Type _____ Amt/day _____

- ☐ Vitamins   ☐ Iron   ☐ Other:

Elimination: **Sleep:**
stools:
voids:

Caregivers:

ROS:

Developmental Screen
- ☐ prone—lifts head
- ☐ regards face
- ☐ responds to noise
- ☐ follows to midline
- ☐ Breast: latches on/positions

Physical Examination   (☑ NL)   **Abnormalities**
- ☐ Vision   ☐ Hearing

Skin	
Head	
Eyes	
ENT	
Chest	
Heart	
Pulses	
Abdomen	
Umbilicus	
Ext gen/GU	
Back/Hip	
Extremities	
Neuro/reflexes	

Assessment and Plan

Guidance
- ☐ no solids; no honey × 1 yr
- ☐ breast/bottle techniques/tips
- ☐ car seat/safety issues
- ☐ no smoking around baby
- ☐ caregivers: both parents
- ☐ fever, diarrhea, congestion
- ☐ never punish, shake, or jerk
- ☐ smoke detectors
- ☐ sun protection
- ☐ skin care
- ☐ sleep on back
- ☐ pacification
- ☐ family planning
- ☐ when to call office

☐ Hep B #1 (☐ done in hospital)

Signed: _____

2 months

Date _____ Age _____
Length _____ Wt _____ HC _____
Temp _____ Pulse _____ Resp _____

Recent Problems: **Meds:** ☐ Yes ☐ No

Nutrition:
- ☐ Breast: Freq _____ min/feeding _____
- ☐ Formula: Type _____ Amt/day _____

- ☐ Vitamins   ☐ Iron   ☐ Other:

Elimination: **Sleep:**
stools:
voids:

Caregivers:

ROS:

Developmental Screen
- ☐ prone—lifts head 45°
- ☐ vocalizes
- ☐ follows to midline
- ☐ smiles responsively
- ☐ Breast: begins to position self
- ☐ responds to noise

Physical Examination   (☑ NL)   **Abnormalities**
- ☐ Vision   ☐ Hearing

Skin	
Head	
Eyes	
ENT	
Nodes	
Chest	
Heart	
Pulses	
Abdomen	
Ext gen/GU	
Back/Hip	
Extremities	
Neuro/reflexes	

Assessment and Plan

Guidance
- ☐ delay solids until 4-6 mo
- ☐ BF on demand
- ☐ safety: rolling over, safe crib
- ☐ car seat
- ☐ no smoking around baby
- ☐ show affection; talk to baby
- ☐ fever, diarrhea, colds
- ☐ smoke detectors
- ☐ breast milk supply
- ☐ sun protection
- ☐ no walker
- ☐ sleep on back
- ☐ skin care
- ☐ caregiver concerns

☐ Hep B #2 ☐ DtaP #1 ☐ HIB #1 ☐ IPV #1 ☐ PCV #1

Signed: _____

4 months

Date _____ Age _____
Length _____ Wt _____ HC _____
Temp _____ Pulse _____ Resp _____

Recent Problems: **Meds:** ☐ Yes ☐ No

Nutrition:
- ☐ Breast: Freq _____ min/feeding _____
- ☐ Formula: Type _____ Amt/day _____

- ☐ Vitamins   ☐ Iron   ☐ Other:

Elimination: **Sleep:**
stools:
voids:

Caregivers:

ROS:

Developmental Screen
- ☐ prone—lifts head 90°
- ☐ laughs
- ☐ follows 180°
- ☐ chest up with arm support
- ☐ Breast: efficiently nurses
- ☐ regards own hand
- ☐ grasps rattle
- ☐ rolls over one way

Physical Examination   (☑ NL)   **Abnormalities**
- ☐ Vision   ☐ Hearing

Skin	
HEENT	
Nodes	
Chest	
Heart	
Pulses	
Abdomen	
Ext gen/GU	
Back/Hip	
Extremities	
Neuro/reflexes	

Assessment and Plan

Guidance
- ☐ juice, cereal gradual 4-6 mo
- ☐ breast milk storage
- ☐ safety: toys, no strings, falls
- ☐ car seat, safe crib
- ☐ no smoking around baby
- ☐ never leave unattended
- ☐ fever, teething
- ☐ smoke detectors
- ☐ never prop bottle
- ☐ bath/water safety
- ☐ no walker
- ☐ interacting with baby
- ☐ spitting up/vomiting
- ☐ caregiver concerns

☐ DtaP #2 ☐ HIB #2 ☐ IPV #2 ☐ PCV #2

Signed: _____

Well-Child Visit: 6 to 12 Months

Name: _____ Birth Date: _____

6 months:	**9 months:**	**12 months:**
Date _____ Age _____	Date _____ Age _____	Date _____ Age _____
Length _____ Wt _____ HC _____	Length _____ Wt _____ HC _____	Length _____ Wt _____ HC _____
Temp _____ Allergy _____	Temp _____ Allergy _____	Temp _____ Allergy _____
Recent Problems: **Meds:** ☐ Yes ☐ No	***Recent Problems:*** **Meds:** ☐ Yes ☐ No	***Recent Problems:*** **Meds:** ☐ Yes ☐ No

6 months:

☐ Assess lead risk
Nutrition:
☐ Breast: Freq _____ min/feeding _____
☐ Formula: Type _____ Amt/day _____
☐ Solids:

☐ Vitamins ☐ Iron ☐ Fluoride:
Elimination: **Sleep:**

Caregivers:

ROS:
Immunization reaction: ☐ Yes ☐ No

Developmental Screen
☐ pulls to sit–no head lag ☐ feeds self
☐ turns to voice ☐ reaches for objects
☐ babbles ☐ rolls over
☐ smiles spontaneously

Physical Examination (☑ NL) **Abnormalities**
☐ Vision ☐ Hearing

Skin	
HEENT	
Nodes	
Chest	
Heart	
Pulses	
Abdomen	
Ext gen/GU	
Back/Hip	
Extremities	
Neuro/reflexes	

Assessment and Plan

☐ Fluoride
Guidance
☐ breast/formula × 1 yr ☐ solids, finger foods
☐ introduce cup ☐ no bottle in bed
☐ safety: toys, cords, pets ☐ gates, stairs
☐ car seat, safe crib ☐ choking prevention
☐ plastic bags, plants, lead ☐ no walker
☐ no smoking around baby ☐ separation anxiety
☐ teething, OTC meds ☐ daycare concerns

☐ Hep B #3 ☐ DtaP #3 ☐ HIB #3 ☐ IPV #3
☐ PCV #3

Signed: _____

9 months:

☐ Assess lead risk
Nutrition:
☐ Breast: Freq _____ min/feeding _____
☐ Formula: Type _____ Amt/day _____
☐ Solids:

☐ Vitamins ☐ Iron ☐ Fluoride:
Elimination: **Sleep:**

Caregivers:

ROS:
Immunization reaction: ☐ Yes ☐ No

Developmental Screen
☐ pulls to stand ☐ stands holding on
☐ sits–no support ☐ finger-thumb grasp
☐ passes cube ☐ dada/mama nonspecific
☐ works for toy ☐ imitates speech

Physical Examination (☑ NL) **Abnormalities**
☐ Vision ☐ Hearing

Skin	
HEENT	
Nodes	
Chest	
Heart	
Pulses	
Abdomen	
Ext gen/GU	
Back/Hip	
Extremities	
Neuro/reflexes	

Assessment and Plan

☐ Fluoride
Guidance
☐ breast/formula × 1 yr
☐ begin weaning to cup ☐ thumbsucking NL
☐ safety: heaters, sockets, ☐ table food with texture
  bath, stairs, small toys ☐ childproof home
☐ car seat, never leave alone ☐ choking prevention
☐ plastic bags, balloons ☐ teach 'no', distraction
☐ poison control tel# ☐ no walker
   ☐ daycare concerns

☐ Hep B #3 ☐ Blood Lead Level (once 9-12 mo)

Signed: _____

12 months:

☐ Assess lead risk
Nutrition:
☐ Breast: ☐ Whole milk
☐ Solids:

☐ Vitamins ☐ Iron ☐ Fluoride:
Elimination: **Sleep:**

Caregivers:

ROS:
Immunization reaction: ☐ Yes ☐ No

Developmental Screen
☐ pulls to stand ☐ stands 2 seconds
☐ plays pat-a-cake ☐ indicates wants
☐ bangs 2 cubes ☐ dada/mama nonspecific
☐ combines syllables ☐ jabbers

Physical Examination (☑ NL) **Abnormalities**
☐ Vision ☐ Hearing

Skin	
HEENT	
Nodes	
Chest	
Heart	
Pulses	
Abdomen	
Ext gen/GU	
Back/Hip	
Extremities	
Neuro/reflexes	

Assessment and Plan

☐ Fluoride
Guidance
☐ cont breast to age 2 yr prn ☐ teething, teeth
☐ wean off bottle, use cup   brushing
☐ safety: stove, sockets, ☐ table food, feed self
  stairs, windows, climbing ☐ whole milk
☐ car seat, never leave in car ☐ choking rescue
☐ plastic bags, plants, lead, ☐ read books
  toys–small parts, bath ☐ daycare concerns
☐ discipline/consistency

☐ Blood Lead Level (once 9-12 mo) ☐ Varicella
☐ MMR (12-15 mo)

Signed: _____

Well-Child Visit: 15 Months to 2 Years

Name: _____ Birth Date: _____

15 months:

Date _____ Age _____
Length _____ Wt _____ HC _____
Temp _____ Allergy _____
Recent Problems: **Meds:** ☐ Yes ☐ No

☐ Assess lead risk
Nutrition:
☐ Breast: ☐ Whole milk
☐ Solids:

☐ Vitamins ☐ Iron ☐ Fluoride:
Elimination: **Sleep:**

Caregivers:

ROS:
Immunization reaction: ☐ Yes ☐ No

Developmental Screen
☐ walks without support ☐ drinks from cup
☐ walks backwards ☐ stoops and recovers
☐ imitates activities ☐ puts block in cup
☐ scribbles ☐ 2-6 words

Physical Examination (☑ NL) **Abnormalities**
☐ Vision ☐ Hearing

Skin	
HEENT	
Nodes	
Chest	
Heart	
Pulses	
Abdomen	
Ext gen/GU	
Back	
Extremities	
Neuro	

Assessment and Plan

☐ Fluoride
Guidance
☐ cont breast to age 2 yr prn ☐ aggressive behavior
☐ cup, no bottle ☐ teeth brushing
☐ safety: toys-small parts, ☐ self-feeding, snacks
   bath, household products ☐ decreased appetite NL
☐ car seat, crib climbing, ☐ consistent schedule
   lead, sunscreen ☐ read books, talk, sing
☐ choking prevention ☐ safe childcare

☐ DtaP #4 ☐ HIB #4 ☐ PCV #4 ☐ MMR (12-15 mos)

Signed: _____

18 months:

Date _____ Age _____
Length _____ Wt _____ HC _____
Temp _____ Allergy _____
Recent Problems: **Meds:** ☐ Yes ☐ No

☐ Assess lead risk
Nutrition:
☐ Breast: ☐ Whole milk
☐ Solids:

☐ Vitamins ☐ Iron ☐ Fluoride:
Elimination: **Sleep:**

Caregivers:

ROS:
Immunization reaction: ☐ Yes ☐ No

Developmental Screen
☐ throws ball ☐ walks backwards
☐ runs ☐ uses spoon and cup
☐ removes garment ☐ makes tower of 3 cubes
☐ says 6-20 words ☐ listens to story

Physical Examination (☑ NL) **Abnormalities**
☐ Vision ☐ Hearing

Skin	
HEENT	
Nodes	
Chest	
Heart	
Pulses	
Abdomen	
Ext gen/GU	
Back	
Extremities	
Neuro	

Assessment and Plan

☐ Fluoride
Guidance
☐ toddler nursing ☐ self-feeding; avoid conflicts
☐ family meals ☐ first aid; street safety
☐ childproof home ☐ poison control #
☐ car seat ☐ choking prevention
☐ family outings ☐ ignore temper tantrums
☐ toilet training ☐ fears/nightmares
☐ sharing toys ☐ sibling relationships
☐ daycare concerns ☐ curiosity about genitalia

Signed: _____

2 years:

Date _____ Age _____
Length _____ Wt _____ HC _____
Temp _____ Allergy _____
Recent Problems: **Meds:** ☐ Yes ☐ No

☐ Assess lead risk   ☐ Assess TB risk
Nutrition:

☐ Vitamins ☐ Iron ☐ Fluoride:
Sleep: **Exercise:**

Preschool/Daycare/Recreation:

ROS:

Developmental Screen
☐ walks up stairs ☐ kicks ball forward
☐ jumps up ☐ makes tower of 6 cubes
☐ removes garment ☐ uses at least 6-20 words
☐ two-word sentences ☐ points to 2 pictures

Physical Examination (☑ NL) **Abnormalities**
☐ Vision ☐ Hearing

Skin	
HEENT	
Nodes	
Chest	
Heart	
Pulses	
Abdomen	
Ext gen/GU	
Back	
Extremities	
Neuro	

Assessment and Plan

☐ Fluoride
Guidance
☐ healthy meals & snacks ☐ close supervision
☐ childproof home ☐ car seat
☐ smoke-free environment ☐ exploration/exercise
☐ playmates, difficulty sharing ☐ toilet training
☐ choices, limits, time out ☐ help express feelings
☐ praise, individual attention ☐ reads books, sing
☐ teeth care ☐ daycare concerns

☐ Blood Lead Level (optional)

Signed: _____

Well-Child Visit: 3 to 5 Years

Name: _____ Birth Date: _____

3 years:

Date _____ Age _____
Length _____ Wt _____ BP _____
Temp _____ Allergy _____
Recent Problems: **Meds:** ☐ Yes ☐ No

☐ Assess lead risk ☐ Assess TB risk
Nutrition:

☐ Vitamins ☐ Iron ☐ Fluoride:
Sleep: **Exercise:**

Preschool/Daycare/Recreation:

ROS:

Developmental Screen
☐ throws ball overhand ☐ balances on each
☐ copies circle, cross foot 1 sec
☐ points to 6 body parts ☐ makes tower of
☐ washes & dries hands 8 cubes
☐ knows name, age, sex ☐ names 4 pictures

Physical Examination (☑ NL) **Abnormalities**
☐ Vision ☐ Hearing

Skin	
HEENT	
Nodes	
Chest	
Heart	
Pulses	
Abdomen	
Ext gen/GU	
Back	
Extremities	
Neuro	

Assessment and Plan

☐ Fluoride
Guidance
☐ healthy meals & snacks ☐ limit TV
☐ safety: playground, strangers ☐ car seat
☐ dental referral: prophylaxis ☐ adequate sleep
☐ matches, poisons, guns ☐ curiosity about sex
☐ socialization, playmates ☐ fears/nightmares
☐ choices, limits, time-out ☐ read books, talk, sing
☐ listen, respect, praise ☐ childcare/preschool

Signed: _____

4 years:

Date _____ Age _____
Length _____ Wt _____ BP _____
Temp _____ Allergy _____
Recent Problems: **Meds:** ☐ Yes ☐ No

☐ Assess lead risk ☐ Assess TB risk
Nutrition:

☐ Vitamins ☐ Iron ☐ Fluoride:
Sleep: **Exercise:**

Preschool/Daycare/Recreation:

ROS:

Developmental Screen
☐ hops on one foot ☐ balances on each foot
☐ builds 10-block tower 3 sec
☐ knows 3 adjectives ☐ names 1-2 colors
☐ knows first & last name ☐ speech all understand-
☐ puts on T-shirt able

Physical Examination (☑ NL) **Abnormalities**
☐ Vision ☐ Hearing

Skin	
HEENT	
Nodes	
Chest	
Heart	
Pulses	
Abdomen	
Ext gen/GU	
Back	
Extremities	
Neuro	

Assessment and Plan

☐ Fluoride
Guidance
☐ healthy meals & snacks ☐ limit TV
☐ safety: playgd, strangers ☐ car seat
☐ matches, poisons, guns ☐ bike helmet/pads
☐ adequate sleep/exercise ☐ siblings, peer play
☐ choices, limits, time-out ☐ household chores
☐ listen, respect, praise ☐ read books, talk, sing
☐ dental referral: prophylaxis ☐ childcare/preschool

☐ DtaP #5 ☐ IPV #4 ☐ MMR #2
☐ UA (optional) ☐ lead (if not done before)

Signed: _____

5 years:

Date _____ Age _____
Length _____ Wt _____ BP _____
Temp _____ Allergy _____
Recent Problems: **Meds:** ☐ Yes ☐ No

☐ Assess lead risk ☐ Assess TB risk
Nutrition:

☐ Vitamins ☐ Iron ☐ Fluoride:
Sleep: **Exercise:**

School/Recreation:

ROS:

Developmental Screen
☐ balances on each foot 5 sec ☐ heel-to-toe walk
☐ draws person with 6 parts ☐ copies square
☐ able to define 5 words ☐ counts 5 blocks
☐ dresses without help ☐ plays board games

Physical Examination (☑ NL) **Abnormalities**
☐ Vision ☐ Hearing

Skin	
HEENT	
Nodes	
Chest	
Heart	
Pulses	
Abdomen	
Ext gen/GU	
Back	
Extremities	
Neuro	

Assessment and Plan

☐ Fluoride
Guidance
☐ food choices: fruit, veg, grains ☐ limit TV
☐ safety: playground, strangers ☐ car seat/helmet
☐ dental referral: prophylaxis ☐ safe after school
☐ matches, poisons, guns ☐ adequate sleep/exercise
☐ siblings, peer play ☐ household chores
☐ family rules, respect ☐ read books, talk, sing
☐ school readiness ☐ conflict resolution

☐ DtaP #5 ☐ IPV #4 ☐ MMR #2
☐ UA (optional) ☐ lead (if not done before)

Signed: _____

Well-Child Visit: 6 to 11 Years

Name: _____   Birth Date: _____

6-7 years:

Date _____ Age _____
Length _____ Wt _____ BP _____
Temp _____ Allergy _____
Recent Problems: **Meds:** ☐ Yes ☐ No

☐ Assess TB risk
Nutrition:

☐ Vitamins
Sleep: **Exercise:**

Recreation:

ROS:

Developmental Screen
School performance: _____
Age-appropriate tasks: _____
Peer relationships: _____
Family/Social: _____

Physical Examination   (☑ **NL)**   **Abnormalities**
☐ Vision   ☐ Hearing

Skin	
HEENT	
Nodes	
Chest	
Heart	
Pulses	
Abdomen	
Ext gen/GU	
Back	
Extremities	
Neuro	

Assessment and Plan

Guidance
☐ food choices: fruit, veg, grains   ☐ limit TV
☐ adequate sleep/exercise   ☐ household chores
☐ safety: seat belt/helmet   ☐ safe after school
☐ matches, poisons, guns   ☐ fire drills
☐ questions about sex   ☐ siblings, peer play
☐ family rules, respect   ☐ praise, affection
☐ dental referral: prophylaxis

☐ lead (up to 6 years if not done before)

Signed: _____

8-9 years:

Date _____ Age _____
Length _____ Wt _____ BP _____
Temp _____ Allergy _____
Recent Problems: **Meds:** ☐ Yes ☐ No

☐ Assess TB risk
Nutrition:

☐ Vitamins
Sleep: **Exercise:**

Recreation:

ROS:

Developmental Screen
School performance: _____
Age-appropriate tasks: _____
Peer relationships: _____
Family/Social: _____
Team: _____

Physical Examination   (☑ **NL)**   **Abnormalities**
☐ Vision   ☐ Hearing

Skin	
HEENT	
Nodes	
Chest	
Heart	
Pulses	
Abdomen	
Ext gen/GU	
Back	
Extremities	
Neuro	

Assessment and Plan

Guidance
☐ food choices: fruit, veg, grains   ☐ limit TV, video
☐ adequate sleep/exercise   ☐ household chores
☐ dental referral; prophylaxis   ☐ personal hygiene
☐ safety: seat belt/helmet,   ☐ discuss puberty
  water, sports, weapons   ☐ reading, hobbies
☐ home alone, strangers   ☐ adult interactions
☐ family activities, rules   ☐ personal space
☐ conflict resolution   ☐ parental expectations

Signed: _____

10-11 years:

Date _____ Age _____
Length _____ Wt _____ BP _____
Temp _____ Allergy _____
Recent Problems: **Meds:** ☐ Yes ☐ No

☐ Assess TB risk
Nutrition:

☐ Vitamins
Sleep: **Exercise:**

Recreation:

ROS:

Developmental Screen
School performance: _____
Age-appropriate tasks: _____
Peer relationships: _____
Family/Social: _____
Team: _____
☐ Adolescent risk assessment screen

Physical Examination   (☑ **NL)**   **Abnormalities**
☐ Vision   ☐ Hearing

Skin	
HEENT	
Nodes	
Chest	
Heart	
Pulses	
Abdomen	
Ext gen/GU	
Back	
Extremities	
Neuro	
Tanner stage:	

Assessment and Plan

Guidance
☐ food choices/weight issues   ☐ limit TV, video
☐ adequate sleep/exercise   ☐ dental care
☐ safety: seat belt/helmet,   ☐ personal hygiene
  water, sports, weapons   ☐ discuss puberty
☐ home alone, strangers   ☐ family activities
☐ reading, hobbies, talents   ☐ stress
☐ alcohol, tobacco, drugs   ☐ adult interactions
☐ parental bond, communication   ☐ peer group

☐ Td   ☐ Varicella (if not prior)

Signed: _____

Well-Adolescent Visit: 12 to 18 Years

Name: _____   Birth Date: _____

12-13 years:

Date _____ Age _____
Length _____ Wt _____ BP _____
Temp _____ Allergy _____
Recent Problems: **Meds:** ☐ Yes ☐ No

☐ Assess TB risk
Nutrition:

☐ Vitamins
Sleep: ***Exercise:***

Recreation:

ROS:

Developmental Screen
School: _____
Age-appropriate tasks: _____
Peer relationships: _____
Family/Social: _____
Team: _____
☐ Adolescent risk assessment screen

Physical Examination   *(☑ NL)*   ***Abnormalities***
☐ Vision ☐ Hearing

Skin	
HEENT	
Nodes	
Chest	
Heart	
Pulses	
Abdomen	
Ext gen/GU	
Back	
Extremities	
Neuro	
Tanner stage:	

♀ **pelvic:**

Assessment and Plan

Guidance
☐ food choices/weight issues
☐ adequate sleep/exercise
☐ safety: seat belt/helmet, water, sports, weapons
☐ reading, hobbies, talents
☐ parental bond, communication
☐ alcohol, tobacco, drugs
☐ sexual information
☐ family meals, time
☐ dental care
☐ personal hygiene
☐ athletic training
☐ stress, sadness
☐ peer pressure
☐ responsibilities
☐ social activities

☐ Td (if not prior)   ☐ urine/Hb (once in adolescence)

Signed: _____

14-15 years:

Date _____ Age _____
Length _____ Wt _____ BP _____
Temp _____ Allergy _____
Recent Problems: **Meds:** ☐ Yes ☐ No

☐ Assess TB risk
Nutrition:

☐ Vitamins
Sleep: ***Exercise:***

Recreation:

ROS:

Developmental Screen
School: _____
Age-appropriate tasks: _____
Peer relationships: _____
Family/Social: _____
Team: _____
☐ Adolescent risk assessment screen

Physical Examination   *(☑ NL)*   ***Abnormalities***
☐ Vision ☐ Hearing

Skin	
HEENT	
Nodes	
Chest	
Heart	
Pulses	
Abdomen	
Ext gen/GU	
Back	
Extremities	
Neuro	
Tanner stage:	

♀ **pelvic:**

Assessment and Plan

Guidance
☐ food choices/weight issues
☐ adequate sleep/exercise
☐ driving, drinking, accidents
☐ school achievement
☐ alcohol, tobacco, drugs
☐ birth control, STDs, safe sex
☐ parents: communication, privacy
☐ safety: seat belt/helmet, water, sports, weapons
☐ self-protection
☐ dental care
☐ athletic training
☐ stress, sadness
☐ peer pressure
☐ sexual educatn
☐ responsibilities

☐ Td (if not prior)   ☐ urine/Hb (once in adolescence)

Signed: _____

16-18 years:

Date _____ Age _____
Length _____ Wt _____ BP _____
Temp _____ Allergy _____
Recent Problems: **Meds:** ☐ Yes ☐ No

☐ Assess TB risk
Nutrition:

☐ Vitamins
Sleep: ***Exercise:***

Recreation/Driving/Work:

ROS:

Developmental Screen
School: _____
Age-appropriate tasks: _____
Peer relationships: _____
Family/Social: _____
Team: _____
☐ Adolescent risk assessment screen

Physical Examination   *(☑ NL)*   ***Abnormalities***
☐ Vision ☐ Hearing

Skin	
HEENT	
Nodes	
Chest	
Heart	
Pulses	
Abdomen	
Ext gen/GU	
Back	
Extremities	
Neuro	
Tanner stage:	

♀ **pelvic:**

Assessment and Plan

Guidance
☐ food choices/weight issues
☐ adequate sleep/exercise
☐ driving, drinking, accidents
☐ school/future plans
☐ parental communication
☐ alcohol, tobacco, drugs
☐ birth control, STDs, safe sex
☐ safety: seat belt/helmet, water, sports, weapons
☐ self-protection
☐ dental care
☐ athletic training
☐ stress, sadness
☐ peer pressure
☐ sexual educatn
☐ responsibilities

☐ Td (if not prior)   ☐ urine/Hb (once in adolescence)
☐ Meningococcal

Signed: _____

Screening Form
For Early Follow-up of Breastfed Infants

Name: _____   *Date:* ____/____/____ *Days Postpartum*

The following questions are designed to help determine whether you are off to a successful start with breastfeeding. Please complete this form when your infant is 4-6 days old.

If you circle any answers in the right-hand column, call _____ for advice. Breastfeeding problems identified early are easier to correct.

1. Do you feel breastfeeding is going well for you so far?	Yes	No
2. Has your milk come in yet (i.e., did your breasts get firm and full between the 2nd and 4th postpartum days)?	Yes	No
3. Is your baby able to latch on to both breasts without difficulty?	Yes	No
4. Is your baby able to sustain rhythmic suckling for at least 10 minutes total per feeding?	Yes	No
5. Does your baby usually demand to feed? (Answer No if you have a sleepy baby who needs to be awakened for most feedings.)	Yes	No
6. Does your baby usually nurse at both breasts at each feeding?	Yes	No
7. Does your baby nurse approximately every 2-3 hrs, with no more than one long interval of up to 5 hrs at night (at least 8 feedings each 24 hrs)?	Yes	No
8. Do your breasts feel full before feedings?	Yes	No
9. Do your breasts feel softer after feedings?	Yes	No
10. Are your nipples extremely sore (i.e., causing you to "dread" feedings)?	Yes	No
11. Is your baby having yellow bowel movements that resemble a mixture of cottage cheese and mustard?	Yes	No
12. Is your baby having at least 4 good-sized bowel movements each day (i.e., more than a "stain" on the diaper)?	Yes	No
13. Is your baby wetting his/her diaper at least 6 times each day?	Yes	No
14. Does your baby appear hungry after most feedings (i.e., sucking hands, rooting, crying, often needing a pacifier, etc.)?	Yes	No
15. Do you hear rhythmic suckling & frequent swallowing while your baby nurses?	Yes	No

Breastfeeding Infant Triage Form

Date _____ Mother's Name _____ Infant's Name _____

Routinely complete this questionnaire for all breastfeeding dyads during the first week of life, either by phone or during the first clinic visit. Subsequently, this form can be used as needed to triage phone calls or for office visits pertaining to breastfeeding-related problems or consults.

COMPLETE BY FILLING IN THE BLANKS, CHECKING BOXES, AND/OR CIRCLING THE ANSWERS.

	NORMALS	RISK FACTORS
SUBJECTIVE HISTORY: ☐ Phone ☐ Office Visit **Chief Complaint:** _____ Infant's Age: _____ days/weeks Gestational age: _____ weeks _____	38-42 gestational weeks.	37-38 weeks with any of the below risk factors, or less than 37 weeks.
Perinatal History: 1. *Birth:* ☐ Single ☐ Multiple # _____ ☐ Vaginal ☐ Cesarean 2. *Pregnancy, birth, maternal, or infant complications?* ☐ NONE or _____ 3. *Medication usage during labor?* ☐ NONE ☐ IV Analgesia ☐ Epidural<5 Hrs or >5 Hrs ☐ Pitocin ☐ Mg Sulfate ☐ Spinal ☐ OTHER _____ 4. *Medication usage in mother/child** ☐ Vitamins ☐ _____ 5. *Any history of jaundice?* ☐ NO ☐ YES If yes, is it improved? _____ *Infant's* ☐ Normal or ☐ Rash ☐ Jaundice ☐ Dusky of *skin color:* ☐ Face ☐ Arms ☐ Hands ☐ Chest ☐ Abdomen ☐ Legs ☐ Feet ☐ Groin	NSVD of a single child. No complications. No medication usage during labor. Infant skin is pink and undamaged. Routinely check for jaundice in the first few days of life. Jaundice normally improves gradually over several days or weeks. *Other than prenatal vitamins in mother or vitamin D in the child, no medication usage after delivery. Ask about hormonal birth control and keep in mind that vitamins or iron can cause colic. Consider asking about herbal or cultural practices as well.	Risks causing impaired milk supply, delayed lactogenesis II (i.e., milk coming in) +/or sucking dysfunction: • precipitous, instrumental, or cesarean delivery • stressful or medicated labor including epidurals and Mg sulfate • hormones, cold remedies, diuretics • diabetes, hypothyroidism, ovarian cyst • jaundice **PROMPTLY EVALUATE any new or worsening jaundice.**
Intake and Feeding: 1. Number of feedings in 24 hrs: _____ 2. Usual feeding interval is every _____ hours. 3. Are feedings scheduled? YES / NO Cluster feeding? YES / NO 4. Is your milk in and is the supply ample? YES / NO How long do you hear the infant swallowing during the feeding? _____ min. 5. Who ends the feeding? ☐ Baby ends ☐ Mom ends ☐ It varies 6. Pumps _____ oz _____ times per day Bottle-fed _____ times per day with _____ oz of ☐ EBM* ☐ Formula ☐ Juice ☐ Water. *EBM: Expressed breast milk	8-12 feedings in 24 hours; frequency may increase to 16 during growth spurts ■ There may be one 5-hour stretch between feedings per day and clusters of feedings at other times ■ Feeds on cue or when infant first starts to lick lips, suck fingers, look around, and/or fuss ■ Lactogenesis II occurs by day 5 ■ Once milk is in, swallowing is heard for at least 10 minutes of feed ■ Baby ends feeding ■ No supplements	Less than 8 or more than 16 feedings ■ More than one 4-5 hour sleeping period per day ■ Several recurring feeding intervals shorter than 45 min ■ Scheduled feedings ■ Failure of Lactogenesis II to occur by day 5 ■ Swallowing not heard or heard consistently less than 10 minutes ■ Use of supplements
Output: **Easy to miss voids with paper diapers 1. Birth weight _____lb_____oz Last weight: ☐ Unknown _____ lb _____ oz on _____ (date) Today's weight: ☐ Unknown _____ lb _____oz 2. # of Wet Cloth or Paper diapers** per 24 hours_____ Urine is: ☐ Clear ☐ Yellow ☐ Brick Red 3. How many **substantial** stools (not smears) in 24 hours?_____ 4. Stool Character: ☐ Meconium ☐ Transitional ☐ Yellow/Seedy ☐ Green ☐ Constipated ☐ Watery ☐ Bloody ☐ OTHER	Loss of less than 8% of birth weight, which is regained by day 14 ■ Weight gain rate then continues at an average of ¾ to 2 oz per day ■ Urine and Stool: One wet diaper per day of age **and** 2 or more stools per 24 hours prior to Lactogenesis II ■ Stools should be substantial; smears don't count ■ Stools progress from meconium to yellow and seedy as the milk comes in ■ Once lactogenesis II occurs, there should be 6-8 clear colored wet diapers and 3 or more stools per day	Weight loss at or greater than 8% ■ Less than birth weight at 2 weeks or gaining on average less than ¾ oz per day ■ Less than 5 wet diapers by day 5 +/or brick red–colored urine ■ Less than 3 stools per day, only smears of stool, stools not progressing or no stooling. **NOTE:** It is important to look at the overall picture of weight gain to determine adequate growth.
Comfort: 1. *Mother:* ☐ Comfortable Symptoms: ☐ Sad/anxious ☐ Tender/Sore ☐ Aching ☐ Sores ☐ Burning ☐ Redness *Location:* ☐ with Latch-on ☐ L / R Breast ☐ L / R Nipple *Frequency:* ☐ Constantly ☐ During feedings ☐ Between feedings ☐ _____ *Pain rating:* _____ scale of 1 (none)-10 (severe) 2. *Infant:* ☐ Comfortable ☐ Sleepy ☐ Crying ☐ Fussing ☐ Vomits 3. *Fever in:* ☐ Mother ☐ Child ☐ Both ☐ Neither	It is common to have 60 seconds or less of latch-on soreness for 1-2 weeks post partum ■ No postpartum depression ■ Breasts/Nipples feel comfortable during and after breastfeeding ■ Skin of breasts and nipples is intact ■ Infant comfortable during/after feedings ■ Infant is alert during feeds ■ Spitting up without discomfort ■ Both are afebrile	• Any pain or sadness that is hindering nursing, eliciting the desire to cease nursing, or interfering with caring for infant • Infant crying inconsolably, drawing legs up, having difficulty feeding, or vomiting

Other: _____

ASSESSMENT: NORMAL or ABNORMAL BREASTFEEDING DYAD SECONDARY TO: _____	☐ Burp/Stimulate Baby ☐ Improve Latch ☐ Use Breast Compression ☐ Use a _____ type pump ☐ after BF or ☐ in lieu of BF _____ times/day
PLAN: 1. EDUCATION: ☐ BF +/or Infant Normals ☐ Breast or Nipple Care ☐ Positioning & Latch-on ☐ Intake & Output ☐ Sleep Cycles ☐ Growth Spurts ☐ Co-sleeping ☐ Hindmilk: Foremilk ☐ Cluster Feeds ☐ Signs of Hunger & Satiation ☐ Jaundice ☐ Exclusive BF for 6 Months ☐ Pumping & Milk Storage ☐ Benefits of BF ☐ Other _____ **2. INSTRUCTIONS:** ☐ Continue Present Routine ☐ Increase Feeding Frequency +/or Feeding Duration ☐ Feed on One Breast per Feeding	for _____ min ☐ Supplement with EBM or Formula _____oz ☐ Feed Supplement via _____ ☐ Other _____ _____ _____ _____ **APPOINTMENT:** ☐ prn ☐ TODAY or within _____ DAYS/WEEK(S) **with** ☐ MD ☐ NP ☐ PA ☐ Lactation Specialist ☐ _____

Copyright Christine Betzold NP, IBCLC, MSN 3/03

Signature: _____

Periodic Blood Lead Screening Risk Questionnaire

Patient Name: _____

Medical Record #: _____

Home/Business Telephone: _____

Date of Birth: _____ Age: _____ Gender: Male Female

Please check the correct response to the following questions:	Date:			Date:			Date:			Date:			Date:		
	Yes	No	Not sure	Yes	No	Not sure	Yes	No	Not sure	Yes	No	Not sure	Yes	No	Not sure
Does your child live in or regularly visit a house built before 1950? This includes a home day-care center or home of a babysitter or relative.															
Does your child live in or regularly visit a house or child care facility built before 1978 with recent or ongoing renovations or remodeling (within the last 6 months)?															
Does your child have a brother, sister, housemate or playmate who has or did have lead poisoning?															

Blood Lead Level Screening Results*

Date	Age of Child	Results

<10 μg/dL - acceptable range

10-19 μg/dL - mild lead toxicity; confirm test within 1 month

20-44 μg/dL - moderate lead toxicity; confirm test within 1 week;

45-69 μg/dL - significant lead toxicity; confirm test within 48 hours

>70 μg/dL - critical lead toxicity; confirm test immediately

*From American Academy of Pediatrics Committee on Environmental Health: Screening for elevated blood levels, *Pediatrics* 101:1072-1078, 1998.

Tuberculosis Risk Questionnaire

Child's Name:_____   Today's Date: _____

Date of Birth: _____   Age: _____   Gender: Male   Female

Tuberculosis (TB) is a disease caused by TB germs and is usually transmitted by an adult person with active TB lung disease. It is spread to another person by coughing or sneezing TB germs into the air. These germs may be breathed in by the child.

A person can have TB germs in his or her body but not have active TB disease (this is called *latent TB infection* or *LTBI*).

Tuberculosis is preventable and treatable. TB skin testing (often called the *PPD* or *Mantoux test*) is used to determine whether your child has been infected with TB germs. The skin test is not a vaccination against TB.

Please answer the following questions to help us determine whether your child needs TB skin testing.

Please check the appropriate box in response to these questions:	Yes	No	Don't Know
Has your child lived with or spent time with anyone who possibly or definitely had TB?			
Were any household members, including your child, born in or have traveled to areas where TB is common (Africa, Asia except Japan, Latin America, Caribbean, Eastern Europe, Middle East)? If so, which countries?			
Does your child have regular (e.g., daily) contact with adults at high risk for TB (i.e., those who are HIV-infected, homeless, incarcerated, and/or illicit drug users?			
Has anyone living in your household had a positive skin test result for TB?			
Does your child have HIV infection?			

Has your child been tested for TB?   Yes _____ (if yes, specify date _____ / _____)
                                           No _____

Has your child ever had a positive TB skin test result?   Yes _____ (if yes, specify date _____ / _____)
                                           No _____

****

FOR HEALTH CARE PROVIDER USE ONLY
****

PPD/Mantoux test administered: Yes _____   No _____

Date administered _____/_____/_____   by _____   _____
Lot # _____   Printed name   Signature

Date read _____/_____/_____   by _____   _____
                                             Printed name   Signature

Result of PPD/Mantoux test: _____ mm   Follow-up Plan: _____

Adolescent Risk Monitoring Log

Patient's Name: _____

Medical Record #: _____

Home/Business Telephone: _____

Date of Birth: _____ Age: _____ Gender: Male Female

Complete for Each Adolescent Well Visit →	Date: Age:	Date: Age:	Date: Age:	Date: Age:
NUTRITION				
Underweight, anorexia, bulimia, overweight	Risks:	Risks:	Risks:	Risks:
Education (circle)	Support group; Ideal ht/wt; exercise; Balanced diet Referral:	Support group; Ideal ht/wt; exercise; Balanced diet Referral:	Support group; Ideal ht/wt; exercise; Balanced diet Referral:	Support group; Ideal ht/wt; exercise; Balanced diet Referral:
SCHOOL				
Academics, attendance, peers	Risks:	Risks:	Risks:	Risks:
SAFETY				
Seatbelts/helmets/drinking & driving/sports/firearms/weapons	Risks:	Risks:	Risks:	Risks:
Education (circle)	Use seatbelt/helmet; designated driver; protective sports gear; weapons risks	Use seatbelt/helmet; designated driver; protective sports gear; weapons risks	Use seatbelt/helmet; designated driver; protective sports gear; weapons risks	Use seatbelt/helmet; designated driver; protective sports gear; weapons risks
SUBSTANCE ABUSE				
Smoking	Yes Amt: No	Yes Amt: No	Yes Amt: No	Yes Amt: No
Alcohol	Yes Amt: No	Yes Amt: No	Yes Amt: No	Yes Amt: No
Street Drugs	Yes Type: No	Yes Type: No	Yes Type: No	Yes Type: No
Education (circle)	Health risks; ↓ use; avoid exposure; help resources:	Health risks; ↓ use; avoid exposure; help resources:	Health risks; ↓ use; avoid exposure; help resources:	Health risks; ↓ use; avoid exposure; help resources:
SEXUALITY				
Birth control method today				
Back-up method				
Emergency birth control info	Yes No	Yes No	Yes No	Yes No
Condom use info	Yes No	Yes No	Yes No	Yes No
Sexual orientation				
STD/HIV: Multiple partners, new partner, previous STD, drug use	Risks:	Risks:	Risks:	Risks:
Education (circle)	Safe sex; condoms; limit partners; abstain; HIV testing	Safe sex; condoms; limit partners; abstain; HIV testing	Safe sex; condoms; limit partners; abstain; HIV testing	Safe sex; condoms; limit partners; abstain; HIV testing
VIOLENCE/ABUSE				
Domestic violence; rape; incest; suicide attempt; gangs; fights; trouble with law				
Education (circle)	Support group; shelter; help resources:	Support group; shelter; help resources:	Support group; shelter; help resources:	Support group; shelter; help resources:
SPECIAL CIRCUMSTANCES				
Homeless; previous runaway; foster care; jail/detention	Risks:	Risks:	Risks:	Risks:

Adolescent Questionnaire

Patient Name: _____

Date: _____

Date of Birth: _____ *Gender:* Male   Female

Age: _____ Grade in School: _____

This form will not be shared with your parents unless we feel there is a life-threatening concern. We will discuss it with you before speaking to your parents.

Do you have any health concerns? _____

These questions will help us get to know you better. Choose the answer that best describes what you feel or do. Your answers will be seen only by your health care provider and his/her assistant.

Eating/Weight/Body

1. Do you eat fruits and vegetables every day? . . . . ☐ Yes   ☐ No
2. Do you drink milk and/or eat milk products every day? . . . . ☐ Yes   ☐ No
3. Do you spend a lot of time thinking about your weight? . . . . ☐ Yes   ☐ No
4. In the past year, have you tried to lose weight or control your weight by vomiting, taking diet pills or laxatives, or starving yourself? . . . . ☐ Yes   ☐ No
5. Do you ever eat in secret? . . . . ☐ Yes   ☐ No
6. Do you work, play, or exercise enough to make you sweat or breathe hard at least 3 times a week? . . . . ☐ Yes   ☐ No

School

7. Is doing well in school important to you? . . . . ☐ Yes   ☐ No
8. Are your grades this year worse than last year? . . . . ☐ Yes   ☐ No   ☐ Not Sure
9. Are you attending school regularly? . . . . ☐ Yes   ☐ No
10. Have you ever been suspended from school this year? . . . . ☐ Yes   ☐ No

Friends & Family

11. Do you know at least one person you really like and feel you can talk with? . . . . ☐ Yes   ☐ No
12. Do you think your parent(s) or guardian(s) usually listen to you and take your feelings seriously? . . . . ☐ Yes   ☐ No   ☐ Not Sure
13. In your opinion, is there a lot of tension or conflict in your home? . . . . ☐ Yes   ☐ No

Weapons/Violence/Safety

14. Is there a gun, rifle, or other firearm where you live? . . . . ☐ Yes   ☐ No   ☐ Not Sure
15. Have you ever carried a gun, knife, club, or other weapon to protect yourself? . . . . ☐ Yes   ☐ No
16. Have you ever been in a physical fight where you or someone else got hurt? . . . . ☐ Yes   ☐ No
17. Have you ever seen a violent act take place at home, school, or in your neighborhood? . . . . ☐ Yes   ☐ No
18. Are you worried about violence or your safety? . . . . ☐ Yes   ☐ No
19. Are you concerned about being physically hurt by a parent or anyone in your home? . ☐ Yes   ☐ No
20. Do you use a seatbelt when driving or riding as a passenger in a car, truck, or van? . . ☐ Yes   ☐ No
21. Do you use a helmet and/or protective gear when you ride a motorcycle, bicycle, skateboard, or rollerblade? . . . . ☐ Yes   ☐ No

Alcohol

22. Do you drink beer, wine, wine coolers, or other alcohol? . . . . ☐ Yes   ☐ No
23. Do any of your friends drink beer, wine, wine coolers, or other alcohol? . . . . ☐ Yes   ☐ No
24. Have you ever ridden in a car driven by someone who had been drinking or using drugs? . . . . ☐ Yes   ☐ No   ☐ Not Sure
25. Have you ever driven a car after drinking or using drugs? . . . . ☐ Yes   ☐ No
26. Does anyone in your family drink or use drugs so much that it worries you? . . . . ☐ Yes   ☐ No

PLEASE FILL OUT BOTH SIDES OF THIS QUESTIONNAIRE

Tobacco

27. Have you ever tried cigarettes or chewing tobacco? .... ☐ Yes ☐ No
28. Do any of your friends ever smoke cigarettes or chew tobacco? .... ☐ Yes ☐ No
29. Does anyone you live with smoke cigarettes/cigars or chew tobacco? .... ☐ Yes ☐ No

Drugs

30. Have you ever used marijuana, cocaine, acid, other drugs or inhalants
    (glue, lighter fluid, paint, etc)? .... ☐ Yes ☐ No ☐ Not Sure
31. Do any of your close friends ever use marijuana, other drugs, or inhalants? .... ☐ Yes ☐ No ☐ Not Sure
32. Some drugs can be bought at a store without a prescription. Do you ever use
    nonprescription drugs to get to sleep, stay awake, calm down, or get high? .... ☐ Yes ☐ No
33. Have you ever used steroids ("roids" or "juice")? .... ☐ Yes ☐ No

Relationships

34. Have you ever had sexual intercourse? .... ☐ Yes ☐ No ☐ Not Sure
35. If so, the last time you had sex, did you or your partner use a condom (rubber)? ..... ☐ Yes ☐ No
36. Have any of your friends ever had sexual intercourse? .... ☐ Yes ☐ No ☐ Not Sure
37. Have you ever felt pressured by anyone to have sex or had sex when you did
    not want to? .... ☐ Yes ☐ No ☐ Not Sure
38. Have you ever had a sexually transmitted disease (STD) such as herpes, gonorrhea,
    chlamydia, trichomonas, genital warts, or others? .... ☐ Yes ☐ No ☐ Not Sure
39. Have you ever been pregnant or ever gotten someone pregnant? .... ☐ Yes ☐ No
40. Do you have any questions or concerns about sex or relationships with
    the opposite sex? .... ☐ Yes ☐ No
41. Do you have any questions or concerns about sex or relationships with a
    partner of the same sex? .... ☐ Yes ☐ No
42. Would you like to receive information or supplies today to prevent pregnancy
    or sexually transmitted diseases? .... ☐ Yes ☐ No ☐ Not Sure
43. Do you know how to avoid getting HIV/AIDS and other sexually transmitted diseases? .. ☐ Yes ☐ No ☐ Not Sure
44. Have you ever been physically hurt in any way by a person you have gone out with? .. ☐ Yes ☐ No

Emotions

45. Have you done something fun during the past two weeks? .... ☐ Yes ☐ No
46. Do you have activities that you enjoy or are good at outside of school? .... ☐ Yes ☐ No
47. When you get angry, do you do violent things? .... ☐ Yes ☐ No
48. During the past few weeks, have you felt very sad or down as though you have
    nothing to look forward to? .... ☐ Yes ☐ No
49. Have you ever seriously thought about killing yourself, made a plan, or tried to
    kill yourself? .... ☐ Yes ☐ No
50. Have you ever been physically, emotionally, or sexually abused? .... ☐ Yes ☐ No ☐ Not Sure

Special Circumstances

51. In the past year, did you ever run away from home overnight? .... ☐ Yes ☐ No
52. In the past year, have you stayed overnight in a homeless shelter, jail,
    or detention center? .... ☐ Yes ☐ No
53. Have you ever lived in foster care, a group home, or an institution? .... ☐ Yes ☐ No

Self

54. What do you like about yourself? _____

55. What do you do best? _____

56. If you could, what would you change about your life and yourself? _____

Thank you for completing this form.

****

FOR CLINICIAN USE ONLY

Risk-taking behaviors discussed? .... ☐ Yes ☐ No

☐ High ☐ Low

****

Adapted with permission, Younger and Older Adolescent Questionnaires. In: Levenberg PB, Elster AB: Guidelines for adolescent preventive services (GAPS): *Clinical evaluation and management handbook.* Chicago, 1995, American Medical Association.

CHAPTER 4

Sports History and Physical Examination Forms

Chapter Contents

TOOL	DESCRIPTION	LOCATION OF TOOLS	FORMAT
Preparticipation Physical Evaluation Form	p. 106	p. 111-112	📄 ✐
Preparticipation Physical Evaluation Clearance Form	p. 108	p. 113	📄 ✐
Medical Conditions and Sports Participation	p. 108	p. 114-115	📄
Classification of Sports by Contact	p. 108	p. 116	📄
Physical Activity Readiness Questionnaires	p. 108		**i**
Patient-Runner History Form	p. 108	p. 117-118	📄 ✐
Sample Special Olympics Athlete Appication for Participation	p. 109	p. 119	📄

ICON KEY: 📄 Tool Printed   ✐ Tool on CD-ROM   ∞ Customizable Tool   **i** Information and Resources Provided for Further Acquisition

Introduction and Contents

Development and Content of the Preparticipation Physical Evaluation

The preparticipation physical evaluation (PPE) is a method of screening children and adolescents for conditions that may preclude their safe participation in sports. Originally, the evaluation was designed to screen primarily for congenital heart disease in an effort to protect affected children by restricting them from sports activity. The PPE has grown to encompass evaluation of personal and family medical history, as well as physical examination with attention to body systems most likely to be affected by athletic activities.

Objectives of the PPE, as determined by physician organizations, are summarized in Box 4-1. Screening of the school-age athlete helps ensure his or her safe participation in sports activities. Although the PPE only denies clearance to 1% to 2% of athletes, another 3% to 14% require further evaluation, follow-up, counseling, or treatment for disclosed conditions or injuries. The PPE offers many children their only chance for health evaluation and is viewed by many as an opportunity for anticipatory guidance and health promotion for adolescent patients. Education regarding sports-related injury prevention, conditioning programs, and appropriate equipment or training modifications that decrease the rate of injury can be accomplished at the time of the PPE. The athlete and parents can be encouraged to understand and accept the risks involved with participation. If professional advice against participation is not accepted by an athlete's family, the clinician has the option of asking parents, guardians, and the athlete to sign a written consent form indicating that they understand the potential dangers of participation.

As of 2000, the PPE was mandated in 49 of 50 states, with Rhode Island being the exception (Metzl, 2000). Despite the widespread use of the evaluation process, there is no standardized form for the PPE. There is wide variability in the required elements of the PPE at state and school district levels. Physician organizations that have issued position statements regarding the PPE process or have developed guidelines for the PPE assert that the responsibility for the PPE should fall to a physician with an MD or DO degree (Metzl, 2001). These views are reflected in the format of the signature area in the PPE

Goals of the Sports Preparticipation Physical Evaluation (PPE) in Young Athletes

- To prevent the occurrence of sudden cardiac death
- To prevent cardiovascular disease progression
- To identify clinically relevant and preexisting cardiovascular abnormalities
- To determine the eligibility of a young athlete to participate in a particular sport
- To detect conditions that may predispose an athlete to injury or illness
- To detect conditions that may be life-threatening or disabling
- To meet legal and insurance requirements
- To determine general health and screen for underlying illness
- To provide counseling on health-related issues
- To assess fitness level for specific sports
- To recognize preexisting injury patterns from previous sports season(s) and devise rehabilitation programs to prevent recurrence

Lyznicki et al, 2000; Maron et al, 1996; Metzl, 2001 (Part 1); Smith et al, 1997.

and medical clearance forms reprinted here. Despite these views, in nearly half of 50 states, advanced practice nurses or physician assistants can complete the PPE; 11 states allow chiropractors to clear young athletes for competition (American Academy of Family Physicians, et al, 1997). Clinical expertise, specialty training, and ability to manage care for the athlete-patient are clearly qualifying criteria for performing the PPE for the physician and other health care professionals alike. See Box 4-2 for a list of professional organizations involved in development or endorsement of recommendations for the PPE.

The Preparticipation Physical Evaluation Task Force recommends that the PPE be performed at least 6 weeks before preseason practice (American Academy of Family Physicians, et al, 1997). There is no consensus on how frequently the evaluation should be performed. Frequency is often determined by local standards, school district regulations, degree of risk of the sport, cost of the evaluation, and availability of qualified health professionals. After an

Professional Organizations Developing or Endorsing Student Athlete Screening Recommendations

- American Academy of Family Physicians
- American Academy of Pediatrics
- American College of Cardiology
- American College of Sports Medicine
- American Heart Association
- American Medical Society for Sports Medicine
- American Orthopedic Society for Sports Medicine
- American Osteopathic Academy of Sports Medicine

initial PPE has been completed, a limited annual reevaluation can meet sports clearance objectives. Findings of problems during interim evaluations should trigger an assessment of the affected area or area(s).

Essential components of the PPE are listed in Box 4-3. If the reader is unfamiliar with the rationale for any evaluation component or the implications of positive findings, he or she is encouraged to consult one of the many resources in the reference list and collaborate with an experienced clinician before initiating preparticipation evaluations.

The American Academy of Pediatrics (AAP) Committee on Sports Medicine and Fitness stresses that "the physician's clinical judgment is essential for applying the participation recommendations to individual patients. This judgment involves the available published information on the risks of participation, the advice of knowledgeable experts, the current health status of the athlete, the level of competition, the position played, the sport in which the athlete participates, the maturity of the competitor, the availability of effective protective equipment that is acceptable to the athlete, the availability and efficacy of treatment, whether treatment (e.g., rehabilitation of an injury) has been completed, whether the sport can be modified to allow safer participation, and the ability of the athlete and parents to understand and accept risks involved in participation. Potential dangers of associated training activities should also be considered" (American Academy of Pediatrics, 2001).

Positive findings in certain areas of the PPE will affect the level of clearance for different sports activities. Findings in the medical history that may require further assessment or result in qualified participation or denial of clearance are listed in Box 4-4.

Preparticipation Physical Evaluation Form

This two-page form is reprinted from the *Preparticipation Physical Evaluation Second Edition* monograph authored by the Preparticipation Physical Evaluation Task Force, chaired by David M. Smith, MD, FAAFP. This monograph is produced in cooperation with the AAP, American Academy of Family Physicians, American Medical Society for Sports Medicine, American Orthopedic Society for Sports Medicine, and American Osteopathic Society for Sports Medicine. The *Third Edition* monograph was scheduled for release concurrent with printing for our text, thus updated forms were unable to be featured in this chapter.

Included on this form are most of the essential components of the PPE, as outlined previously. Absent from this form are three items recommended by the American Heart Association: family history of heart disease, a specific item for recognition of a heart murmur in the physical examination, and a specific item for recognition of the physical stigmata of Marfan syndrome (Maron, 1996, 1999). Readers are advised to consult the *Third Edition* monograph for updated forms and information.

Box 4-3 Preparticipation Physical Evaluation: Essential Components

GENERAL HISTORY

- Past medical illnesses or injuries since last medical exam
- Chronic illnesses and conditions
- Past hospitalizations and surgeries
- Childhood illnesses and immunization status
- Past medical restriction in sports participation

CARDIOVASCULAR HISTORY

- Heart murmur
- Systemic hypertension
- Excessive fatigability
- Syncope, dizziness, excessive/progressive shortness of breath or chest pain/discomfort, particularly with exertion
- Tachycardia
- Arrhythmia
- Hypercholesterolemia

MEDICATIONS

- Current and recently prescribed and nonprescription medications
- Vitamin and supplement use to alter weight or improve performance
- Protective or corrective equipment or devices: braces, orthotics, corrective lenses, protective eyewear, dental retainer, hearing aid

FAMILY HISTORY

- Family occurrence of premature death (sudden or otherwise)
- Family occurrence of heart disease in surviving relatives
- Family occurrence of cardiovascular conditions such as hypertrophic cardiomyopathy, long QT syndrome, Marfan syndrome, significant dysrhythmias
- Significant disability from cardiovascular disease in close relatives younger than 50 years

SOCIAL HISTORY

- Caffeine and other stimulant use
- Tobacco and alcohol use
- Recreational drug use
- Steroid and other sports performance enhancer use
- Diet during season and off season
- Sleep and exercise habits
- Stress and coping patterns

ALLERGIES

- Medications
- Environmental allergens
- Stinging insects
- Foods
- Rash or hives after exercise

REVIEW OF SYSTEMS

- General: Recent viral infections, other infections and blood-borne pathogens, history of heat illness, weight loss or gain
- Dermatologic: Infectious conditions
- HEENT: Headache, vision impairment, hearing change, chronic allergies, dental appliance
- Pulmonary: Exercise-induced asthma
- Cardiovascular (as noted above)
- Gastrointestinal: Infectious conditions
- Genitourinary: Kidney disease, absence of gonad, menstrual history, pregnancy
- Hematologic: SCA, bleeding disorder
- Orthopedic: Sprains, strains, fractures, congenital condition
- Neurologic: Concussion, loss of consciousness, seizure, extremity paresthesias, stinger/burner/pinched nerve
- Psychiatric: Eating disorder, anxiety, irritability

PHYSICAL EXAMINATION

Objective findings on physical examination with particular attention to the following systems:

- General appearance, vital signs with seated brachial artery blood pressure, height, weight, visual acuity
- Eyes, ears, nose, throat
- Pulmonary
- Cardiovascular
  - Precordial auscultation in supine and standing positions
  - Femoral and radial artery pulses
  - Exam for physical stigmata associated with Marfan syndrome
- Abdomen: Presence of organomegaly
- Genitalia (males only)
- Musculoskeletal
- Skin

CLEARANCE

- Cleared for sports without restrictions
- Clearance only after completion of further evaluation or rehabilitation
- No clearance with reason stated

PLAN

- Treatment plan for active disease, infection, or injury
- Diagnostic tests or studies to be performed on the basis of examination findings; routine screening laboratory tests and special procedures are not indicated
- Referral for specialist evaluation
- Referral or plan for rehabilitation

Smith et al, 1997; Lyznicki et al, 2000; Maron et al, 1996 ; Kurowski and Chandran, 2000.
HEENT, Head, ears, eyes, nose, and throat; *SCA,* sickle cell anemia.

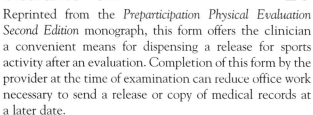

Box **4-4**   Specific Significant Findings in Medical History

PERSONAL MEDICAL HISTORY
- Subjective feeling of faintness, weakness, or frank syncope during exercise
- Wheezing during sports
- Concussion
- Recent mononucleosis
- Unilateral organ
- Current medications
- Menstrual history
- Seizure disorder
- Past cardiac abnormality
- Past history of injury
- Ergogenic aids

FAMILY HISTORY
- Cardiac-related death in a first-degree relative younger than 50 years of age
- Family occurrence of heart disease in surviving relatives
- Family occurrence of cardiovascular conditions such as hypertrophic cardiomyopathy, long QT syndrome, Marfan syndrome, significant dysrhythmias
- Family history of chronic disease

Metzl, 2001 (Part 1); Maron et al, 1996; Lyznicki, et al, 2000.

Preparticipation Physical Evaluation Clearance Form

Reprinted from the *Preparticipation Physical Evaluation Second Edition* monograph, this form offers the clinician a convenient means for dispensing a release for sports activity after an evaluation. Completion of this form by the provider at the time of examination can reduce office work necessary to send a release or copy of medical records at a later date.

Medical Conditions and Sports Participation

This table is included in this chapter to guide the clinician in authorizing clearance for sports participation based on the examination findings. These participation guidelines are the current consensus of the AAP Committee on Sports Medicine and Fitness. The position statement on medical conditions that affect sports participation in children and adolescents appeared in the May 2001 issue of *Pediatrics*, available online at http://aappolicy.aappublications.org/cgi/content/full/pediatrics;107/5/1205. The reader is encouraged to consult this publication for the current information and recommendations which include the classification of sports by contact and strenuousness, and legal implications of medical clearance. Additional information on specific risks and injuries affecting sports participation may be found in the References and Suggested Readings section.

Classification of Sports by Contact

This table, also from the policy statement by the AAP Committee on Sports Medicine and Fitness, categorizes sports by their probability for "collision" (very forceful contact) or "contact" (less forceful contact) (American Academy of Pediatrics, 2001). By categorizing sports in this manner, relative risk for acute traumatic injuries resulting from blows to the body may be estimated. Collision and contact sports are grouped together because there is no clear dividing line between them. "Limited-contact" sports involve infrequent or inadvertent contact with other athletes or inanimate objects. "Noncontact" sports do not involve risk of acute contact injury.

Not all injuries can be prevented by avoidance of contact or collision sports. The policy authors point out that some limited-contact sports, such as downhill skiing and gymnastics, and noncontact sports, such as power lifting, can result in serious traumatic or overuse injuries. Although the categorization of sports by contact is insufficient in reflecting all the relative risks of injury, it may serve as a guide when recommending nonparticipation to athletes with qualified medical conditions.

Physical Activity Readiness Questionnaires

The Physical Activity Readiness (PAR) Questionnaires (Par-Q and You, PARmed-X, and PARmedX for Pregnancy) are available online through the Canadian Society for Exercise Physiology (CSEP). These three useful tools, originally developed by the British Columbia Ministry of Health, are used extensively in Canada. The PAR-Q and You was revised in 1992 (Thomas, Reading, Shepard, 1992), and all three forms were revised again in 2002, by an Expert Advisory Committee of the Canadian Society for Exercise Physiology. The tools screen for health indicators that may compromise a person's ability to safely participate in physical activity.

The PAR-Q and You is a two-page form that persons aged 15-69 can complete to see if they should consult with their healthcare provider before becoming more physically active. The PARmed-X is four-page physical activity-specific checklist to be used by a clinician with patients who have had positive responses to the PAR-Q and You. The PARmed X for Pregnancy, reflecting a collaboration of CSEP and Canadian obstetricians, is a four-page guideline for health screening prior to participation in a prenatal fitness class or other exercise.

There are no restrictions or fees for use of the forms. The PDF formatted forms may be downloaded from: http://www.csep.ca/forms.asp.

Patient-Runner History Form

This questionnaire was developed from a published article that provided a list of questions, with rationale, for the runner-patient (Kirby, Valmassy, 1983). The questions are detailed and focus on areas of training history, racing history, running shoe history, pre-run and post-run activities, and injury-related history. Answers to these questions provide the clinician with specific information to individualize treatment and implement modifications to running-related habits to reduce further injuries. If unfamiliar with the implications of each of the runner-patient questions, the reader is encouraged to consult this original article or other sports medicine publications for further information.

Special Olympics Guidelines and Resources

Special Olympics is an international organization dedicated to empowering individuals with intellectual disabilities to become physically fit, productive, and respected members of society through sports training and competition. Special Olympics offers children and adults with intellectual disabilities year-round training and competition in 26 Olympic-type summer and winter sports.

The international program serves more than 1 million persons who have intellectual or developmental disabilities in more than 150 countries; that number is expected to double by the year 2005. There is no cost for participation in the program.

Eligibility for participation in a Special Olympics competition, as stated on the Special Olympics website, includes:

- Participants must be at least eight years old, and
- Participants must be identified by an agency or professional as having intellectual disabilities as determined by their localities; or
- The participant has a cognitive delay, as determined by standardized measures such as intelligent quotient or IQ testing or other measures that are generally accepted within the professional community in that Accredited Program's nation as being a reliable measurement of the existence of a cognitive delay; or
- The participant has a closely related developmental disability. A "closely related developmental disability" means having functional limitations in both general learning (such as IQ) and in adaptive skills (such as in recreation, work, independent living, self-direction, or self-care).

Special Olympics Official General Rules (2004) have been revised and restated in order to provide current and consolidated guidance to all accredited Special Olympics programs. Adopted by the Special Olympics International (SOI) board of directors on July 22, 1997, amendments by the SOI board of directors were approved in 1999, 2001, and 2003. Of note, the General Rules uses the phrase "persons with mental retardation" when describing the individuals eligible for participation in Special Olympics. Alternate recommended terminology for this phrase that may be recognized by local accredited programs includes "mental handicap," "mental disability," and "intellectual disability," as provided in Section 10.01 of the General Rules. Special Olympics sub-programs, or accredited programs, operate as a division or branch of the accrediting National Program [section 4.01]. In the United States, accredited sub-programs are state based. Requirements for registration and medical certification of participants

follow national guidelines; however, each state accredited program may create their own forms for athlete registration for use within their own jurisdiction [section 6.02].

Registration forms include the following [section 6.02]:

- A completed Athlete Data Form, which contains athlete identifying information
- A completed Athlete Medical Form detailing the athlete's medical background that pertains to participation in Special Olympics, which includes a licensed medical professional's report and certification
- A completed Athlete Release Form, signed by the athlete or the parent/guardian of a minor athlete, concerning medical matters and publicity permissions

Additional forms may include the following:

- A Religious Objections Release Form, for athletes or parents/guardians objecting on religious grounds to certain emergency medical treatment as described in the Athlete Release Form
- A Special Release for Athletes with Atlanto-Axial Instability Form, concerning the potential risks of atlanto-axial instability in athletes with Down syndrome.

Each accredited program is responsible for developing procedures to confirm that all registered athletes have obtained the required medical examination. Because each U.S. accredited program does "personalize" the registration and medical certification forms, SOI has recommended that people seeking this information should contact the Special Olympics program within their state (personal communication, Jill Kauffman, Special Olympics Risk Manager, Washington, D.C., 10/11/02). State contact information can be accessed online at http://www.specialolympics.org/, and clicking on "Find a Location." An example of a state medical certification form is included in this chapter for informational purposes only.

SOI requires that all medical certification examinations be performed by a licensed physician or trained medical professional "who is not a physician, but who is authorized or licensed under the laws of the accredited programs' jurisdiction to perform medical examinations and make medical diagnoses (collectively a 'licensed medical professional')" [section 6.02 (f)(1)].

Physical examination requirements for Special Olympics participants include the following (General Rules section 6.02 [f-g]):

- First time registrants for participation in Special Olympics must be examined before registration by a licensed medical professional, who must complete the "medical certification" section of the Athlete Registration Form.
- Subsequent medical examinations may be required for athletes at the discretion of the directors of the accredited program, if participation continues for more than one year. If examination is required, the accredited program directors will have a reasonable

Box 4-5 Excluded Activities for Special Olympics Participants with Atlanto-Axial Instability

Swimming: Butterfly stroke
Swimming: Diving starts
Diving
Pentathlon
High jump
Squat lifts
Equestrian sports
Artistic gymnastics
Football (soccer)
Alpine skiing
Warm-up exercise placing undue stress on the head and neck

Special Olympics Official General Rules, 2004.

basis for believing that there has been a significant change in the athlete's health since the initial medical examination.

- Participation by individuals with Down syndrome excludes activities listed in Box 4-5, unless the participant meets the following requirements:
  1. Certification, based on examination by a physician, that the participant does not have atlanto-axial instability, and
  2. Radiographs of full extension and flexion of the neck
- Individuals with Down syndrome who have atlanto-axial instability will be excluded from participation in activities listed in Box 4-5 unless:
  1. The athlete or parent/guardian of a minor athlete confirm in writing the decision to proceed despite the risks created by atlanto-axial instability, and
  2. Two licensed medical professionals certify that they have explained the risks to the athlete and his or her guardian, and that the athlete's condition does not, in their judgment, preclude the athlete from participation in Special Olympics.

Further information regarding Special Olympics can be obtained on the website: http://www.specialolympics.org/.

References and Suggested Readings

American Academy of Family Physicians, et al: *Preparticipation physical evaluation task force, DM Smith, chairman, et al*: ed 2. American Academy of Pediatrics, American Academy of Family Physicians, American Academy of Pediatrics, American Medical Society for Sports Medicine, American Orthopedic Society for Sports Medicine, American Osteopathic Society for Sports Medicine. Minneapolis, Minn, 1997, McGraw Hill.

American Academy of Pediatrics: Committee on Sports Medicine and Fitness: medical conditions affecting sports participation, *Pediatrics* 107:1205-1209, 2001. Available at: http://aappolicy.aappublications.org/cgi/content/full/pediatrics;107/5/1205.

Carek PJ: Physical examination for the Special Olympics, *Am Fam Physician* 65:1516, 1518, 2002.

Dec KL, Sparrow KJ, McKeag DB: The physically-challenged athlete: medical issues and assessment, *Sports Med* 29:245-258, 2000.

Kirby KA, Valmassy RL: The runner-patient history: what to ask and why, *J Am Podiatry Assoc* 73:39-43, 1983.

Kurowski K, Chandran S: The preparticipation athletic evaluation, *Am Fam Physician* 61:2683-2690, 2696-2698, 2000.

Lai AM, Stanish WD, Stanish HI: The young athlete with physical challenges, *Clin Sports Med* 9:793-819, 2000.

Luckstead EF Sr: Cardiac risk factors and participation guidelines for youth sports, *Pediatr Clin North Am* 49:681-707, 2002.

Lyznicki JM, Nielsen NH, Schneider JF: Cardiovascular screening of student athletes, *Am Fam Physician* 62:765-784, 2000.

Magee DJ: Preparticipation examination. In Magee DJ, editor: *Orthopedic physical assessment*, ed. 4, Philadelphia, 2002, WB Saunders.

Maron BJ, et al: Cardiovascular preparticipation screening of competitive athletes. A statement for health professionals from the Sudden Death Committee (clinical cardiology) and Congenital Cardiac Defects Committee (cardiovascular disease in the young), American Heart Association, *Circulation* 94:850-856, 1996 [Addendum published in *Circulation* 1998;97:2294].

Maron BJ: Comprehensive cardiac PPE, *Phys Sportsmed* 27:118, 1999 (reply to letter).

Martin TJ, Martin JS: Special issues and concerns for the high school- and college-aged athletes, *Pediatr Clin North Am* 49:533-552, 2002.

Metzl JD: The adolescent preparticipation physical examination. Is it helpful? *Clin Sports Med* 19:577-592, 2000.

Metzl JD: Preparticipation examination of the adolescent athlete: part 1, *Pediatr Rev* 22:199-204, 2001.

Metzl JD: Preparticipation examination of the adolescent athlete: part 2, *Pediatr Rev* 22:227-239, 2001.

Patel DR, Greydanus DE: The pediatric athlete with disabilities, *Pediatr Clin North Am* 49:803-827, 2002.

Reider B: *The orthopedic physical examination*, Philadelphia, 1999, WB Saunders.

Reider B: *Sports medicine: The school-age athlete*, ed 2, Philadelphia, 1996, WB Saunders.

Rockwell PG, Alvarez DJ: Adolescent sports injuries and the preparticipation physical evaluation, *Clin Fam Pract* 2:837-862, 2000.

Special Olympics Official General Rules: Available at: http://www.specialolympics.org/special+olympics+public+website/english/aboutus/general+rules.htm (accessed March 4, 2004).

Stanitski CL: Pediatric and adolescent sports injuries, *Clin Sports Med* 16:613-633, 1997.

Stanitski CL, DeLee JC, Drez D Jr: *Pediatric and adolescent sports medicine, vol 3*, Philadelphia, 1994, WB Saunders.

Sullivan JA, Anderson SJ, editors. *Care of the young athlete*, Elk Grove Village, IL, 2000, American Academy of Pediatrics.

Thomas S, Reading J, Shepard RJ: Revision of the Physical Activity Readiness Questionnaire (PAR-Q), *Can J Spt Sci* 17:338-345, 1992.

Preparticipation Physical Evaluation

HISTORY

DATE OF EXAM _____

Name _____ Sex _____ Age _____ Date of birth _____

Grade ____ School _____ Sport(s) _____

Address _____ Phone _____

Personal physician _____

In case of emergency, contact

Name _____ Relationship _____ Phone (H) _____ (W) _____

**Explain "Yes" answers below.
Circle questions you don't know the answers to.**

Yes No

1. Have you had a medical illness or injury since your last check up or sports physical?
   Do you have an ongoing or chronic illness?
2. Have you ever been hospitalized overnight?
   Have you ever had surgery?
3. Are you currently taking any prescription or nonprescription (over-the-counter) medications or pills or using an inhaler?
   Have you ever taken any supplements or vitamins to help you gain or lose weight or improve your performance?
4. Do you have any allergies (for example, to pollen, medicine, food, or stinging insects)?
   Have you ever had a rash or hives develop during or after exercise?
5. Have you ever passed out during or after exercise?
   Have you ever been dizzy during or after exercise?
   Have you ever had chest pain during or after exercise?
   Do you get tired more quickly than your friends do during exercise?
   Have you ever had racing of your heart or skipped heartbeats?
   Have you had high blood pressure or high cholesterol?
   Have you ever been told you have a heart murmur?
   Has any family member or relative died of heart problems or of sudden death before age 50?
   Have you had a severe viral infection (for example, myocarditis or mononucleosis) within the last month?
   Has a physician ever denied or restricted your participation in sports for any heart problems?
6. Do you have any current skin problems (for example, itching, rashes, acne, warts, fungus, or blisters)?
7. Have you ever had a head injury or concussion?
   Have you ever been knocked out, become unconscious, or lost your memory?
   Have you ever had a seizure?
   Do you have frequent or severe headaches?
   Have you ever had numbness or tingling in your arms, hands, legs, or feet?
   Have you ever had a stinger, burner, or pinched nerve?
8. Have you ever become ill from exercising in the heat?
9. Do you cough, wheeze, or have trouble breathing during or after activity?
   Do you have asthma?
   Do you have seasonal allergies that require medical treatment?

Yes No

10. Do you use any special protective or corrective equipment or devices that aren't usually used for your sport or position (for example, knee brace, special neck roll, foot orthotics, retainer on your teeth, hearing aid)?
11. Have you had any problems with your eyes or vision?
    Do you wear glasses, contacts, or protective eyewear?
12. Have you ever had a sprain, strain, or swelling after injury?
    Have you broken or fractured any bones or dislocated any joints?
    Have you had any other problems with pain or swelling in muscles, tendons, bones, or joints?
    If yes, check appropriate box and explain below.
    ☐ Head ☐ Elbow ☐ Hip
    ☐ Neck ☐ Forearm ☐ Thigh
    ☐ Back ☐ Wrist ☐ Knee
    ☐ Chest ☐ Hand ☐ Shin/calf
    ☐ Shoulder ☐ Finger ☐ Ankle
    ☐ Upper arm ☐ Foot
13. Do you want to weigh more or less than you do now?
    Do you lose weight regularly to meet weight requirements for your sport?
14. Do you feel stressed out?
15. Record the dates of your most recent immunizations (shots) for:
    Tetanus _____ Measles _____
    Hepatitis B _____ Chickenpox _____

FEMALES ONLY

16. When was your first menstrual period? _____
    When was your most recent menstrual period? _____
    How much time do you usually have from the start of one period to the start of another? _____
    How many periods have you had in the last year? _____
    What was the longest time between periods in the last year? _____

Explain "Yes" answers here: _____
_____
_____
_____
_____
_____
_____
_____

I hereby state that, to the best of my knowledge, my answers to the above questions are complete and correct.

Signature of athlete _____ Signature of parent/guardian _____ Date _____

© 1997 *American Academy of Family Physicians, American Academy of Pediatrics, American Medical Society for Sports Medicine, American Orthopaedic Society for Sports Medicine, and American Osteopathic Academy of Sports Medicine.*

Preparticipation Physical Evaluation

Name _____ **Date of birth** _____

Height _____ **Weight** _____ **% Body fat (optional)** _____ **Pulse** _____ **BP** ___/____ (___/___ , ___/___)

Vision   R 20/ _____ **L 20/** _____   **Corrected: Y N**   **Pupils: Equal** _____ **Unequal** _____

	NORMAL	ABNORMAL FINDINGS	INITIALS*
MEDICAL			
Appearance			
Eyes/Ears/Nose/Throat			
Lymph Nodes			
Heart			
Pulses			
Lungs			
Abdomen			
Genitalia (males only)			
Skin			
MUSCULOSKELETAL			
Neck			
Back			
Shoulder/arm			
Elbow/forearm			
Wrist/hand			
Hip/thigh			
Knee			
Leg/ankle			
Foot			

* Station-based examination only

❑ **Cleared**

❑ **Cleared after completing evaluation/rehabilitation for:** _____

_____

_____

_____

❑ **Not cleared for:** _____ **Reason:** _____

Recommendations: _____

_____

_____

_____

Name of physician (print/type) _____ **Date** _____

Address _____ **Phone** _____

Signature of physician _____ **, MD or DO**

Preparticipation Physical Evaluation

Clearance Form

❏ **Cleared**

❏ **Cleared after completing evaluation/rehabilitation for:** _____

_____

_____

_____

❏ **Not cleared for:** _____ **Reason:** _____

Recommendations: _____

_____

_____

_____

Name of physician (print/type) _____ **Date** _____

Address _____ **Phone**_____

Signature of physician _____ **, MD or DO**

© 1997 *American Academy of Family Physicians, American Academy of Pediatrics, American Medical Society for Sports Medicine, American Orthopaedic Society for Sports Medicine, and American Osteopathic Academy of Sports Medicine.*

Preparticipation Physical Evaluation

Clearance Form

❏ **Cleared**

❏ **Cleared after completing evaluation/rehabilitation for:** _____

_____

_____

_____

❏ **Not cleared for:** _____ **Reason:** _____

Recommendations: _____

_____

_____

_____

Name of physician (print/type) _____ **Date** _____

Address _____ **Phone**_____

Signature of physician _____ **, MD or DO**

© 1997 *American Academy of Family Physicians, American Academy of Pediatrics, American Medical Society for Sports Medicine, American Orthopaedic Society for Sports Medicine, and American Osteopathic Academy of Sports Medicine.*

Medical Conditions and Sports Participation*

CONDITION	MAY PARTICIPATE?
Atlantoaxial instability (instability of the joint between cervical vertebrae 1 and 2)	Qualified yes
Explanation: Athlete needs evaluation to assess risk of spinal cord injury during sports participation.	
Bleeding disorder	Qualified yes
Explanation: Athlete needs evaluation.	
Cardiovascular disease	
Carditis (inflammation of the heart)	No
Explanation: Carditis may result in sudden death with exertion.	
Hypertension (high blood pressure)	Qualified yes
Explanation: Those with significant essential (unexplained) hypertension should avoid weight and power lifting, body building, and strength training. Those with secondary hypertension (hypertension caused by a previously identified disease) or severe essential hypertension need evaluation. The National High Blood Pressure Education Working group defined significant and severe hypertension.	
Congenital heart disease (structural heart defects present at birth)	Qualified yes
Explanation: Those with mild forms may participate fully; those with moderate or severe forms or who have undergone surgery need evaluation. The 26th Bethesda Conference defined mild, moderate, and severe disease for common cardiac lesions.	
Dysrhythmia (irregular heart rhythm)	Qualified yes
Explanation: Those with symptoms (chest pain, syncope, dizziness, shortness of breath, or other symptoms of possible dysrhythmia) or evidence of mitral regurgitation (leaking) on physical examination need evaluation. All others may participate fully.	
Heart murmur	Qualified yes
Explanation: If the murmur is innocent (does not indicate heart disease), fully participation is permitted. Otherwise, the athlete needs evaluation (see congenital heart disease and mitral valve prolapse).	
Cerebral palsy	Qualified yes
Explanation: Athlete needs evaluation.	
Diabetes mellitus	Yes
Explanation: All sports can be played with proper attention to diet, blood glucose concentration, hydration, and insulin therapy. Blood glucose concentration should be monitored every 30 minutes during continuous exercise and 15 minutes after completion of exercise.	
Diarrhea	Qualified no
Explanation: Unless disease is mild, no participation is permitted, because diarrhea may increase the risk of dehydration and heat illness. See fever.	
Eating disorders	Qualified yes
Anorexia nervosa	
Bulimia nervosa	
Explanation: Patients with these disorders need medical any psychiatric assessment before participation.	
Eyes	Qualified yes
Functionally one-eyed athlete	
Loss of an eye	
Detached retina	
Previous eye surgery or serious eye injury	
Explanation: A functionally one-eyed athlete has a best-corrected visual acuity of less than 20/40 in the eye with worse acuity. These athletes would suffer significant disability if the better eye were seriously injured, as would those with loss of an eye. Some athletes who previously have undergone eye surgery or had a serious eye injury may have an increased risk of injury because of weakened eye tissue. Availability of eye guards approved by the American Society for Testing and Materials and other protective equipment may allow participation in most sports, but this must be judged on an individual basis.	
Fever	No
Explanation: Fever can increase cardiopulmonary effort, reduce maximum exercise capacity, make heat illness more likely, and increase orthostatic hypertension during exercise. Fever may rarely accompany myocarditis or other infections that may make exercise dangerous.	
Heat illness, history of	Qualified yes
Explanation: Because of the increased likelihood of recurrence, the athlete needs individual assessment to determine the presence of predisposing conditions and to arrange a prevention strategy.	
Hepatitis	Yes
Explanation: Because of the apparent minimal risk to others, all sports may be played that the athlete's state of health allows. In all athletes, skin lesions should be covered properly, and athletic personnel should use universal precautions when handling blood or body fluids with visible blood.	

*This table is designed for use by medical and nonmedical personnel. "Needs evaluation" means that a physician with appropriate knowledge and experience should assess the safety of a given sport for an athlete with the listed medical condition. Unless otherwise noted, this is because of variability of the severity of the disease, the risk of injury for the specific sports listed in Table 1, or both.

Medical Conditions and Sports Participation—cont'd

CONDITION	MAY PARTICIPATE?
Human immunodeficiency virus infection	Yes
Explanation: Because of the apparent minimal risk to others, all sports may be played that the athlete's state of health allows. In all athletes, skin lesions should be covered properly, and athletic personnel should use universal precautions when handling blood or body fluids with visible blood.	
Kidney, absence of one	Qualified yes
Explanation: Athlete needs individual assessment for contact, collision, and limited-contact sports.	
Liver, enlarged	Qualified yes
Explanation: If the liver is acutely enlarged, participation should be avoided because of risk of rupture. If the liver is chronically enlarged, individual assessment is needed before collision, contact, or limited-contact sports are played.	
Malignant neoplasm	Qualified yes
Explanation: Athlete needs individual assessment.	
Musculoskeletal disorders	Qualified yes
Explanation: Athlete needs individual assessment.	
Neurologic disorders	
History of serious head or spine trauma, severe or repeated concussions, or craniotomy.	Qualified yes
Explanation: Athlete needs individual assessment for collision, contact, or limited-contact sports and also for noncontact sports if deficits in judgment or cognition are present. Research supports a conservative approach to management of concussion.	
Seizure disorder, well-controlled	Yes
Explanation: Risk of seizure during participation is minimal.	
Seizure disorder, poorly controlled	Qualified yes
Explanation: Athlete needs individual assessment for collision, contact, or limited-contact sports. The following noncontact sports should be avoided: archery, riflery, swimming, weight or power lifting, strength training, or sports involving heights. In these sports, occurrence of a seizure may pose a risk to self or others.	
Obesity	Qualified yes
Explanation: Because of the risk of heat illness, obese persons need careful acclimatization and hydration.	
Organ transplant recipient	Qualified yes
Explanation: Athlete needs individual assessment.	
Ovary, absence of one	Yes
Explanation: Risk of severe injury to the remaining ovary is minimal.	
Respiratory conditions	
Pulmonary compromise, including cystic fibrosis	Qualified yes
Explanation: Athlete needs individual assessment, but generally, all sports may be played if oxygenation remains satisfactory during a graded exercise test. Patients with cystic fibrosis need acclimatization and good hydration to reduce the risk of heat illness.	
Asthma	Yes
Explanation: With proper medication and education, only athletes with the most severe asthma will need to modify their participation.	
Acute upper respiratory infection	Qualified yes
Explanation: Upper respiratory obstruction may affect pulmonary function. Athlete needs individual assessment for all but mild disease. See fever.	
Sickle cell disease	Qualified yes
Explanation: Athlete needs individual assessment. In general, if status of the illness permits, all but high exertion, collision, and contact sports may be played. Overheating, dehydration, and chilling must be avoided.	
Sickle cell trait	Yes
Explanation: It is unlikely that persons with sickle cell trait have an increased risk of sudden death or other medical problems during athletic participation, except under the most extreme conditions of heat, humidity, and possibly increased altitude. These persons, like all athletes, should be carefully conditioned, acclimatized, and hydrated to reduce any possible risk.	
Skin disorders (boils, herpes simplex, impetigo, scabies, molluscum contagiosum)	Qualified yes
Explanation: While the patient is contagious, participation in gymnastics with mats; martial arts; wrestling; or other collision, contact, or limited-contact sports is not allowed.	
Spleen, enlarged	Qualified yes
Explanation: A patient with an acutely enlarged spleen should avoid all sports because of risk of rupture. A patient with a chronically enlarged spleen needs individual assessment before playing collision, contact, or limited-contact sports.	
Testicle, undescended or absence of one	Yes
Explanation: Certain sports may require a protective cup.	

From American Academy of Pediatrics, Committee on Sports Medicine and Fitness: Medical conditions affecting sports participation, *Pediatrics* 107:1205-1209, 2001, with permission.

Classification of Sports by Contact

Contact or Collision	Limited Contact	Noncontact
Basketball	Baseball	Archery
Boxing[1]	Bicycling	Badminton
Diving	Cheerleading	Body building
Field hockey	Canoeing or kayaking (white water)	Bowling
Football	Fencing	Canoeing or kayaking (flat water)
Tackle	Field events	Crew or rowing
Ice hockey[2]	High jump	Curling
Lacrosse	Pole vault	Dancing[4]
Martial arts	Floor hockey	Ballet
Rodeo	Football	Modern
Rugby	Flag	Jazz
Ski jumping	Gymnastics	Field events
Soccer	Handball	Discus
Team handball	Horseback riding	Javelin
Water polo	Racquetball	Shot put
Wrestling	Skating	Golf
	Ice	Orienteering[5]
	In-line	Power lifting
	Roller	Race walking
	Skiing	Riflery
	Cross-country	Rope jumping
	Downhill	Running
	Water	Sailing
	Skateboarding	Scuba diving
	Snowboarding[3]	Swimming
	Softball	Table tennis
	Squash	Tennis
	Ultimate frisbee	Track
	Volleyball	Weight lifting
	Windsurfing or surfing	

[1]Participation not recommended by the American Academy of Pediatrics.

[2]The American Academy of Pediatrics recommends limiting the amount of body checking allowed for hockey players 15 years and younger to reduce injuries.

[3]Snowboarding has been added since previous statement was published.

[4]Dancing has been further classified into ballet, modern, and jazz since previous statement was published.

[5]A race (contest) in which competitors use a map and compass to find their way through unfamiliar territory.

From American Academy of Pediatrics, Committee on Sports Medicine and Fitness: Medical conditions affecting sports participation, *Pediatrics* 107:1205-1209, 2001, with permission.

RUNNING HISTORY

Name _____

Date _____

Please answer the following questions to the best of your ability. Your answers will provide valuable information to better assess your injury status and risks. Your answers will also allow us to advise changes to your training habits to prevent further injuries.

Training History

1. How long have you been running (in years)? _____

2. How many miles per day do you average? _____

3. How many days per week do you run? _____

4. How far is your longest run during the week? _____

5. What pace (minutes per mile) do you average in your workouts? _____

6. Which of the following do you do in your workouts? (check all that apply and indicate days per week for each checked box)

   ☐ Intervals _____ ☐ Long slow distance _____

   ☐ Fartleck _____ ☐ Long fast distance _____

7. On what type of terrain do you usually run? (check all that apply)

   ☐ grass   ☐ sand

   ☐ dirt   ☐ hills

   ☐ concrete   ☐ flat

   ☐ asphalt   ☐ other _____

8. Do you run on any canted surfaces? (i.e. on one side of the road, on beaches, or always around the track in the same direction)

   _____

9. What time of day do you normally run?

   ☐ Morning   ☐ Afternoon   ☐ Night

Racing History

10. How often do you race? _____

11. What distances do you normally race? _____

Running Shoe History

12. What model(s) of running shoes do you train in and/or race in?

    _____

13. How long have you had your present pair(s) of shoes? _____

14. Do you wear any orthotic devices, special arch supports, etc, in your shoes? _____

15. Do any of your shoes make the problem better or worse? _____

16. Do you "build up" your running shoes to keep the outsoles from wearing out too quickly?

    _____

17. Where does the most outsole wear occur on your running shoes? _____

(continued on other side)

18. How do your shoes fit?

☐ Too long   ☐ Too wide

☐ Too short   ☐ Too loose in heel

☐ Too narrow   ☐ Other _____

19. Do you wear socks when you run? ☐ yes ☐ no how many pairs? _____

Pre-/Post-run Activities

20. Do you stretch?

☐ Before run: how long _____   ☐ After run: how long _____

21. What type of stretching exercises do you do?

_____

22. Do you warm up/cool down for your runs?

☐ Before run: how long _____   ☐ After run: how long _____

23. Do you do any muscle strengthening exercises? _____

24. Do you participate in any other sports or any other physical activities? Please list: _____

_____

Injury-related History

25. Did you change your training/racing schedule prior to your injury? _____

26. Did you run a particularly hard race or have a hard workout immediately prior to your injury? _____

27. Did you switch to another pair of running shoes prior to your injury? _____

28. Did you modify your shoes prior to your injury? _____

29. Was there any direct trauma associated with your injury? _____

30. Did you have another injury or any discomfort in your feet, legs, hips or back prior to your injury that you tried to train through?

_____

31. Have you cut back in your mileage or pace since your injury? ☐ yes ☐ no

If yes, has it produced any results? _____

32. Do you take any medications as self-treatment for your injury? ☐ yes ☐ no

If yes, please give name of medication, dosage, and frequency:

_____

33. Have you done any other home treatment for your injury, or had professional treatment elsewhere? ☐ yes ☐ no

If yes, please describe: _____

Adapted from Kirby KA, Valmassey RL. The patient-runner history: what to ask and why. *J Am Podiatry Assoc* 73:29-43, 1983, with permission.

Athlete Application for Participation
(Valid for 3 Years from the Date of the Physical Exam)

Special Olympics
Massachusetts

Area and Local Program _____

Please print clearly. All information is required.

Name
☐☐☐☐☐☐☐☐☐☐☐☐☐☐☐☐☐☐☐☐☐☐☐☐☐☐

Social Security Number (optional) Male ☐ Female ☐ Date of Birth __/__/__ Phone # ___-___-____

Street Address or PO Box ☐☐☐☐☐☐☐☐☐☐☐☐☐☐☐☐☐☐ Apt # ☐☐

City/Town ☐☐☐☐☐☐☐☐☐☐☐☐ State ☐☐ Zip Code + 4 ☐☐☐☐☐

Emergency Contact Name ☐☐☐☐☐☐☐☐☐☐☐☐ Emergency Contact Phone #

HEALTH HISTORY: TO BE COMPLETED BY PARENT/CAREGIVER

Yes	No		Yes	No	
☐	☐	Allergies:	☐	☐	Easy bleeding
☐	☐	*Environmental:* _____	☐	☐	Emotional/psychiatric/behavioral
☐	☐	*Food:* _____	☐	☐	Heart disease/heart defect*
☐	☐	*Insect stings/bites:* _____	☐	☐	Hernia
☐	☐	*Medicines:* _____	☐	☐	High blood pressure*
☐	☐	Asthma*	☐	☐	Immunizations up-to-date
☐	☐	Blind*	☐	☐	Date of last tetanus immun. __/__/__
☐	☐	*Visually impaired*	☐	☐	Needs medication (see "Medications" table below)
☐	☐	Bone or joint problem	☐	☐	Requires extra supervision
☐	☐	Concussion or serious head injury*	☐	☐	Seizures/epilepsy/fainting spells*
☐	☐	Deaf	☐	☐	Sickle cell
☐	☐	*Hearing impaired*	☐	☐	Special diet
☐	☐	Diabetes*	☐	☐	Tobacco
☐	☐	Down Syndrome (see below)	☐	☐	Other: _____

(*) Requires physical examination if new problem

Medications (if applicable): Please print medication name, amount, date prescribed and number of times per day medication is given.

Medication Name	Dosage	Date Presc.	Times per day	Medication Name	Dosage	Date Presc.	Times per day

Special Olympics Massachusetts (SOMA) specifically has my permission (both during participation and anytime thereafter) to use my/my child's/my ward's likeness, name, voice, and words in television, radio, film, newspapers, magazines, and any other media, and in any form, for the purpose of advertising or communicating the purposes and activities of Special Olympics Massachusetts.

I understand that if a medical emergency should arise during my/my child's/my ward's participation in any SOMA activity and I am not able to give my consent for treatment, that SOMA is authorized to take whatever measures are necessary to protect my health and well-being including hospitalization.

Signature of parent/legal guardian/adult athlete (over 18) _____ Date ___/___/___

SECTION BELOW TO BE COMPLETED BY EXAMINING PHYSICIAN:

For Athletes with Down Syndrome: Persons with Down syndrome should have a lateral x-ray of the cervical spine in hyper flexion and hyperextension. The interpretation of the radiographs should include measurements of the atlanto-dens interval.

Yes	No	
☐	☐	Has an x-ray examination for atlantoaxial instability been done? Date of x-ray: ___/___/___
☐	☐	If yes, was it positive for atlantoaxial instability? (positive indicates that the atlanto-dens interval is 5mm or more)

I have reviewed the above health information and have performed the above examination on this athlete within the past 6 months and certify that the athlete can participate in Special Olympics. **RESTRICTIONS:** _____

Signature of Examiner _____ Exam Date ___/___/___
(no office stamps accepted without provider's signature)

Examiner's Name ☐☐☐☐☐☐☐☐☐☐☐☐☐☐☐☐☐☐☐☐☐☐☐☐☐☐

Street Address or P.O. ☐☐☐☐☐☐☐☐☐☐☐☐☐☐☐☐☐☐☐☐☐☐☐☐☐☐

City/Town ☐☐☐☐☐☐☐☐☐☐☐☐ State ☐☐ ZIP ☐☐☐☐☐ Phone # ___-___-____

A COPY OF THIS APPLICATION MUST BE FILED AT THE SOMA HEADQUARTERS & EITHER THE AREA OR SECTIONAL OFFICE   3/02

Last Name, First Name:

Form Expiration Date ___/___/___

SAMPLE

COACHES WILL BE RESPONSIBLE FOR HAVING UP-TO-DATE ATHLETE MEDICAL FORMS IN THEIR POSSESSION AT TRAINING AND COMPETITION EVENTS. THE COACH'S COPIES OF MEDICAL FORMS WILL BE UTILIZED AT ALL QUALIFYING COMPETITIONS AND AREA EVENTS.

Medical forms are evaluated for completeness using the following required information as criteria:
- on the correct form
- area and local program
- full first and last name
- gender
- date of birth
- street address
- city
- home phone number, including area code
- parent/guardian name (if under 18)
- emergency contact name and phone number, including area code
- signature of athlete (18 or older) or signature of parent/guardian
- "history of" medical information on the medical unless supplemented by an attachment which contains the same info
- doctor's/physician's assistant/nurse practitioner's signature (no office stamps allowed)
- date of physical examination
- no fax copies accepted

OVERNIGHT EVENTS
- If medication is to be dispensed by SOMA medical volunteers, it must be accompanied by a medication form *(supplemental medication form)*
- Medication must be in its original container

CHAPTER 5

Psychiatric Histories and Related Forms

Chapter Contents

ICON KEY: 📄 Tool Printed ⊘ Tool on CD-ROM ∞ Customizable Tool i Information and Resources Provided for Further Acquisition

Introduction and Contents

In addition to gathering information on the general health status of a patient, the primary care clinician may wish to document specific information regarding mental status. This chapter contains history and physical exam forms and specialized history questionnaires with a psychiatric or spiritual health focus. Structured and semistructured interviews and questionnaires may improve the accuracy of information and assist in documentation of observations regarding mental health status. With specific psychologic and spiritual information, the clinician may better interpret physiologic findings and responses to treatment interventions. Mental health information may also lead to improved referral patterns for specialty psychiatric care.

In collecting information on psychologic issues, the *Diagnostic and Statistical Manual of Mental Disorders (DSM)*

may be used to categorize diagnoses. The *DSM* is the standard classification system of mental disorders used by mental health professionals in the United States. The *Diagnostic and Statistical Manual of Mental Disorders, Fourth Edition* (*DSM-IV*) was the last major revision of the *DSM*, released in 1994. Major revisions involve changes to the classification of disorders, diagnostic criteria, and descriptive text based on current research information. A minor revision to the *DSM-IV*, the *DSM-IV-Text Revision* (*DSM-IV-TR*), was published in July 2000 (American Psychiatric Association, 2000). In the *DSM-IV-TR* descriptive text has been modified to be consistent with the most recent literature, errors in criteria listings have been corrected, and diagnostic codes have been updated to conform to the *International Classification of Diseases, 10th Revision* (*ICD-10-CM*) coding system (World Health Organization, 1992).

The *DSM-IV* categorizes disorders on the basis of criteria sets with defining symptoms or features. The system uses five axes (Box 5-1) to classify general medical and psychiatric diagnoses, distinguish environmental and psychosocial aspects, and score overall functioning. Axes I and II contain the entire classification system for psychiatric disorders. Each disorder includes a set of inclusion and exclusion diagnostic criteria and a description. Axis III identifies physical disorders. Multiple diagnoses may be listed on axes I, II, and III by using the *ICD-10-CM* for coding purposes. Axis IV identifies psychosocial and environmental problems that may influence the diagnosis, treatment, and prognosis of psychiatric disorders. Axis V is used to report the overall level of functioning as assessed with the Global Assessment of Functioning Scale.

PSYCHIATRIC HISTORY AND PHYSICAL EXAMINATION FORMS

Mental Health Assessment Form

This two-page form, adapted from Varcarolis 1998, contains adult history information specific to mental health issues. The form is divided into two main areas: "Client History" and "Mental and Emotional Status." Client History includes a general social history, presenting

problem, personal psychosocial history, and family psychosocial history. Mental and Emotional Status includes sections for appearance, behavior, speech, mood, affect, thought process, thought content, reality orientation, and level of anxiety.

Child Psychiatry Emergency Consultation Mental Status Examination Checklist

This three-page form is designed to evaluate the mental status of children and adolescents on an emergency basis (Lewis, 1996). The first half of the form lists indicators for behavior, speech, self-reported mood, observed affect, neurovegetative symptoms, substance use, thought processes and suicidality. Space is available for comments after each heading. The second half contains focused exploration of suicidality with 19 components detailing episode features and outcome.

Substance Use History and Physical Examination Form

The Substance Use History and Physical Examination form was developed by Nordsey and Smith (1989) for the Project Cork Program and was revised in July 2002. This standardized form may be used for history and physical exam documentation when substance use is known or suspected. The form contains sections for past medical history, family history, social history, review of systems (general; head ears, eyes, nose, and throat [HEENT]; cardiovascular; gastrointestinal; genitourinary; neuropsychiatric), substance use history, and physical examination documentation. Each of the preceding sections targets indicators, signs, and symptoms that are specific to substance abuse. Additionally, the form incorporates a substance use screening test and provides space for assessment of alcohol or drug use and withdrawal risk. The form, reprinted in this text, is also available in PDF format at http://www.projectcork.org/clinical_tools/index.html and is suitable for duplication for use in clinical settings. No permission is required for noncommercial use.

Brief Substance Abuse History Form i

The Brief Substance Abuse History Form is intended as a standardized measure of lifetime and current substance abuse, including both injection and noninjection routes of administration. Developed by Huba et al (1997), the form may be downloaded from http://www.themeasurement-group.com/modules/module24.htm. The Brief Substance Abuse History Form is intended to be used during an interview rather than for self-report. Permission is granted by The Measurement Group for noncommercial use so long as the form is not altered, the copyright is not removed, and a proper citation to the instrument is made.

Form content includes check-off boxes for information pertaining to "ever used," "age at first use," "ever injected," "used in the last 6 months," "days used in last 30 days," "days injected in last 30 days," and "times injected in last

---

Box **5-1** *DSM-IV* Multiaxial System

Axis I:
Clinical disorders and other conditions that may be a focus of clinical attention
Axis II:
Personality disorders and mental handicap
Axis III:
General medical conditions
Axis IV:
Psychosocial and environmental problems
Axis V:
Global assessment of functioning

From American Psychiatric Association, 2000.

30 days" for alcohol, marijuana, crack, cocaine, heroin, speedballs, amphetamines, and other drugs (PCP, LSD, other hallucinogens, barbiturates). Age at first injected drug use is also included.

Daily Mood Chart   **i**

In addition to documenting behavioral history elicited by the clinician, it may be advantageous to have the patient keep a record of mood changes. A daily mood log is available for downloading at http://healthnet.umassmed.edu/mhealth/NewMoodWksheet.pdf. This chart permits the patient to check boxes on a daily basis that reflect levels of elevated or depressed mood, hours slept, and presence of anxiety or irritability. Examination of mood changes over time will provide more detailed information, allowing the provider and patient to arrive at a mutually acceptable and understandable treatment plan.

DOMESTIC VIOLENCE QUESTIONNAIRES

Partner violence is a serious health risk. The recommendation that all women and adolescent girls in primary care be screened for past and present intimate partner violence is endorsed by numerous groups such as the American Medical Association, the American College of Obstetricians and Gynecologists, the U.S. Preventive Services Task Force, the American Nursing Association, and the American Academy of Pediatrics (Kimberg, 2001). As domestic violence screening becomes more widely implemented in primary care practice, earlier detection and intervention efforts may result in improved safety and education for all families.

The primary care setting provides a safe and confidential venue for screening for intimate partner violence with the opportunity to discuss abuse as an important health care issue. When incorporating routine screening for domestic violence into a practice, clinicians need to be aware of any state mandatory reporting laws and make any limits of confidentiality known to patients before screening. In an established relationship with a provider, a patient has developed trust, which allows truthful, nonjudgmental inquiry and response. It has been demonstrated that women and girls respond positively to very direct questions about abuse in the health care setting (Kimberg, 2001). Using direct questions with specific behavioral examples is far preferable to indirect questions regarding "abuse."

The five tools in this section reflect the need for direct questioning and assist the clinician in choosing appropriate terms for inquiry. Use of one of these brief tools for guidance in routine screening for domestic violence provides a standardized and rapid assessment process that can be integrated into daily practice.

Abuse Assessment Screen

The Abuse Assessment Screen was developed by the Nursing Consortium on Violence and Abuse for pregnant and nonpregnant women (Parker & McFarlane, 1991). A five-question format and a three-question format are available; the three-question form is reproduced here.

This screening tool has been found to be reliable in detecting family violence during pregnancy (McFarlane et al, 1992; Soeken et al, 1998). Validity was assessed using the Conflict Tactics Scale (Straus, 1979), the Index of Spousal Abuse (Hudson & MacIntosh, 1981), and the Danger Assessment instrument (Campbell, 1986) as comparison models, with high agreement among them in detecting domestic abuse (Soeken et al, 1998).

Soeken et al (1998) offer a seven-step protocol for use of the Abuse Assessment Screen, which may be summarized as follows:

1. Provide a private and confidential place for the assessment.
2. Tell each woman that all women are assessed for abuse.
3. Read the Abuse Assessment Screen to the woman.
4. Record the abuse.
5. Respect the woman's response.
6. Document findings.
7. Provide appropriate intervention.

Partner Violence Screen

A brief, three-question screening instrument was designed by Feldhaus et al (1997) to detect partner violence (Box 5-2). Three questions about past physical violence and perceived personal safety are intended to identify a large number of women who have a history of partner violence. A positive response to any of the three questions represents a positive screen for partner violence. The Partner Violence Screen was validated against the Index of Spouse Abuse (ISA) and the Conflict Tactics Scale (CTS); sensitivities ranged from 64.5% to 71.4% and specificities ranged from 80.3% to 84.4% when compared with these validated instruments. Positive predictive values ranged from 51.3% to 63.4%, and negative predictive values ranged from 87.6% to 88.7%.

Spouse Abuse: Assessing Level of Violence in the Home

Because each cycle of violence may escalate the degree of intensity, assessment for the level of violence in the home is essential for protection of the lives of the spouse and children. Jezierski (1994) describes interview questions

---

Box 5-2   **Partner Violence Screen**

1. Have you been hit, kicked, punched or otherwise hurt by someone within the last year?
2. Do you feel safe in your present relationship?
3. Is there a partner from a previous relationship who is making you feel unsafe now?

With permission from Feldhaus K et al: Accuracy of three brief screening questions for detecting partner violence in the emergency department. *JAMA* 277:1357-1361, 1997.

Box **5-3** Spouse Abuse: Assessing Level of Violence in the Home

1. Does the client feel safe?
2. Has there been a recent increase in violence?
3. Has the client been choked?
4. Is there a weapon in the house?
5. Has the abuser used/threatened to use a weapon?
6. Has the abuser threatened to harm the children?
7. Has the abuser threatened to kill the client?

From Jezierski M: Abuse of women by male partners: basic knowledge for emergency nurses. *J Emerg Nurs* 20(5):361-368, 1994. Reprinted with permission from the Emergency Nurses Association.

designed to detect violence that may be increasing in intensity (Box 5-3).

SAFE Technique

This Screening for Domestic Violence online resource lists the SAFE technique for routine screening for domestic violence in all patients (Box 5-4). For more detailed guidance on screening for domestic violence with the SAFE technique, please see the following website: http://www.continuingeducation.com/emt/domesticviolence/domesticviolence.pdf.

RADAR Screening Tool

The RADAR action steps were developed by the Massachusetts Medical Society (Box 5-5). This five-letter mnemonic cues the provider to screen every female patient for domestic violence using standard recommended guidelines from domestic violence professionals. Remembering to routinely screen female patients is the first step in increasing detection of domestic violence situations. The second step is to ask direct questions. Numerous studies have demonstrated that asking directed, specific questions about personal safety at home results in

Box **5-4** SAFE Technique

S = Inquire about **S**tress and **S**afety
A = **A**sk if she is **A**fraid or **A**bused
F = Inquire about **F**riends and **F**amily
E = Inquire about an **E**mergency Plan

Box **5-5** RADAR Screening Tool

R = **R**outinely Screen Female Patients
A = **A**sk Direct Questions
D = **D**ocument Your Findings
A = **A**ssess Patient Safety
R = **R**eview Options and **R**eferrals

Used with permission from *Use Your "RADAR"—Recognizing and treating partner violence screening tool.* Copyright 1992, 1996, 1999 Massachusetts Medical Society.

increased detection of intimate partner violence. Once the questions are asked and answered, the clinician must document any findings with an accurate description of the abuse. All pertinent physical findings should be recorded, and any physical evidence of serious injury or sexual abuse should be preserved. Assessment of patient safety should be done before the patient leaves the clinical setting. Lastly, the clinician should review options and make appropriate referrals for follow-up care or shelter. More detailed guidance on screening for domestic violence with the RADAR action steps may be found at the following website: http://www.opdv.state.ny.us/health_humsvc/health/radar.html.

Domestic Violence Online Resources

Measuring Violence-Related Attitudes, Beliefs, and Behaviors Among Youths: A Compendium of Assessment Tools: Website: http://www.cdc.gov/ncipc/pub-res/measure.htm

This publication is provided in electronic format by the Centers for Disease Control's National Center for Injury Prevention and Control. This compendium contains a set of tools that evaluate youth violence. More than 100 measures are included, most of which are intended for use with youths between 11 and 20 years, to assess factors such as attitudes toward violence, aggressive behavior, conflict resolution strategies, self-esteem, self-efficacy, and exposure to violence. The compendium also contains a number of scales and assessments developed for use with children between the ages of 5 and 10 years, to measure factors such as aggressive fantasies, beliefs supportive of aggression, attributional biases, prosocial behavior, and aggressive behavior.

Nursing Network on Violence Against Women (NNVAW): Website: http://www.nnvawi.org/assessment.htm

The Nursing Network on Violence Against Women (NNVAW) was formed in 1985 to encourage the development of a nursing practice that focuses on health issues relating to the effects of violence on women's lives. This website offers the current NNVAW newsletter, conferences, information on research and political action, and other information of interest to members. Domestic violence assessment tools are available on the website; the reader is encouraged to reproduce and use the tools in clinical practice. Available tools include the Abuse Assessment Screen, Campbell's Danger Assessment instrument, and the Domestic Violence Survivor Assessment.

Partnerships Against Violence Network (PAVNET): Website: http://www.pavnet.org/

Partnerships Against Violence Network (PAVNET) is a "virtual library" of information about violence and youth at risk, representing data from seven different federal agencies. Resources for violence prevention professionals include an online, searchable database for information about current, federally funded research on violence; programs, curricula, and technical assistance menus; links to an extensive network of violence prevention services; and a PAVNET users' mail group.

Peace at Home: Website: http://www.peaceathome.org/

Peace at Home is a human rights agency dedicated to stopping domestic violence. The agency is based in Massachusetts, and its website provides links to local and national resources for all aspects of domestic violence. Several programs and publications are available to assist with educating the public about domestic violence.

Sexual Assault Resource Service (SARS): Website: http://www.sanesart.com/Default.asp

This guide is designed for nursing professionals involved in providing evaluations of victims of sexual abuse. Sexual Assault Nurse Examiner (SANE) and Sexual Assault Response Team (SART) program information is available, as well as other related resources for clinicians.

Substance Abuse Treatment and Domestic Violence-Treatment Improvement Protocol (TIP) Series 25: Website: http://ncadi.samhsa.gov/govpubs/BKD239/

One of a series of TIP documents published by the Department of Health and Human Services, this TIP presents an introduction to domestic violence. It includes information about the role of substance abuse in domestic violence, techniques for detecting and eliciting information, and treatment/safety advice. Appendix C of this document includes four tools that may be reproduced: Abuse Assessment Screen (in English and Spanish), Danger Assessment, Psychological Maltreatment of Women Inventory (PMWI), and the Revised Conflict Tactics Scale (CTS2).

MENTAL HEALTH, SPIRITUAL, AND CULTURAL HISTORIES

This section contains specialized tools for taking histories involving mental health, spiritual, and cultural concepts. Focused mental health histories provide information that the provider can use to assist in diagnosis of behavioral conditions. The relationship between spirituality and beliefs with physical health has been an increasingly examined variable in the study of total well-being; these tools provide reminders for key concepts in exploration of spirituality. Cultural beliefs have also long been known to influence outcomes and acceptance of treatment interventions; cultural influences may be explored by using a structured interview.

These tools include mnemonic devices to promote recall of key words or concepts. For each key word, questions that explore that concept are suggested. The clinician may choose to ask more questions that assess an issue more fully or to use the overall information to diagnose and propose treatment options or refer for further specialty care.

SIG E CAPS System

The mood mnemonic SIG E CAPS serves as a reminder of eight criteria for major depression. The term *SIG E CAPS* may be remembered as "a prescription for 'energy capsules.'" The letters stand for changes in sleep, interest, guilt, energy, concentration, appetite, and psychomotor activity and the presence of suicidal ideation. The SIG E CAPS criteria parallel the *DSM-IV* criteria for major depression; guidelines suggest that a patient must exhibit five of nine symptoms (eight symptoms from SIG E CAPS plus depressed mood permeating daily life for 2 weeks or more) to meet criteria for a diagnosis of major depression (Box 5-6).

SALSA: Depression Screening

The SALSA mnemonic device originated as a result of a study by Brody et al (1998), which was done to determine whether there was a core subset of depressive symptoms that could be used to efficiently diagnose depression following the use of a two-item depression screener (Box 5-7). Four symptoms (sleep disturbance, anhedonia, low self-esteem, and decreased appetite) accounted for virtually all the depression symptom–related variance in functional status and well-being among 1000 study subjects. The authors concluded that evaluation of four core depressive symptoms after the use of a two-item depression screener effectively identified primary care patients with depression in need of clinical attention.

Box 5-6 SIG E CAPS System

MNEMONIC	SYMPTOM
S	**Sleep** changes: difficulty falling asleep and early morning awakening; increased sleep. Decrease in **sexual** desire, though not a major criteria, may also be considered.
I	Decreased **interest** or pleasure in previously enjoyed activities.
G	Inappropriate **guilt** or feelings of worthlessness/hopelessness.
E	Decreased **energy** or fatigue.
C	Impaired **concentration;** difficulty performing tasks from start to finish.
A	Increased or decreased **appetite** with weight gain or loss.
P	**Psychomotor** agitation or retardation; there may be a flat affect with little gesturing. Crying may occur often and unexpectedly.
S	**Suicidal** ideation, plan, or attempt.

Box 5-7 SALSA Depression Screening

Sleep disturbance
Anhedonia
Low **S**elf esteem
Appetite decreased

From Brody DS, et al: Identifying patients with depression in the primary care setting: a more efficient method. *Arch Intern Med* 158:2469-2475, 1998.

BATHE Technique

The BATHE technique frames the patient interview with the purpose of understanding the patient in the context of his or her total life situation (Box 5-8). By enabling primary care practitioners to recognize patients who have mental health problems, the BATHE technique allows for the unmasking of psychosocial problems and lends support to patients as they face these issues (Lieberman, 1997). Five areas are addressed by using the mnemonic *BATHE* to recall each core concept.

HOPE Questionnaire: A Framework for Spiritual Assessment

Clinicians may choose to incorporate a spiritual assessment into the medical interview in the interest of exploring an individual's spiritual resources, concerns, and support (Anandarajah & Hight, 2001). Spiritual factors may play a role in a patient's response to illness and treatment; knowledge of such factors may assist the clinician in recruiting further resources for patient support.

Box 5-8 BATHE Technique

MNEMONIC	QUESTIONS
B: Background	What is going on in your life?
	What is going on right now
	Has anything changed recently?
A: Affect	How do you feel about that?
	What is your mood?
T: Trouble	What about the situation troubles you most?
	What worries or concerns you?
H: Handling	How are you handling that?
	How are you coping?
E: Empathy	That must be very difficult for you.
	I can understand that you would feel that way.

From Lieberman JA III: BATHE: an approach to the interview process in the primary care setting, *J Clin Psychiatry* 58(suppl 3): 3-6, 1997.

The HOPE Questionnaire is a mnemonic device that cues the clinician to concepts involving spiritual health (Box 5-9). The letters in the mnemonic stand for the following: H–sources of hope, strength, comfort, meaning, peace, love, and connection; O–the role of organized religion for the patient; P–personal spirituality and practices; E–effects on medical care and end-of-life issues (Anandarajah & Hight, 2001).

Suggestions by Anandarajah and Hight (2001) for medical management after a spiritual interview follow four principles for care:

1. Take no further medical action; offer your presence, understanding, acceptance, and compassion.
2. Incorporate spirituality into preventive health care.
3. Include spirituality in adjuvant care.
4. Modify the treatment plan.

SPIRIT: A Framework for Spiritual Assessment

The SPIRIT questionnaire uses a mnemonic to recall cues to questions regarding spiritual beliefs, practices, and

Box 5-9 HOPE Questionnaire: A Framework for Spiritual Assessment

MNEMONIC	QUESTIONS
H: Hope—sources of hope, meaning, comfort, strength, peace, love, and connection	We have been discussing your support systems. I was wondering, what is there in your life that gives you internal support?
	What are your sources of hope, strength, comfort, and peace?
	What do you hold on to during difficult times?
	What sustains you and keeps you going?
	For some people, their religious or spiritual beliefs act as a source of comfort and strength in dealing with life's ups and downs; is this true for you?
	If the answer is yes, go on to O and P questions. If the answer is no, consider asking, "Was it ever?" If the answer is yes, ask, "What changed?"
O: Organized religion	Do you consider yourself part of an organized religion? How important is this to you?
	What aspects of your religion are helpful and not so helpful to you?
	Are you part of a religious or spiritual community? Does it help you? How?
P: Personal spirituality/practices	Do you have personal spiritual beliefs that are independent of organized religion? What are they?
	Do you believe in God? What kind of relationship do you have with God?
	What aspects of your spirituality or spiritual practices do you find most helpful to you personally? (Examples include prayer, meditation, reading scripture, attending religious services, listening to music, hiking, communing with nature.)
E: Effects on medical care and end-of-life issues	Has being sick (or your current situation) affected your ability to do the things that usually help you spiritually (or affected your relationship with God)?
	As a doctor, is there anything that I can do to help you access the resources that usually help you?
	Are you worried about any conflicts between your beliefs and your medical situation/care/decisions?
	Would it be helpful for you to speak to a clinical chaplain/community spiritual leader?
	Are there any specific practices or restrictions I should know about in providing your medical care (e.g., dietary restrictions, use of blood products)?
	If the patient is dying: How do your beliefs affect the kind of medical care you would like me to provide over the next few days/weeks/months?

From Anandarajah G, Hight, E: Spirituality and medical practice: using the HOPE questions as a practical tool for spiritual assessment. *Am Fam Physician* 63(1):81-89, 2001.

Box **5-10** SPIRIT: A Framework for Spiritual Assessment

MNEMONIC	QUESTIONS
S: Spiritual belief system	What is your formal religious affiliation?
	Name or describe your spiritual belief system.
P: Personal spirituality	Describe the beliefs and practices of your religion or spiritual system that you personally accept.
	Describe the beliefs or practices you do not accept.
	Do you accept or believe (specific tenet or practice)?
	What does your spirituality/religion mean to you?
	What is the importance of your spirituality/religion in daily life?
I: Integration with a spiritual community	Do you belong to any spiritual or religious group or community? What is your position or role?
	What importance does this group have to you? Is it a source of support? In what ways?
	Does or could this group provide help in dealing with health issues?
R: Ritualized practices and restrictions	Are there specific practices that you carry out as part of your religion/spirituality (e.g., prayer or meditation)?
	Are there certain lifestyle activities or practices that your religion/ spirituality encourages or forbids? Do you comply? What significance do these practices and restrictions have to you?
	Are there specific elements of medical care that you forbid on the basis of religious/spiritual grounds?
I: Implications for medical care	What aspects of your religion/spirituality would you like me to keep in mind as I care for you?
	Would you like to discuss religious or spiritual implications of health care?
	What knowledge or understanding would strengthen our relationship as physician and patient?
	Are there any barriers to our relationship based on religious or spiritual issues?
T: Terminal events planning	As we plan for your care near the end of life, how does your faith affect your decisions?
	Are there particular aspects of care that you wish to forgo or have withheld because of your faith?

From Maugans TA: The SPIRITual history, *Arch Fam Med* 5(1):11-16, 1996.

incorporation of such into a medical care plan (Box 5-10) (Maugans, 1996). It is slightly more focused on specific religious affiliation, beliefs, and practices than the HOPE Questionnaire. Answers elicited with the SPIRIT Questionnaire offer the clinician an opportunity to implement treatment consistent with a patient's spiritual and religious beliefs. The letters stand for the following: S–spiritual belief system; P–personal spirituality; I–integration with a spiritual community; R–ritualized practices and restrictions; I–implications for medical care; T–terminal events planning.

ETHNIC: A Framework for Culturally Competent Clinical Practice

This mnemonic device is designed to elicit information regarding a patient's cultural beliefs and practices (Levin, et al, 2003). Although it is not a spiritual or mental health assessment, the ETHNIC questionnaire permits exploration of a patient's cultural background and the effect it may have on his or her acceptance of interventions for care (Box 5-11). The questionnaire contains three sections for elicitation of cultural information and three areas cueing treatment planning. The letters stand for the following: E–explanation; T–treatment; H–healers; N–negotiate; I–intervention; C–collaboration.

References

American Psychiatric Association: *Diagnostic and statistical manual of mental disorders*, ed 4, text revision, Washington, DC, 2000, American Psychiatric Publishing, Inc.

Anandarajah G, Hight E: Spirituality and medical practice: using the HOPE questions as a practical tool for spiritual assessment, *Am Fam Physician* 63:81-89, 2001.

Brody DS et al: Identifying patients with depression in the primary care setting: a more efficient method, *Arch Intern Med* 158:2469-2475, 1998.

Campbell JC: Nursing assessment for risk of homicide with battered women, *Adv Nurs Sci* 8:36-51, 1986.

Feldhaus K et al: Accuracy of three brief screening questions for detecting partner violence in the emergency department, *JAMA* 277:1357-1361, 1997.

Huba GJ, Melchior LA, Staff of The Measurement Group, HRSA/ HAB's SPNS Cooperative Agreement Steering Committee: *Module 24: Brief Substance Abuse History Form. Adapted from work used in the*

Box 5-11 ETHNIC: A Framework for Culturally Competent Clinical Practice

MNEMONIC	QUESTIONS
E: Explanation	Why do you think you have these symptoms? What do friends, family, and others say? Do you know others with this problem? Have you seen it on TV, heard about it on the radio, or read about it in the newspaper?
T: Treatment	Do you take any treatments, medicines, or home remedies to treat the illness or to stay healthy? What kinds of treatment are you seeking from me?
H: Healers	Have you sought advice from friends, alternative folk healers, or other nondoctors?
N: Negotiate	Negotiate mutually acceptable options; incorporate patient's beliefs. Ask results patient hopes to achieve from intervention.
I: Intervention	Determine an intervention with your patient. May include incorporation of alternative treatments, spirituality, healers, or other cultural practices (e.g., foods to be eaten or avoided).
C: Collaborate	Collaborate with the patient, family, health team members, healers, and community resources.

Developed by Steven Levin, MD; Robert Like, MD, MS; Jan Gottlieb, MPH: Department of Family Medicine, University of Medicine and Dentistry of New Jersey, Robert Wood Johnson Medical School, 1997.

NIDA Risk Behavior Assessment (RBA). Culver City, CA, 1997, The Measurement Group. Available from http://www.themeasurementgroup.com/modules/module24.htm.

Hudson WW, McIntosh SR: The assessment of spouse abuse: two quantifiable dimensions, *J Marriage Family* 43:873-888, 1981.

Jezierski M: Abuse of women by male partners: basic knowledge for emergency nurses, *J Emerg Nurs* 20:361-368, 1994.

Kimberg L: Addressing intimate partner violence in primary care practice, *Medscape Womens Health* 6:E1, 2001. Available from http://www.medscape.com/viewarticle/408937.

Levin S, Like R, Gottlieb J: ETHNIC: a framework for culturally competent clinical practice. In Seidel HM et al, editors: *Mosby's physical examination handbook*, ed 3, St Louis, Mo, 2003, Mosby, Inc, p. 318.

Lewis M: Psychiatric assessment of infants, children, and adolescents. In Lewis M, editor: *Child and adolescent psychiatry: a comprehensive textbook*, ed 2, Baltimore, MD, 1996, Williams & Wilkins, pp. 440-457.

Lieberman JA III: BATHE: an approach to the interview process in the primary care setting, *J Clin Psychiatry* 58(suppl 3):3-6, 1997.

Little KJ: Screening for domestic violence. Identifying, assisting, and empowering adult victims of abuse. *Postgrad Med* online 108(2), 2000. Available from http://www.postgradmed.com/issues/2000/08_00/little.htm.

Maugans TA: The SPIRITual history, *Arch Fam Med* 5:11-16, 1996.

McFarlane J et al: Assessing for abuse during pregnancy: severity and frequency of injuries and associated entry into prenatal care, *JAMA* 267:3176-3178, 1992.

Nordsey D, Smith N: *Protocol for medical assessment. Project Cork Weekend Program*. Hanover, NH, 1989. http://www.projectcork.org/.

Parker B, McFarlane J: Identifying and helping battered pregnant women, *MCN Am J Maternal Child Nurs* 16:161-164, 1991.

Soeken KL et al: The abuse assessment screen: a clinical instrument to measure frequency, severity and perpetrator of abuse against women. In Campbell JC, editor: *Empowering survivors of abuse: health care for battered women and their children*, Thousand Oaks, CA, 1998, Sage Publications, Inc. Available from http://www.nnvawi.org/abusescreen.pdf.

Straus MA: Measuring intrafamily conflict and violence: the Conflict Tactics (CT) Scale, *J Marriage Family* 41:75-78, 1979.

Varcarolis E: *Foundations of psychiatric mental health nursing*, ed 3, Philadelphia, 1998, WB Saunders, pp. 996-998.

World Health Organization: *International statistical classification of diseases and related health problems*, 10th revision, Geneva, 1992, World Health Organization.

Mental Health Assessment Form

Patient name: _____

Date: _____

1. Client History

I. GENERAL HISTORY OF CLIENT

Name _____ Age _____ Sex _____

Racial and ethnic data _____ Marital status _____

Number and ages of children/siblings_____

Living arrangements _____ Occupation _____

Education _____ Spiritual beliefs and affiliations_____

II. PRESENTING PROBLEM

A. Statement in the client's own words of why he or she is hospitalized or seeking help _____

B. Recent difficulties/alterations in	C. Increased feelings of	D. Somatic changes, such as
1. Relationships	1. Depression	1. Constipation
2. Usual level of functioning	2. Anxiety	2. Insomnia
3. Behavior	3. Hopelessness	3. Lethargy
4. Perceptions or cognitive abilities	4. Being overwhelmed	4. Weight loss or gain
	5. Suspiciousness	5. Palpitations
	6. Confusion	

III. RELEVANT HISTORY—PERSONAL

A. Previous hospitalizations and illnesses _____

B. Educational background _____

C. Occupational background _____

    1. If employed, where? _____

    2. How long at that job?_____

    3. Previous positions and reasons for leaving _____

    4. Special skills _____

D. Social patterns

    1. Describe friends _____

    2. Describe a usual day_____

E. Sexual patterns

    1. Sexually active?_____

    2. Sexual orientation _____

    3. Sexual difficulties_____

F. Interests and abilities

    1. What does the client do in his or her spare time? _____

    2. What is the client good at? _____

    3. What gives the client pleasure? _____

G. Substance use and abuse

    1. What nonprescription drugs does the client take?_____

        How often? _____ How much? _____

    2. How many drinks of alcohol does the client take per day? _____

        Per week? _____

    3. What meds (prescription and OTC) is the client taking? _____

        How often? _____ How much? _____

Mental Health Assessment Form-2

III. RELEVANT HISTORY—PERSONAL—cont'd

H. How does the client cope with stress?

    1. What does the client do when he or she gets upset? _____

    2. Whom can the client talk to? _____

    3. What usually helps to relieve stress? _____

    4. What did the client try this time? _____

IV. RELEVANT HISTORY—FAMILY

A. Childhood

    1. Who was important to the client growing up? _____

    2. Was there physical or sexual abuse? _____

    3. Did the parents drink or use drugs? _____

    4. Who was in the home when the client was growing up? _____

B. Adolescence

    1. How would the client describe his or her feelings in adolescence? _____

    2. Describe the client's peer group at that time. _____

C. Use of drugs

    1. Was there use or abuse of drugs by any family member? _____

        Prescription _____ Street _____ By whom? _____

    2. What was the effect on the family? _____

D. Family physical or mental problems

    1. Who in the family had physical or mental problems? _____

    2. Describe the problems. _____

    3. How did it affect the family? _____

E. Was there an unusual or outstanding event the client would like to mention? _____

2. Mental and Emotional Status

A. Appearance

    Physical handicaps _____

    Dress appropriate _____ Sloppy _____

    Grooming neat _____ Poor _____

    Eye contact held _____ Describe posture _____

B. Behavior

    Restless _____ Agitated _____ Lethargic _____

    Mannerisms _____ Facial expressions _____ Other _____

C. Speech

    Clear _____ Mumbled _____ Rapid _____ Slurred _____

    Constant _____ Mute or silent _____ Barriers to communication _____

    Specify (e.g., client has delusions or is confused, withdrawn, or verbose) _____

D. Mood

    What mood does the client convey? _____

E. Affect

    What is the client's affect? (bland, apathetic, dramatic, bizarre, or appropriate?)

    Describe _____

Mental Health Assessment Form-3

IV. RELEVANT HISTORY—FAMILY—cont'd

2. Mental and Emotional Status—cont'd

F. Thought process

1. Characteristics

Describe the characteristics of the person's responses:

Looseness of association _____ Blocking _____ Concrete _____

Confabulation _____ Tangential _____ Flights of ideas _____

Describe _____

2. Cognitive ability

Proverbs: Concrete _____ Abstract _____

Serial sevens: How far does the client go? _____

Can the client do simple math? _____

What seems to be the reason for poor concentration? _____

G. Thought content

1. Central theme: What is important to the client? _____

Describe _____

2. Self-concept: How does the client view him- or herself? _____

What does the client want to change about him- or herself? _____

3. Insight? Does the client realistically assess his or her symptoms? _____

Realistically appraise his or her situation? _____

4. Suicidal or homicidal ideation? _____ What is suicide potential? _____

Family history of suicide or homicide attempt or successful completion? _____

_____

Explain _____

Preoccupations: does the client have hallucinations? _____

Delusions _____ Obsessions _____ Rituals _____ Phobias _____

Grandiosity _____ Religiosity _____ Worthlessness _____

Describe _____

H. Reality orientation

Time: _____

Place: _____

Person: _____

Memory: _____

I. Level of anxiety

Mild   Data _____

Moderate   Data _____

Severe   Data _____

Panic   Data _____

Completed by: _____

Date: _____

Adapted from Varcarolis, E. (1998). Foundations of Psychiatric Mental Health Nursing, 3rd ed. Philadelphia: W.B. Saunders Co., pp. 996-998; reprinted with permission.

Child Psychiatry Emergency Consultation
Mental Status Examination Checklist

Patient name: _____ Age: _____ Sex: _____ Examination date: _____

Behavior:	Yes	No	No Info	Comments
Alert	☐	☐	☐	
Cooperative	☐	☐	☐	
Agitated	☐	☐	☐	
Belligerent	☐	☐	☐	
Reliable Historian	☐	☐	☐	

Speech:	Yes	No	No Info	Comments
Slowed	☐	☐	☐	
Pressured	☐	☐	☐	
Monotone	☐	☐	☐	
Ataxic	☐	☐	☐	

Mood (Self-Report):	Yes	No	No Info	Comments
Sad	☐	☐	☐	
So-so	☐	☐	☐	
Happy	☐	☐	☐	
Angry	☐	☐	☐	
Nervous	☐	☐	☐	

Affect (Observed):	Yes	No	No Info	Comments
Congruent	☐	☐	☐	
Euthymic	☐	☐	☐	
Expansive	☐	☐	☐	
Dysphoric	☐	☐	☐	
Anxious	☐	☐	☐	
Irritable	☐	☐	☐	
Angry	☐	☐	☐	

Neurovegetative Symptoms:	Yes	No	No Info	Comments
Poor Sleep	☐	☐	☐	
Poor Appetite	☐	☐	☐	
Anhedonic (loss of interests)	☐	☐	☐	
Guilty/Worthless Feelings	☐	☐	☐	
Decreased Energy	☐	☐	☐	
Impaired Concentration	☐	☐	☐	
Psychomotor Agitation	☐	☐	☐	
Psychomotor Slowing	☐	☐	☐	
Recurrent Thoughts of Death (SI is below)	☐	☐	☐	

Substance Use:	Yes	No	No Info	Comments
Tobacco	☐	☐	☐	
Alcohol	☐	☐	☐	
Marijuana	☐	☐	☐	
Stimulants	☐	☐	☐	
Narcotics	☐	☐	☐	
Hallucinogens	☐	☐	☐	
Other	☐	☐	☐	

Detail Any "Yes" Responses: _____

Child Psychiatry Emergency Consultation
Mental Status Examination Checklist - 2

Thought Processes:	Yes	No	No Info	Comments
Circumstantial	☐	☐	☐	
Loosened Associations	☐	☐	☐	
Paranoid	☐	☐	☐	
Delusional	☐	☐	☐	
Auditory Hallucinations	☐	☐	☐	
Visual Hallucinations	☐	☐	☐	
Ideas of Reference	☐	☐	☐	
Grandiosity	☐	☐	☐	

Suicidality:	Yes	No	No Info	Comments
Presenting Suicidal Ideation	☐	☐	☐	
Previous Suicidal Ideation	☐	☐	☐	
Presenting Suicidal Behavior	☐	☐	☐	
Previous Suicidal Behavior	☐	☐	☐	(If yes, # of times:_____)

N.B. If "yes" to presenting suicidality questions, then complete the following:

1. Type of Present Episode: Specify:
   - None   ☐ (0) _____
   - Ideation without plan   ☐ (1) _____
   - Ideation with plan   ☐ (2) _____
   - Threat (Verbal)   ☐ (3) _____
   - Gesture (e.g. only brandishes knife or pills) ☐ (4) _____
   - Attempt (deliberate self-injurious)   ☐ (5) _____

2. Method of Attempt:
   - Overdose/Ingestion   ☐ Type/Amount: _____
   - Cutting/Slashing   ☐ _____
   - Firearms   ☐ _____
   - Hanging   ☐ _____
   - Other   ☐ _____

3. Alcohol or drug use prior to episode:
   ☐ No (0)   ☐ Yes (2)   ☐ Don't Know   ☐ Type/Amount: _____

4. Intent Rating: ☐ No data
   - ☐ Wanted to die   ☐ _____
   - ☐ Did not want to die   ☐ _____
   - ☐ Ambivalent; did not care whether lived or died ☐ _____

5. Premeditation Rating:
   - ☐ Impulsive act; no premeditation—less than one hour ☐ _____
   - ☐ Less than 1 day   ☐ _____
   - ☐ Longer than 1 day   ☐ _____

6. Suicide Note: ☐ No data
   - ☐ Absence of note   ☐ _____
   - ☐ Note written but torn up, or note just thought about ☐ _____
   - ☐ Presence of note   ☐ _____

7. Degree of Planning: ☐ No data
   - ☐ No preparation   ☐ _____
   - ☐ Minimal/moderate preparation   ☐ _____
   - ☐ Extensive preparation   ☐ _____

8. Preparation (Arrangements made while thinking he/she was going to die; giving things away, etc.)   ☐ No data
   - ☐ None   ☐ _____
   - ☐ Partial preparation or ideation   ☐ _____
   - ☐ Definite plans made   ☐ _____

Child Psychiatry Emergency Consultation
Mental Status Examination Checklist - 3

9. Precautions: ☐ No data
   - ☐ No precautions
   - ☐ Passive precautions (such as avoiding others but doing nothing to prevent their intervention, e.g., alone in room, door unlocked)
   - ☐ Active precautions (e.g., locking doors)

   ☐ _____
   ☐ _____
   ☐ _____

10. Proximity of other people: ☐ No data
    - ☐ Somebody present—Who? _____
    - ☐ Somebody nearby or in contact—Who? _____
    - ☐ No one nearby or in contact

11. Intervention Rating: ☐ No data
    - ☐ Intervention was probable
    - ☐ Intervention was not likely, or uncertain
    - ☐ Intervention was highly unlikely

12. Notification: Did pt. let anyone know what he/she had done? ☐ Yes ☐ No
    Who? _____
    - ☐ Key person
    - ☐ Professional
    - ☐ Passerby

13. Notification Cont.
    How did pt. let them know?
    - ☐ Notified potential helper regarding attempt
    - ☐ Contacted but did not specifically notify potential helper regarding the attempt
    - ☐ Other _____

14. Delay until discovery: ☐ No data
    - ☐ Immediate—1 hour
    - ☐ Less than 4 hours
    - ☐ Greater than 4 hours

15. Did pt. pass out or get confused?
    - ☐ No
    - ☐ Confusion, semicoma
    - ☐ Coma, deep coma

16. Medical Treatment: (if any)   If cutting: ☐ Sutures
    - ☐ None   ☐ No sutures
    - ☐ First Aid, E. care
    - ☐ House admission, routine treatment
    - ☐ Intensive care, special treatment

17. Patient's statement of lethality: ☐ No data
    - ☐ Thought it would not kill him/her
    - ☐ Unsure whether it would kill him/her
    - ☐ Believed that it would kill him/her

18. Risk Rating (Medical Estimate):
    - ☐ No risk
    - ☐ Small risk—probability of only minor injury
    - ☐ Medium risk—possibility of significant physical injury, low probability
    - ☐ Large risk—significant risk of death or disability
    - ☐ Extreme risk—high probability of death

19. Patient's feelings about episode: ☐ No data
    - ☐ Glad he/she recovered
    - ☐ Uncertain whether he/she is glad or sorry
    - ☐ Sorry he/she recovered

Clinician Signature _____   Date _____

Modified from unpublished working draft. Reprinted with permission from Brad Peterson MD, Melvin Lewis MD, and Robert King MD. Lewis M: Psychiatric assessment of infants, children, and adolescents. In Lewis M, editor: *Child and adolescent psychiatry: a comprehensive textbook*, ed 2, Baltimore, MD, 1996, Williams & Wilkins.

Substance Use History and Physical Examination

Name _____ Age _____

Height _____ Weight _____ BAC (if known/applicable) _____

I. Past Medical History

Have you ever been told that you had:

Gastritis_____	Hepatitis_____
Pancreatitis _____	Cirrhosis_____
Abnormal liver tests _____	Diabetes_____
High blood pressure _____	Delirium tremens _____
Gout _____	Anemia_____
Do you use tranquilizers? _____	Sedatives _____
Do you smoke?_____	History: Packs/day _____ Pack Years _____

Comments_____

II. Family History

High blood pressure _____   Alcohol dependence/drug dependence

Diabetes _____   Mother ____ / ____   Father ____ / ____

Liver disease_____   Siblings ____ / ____   Aunts/Uncles ____ / ____

                                                                          Grandparents ____ / ____

Comments_____

III. Social History

Occupation _____   Marital Status _____

Lives with whom _____

Children?_____

IV. Review of Systems

	Yes	No	Explain
Fatigue	_____	_____	_____
Anxiety	_____	_____	_____
Fever, Sweating	_____	_____	_____
HEENT			
Head Trauma	_____	_____	_____
Headaches	_____	_____	_____
Epistaxis	_____	_____	_____
Hoarseness	_____	_____	_____
Vision changes	_____	_____	_____
Cardiovascular			
Change in exercise tolerance	_____	_____	_____
Shortness of breath	_____	_____	_____
Chest pain/discomfort	_____	_____	_____
Palpitations	_____	_____	_____
Dizziness	_____	_____	_____

Substance Use History and Physical Examination - 2

IV. Review of Systems—cont'd   Yes   No   Explain

Gastrointestinal

Ingestion or nausea (especially A.M.) _____ _____ _____

Heavy retching _____ _____ _____

Vomiting (with blood?) _____ _____ _____

Abdominal pain _____ _____ _____

Jaundice _____ _____ _____

Diarrhea _____ _____ _____

Black "tarry" stools _____ _____ _____

Genitourinary

Trouble getting an erection _____ _____ _____

Polyuria _____ _____ _____

Amenorrhea _____ _____ _____

Neuropsychiatric

Tremors (especially A.M.) _____ _____ _____

Blackouts _____ _____ _____

Memory problems/changes _____ _____ _____

Periods of confusion _____ _____ _____

Hallucinations _____ _____ _____

Staggering/balance problems _____ _____ _____

Paresthesias _____ _____ _____

Muscle weakness _____ _____ _____

Depressed? Down mood _____ _____ _____

Change in appetite _____ _____ _____

Decreased energy level _____ _____ _____

Decreased activity level _____ _____ _____

Suicide attempts/ideation _____ _____ _____

Sleep (hrs.) _____   EMA _____   MCA _____   TFA _____   Changes _____

V. Substance Use History

Alcohol

Do you use alcohol? _____

How often (days per week) do you drink?_____

What do you prefer? _____ How much do you drink per day? _____

How many drinks until you feel happy? _____ How many until you feel drunk? _____

Is this more than it has taken in the past? _____

Has there been any change in your pattern over the past 6 months or 1 year? _____

What age did you begin using alcohol? _____

Have you ever drunk (in one day): Case of beer? _____ Fifth of liquor _____ Gallon of wine? _____

Have you ever used non-beverage alcohol? _____

Longest period without alcohol? _____

Why did you stop?_____

Did you experience any discomfort? (hallucinations, tremors, fever) _____

Substance Use History and Physical Examination - 3

V. Substance Use History—cont'd

Drugs

What drugs other than alcohol have you used? _____ How much _____

_____ _____

_____ _____

_____ _____

When did you last use these drugs? _____

When using, how much do you spend on drugs in a week? _____

Consequences of Use

Has drinking or drug use ever caused you to miss or be late for work? _____

Has drinking or drug use ever affected your relationships or home life? _____

How do you feel about your drinking or drug use? _____

Has your physician ever told you to cut down or quit? _____

Have you ever attended an AA meeting? _____ Why? _____

CAGE Screening Test

C _____ Have you ever felt the need to **C**ut down on your drinking?

A _____ Have you ever felt **A**nnoyed when others criticize your drinking?

G _____ Have you ever felt **G**uilty about your drinking?

E _____ Have you ever had a drink as an **E**ye opener to get going in the morning or to stop tremors?

When was your last drink? _____ How much? _____ What? _____

When was your last drug use? _____ What? _____ How much? _____

VI. PHYSICAL EXAMINATION

General

Appearance (dress, cleanliness, etc.) _____

Blood pressure _____ Respiratory rate _____ / minute

Pulse _____ Regular _____ Irregular _____ Explain _____

Behavior	Yes	No	Explain
Trouble getting an erection	___	___	_____
Anxious	___	___	_____
Irritable	___	___	_____
Uncooperative	___	___	_____
Hyperactive	___	___	_____
Alcohol on breath	___	___	_____

Dermatology

	Yes	No	
Vascular dilation	___	___	_____
Clubbing/edema	___	___	_____
Dupuytren's contractures	___	___	_____
Rhinophyma	___	___	_____
Palmar erythema	___	___	_____
Cigarette burns	___	___	_____
Spider nevi	___	___	_____
IV drug needle marks	___	___	_____

Other burns/scars not attributable to surgery? Where _____

Substance Use History and Physical Examination - 4

HEENT

Evidence of head trauma _____

Extraocular movements intact _____   Explain _____

Pupil Size _____   PERRLA _____   Sclera Clear _____   Icteric_____

Nasal septum: Intact _____

Periodontal Disease   Yes _____   No _____

Swollen Parotids   Yes _____   No _____

Chest

Gynecomastia _____

Lungs: Clear to A&P _____   Dullness _____   Rales _____   Rhonchi _____   Wheezes _____

Heart: PMI: size and location _____

Rhythm: Regular _____   Irregular _____   Explain _____

Sounds: S1 _____   S2 _____   Others? (S3, S4, Rubs, Gallops) _____

Murmur: (describe if possible) _____

Abdominal Examination

Bowel sounds (+ / −) _____

Ascites _____   Tenderness _____   Masses _____

Liver (size @ MCL) _____   Palpable? _____   Splenomegaly_____

Neuropsychiatric

Cranial nerves intact? _____

Cerebellar: Tremor _____   Tandem Walk _____   F to N _____   Romberg + /−? _____

Extremities

Sensory (upper + lower) intact_____

Symmetrical _____

Motor (upper + lower) intact_____

Symmetrical _____

Cognition

Object Retention   3@ _____ minute

World → _____   ←_____

Serial Sevens _____   _____   _____   _____   _____   _____   _____

Assessment of Alcohol Use/Drug Use _____

_____

_____

_____

Withdrawal Risk _____

_____

Interviewer's Name _____   Date_____

From Nordsey D, Smith N. (1989). Protocol for medical assessment, Project Cork Weekend Program. Hanover, NH. www.ProjectCork.org

Abuse Assessment Screen

Patient Name: _____

Date: _____

1. **WITHIN THE LAST YEAR,** have you been hit, slapped, kicked, or   YES   NO
   otherwise physically hurt by someone?
   If YES, by whom? _____
   Total number of times _____

2. **SINCE YOU'VE BEEN PREGNANT,** have you been hit, slapped,   YES   NO
   kicked, or otherwise physically hurt by someone?
   If YES, by whom? _____
   Total number of times _____

**MARK THE AREA OF INJURY ON THE BODY MAP. SCORE EACH INCIDENT
ACCORDING TO THE FOLLOWING SCALE:**

SCORE

1 = Threats of abuse including use of a weapon   _____
2 = Slapping, pushing; no injuries and/or lasting pain   _____
3 = Punching, kicking, bruises, cuts and/or continuing pain   _____
4 = Beating up, severe contusions, burns, broken bones   _____
5 = Head injury, internal injury, permanent injury   _____
6 = Use of weapon; wound from weapon   _____

If any of the descriptions for the higher number apply, use the higher number.

3. **WITHIN THE LAST YEAR,** has anyone forced you to have   **YES**   **NO**
   sexual activities?
   If YES, by whom? _____
   Total number of times _____

Completed by: _____
Date: _____

Developed by the Nursing Research Consortium on Violence and Abuse, Sockenk L et al, 2003.

Nutrition Forms

Chapter Contents

ICON KEY: 🗎 Tool Printed ✐ Tool on CD-ROM ∞ Customizable Tool **i** Information and Resources Provided for Further Acquisition

Nutritional Assessment

Nutritional screening may be completed periodically in the primary care setting and is recommended for all individuals. Screening forms may include questions about food and supplement intake patterns, current physical health issues, social factors that may influence food choices, eating habits, and environment. Individuals identified to be at nutritional risk and those who are likely to become at nutritional risk may be assessed further by the primary care clinician or referred to a registered dietician for comprehensive nutritional assessment and plan for care. The clinician should consider the reliability and validity of food frequency patterns that the patient recalls. If there are concerns regarding the accuracy of the reported intake, the clinician may consider using a food diary for a more factual survey. Many general nutritional screening forms are available; the clinician may choose from several included in this chapter.

GENERAL NUTRITIONAL ASSESSMENT FORMS

Nutritional Screening Initiative Forms

These forms were created by the Nutritional Screening Initiative, a joint project of the American Academy of Physicians, The American Dietetic Association, and the

National Council on the Aging, Inc. (Nutrition Interventions Manual, 1991):

- Level I Screen
  This nutritional screen may be used for adults or healthy older adults. The form includes questions on body weight, eating habits, and functional status. A nomogram for body mass index is included in this form.
- Level II Screen
  This screening and assessment tool is used for older adults or those at nutritional risk. The form includes all information in the Level I Screen, plus sections for anthropometric data, laboratory data, and indicators for medication use, physical impairments that may limit eating, conditions of the living environment, and mental/cognitive status.
- Determine Your Nutritional Health
  This quick and easy screening tool provides a "nutritional score," which indicates individual nutritional risk. Warning signs of nutritional risk are explained, and the completed form may be given to the patient for educational purposes.
- Medications Use Checklist
  This checklist provides a simple scoring method to determine whether an individual is at increased risk for adverse interactions related to food/nutrients and use of prescribed medications or over-the-counter drugs

Nutrition History

This form records the daily or weekly frequency of intake from the various food groups, beverage intake, and meals away from home (frequency and type). Daily frequencies of meals and snacks and television snacking habits are also addressed.

General Food Frequency Questionnaire

This form includes questions regarding frequency of intake from the various food groups with more specific foods listed, beverage consumption, sugar/sugar substitute intake, salt use, and snacking habits.

Food Intake Record

This form allows the user to record recalled intake from a comprehensive list of food types with three choices: less than once a week, not daily but at least once a week, and daily. Specific amounts are not recorded. A brief table to record the usual daily eating pattern is included at the bottom of the page.

Nutrition History Form

This form is geared toward weight management and includes an area for anthropomorphic data (height and weight) and goal weight/body mass index. Questions pertain to eating habits, use of beverages and gum, chewing problems, supplements, food tolerances, special diet history, and meals away from home. The form does not address frequency of intake from various food groups.

Initial Nutrition Assessment

This form provides a more comprehensive general assessment in preparation for nutrition counseling. It includes current and past medical history; brief family and social history; space for results of relevant laboratory tests; medications: and use of laxatives, diuretics, insulin, and supplements. Also included are weight history, activities, food allergies and aversions, appetite and related issues, and psychosocial factors affecting eating habits. At the bottom of the form are areas for nutritional diagnosis and dietary intake analysis. This form does not include frequency of intake from various food groups.

FOOD DIARIES

In contrast to the food frequency forms described previously, the food diaries are used to record dietary intake as it occurs. Food diaries recorded on the same day as the food is eaten are considered to be more accurate than a food frequency questionnaire, which depends on retrospective recall. The dietary record allows the clinician to evaluate the nutrient intake over a certain time period. Dieticians recommend a period of 3 to 7 days for record keeping, after which the nutrient intake may be calculated and averaged. Comparison with standardized guidelines, such as Recommended Dietary Allowances (RDAs) or food pyramids, may then be made.

Food Diary

This food diary allows the individual to record all food intake without assigning the foods to a particular meal or snack. The table allows the individual to record where the food is eaten, with whom it is eaten, other activities done while eating, and emotional feelings at the time of eating. This survey may be open-ended in that patients may be given any number of copies of this form for a predetermined period for dietary analysis or for home use in dietary management.

One-Day (24-Hour) Record of Food Intake

This three-page form provides the user with more specific food choices for the standard three daily meals and snacks. The recording individual may check off the foods eaten, list the method of preparation, and indicate amounts. Each standard meal offers traditional North American food choices for that meal. Although there is space at the bottom of each page to record other foods eaten, consideration should be given to the suitability of this form for individuals who do not follow the typical North American diet.

SPECIFIC NUTRITIONAL ASSESSMENT FORMS

Comprehensive nutritional assessment is recommended for all persons at nutritional risk (Box 6-1). Initial nutritional screening allows for identification of such individuals, and referral for comprehensive nutritional assessment and a care plan may be made. Comprehensive assessment, as performed by a registered dietician, includes complete medical history, physical examination, anthropometric data, and laboratory data. For primary care purposes, initial nutritional assessment may be completed for certain patient populations before referral for specialized plans. Forms for two such populations, perinatal mothers and patients with eating disorders, are included here.

Use of herbal, botanical, and dietary supplements has increased as the public has become more educated about disease prevention and health promotion. Self-treatment trials and regular use of such products are implemented by consumers who may not inform their health care providers of their practices. There are potential risks for interactions between supplements and prescribed medications. Data obtained by the primary care provider regarding supplement use provide information for subsequent counseling to reduce the risk of untoward interactions or effects from use of such products.

Perinatal Nutrition Screening/Assessment Form

This screening and assessment tool is designed to identify women at nutritional risk during the perinatal period. Screening criteria include antepartum, postpartum, and breastfeeding risk factors. Below screening criteria are boxes to record assessment data pertinent to perinatal nutritional health. The last box provides the clinician with a space to record the estimated nutritional needs, the adequacy of intake, and evaluation of nutritional status.

Box **6-1**	Conditions with Potential for Nutritional Risk

Acute illnesses
Chronic diseases
Use of certain medications
Obesity
Disordered eating diagnoses
Substance abuse
Hospitalization for more than 2 weeks
Trauma
Cachexia
Advanced age
Infancy and childhood
Pregnancy
Lower economic status
Social isolation

From Mahan LK, Escott-Stump DD, 2004; Hensrud DD, 1999.

Eating Disorder Nutritional Assessment Form

This form focuses on topics pertinent to the patient with a diagnosed eating disorder. There are sections to record weight history, anthropometric data, body image information, food allergies, menstrual history, medications, and bowel function. Dietary intake documentation includes a 24-hour recall, fluid intake, vitamin/mineral/other supplement use, and consumption of sugar/fat substitutes and miscellaneous products. Disordered eating practices including binging, self-induced vomiting, and use of laxatives and diuretics as well as exercise practices are addressed.

Herbal, Botanical, and Dietary Supplement Intake Form

This patient questionnaire contains numbered questions with check-off boxes on the topics of supplement use history, medical conditions, use of over-the-counter and prescription medications, use of alcohol or tobacco, allergies, pregnancy status, and current diet/eating plan. Following the questions is a table listing commonly used herbal and nutritional supplements with space to record dosing information.

Resources and References

Online Resources

American Dietetic Association (ADA): http://www.eatright.org/ Professional and public nutrition information including policies and publications from the ADA.

Nutrition Interventions Manual for Professionals Caring for Older Americans. Executive Summary: AAFP, ADA and National Council on Aging, Washington, DC, 1991, Nutrition Screening Initiative: http://www.aafp.org/nsi.xml A summary of this manual with tables, charts, and screening tools is available at : http://www.rosslearningcenter.com/default.asp?pageID=13&itemID=298

The Food and Nutrition Information Center (FNIC), National Agricultural Library, U.S. Department of Agriculture and the Agricultural Research Service: http://www.nal.usda.gov/fnic/ The Food and Nutrition Information Center (FNIC), a division of the United States Department of Agriculture (USDA), provides access to the food and human nutrition collection at the National Agricultural Library, consultation with nutritional staff, and referral to a wide variety of resources on nutrition topics and databases.

Vitamin and Mineral Supplements, MEDLINE Plus Health Information, National Library of Medicine: http://www.nlm.nih.gov/medlineplus/vitaminandmineralsupplements.html

References and Suggested Readings

American Academy of Pediatrics Committee on Adolescence: American Academy of Pediatrics policy statement: identifying and treating eating disorders, *Pediatrics* 111:204-211, 2003.

American Dietetic Association: *Medical nutrition therapy across the continuum*, ed 2, Chicago, 1998, American Dietetic Association.

American Dietetic Association: Standards of professional practice for dietetics professionals, *J Am Diet Assoc* 98:83-87, 1998.

Eisenberg DM et al: Trends in alternative medicine use in the United States, 1990-1997, *JAMA* 280:1569-1575, 1998.

Escott-Stump S: *Nutrition and diagnosis-related care*, ed 5, Philadelphia, 2002, Lippincott, Williams & Wilkins.

Grodner M, Long S, DeYoung S: *Foundations and clinical applications of nutrition, a nursing approach*, ed 3, revised reprint with Nutritrac 3.0 software, St Louis, 2004, Mosby.

Hark L, Deeb D: Taking a nutrition history: a practical approach for family physicians, *Am Family Physician* 59:1521-1528, 1531-1532, 1999.

Hensrud DD: Nutrition screening and assessment, *Med Clin North Am* 83:1525-1546, 1999.

Mahan LK, Escott-Stump S: *Krause's food, nutrition, & diet therapy*, ed 11, Philadelphia, 2004, WB Saunders.

Williams SR, Schlenker E: *Essentials of nutrition and diet therapy*, ed 8, St Louis, 2003, Mosby.

LEVEL I SCREEN

Body Weight

Measure height to the nearest inch and weigh to the nearest pound. Record the values below and mark them on the Body Mass Index (BMI) scale to the right. Then use a straight edge (ruler) to connect the two points and circle the spot where this straight line crosses the center line (body mass index). Record the number below.

Healthy older adults should have a BMI between 24 and 27.

Height (in): _____

Weight (lbs): _____

Body Mass Index: _____
(number from center column)

Check any boxes that are true for the individual:

☐ Has lost or gained 10 pounds (or more) in the past 6 months.

☐ Body mass index < 24

☐ Body mass index > 27

A physician should be contacted if the individual has gained or lost 10 pounds unexpectedly or without intending to during the past 6 months. A physician should also be notified if the individual's body mass index is above 27 or below 24.

For the remaining sections, please ask the individual which of the statements (if any) is true for him or her and place a check by each that applies.

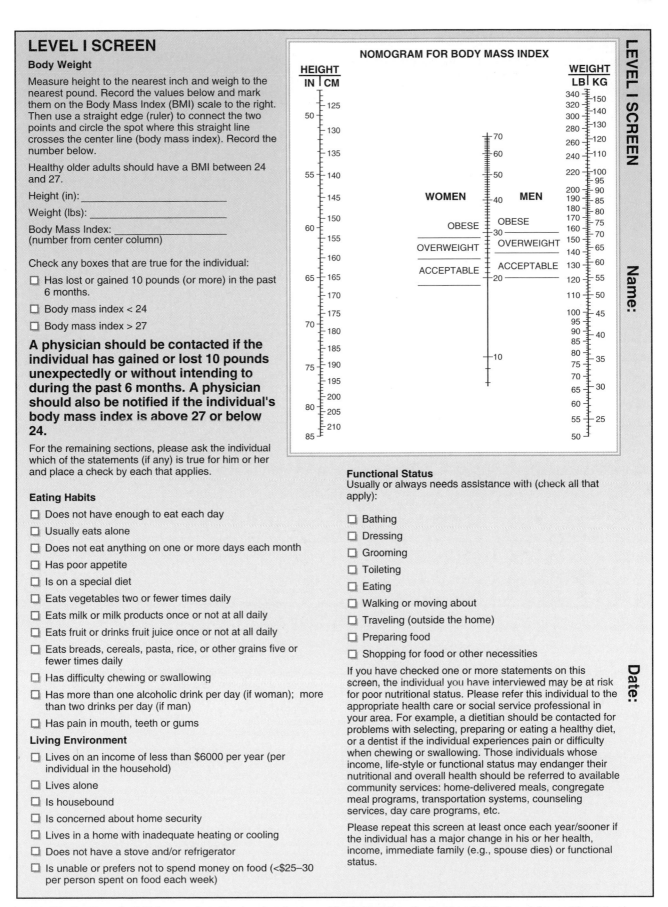

NOMOGRAM FOR BODY MASS INDEX

HEIGHT IN/CM — WEIGHT LB/KG

WOMEN — MEN

OBESE — OBESE
OVERWEIGHT — OVERWEIGHT
ACCEPTABLE — ACCEPTABLE

Eating Habits

☐ Does not have enough to eat each day

☐ Usually eats alone

☐ Does not eat anything on one or more days each month

☐ Has poor appetite

☐ Is on a special diet

☐ Eats vegetables two or fewer times daily

☐ Eats milk or milk products once or not at all daily

☐ Eats fruit or drinks fruit juice once or not at all daily

☐ Eats breads, cereals, pasta, rice, or other grains five or fewer times daily

☐ Has difficulty chewing or swallowing

☐ Has more than one alcoholic drink per day (if woman); more than two drinks per day (if man)

☐ Has pain in mouth, teeth or gums

Living Environment

☐ Lives on an income of less than $6000 per year (per individual in the household)

☐ Lives alone

☐ Is housebound

☐ Is concerned about home security

☐ Lives in a home with inadequate heating or cooling

☐ Does not have a stove and/or refrigerator

☐ Is unable or prefers not to spend money on food (<$25–30 per person spent on food each week)

Functional Status

Usually or always needs assistance with (check all that apply):

☐ Bathing

☐ Dressing

☐ Grooming

☐ Toileting

☐ Eating

☐ Walking or moving about

☐ Traveling (outside the home)

☐ Preparing food

☐ Shopping for food or other necessities

If you have checked one or more statements on this screen, the individual you have interviewed may be at risk for poor nutritional status. Please refer this individual to the appropriate health care or social service professional in your area. For example, a dietitian should be contacted for problems with selecting, preparing or eating a healthy diet, or a dentist if the individual experiences pain or difficulty when chewing or swallowing. Those individuals whose income, life-style or functional status may endanger their nutritional and overall health should be referred to available community services: home-delivered meals, congregate meal programs, transportation systems, counseling services, day care programs, etc.

Please repeat this screen at least once each year/sooner if the individual has a major change in his or her health, income, immediate family (e.g., spouse dies) or functional status.

LEVEL I SCREEN   Name: Date:

From the Nutrition Screening Initiative, a project of the American Academy of Family Physicians, the American Dietetic Association, and the National Council on the Aging, Inc., and funded in part by a grant from Ross Products Division, Abbott Laboratories.

LEVEL II SCREEN

Complete the following screen by interviewing the patient directly and/or by referring to the patient chart. If you do not routinely perform all of the described tests or ask all of the listed questions, please consider including them, but do not be concerned if the entire screen is not completed. Please try to conduct a minimal screen on as many older patients as possible, and please try to collect serial measurements, which are extremely valuable in monitoring nutritional status. Please refer to the manual for additional information.

Anthropometrics

Measure height to the nearest inch and weigh to the nearest pound. Record the values below and mark them on the Body Mass Index (BMI) scale to the right. Then use a straight edge (paper, ruler) to connect the two points and circle the spot where this straight line crosses the center line (body mass index). Record the number below. Healthy older adults should have a BMI between 24 and 27; check the appropriate box to flag an abnormally high or low value.

Height (in): _____

Weight (lbs): _____

Body Mass Index: _____
(number from center column)

Please place a check by any statement regarding BMI and recent weight loss that is true for the patient:

- ☐ Body mass index < 24
- ☐ Body mass index > 27
- ☐ Has lost or gained 10 pounds (or more) in the past 6 months.

Record the measurement of mid-arm circumference to the nearest 0.1 centimeter and of triceps skinfold to the nearest 2 millimeters.

Mid-arm circumference (cm): _____

Triceps skinfold (mm): _____

Mid-arm muscle circumference (cm): _____

Refer to the table and check any abnormal values:

- ☐ Mid-arm muscle circumference < 10th percentile
- ☐ Triceps skinfold < 10th percentile
- ☐ Triceps skinfold > 95th percentile

Note: mid-arm circumference (cm) − {0.314 x triceps skinfold (mm)} = mid-arm *muscle* circumference (cm)

Percentile	Men		Women	
	55–65 y	65–75 y	55–65 y	65–75 y
Arm circumference (cm)				
10th	27.3	26.3	25.7	25.2
50th	31.7	30.7	30.3	29.9
95th	36.9	35.5	38.5	37.3
Arm muscle circumference (cm)				
10th	24.5	23.5	19.6	19.5
50th	27.8	26.8	22.5	22.5
95th	32.0	30.6	28.0	27.9
Triceps skinfold (mm)				
10th	6	6	16	14
50th	11	11	25	24
95th	22	22	22	36

For the remaining sections, please place a check by any statements that are true for the patient.

Laboratory Data

- ☐ Serum albumin below 3.5 g/dL
- ☐ Serum cholesterol below 160 mg/dL
- ☐ Serum cholesterol above 240 mg/dL

Drug Use

- ☐ Three or more prescription drugs, OTC medications, and/or vitamin/mineral supplements daily

Clinical Features

Presence of (check all that apply)

- ☐ Problems with mouth, teeth or gums
- ☐ Difficulty chewing
- ☐ Angular stomatitis
- ☐ Glossitis
- ☐ History of bone pain
- ☐ History of bone fractures
- ☐ Skin changes (dry, loose, nonspecific lesions, edema)

NOMOGRAM FOR BODY MASS INDEX

HEIGHT IN CM		WEIGHT LB KG

WOMEN   MEN

OBESE   OBESE

OVERWEIGHT   OVERWEIGHT

ACCEPTABLE   ACCEPTABLE

Eating Habits

- ☐ Does not have enough to eat each day
- ☐ Usually eats alone
- ☐ Does not eat anything on one or more days each month
- ☐ Has poor appetite
- ☐ Is on a special diet
- ☐ Eats vegetables two or fewer times daily
- ☐ Eats milk or milk products once or not at all daily
- ☐ Eats fruit or drinks fruit juice once or not at all daily
- ☐ Eats breads, cereals, pasta, rice, or other grains five or fewer times daily
- ☐ Has more than one alcoholic drink per day (if woman); more than two drinks per day (if man)

Living Environment

- ☐ Lives on an income of less than $6000 per year (per individual in the household)
- ☐ Lives alone
- ☐ Is housebound
- ☐ Is concerned about home security
- ☐ Lives in a home with inadequate heating or cooling
- ☐ Does not have a stove and/or refrigerator
- ☐ Is unable or prefers not to spend money on food (<$25–30 per person spent on food each week)

Functional Status

Usually or always needs assistance with (check all that apply)

- ☐ Bathing
- ☐ Dressing
- ☐ Grooming
- ☐ Toileting
- ☐ Eating
- ☐ Walking or moving about
- ☐ Traveling (outside the home)
- ☐ Preparing food
- ☐ Shopping for food or other necessities

Mental/Cognitive Status

- ☐ Clinical evidence of impairment (e.g., Folstein < 26)
- ☐ Clinical evidence of depressive illness (e.g., Beck Depression Inventory > 15, Geriatric Depression Scale > 5)

From the Nutrition Screening Initiative, a project of the American Academy of Family Physicians, the American Dietetic Association, and the National Council on the Aging, Inc., and funded in part by a grant from Ross Products Division, Abbott Laboratories.

LEVEL II SCREEN   Name: Date:

DETERMINE YOUR NUTRITIONAL HEALTH

The Warning Signs of poor nutritional health are often overlooked.
Use this checklist to find out if you or someone you know is at nutritional risk.

Read the statements below. Circle the number in the yes column for those that apply to you or someone you know. For each yes answer, score the number in the box. Total your nutrition score.

	YES
I have an illness or condition that made me change the kind and/or amount of food I eat.	2
I eat fewer than 2 meals per day.	3
I eat few fruits or vegetables, or milk products.	2
I have 3 or more drinks of beer, liquor or wine almost every day.	2
I have tooth or mouth problems that make it hard for me to eat.	2
I don't always have enough money to buy the food I need.	4
I eat alone most of the time.	1
I take 3 or more different prescribed or over-the-counter drugs a day.	1
Without wanting to, I have lost or gained 10 pounds in the last 6 months.	2
I am not physically able to shop, cook and/or feed myself.	2
TOTAL	

Total Your Nutritional Score. If it's —

0–2 **Good!** Recheck your nutritional score in 6 months.

3–5 **You are at moderate nutritional risk.** See what can be done to improve your eating habits and lifestyle. Your office on aging, senior nutrition program, senior citizens center or health department can help. Recheck your nutritional score in 3 months.

6 or more **You are at high nutritional risk.** Bring this checklist the next time you see your doctor, dietitian or other qualified health or social service professional. Talk with them about any problems you may have. Ask for help to improve your nutritional health.

Remember that warning signs suggest risk, but do not represent diagnosis of any condition.

The Nutrition Checklist is based on the Warning Signs described below.
Use the word DETERMINE to remind you of the Warning signs.

Disease   Any disease, illness or chronic condition which causes you to change the way you eat, or makes it hard for you to eat, puts your nutritional health at risk. Four out of five adults have chronic diseases that are affected by diet. Confusion or memory loss that keeps getting worse is estimated to affect one out of five or more of older adults. This can make it hard to remember what, when or if you've eaten. Feeling sad or depressed, which happens to about one in eight older adults, can cause big changes in appetite, digestion, energy level, weight and well-being.

Eating Poorly   Eating too little and eating too much both lead to poor health. Eating the same foods day after day or not eating fruit, vegetables, and milk products daily will also cause poor nutritional health. One in five adults skip meals daily. Only 13% of adults eat the minimum amount of fruit and vegetables needed. One in four older adults drink too much alcohol. Many health problems become worse if you drink more than one or two alcoholic beverages per day.

Tooth Loss/Mouth Pain   A healthy mouth, teeth and gums are needed to eat. Missing, loose or rotten teeth, or dentures which don't fit well or cause mouth sores, make it hard to eat.

Economic Hardship   As many as 40% of older Americans have incomes of less than $6,000 per year. Having less—or choosing to spend less— than $25–30 per week for food makes it very hard to get the foods you need to stay healthy.

Reduced Social Contact   One-third of all older people live alone. Being with people daily has a positive effect on morale, well-being and eating.

Multiple Medicines   Many older Americans must take medicines for health problems. Almost half of older Americans take multiple medicines daily. Growing old may change the way we respond to drugs. The more medicines you take, the greater the chance for side effects, such as increased or decreased appetite, change in taste, constipation, weakness, drowsiness, diarrhea, nausea, and others. Vitamins or minerals, when taken in large doses, act like drugs and can cause harm. Alert your doctor to everything you take.

Involuntary Weight Loss/Gain   Losing or gaining a lot of weight when you are not trying to do so is an important warning sign that must not be ignored. Being overweight or underweight also increases your chance of poor health.

Needs Assistance in Self-Care   Although most older people are able to eat, one out of every five has trouble walking, shopping, or buying and cooking food, especially as they get older.

Elder Years Above Age 80   Most older people lead full and productive lives. But as age increases, the risk of frailty and health problems increases. Checking your nutritional health regularly makes good sense.

Reprinted with permission by the Nutrition Screening Initiative, a project of the American Academy of Family Physicians, the American Dietetic Association, and the Nathional Council on the Aging, Inc., and funded in part by a grant from Ross Products Division, Abbott Laboratories.

The Warning Signs of poor nutritional health are often overlooked. Use this checklist to find out if you or someone you know is at nutritional risk because of factors related to over-the-counter drugs or prescribed medications.

MEDICATIONS USE CHECKLIST

Read the statements below. Circle the number in the yes column for those that apply to you or someone you know. For each yes answer, add the number in the box. Write the total in the last box.

	YES
I do not know if I should take my medications before or after eating.	1
I take 3 or more medications each day.	2
I have gained or lost more than 10 lbs. since I started taking my medications.	1
I go to more than one pharmacy or drugstore to get my prescriptions filled.	2
I do not always ask my doctor about the safety of taking prescribed medications or vitamins and minerals.	2
I take one or more of the following medications: (Check the ones you take.) ( ) Digoxin ( ) Lithium ( ) Theophylline ( ) Phenytoin (Dilantin) and my doctor does not check my blood level.	2
I drink 2 or more alcoholic beverages on a daily basis.	2
I take insulin or pills for the control of diabetes and I sometimes skip my supper and/or bedtime snack.	2
I cannot read the labels on my medication.	2
TOTAL	

Total Your Medications Used Score.

If it's more than 2, you may have a problem with your health because of your medications and diet. Talk with your doctor or pharmacist. Bring this checklist the next time you see them. Remember that warning signs suggest risk, but do not represent diagnosis of any condition.

The Nutrition Screening Initiative
1010 Wisconsin Avenue, NW, Suite 800
Washington, DC 20007

These materials developed and distributed by the Nutrition Screening Initiative, a project of:

 AMERICAN ACADEMY
OF FAMILY PHYSICIANS

 THE AMERICAN
DIETETIC ASSOCIATION

 NATIONAL COUNCIL
ON THE AGING

The Nutrition Screening Initiative is funded in part by a grant from Ross Products Division of Abbott Laboratories.

Reprinted with permission by the Nutrition Screening Initiative, a project of the American Academy of Family Physicians, the American Dietetic Association, and the Nathional Council on the Aging, Inc., and funded in part by a grant from Ross Products Division, Abbott Laboratories.

Nutrition History

Date of Visit: _____

Patient Name: _____

Address: _____

*Telephone: (home)*_____ *(business)* _____   *Completed by:* _____

Date of Birth: _____ *Age:* _____ *Gender:* Male Female   *Language* _____ *Interpreter present:* ☐ Yes ☐ No

Provider: _____   *Reliability:* ☐ Adequate   ☐ Inadequate

1. How many meals and snacks do you eat each day?

   Meals _____   Snacks _____

2. How many times a week do you eat the following meals away from home?

   Breakfast _____   Lunch _____   Dinner _____

   What types of eating places do you frequently visit? (Check all that apply)

   Fast-food _____   Diner/cafeteria _____

   Restaurant _____   Other _____

3. On average, how many pieces of fruit or glasses of juice do you eat or drink each day?

   Fresh fruit _____   Juice (8 oz cup) _____

4. On average, how many servings of vegetables do you eat each day? _____

5. On average, how many times a week do you eat a high-fiber breakfast cereal? _____

6. How many times a week do you eat red meat (beef, lamb, veal) or pork? _____

7. How many times a week do you eat chicken or turkey? _____

8. How many times a week do you eat fish or shellfish? _____

9. How many hours of television do you watch every day? _____

   Do you usually snack while watching television?   Yes _____   No _____

10. How many times a week do you eat desserts and sweets? _____

11. What types of beverages do you usually drink? How many servings of each do you drink a day?

    Water _____   Milk: _____   Alcohol: _____

    Juice _____   Whole milk _____   Beer _____

    Soda _____   2% milk _____   Wine _____

    Diet soda _____   1% milk _____   Hard liquor _____

    Sports drinks _____   Skim milk _____

    Iced tea _____

    Iced tea with sugar _____

Reprinted with permission from Hark L, Deeb D: Taking a nutrition history: a practical approach for family physicians, *Am Family Physician* 59: 1521-1528, 1531-1532, 1999.

150

General Food Frequency Questionnaire

Date of Visit: _____

Patient Name: _____

Address: _____

Telephone: (home)_____ (business) _____ Completed by: _____

Date of Birth:_____ Age:____ Gender: Male Female   Language _____ Interpreter present: ☐ Yes ☐ No

Provider: _____   Reliability: ☐ Adequate ☐ Inadequate

1. Do you drink milk? _____ If so, how much? _____ What kind? ☐ Whole ☐ Skim ☐ Low-fat

2. Do you use fat? _____ If so, what kind? _____ How much? _____

3. How many times do you eat meat? _____ Eggs? _____ Cheese? _____ Beans? _____

4. Do you eat snack foods? _____ If so, which ones? _____ How often? _____ How much? _____

5. What vegetables (in each group) do you eat? How often?

   a. broccoli _____ green peppers _____ cooked greens _____ carrots _____ sweet potato _____

   b. tomatoes _____ raw cabbage _____

   c. asparagus _____ beets _____ cauliflower _____ corn _____ cooked cabbage _____ celery _____ peas _____ lettuce _____

6. What fruits (in each group) do you eat? How often?

   a. apples or applesauce _____ apricots _____ bananas _____ berries _____ cherries _____ grapes or grape juice _____ peaches _____ pears _____ pineapple _____ plums _____ prunes _____ raisins _____

   b. oranges _____ orange juice _____ grapefruit _____ grapefruit juice _____

7. Bread and cereal products

   a. How much bread do you usually eat with each meal? _____ How much between meals? _____

   b. Do you eat cereal? _____ ☐ daily ☐ weekly What type: ☐ cooked ☐ dry

   c. How often do you eat foods such as macaroni, spaghetti, noodles, rice, etc.? _____

   d. Do you eat whole grain breads and cereals? _____ How often? _____

8. Do you use salt? _____ Do you salt your food before tasting it? _____ Do you cook with salt? _____
   Do you crave salt or salty foods? _____

9. How many teaspoons of sugar do you use daily? (Please include sugar on cereal, fruit, toast, and in coffee, tea, etc.) _____

10. Do you eat desserts? _____ If so, what kind? _____ How often? _____

11. Do you drink sugar-containing beverages, such as soda pop or sweetened juice drinks? _____ How often? _____
    How much? _____

12. How often do you eat candy or cookies? _____

13. Do you drink water? _____ How often during the day? _____ How much each time? _____
    How much water would you say you drink each day? _____

14. Do you use sugar substitutes in packet form or in drinks? _____ If so, what type do you use? _____ How often? _____

15. Do you drink alcohol? _____ How often? _____ How much? _____ Type: ☐ beer ☐ wine ☐ liquor

16. Do you drink caffeinated beverages? _____ How often? _____ How much per day? _____ Type: ☐ coffee ☐ tea ☐ soda

Record answers with the appropriate time frame (e.g., 1/day, 1/wk, 3/mo) or as accurately as possible. The frequency may need to be recorded as "occasionally" or "rarely" if answers are not more specific.

From General Food Frequency Questionnaire. From Mahan K, Stump S: *Krause's Food Nutrition & Diet Therapy,* ed 11, Philadelphia, 2004, Saunders.

Food Intake Record

Date of Visit: _____

Patient Name: _____

Address: _____

Telephone: (home)_____ (business) _____   *Completed by:* _____

Date of Birth: _____ *Age:* _____ *Gender:* Male Female   *Language* _____ *Interpreter present:* ☐ Yes ☐ No

Provider: _____   *Reliability:* ☐ Adequate ☐ Inadequate

Please indicate which foods you eat.

	Less than once a week	Not daily but at least once a week	Daily
Milk, yogurt			
Cheese			
Red meat			
Poultry			
Fish			
Eggs			
Mixed dishes			
Dried beans, legumes			
Peanut butter			
Nuts			
Breads, cereal			
Potatoes, pasta, rice			
Fruits, juices			
Vegetables			
Margarine, butter			
Cooking oil			
Sour cream, salad dressing			
Ice cream			
Cookies, cake, pie			
Candy			
Soft drink			
Coffee			
Tea, iced tea			
Alcohol			

Describe your usual daily eating pattern (include amount eaten).

Time	Meal	Food/method of preparation	Amount eaten	Calculations (for RD)
	Breakfast			
	Snack			
	Lunch			
	Dinner			
	Snack			

Nutrition History Form

Name: _____

Date: _____

Occupation: _____

Height: _____   Present Weight: _____

To be completed by dietician
GOAL WEIGHT _____ BMI _____

1. How would you generally describe your eating habits? ☐ Good ☐ Fair ☐ Poor

2. Has your appetite changed recently? ☐ Yes ☐ No

3. How many times a day do you eat? _____

4. How long does it usually take to complete a meal? _____

5. When you chew your food, do you: Take your time? _____ Chew a few times, then swallow? _____

6. Do you use a straw to drink beverages? ☐ Yes ☐ No

7. Do you chew gum? ☐ Yes ☐ No If so, how often? _____

8. Number of carbonated beverages daily _____

9. Number of caffeinated beverages daily (coffee, regular colas, and tea)
   _____ cups of coffee (regular)
   _____ cans of cola or other beverage (regular, diet, Tab®, Mellow Yellow®, Red Bull®, Jolt®, Mountain Dew®, Surge®, etc.)
   _____ cups of tea (regular)

10. Do you have dentures? ☐ Yes ☐ No If so, do you wear them at mealtime? ☐ Yes ☐ No

11. Do you have problems chewing? ☐ Yes ☐ No

12. Do you take any vitamin or mineral supplements? ☐ Yes ☐ No Describe: _____

13. List any foods that you do **NOT** tolerate: _____

14. Are you now on or have you ever followed any special diet? ☐ Yes ☐ No
    If so, what type of diet? _____

15. How often do you eat out? _____ times a week. What types of restaurants? _____

Initial Nutrition Assessment (Adult)

Patient Name: _____

Date: _____

Medical Record #: _____

Date of Birth: _____ *Age:* _____ *Gender:* Male Female

Referring Clinician: _____

Diagnoses:
Problems: 1) _____   2) _____   3) _____   4) _____

Vision Problems: _____   **Hearing Problems:** _____   **Ambulation Problems:** _____

Occupation: _____   **Hours of Work:** _____   **Stress Level:** _____

Household Members' Ages/Health: _____

Ethnic Background: _____

Country of Origin: _____   **Years in U.S.:** _____   **Years in School:** _____   **Language:** _____   **Needs Interpreter:** _____

Family Hx: CAD/Athero: _____   HTN: _____   High Chol: _____   DM: _____   CVA: _____

CA: Site _____   **Other:** _____

Medical Hx: Onset of Disease: _____   (mo/yr) Type of Treatment: _____

Previous MNT   Yes _____   No _____   If yes, when: _____   where: _____

Diet Order _____   **Nourishments** _____

Relevant Labs: Gluc   BUN   Creat   Chol   TG   Ca++   Phos   Na++   K+   Alb   Hgb/Hct   I & O _____

   Other: _____

Medications/Interactions: _____

Laxatives: _____   **Diuretics:** _____   **Insulin:** _____

Vitamins/Minerals _____   **Herbs/Botanicals** _____

Weight History:

Height: _____   Current Weight: _____   Usual Weight: _____   Wt Changes over _____ mo/yr

Highest Weight: _____   Lowest Weight: _____   Desired Weight/Why _____

Attempts at Wt Changes. _____

Activity: Type: _____   Duration/Frequency: _____

Food Allergies: _____

Food Aversions: _____

Appetite: good/fair/poor   **Difficulty chewing/swallowing**   **Nausea/vomiting/constipation/diarrhea**

Food Purchase/Prep: _____

Religious, Ethnic, Economic: _____   **Food Assist:** _____

Psychosocial Factors: _____   **Smokes:** _____ ppd

Readiness to Learn: _____

Nutritional Status: _____   Mild protein–calorie malnutrition (weight loss under 5%, albumin 3.2 or higher)

_____   Nutritional marasmus (alb over 3.2 g/dl, weight loss over 10%)

_____   Kwashiorkor (alb below 3.2 g/dl; weight loss under 10%)

_____   Mixed PCM (malnutrition with hypoalbuminemia and weight loss 25% or more)

Dietary Intake Analysis: Meal/Snack Times: _____

Kcal _____   CHO _____ g(_____%)   Pro _____ g(_____%)   Fat _____ g (_____%)   Sat Fat _____   Chol _____ mg

Na _____ g   K _____ g   Ca _____ mg   Fe _____ mg   Folate _____ mg   Mg _____ mg   B6 _____ mg   vit E _____ IU

Fiber _____ g   ETOH _____   Caffeine _____ mg   H2O _____ cc   Findings: _____

ASSESSED NEEDS: Protein _____ g/Kg/day = _____   Kcals _____ kcals/Kg/day = _____   Fluids: _____ cc/Kg/day = _____

Dietitian: _____   **Date of Review:** _____   **Follow-Up Date:** _____

Food Diary

Name: _____

Date: _____

Time	Food type and amount	Where eaten and with whom	Other activity while eating	How you feel before eating (e.g., anxious, bored, tired, angry, depressed)

A One-Day (24-Hour) Record of Food Intake

Name: _____

Date of Record: _____

BREAKFAST: Time Eaten _____

Food/Beverage	Type and/or Method of Preparation (List Ingredients)	Amount
MILK		
FRUIT Fresh, canned, sweetened, etc.		
CEREAL _____ with milk _____ with sugar _____ other	Brand _____	
BREAD _____ margarine/butter _____ mayonnaise _____ other	White _____ Brown _____	
EGGS		
MEAT or OTHER PROTEIN		
BEVERAGE _____ with milk _____ with sugar _____ other		
OTHER FOODS		

Did you eat a mid-morning snack?   Yes _____   No _____   If yes, time? _____
(list foods and beverages eaten)

_____

_____

A One-Day (24-Hour) Record of Food Intake - 2

Noon Meal: Time Eaten _____

Food/Beverage	Type and/or Method of Preparation (List Ingredients)	Amount
SOUP		
BREAD _____ margarine/butter _____ mayonnaise _____ other	White _____ Brown _____	
_____ MEAT _____ EGG _____ FISH _____ CHEESE		
VEGETABLES _____ cooked _____ raw _____ topping/seasoning (butter, white sauce, cheese sauce, etc.)		
SALAD _____ dressing (brand, etc)		
FRUIT Fresh, canned, sweetened, etc.		
MILK		
BEVERAGE _____ with milk _____ with sugar _____ other		
DESSERT		
OTHER FOODS		

Did you eat an afternoon snack?   Yes _____   No _____   If yes, time? _____
(list foods and beverages eaten)

_____

_____

A One-Day (24-Hour) Record of Food Intake - 3

Evening Meal: Time Eaten _____

Food/Beverage	Type and/or Method of Preparation (List Ingredients)	Amount
MAIN DISH _____ meat _____ cheese _____ poultry _____ other protein _____ pasta _____ rice		
VEGETABLES _____ cooked _____ raw _____ topping/seasoning (butter, white sauce, cheese sauce, etc.)		
SALAD _____ dressing (brand, etc)		
BREAD _____ margarine/butter _____ mayonnaise _____ other	White _____ Brown _____	
FRUIT Fresh, canned, sweetened, etc.		
MILK		
BEVERAGE _____ with milk _____ with sugar _____ other		
DESSERT		
OTHER FOODS		

Did you eat an afternoon snack?   Yes _____   No _____   If yes, time? _____
(list foods and beverages eaten)

_____

_____

Perinatal Nutrition Screening/Assessment Form

Date of Visit: _____

Patient Name: _____

Medical Record #: _____

Address: _____

Telephone: (home) _____ *(business)* _____   *Informant/Relationship:* _____

Date of Birth: _____ *Age:* _____ *Gender:* Male Female   *Language* _____ *Interpreter present:* ☐ Yes ☐ No

Provider: _____   *Reliability:* ☐ Adequate ☐ Inadequate

SCREENING CRITERIA FOR POTENTIAL NUTRITIONAL RISK *(full assessment if one checked)*

SCREENING CRITERIA FOR POTENTIAL NUTRITIONAL RISK

ANTEPARTUM

☐ Obstetrical Condition (Multiple Gestation, PIH, IUGR, Diabetes, Hyperemesis, Anemia)
☐ Chronic/Systemic Condition Affecting Nutritional Status or Intake
☐ Adolescence (≤17)   ☐ Inappropriate Weight Change
☐ Albumin ≤2.5   ☐ Therapeutic or Limited Diet
☐ Lack of Knowledge re Pregnancy Diet   ☐ Length of Stay ≥5 days

POSTPARTUM

☐ Gestational Diabetes this Pregnancy   ☐ Albumin ≤2.5   ☐ Hg <8.0

Breastfeeding mother meeting the following criteria:

☐ ≤17 Years Old
☐ Therapeutic or Limited Diet
☐ Lack of Knowledge re Lactation Diet
☐ Multiple Birth with Infants in Special Care Nursery

COMPREHENSIVE ASSESSMENT

SUBJECTIVE

Weight Gain/Expected Weight Gain _____

Cultural/Social Concerns _____

Activity Level_____

Plans to Breastfeed? ☐ Yes ☐ No

Other _____

OBJECTIVE

Diagnosis _____   Parity _____   EGA/EDC _____

Medical/Obstetrical History_____

Age _____   Ht_____   Pregravid Wt _____   BMI/Category _____   Current Wt _____

Medications_____   Vitamin/Mineral Supplements _____

Physical Exam _____   GI Function _____

Food Allergies/Intolerance _____   Diet Order _____

Labs _____

ASSESSMENT

Estimated Energy Needs _____   Protein _____   Other _____

Adequacy of Intake/Evaluation of Nutritional Status_____

_____

_____

_____

_____

Perinatal nutrition screen/assessment form. *PIH,* pregnancy-induced hypertension; *IUGR,* intrauterine growth retardation; *EGA,* estimated gestational age; *EDC,* estimated date of confinement; *BMI,* body mass index; *GI,* gastrointestinal.

Courtesy of Northside Hospital, Atlanta, GA.

Eating Disorder Nutritional Assessment Form

Date of Visit: _____

Patient Name: _____

Medical Record #: _____

Address: _____

Telephone: (home)_____ (business) _____

Date of Birth: _____ Age: _____ Gender: Male Female

Provider: _____

Informant/Relationship: _____

Language _____ Interpreter present: ☐ Yes ☐ No

Reliability: ☐ Adequate ☐ Inadequate

DIAGNOSIS:

Hospitalizations for eating disorder:

☐ Anorexia Nervosa ☐ In-patient

☐ Bulimia Nervosa ☐ Day patient

☐ Eating Disorder NOS ☐ Out-patient

WEIGHT HISTORY

Wt loss: #lb _____ From _____ To _____

Minimum weight at current height _____

Maximum weight at current height_____

IBW: _____ %IBW: _____

%Wt loss: _____ BMI: _____

ANTHROPOMETRIC PROFILE

Skinfolds (mm): _____

Triceps: _____ Biceps: _____ Subscapular: _____

Suprailiac: _____

Sum of sites (mm): _____ % Body fat: _____ TSF%: _____

MAC (cm): _____ MAMC (cm): _____ MAMC%: _____

BODY IMAGE: _____

_____

_____

FOOD ALLERGIES:_____

_____

_____

24-HOUR RECALL: _____

_____

_____

_____

_____

_____

_____

_____

_____

FLUID INTAKE: _____

_____

VITAMIN/MINERAL SUPPLEMENTS:_____

OTHER SUPPLEMENTS: _____

_____

SUGAR AND FAT SUBSTITUTES: _____

_____

MISCELLANEOUS: Chewing gum: _____

Hard candy: _____

Condiments:_____

BINGES: # per day _____ # per week _____

Duration per episode: _____

Binge foods: _____

Approximate kcal/binge: _____

SELF-INDUCED VOMITING:

Times per day: _____ Method: _____

LAXATIVES:

Type/brand: _____ Amount:_____

Duration of use: _____ Frequency of use: _____

DIURETICS:

Type: _____ Amount: _____

Duration of use: _____ Frequency of use: _____

EXERCISE:

Type: _____

Minutes/day: _____ Times/week: _____

Purpose of exercise: _____

MENSTRUAL HISTORY:

Age at menarche: _____

Last menstrual period: _____

MEDICATIONS (prescription and over-the-counter):

_____

_____

_____

BOWEL FUNCTION: _____

_____

_____

_____

From Mahan LK, Escott-Stump S: *Krause's Food, Nutrition & Diet Therapy*, ed 11, Philadelphia, 2004, WB Saunders.

Herbal, Botanical and Dietary Supplement Intake Form

Name: _____ Age: _____ Date: _____

Your health care professional needs the following information about your usual supplement and dietary habits to develop a personal plan for you. Please complete all sections completely and accurately.

1. **What kind of supplements do you use? (Check all that apply.)**
   _____ None
   _____ Multivitamin/mineral supplement
   _____ Herbal or botanical supplement
   _____ Amino acid or protein supplement
   _____ Fiber supplement
   _____ Other (see question 14 checklist at end of this form)

2. **How long have you used this supplement(s)?**
   _____ 1 month or less
   _____ 3 months
   _____ 6 months
   _____ 1 year
   _____ more than 1 year
   (specify):_____

3. **How long do you plan to use this supplement(s)?**
   _____ Indefinitely
   _____ 1 year
   _____ 6 months
   _____ 3 months
   _____ 1 month or less

4. **What are your primary reason(s) for taking this supplement(s)?**
   _____ For its preventive effect against disease/medical condition
   _____ To help treat a disease/medical condition
   _____ General wellness
   _____ Energy
   _____ Weight loss
   _____ Pregnancy/lactation
   _____ Other (specify): _____

If used to *treat* specific medical condition:
What are your medical symptoms? _____

_____

5. **How long have you had these symptoms/medical condition?**
   _____ 1 week or less
   _____ 1 month
   _____ 3 months
   _____ 6 months
   _____ 1 year
   _____ More than 1 year (specify): _____

6. **Have symptoms improved since you started taking this supplement?**
   _____ Yes (specify): _____
   _____ No

7. **Are you currently taking or have you recently taken any over-the-counter or prescription medications, including oral contraceptives?**
   _____ Yes (specify): _____
   _____ No

8. **Do you have any additional illnesses or medical conditions?**
   _____ Yes (specify): _____
   _____ No

9. **Are you pregnant or breastfeeding?**
   _____ Yes   _____ No

10. **Do you drink alcohol?**
    _____ Yes   _____ No

    If yes, how often?
    _____ Rarely
    _____ Occasionally
    _____ Often
    _____ Never

    If yes, how much at one sitting?
    _____ 1 glass
    _____ 2 glasses
    _____ 3 glasses or more

11. **Do you smoke?**
    _____ Yes   _____ No

    If yes, how often and how much?
    _____ 1-5 cigarettes, cigars, pipes per day
    _____ 1 pack per day
    _____ 2 packs per day
    _____ More than 2 packs per day

(over)

Herbal, Botanical and Dietary Supplement Intake Form - 2

12. Are you allergic to any medications, foods, plants, or flowers?

_____ Yes (specify): _____

_____ No

13. Are you on a self- or medically prescribed eating plan/diet?

_____ Yes (specify): _____

_____ No

14. What specific supplement(s) do you take, how much do you take, and how often do you take it?

	Amount/Dose	Number of Doses (per day or week)
Aloe		
Amino acid(s)		
Black cohosh		
Bee pollen		
Calcium		
Cat's claw		
Chondroitin		
Chromium		
Coenzyme Q10		
Creatine		
"Andro"/DHEA		
Dong quai		
Echinacea		
Evening primrose oil		
Feverfew		
Fiber		
Fish oil/DHA		
Folic acid		
Garlic		
Ginger		
Ginkgo biloba		
Ginseng		
Goldenseal		
Grapeseed extract		
Iron		
Kava		
Ma huang/ephedra		
Milk thistle		
Multiple vitamin/mineral		
Peppermint		
Pyruvate		
St John's wort		
Saw palmetto		
SAM-e		
Valerian		
Vitamin B complex		
Vitamin C		
Vitamin D		
Vitamin E		
Other		

CHAPTER 7

Specialized Evaluation Forms

Chapter Contents

ICON KEY: 🗎 Tool Printed   ✐ Tool on CD-ROM   ∞ Customizable Tool   𝐢 Information and Resources Provided for Further Acquisition

Introduction to Specialized Forms

Specialized examination forms are useful for documenting findings of examinations that are needed to meet private agency or government requirements and to convey important examination findings in an efficient manner. This chapter contains three unrelated examination subject areas and provides the reader with documentation forms and standardized criteria for each topic that assist in recording information.

Preoperative evaluation is frequently performed by the primary care provider. The goals of this evaluation are to identify patient factors that may increase the risk of surgery. The clinician may also make recommendations on management of coexisting medical conditions and their associated medication requirements during the perioperative period. Included in this section is updated information on the contents of a preoperative evaluation, indicated laboratory testing, and cardiac risk assessment.

Also included are the American Society of Anesthesiologists (ASA) Physical Status Classification System and customizable adult and pediatric preoperative evaluation forms.

In an effort to reduce the incidence of accidents and injuries involving commercial vehicles, the United States Department of Transportation Federal Motor Carrier Safety Administration (FMCSA) has developed medical standards for qualifying commercial drivers. Applicants for commercial driver's licenses may present to any primary care clinician for examination and qualifying certification. Drivers are certified by means of physical qualification criteria designed to promote safety in operating commercial motor vehicles on national highways. Included in this chapter are the guidelines for driver physical qualifications, report forms required for commercial driver fitness determination, and detailed instructions on completing the required medical examination. Resources for further information regarding these regulations are also provided.

Information regarding medical clearance for immigrants and refugees is of interest to primary care providers who may encounter these patients in the course of practice. Alien patients often have questions regarding medical clearance regulations, examinations, and paperwork required to change their immigrant status. Regulations on these issues were updated in 2003 and are now managed by the United States Citizenship and Immigration Services (USCIS) within the U.S. Department of Homeland Security. This chapter contains useful information pertaining to mandatory medical examinations for all refugees coming to the United States and all applicants outside the United States applying for immigrant visas.

PREOPERATIVE EVALUATION

The primary goal of preoperative data collection is to inform the surgical and anesthesia care teams about the medical history and current condition of the patient undergoing surgery. The concepts of "clearing for anesthesia" or "providing medical clearance" are no longer appropriate; preoperative evaluation is considered to be a *consultation* for evaluation of a patient's clinical status. The preoperative evaluation provides information, laboratory test results, and medical recommendations that assist in the process of risk assessment and guide selection and modification of an appropriate perioperative care plan. Perioperative management of the patient is the responsibility of the anesthesiology and surgical teams, who may base their decisions, in part, on the medical information provided by the primary care clinician (Pasternak, 2003).

Documentation must meet the specific requirements of hospitals, which are driven by the Joint Commission on Accreditation for Healthcare Organizations; insurance organizations; the federal government, generally through the Centers for Medicare and Medicaid Services;

and professional organizations, such as the American Society of Anesthesiologists (ASA). Hospital-based perioperative evaluation forms are designed to be completed by the attending anesthesiologist or anesthetist and are often based, in part, on review of a patient's medical record or preoperative evaluation completed by the primary care provider. This chapter provides the primary care provider with forms containing data necessary for a complete preoperative evaluation, which is done before the anesthesia evaluation.

Contents of the Preoperative Evaluation

Preoperative evaluation centers on documentation of medical history and physical findings that may affect patient outcome during and after surgery. Guidelines have been

---

Box **7-1**	Suggested Parameters for Inclusion in the Preoperative Evaluation

IDENTIFYING AND DEMOGRAPHIC PATIENT DATA
MEDICAL HISTORY:
- Preoperative diagnosis
- Acute medical conditions of cardiac, pulmonary, and neurologic systems and infection.
- Chronic medical conditions: COPD, dementia, depression, parkinsonism, malnutrition
- Medication regimens
- Allergies
- Anesthetic history and complications
- Surgical history
- Familial history of anesthetic complications
- Social habits
- Exercise tolerance/functional capacity
- Pregnancy status
- Focused review of systems

PHYSICAL EXAM:
- Vital signs
- Height and weight
- Airway exam
- Pulmonary examination to include auscultation of the lungs
- Cardiovascular examination
- Neurologic exam
- Regional site
- Recent laboratory testing findings

ASSESSMENT:
- Problem list and concerns
- ASA status

PLAN:
- Recommended preoperative testing
- Discussion of advance directives
- Consideration of preoperative prophylaxis (e.g., antibiotic and anticoagulant)

Data from American Society of Anesthesiologists Task Force on Preanesthesia Evaluation, 2002; Eagle KA et al, 2002; Hefferman JJ, et al, 2001; Pasternak LR, 2003; and Takata MN, 2001. With permission. *ASA,* American Society of Anesthesiologists; *COPD,* chronic obstructive pulmonary disease.

established for the minimal data necessary to allow reduction of risks associated with surgery (American Society of Anesthesiologists Task Force on Preanesthesia Evaluation, 2002; Eagle et al, 2002; Heffernan et al, 2001; Pasternak, 2003). Suggested subjects to be included in the preoperative evaluation are listed in Box 7-1. Data may be derived from review of pertinent medical records, patient interviews, and findings from physical examination and preoperative tests. Preoperative assessment forms included in this chapter are designed to include all suggested parameters; the reader may customize the forms to best suit his or her practice and patient population by using the enclosed CD-ROM.

Routine and Indicated Laboratory Testing

The subject of routine preoperative laboratory testing has been debated and examined extensively. Recommendations for routine testing have changed considerably in the last 2 decades. A routine test is defined as a test ordered in the absence of a specific clinical indication or purpose. Global designations such as *preop status* or *surgical screening* are no longer considered to be appropriate clinical indicators. Preoperative screening tests are now ordered for a specific clinical indication or purpose. Results of preoperative laboratory testing are supplements to the patient's health history and findings from physical examination. Results of such tests are beneficial in that they suggest a change in the care to be provided to an individual patient to improve his or her health or to prevent a potential problem (Roizen et al, 2000).

Tests that are intended to detect a disease or disorder in an asymptomatic patient do not make an important contribution to the process of perioperative assessment and management of the patient by the anesthesiologist (Pasternak, 2003). Additionally, when laboratory tests are ordered without regard to clinical indications in an asymptomatic patient, a range of abnormal results may be encountered. These results may be unrelated to surgical management issues, represent individual variants, or be transient in nature but may oblige the clinician to order more extensive or invasive testing in pursuit of a diagnosis.

The ASA Task Force on Preanesthesia Evaluation (2002) recommends that preoperative tests not be ordered routinely. Preoperative tests may be ordered, required, or performed on a selective basis for purposes of guiding or optimizing perioperative management. The indications for specific testing and their timing should be documented and based on information obtained from medical records, current age, patient history, physical examination findings, presence of comorbid disease, current medications, type and invasiveness of the planned procedure, expected blood loss, anesthesia route and duration, and emergency status.

Clinical characteristics may guide the clinician in making decisions about whether to order, require, or perform preoperative tests. General recommended indications for preoperative testing, as described by Pasternak (2003), are included in Table 7-1. Also included are the additional clinical characteristics to be considered for laboratory testing (ASA Task Force on Preanesthesia Evaluation, 2002). Because there is no consensus regarding preoperative testing, the ASA Task Force emphasizes that these characteristics should not be considered unequivocal indications for testing, but are presented for consideration only.

With regard to the timing of preoperative testing, opinions and preferences have been published by numerous medical groups. The ASA Task Force (2002) believes that test results obtained from the medical record within 6 months of surgery are generally acceptable if the patient's medical history has not changed substantially. If the medical history has changed or test results may play a role in the selection of a specific anesthesia technique, more recent test results may be desirable. Other groups suggest that "normal results from a chest radiograph within 1 year of surgery, normal results from an ECG performed within 6 months of surgery, and normal results from laboratory analyses performed within 6 weeks of surgery can be used if there has been no intervening clinical event" (Shulkin et al, 1996).

Stepwise Approach to Preoperative Cardiac Assessments

Because cardiac perioperative complications are associated with significant morbidity and death, assessment of cardiac risk is imperative in the preoperative evaluation. Cardiac risk level determines the most appropriate cardiac tests and treatments for optimal perioperative patient care.

In 2002, the American College of Cardiology (ACC) and the American Heart Association (AHA) jointly published updated guidelines for perioperative cardiovascular evaluation for noncardiac surgery (Eagle et al, 2002). These guidelines provide a framework for consideration of the cardiac risk of noncardiac surgery in a variety of patients and surgical situations. A stepwise algorithm, reprinted in this chapter, guides the examining clinician in ordering appropriate preoperative cardiac screening tests. This algorithm provides the clinician with major, intermediate, and minor clinical predictors of increased perioperative cardiac risk, with recommendations for preoperative cardiac testing according to risk level.

In addition to clinical predictors, the ACC/AHA guidelines (Eagle et al, 2002) include functional capacity and surgical procedure risk for patients with intermediate or minor predictors. *Functional capacity* is assessed by using metabolic equivalent levels (MET) to represent the aerobic demands for specific activities. As a point of reference, low activity levels (eating, dressing, walking in the house) expend 1 to 4 MET; moderate activity levels (climbing a flight of stairs, running a short distance, or playing a game of golf) expend 4 to 10 MET; and

Table 7-1 Clinical Indications for Preoperative Testing

Recommended Laboratory Testing for Administration of Anesthesia*	Additional Clinical Characteristics for Consideration of Testing†
ELECTROCARDIOGRAM	
Age 50 or older	Respiratory disease
Hypertension	Type or invasiveness of surgery
Current or past significant cardiac disease	Presence of known cardiac risk factors
Current or past circulatory disease	
Diabetes mellitus (age 40 or older)	
Renal, thyroid, or other metabolic disease	
CHEST RADIOGRAPH	
Asthma or COPD that is debilitating or with change of symptoms or acute episode within past 6 months	Smoking
Cardiothoracic procedure	Recent upper respiratory tract infection
	Type or invasiveness of surgery
	Cardiac disease
	Stable COPD
OTHER PULMONARY TESTS (SPIROMETRY, PULSE OXIMETRY, ARTERIAL BLOOD GAS)	
No recommendations	Type or invasiveness of surgery
	Interval from prior evaluation
	Treated or symptomatic asthma
	Symptomatic COPD
	Scoliosis with restrictive function
SERUM CHEMISTRIES	
Renal disease	Perioperative therapies
Adrenal or thyroid disorders	Endocrine disorders
Diuretic therapy	Risk of renal and liver dysfunction
Chemotherapy	Use of certain medications or alternative therapies
	History of anemia
URINALYSIS	
As requested by the surgeon	Presence of urinary tract symptoms
COMPLETE BLOOD COUNT	
Hematologic disorder	Type or invasiveness of surgery
Vascular procedure	Liver disease
Chemotherapy	Extremes of age
	History of anemia
COAGULATION STUDIES	
Anticoagulation therapy	Bleeding disorders
Vascular procedure	Renal dysfunction
	Liver dysfunction
	Type and invasiveness of procedure
PREGNANCY TESTING	
Patients for whom pregnancy might complicate the surgery	History suggestive of current pregnancy
Patients of uncertain status by history	All female patients of childbearing age

COPD, Chronic obstructive pulmonary disease.
*Data from Pasternak LR, 2003.
†Data from American Society of Anesthesiologists Task Force on Preanesthesia Evaluation, 2002.

strenuous sports activity levels (swimming, tennis, football) often exceed 10 MET. *Surgical procedure risk* is related to the type of surgery and degree of hemodynamic stress associated with the procedure. Box 7-2 summarizes the cardiac risk stratification for noncardiac surgical procedures.

Recommendations regarding management of specific preoperative cardiovascular conditions including hypertension, valvular heart disease, myocardial disease, arrhythmias, and presence of pacemakers and implantable cardioverter-defibrillators are also provided in the ACC/AHA guidelines. The full report of the updated guidelines is available on the ACC and AHA websites: http://www.acc.org/clinical/guidelines/perio/update/pdf/perio_update.pdf and http://www.americanheart.org/downloadable/heart/1013454973885perio_update.pdf. In addition to the ACC/AHA guidelines, several preoperative risk indexes that purport to accurately predict

| Box **7-2** | Cardiac Risk* Stratification for Noncardiac Surgical Procedures |

High (Reported cardiac risk often greater than 5%)
- Emergent major operations, particularly in the elderly
- Aortic and other major vascular surgery
- Peripheral vascular surgery
- Anticipated prolonged surgical procedures associated with large fluid shifts and/or blood loss

Intermediate (Reported cardiac risk generally less than 5%)
- Carotid endarterectomy
- Head and neck surgery
- Intraperitoneal and intrathoracic surgery
- Orthopedic surgery
- Prostate surgery

Low† (Reported cardiac risk generally less than 1%)
- Endoscopic procedures
- Superficial procedure
- Cataract surgery
- Breast surgery

Data from Eagle et al (2002), with permission.
*Combined incidence of cardiac death and nonfatal myocardial infarction.
†Does not generally require further preoperative cardiac testing.

| Box **7-3** | American Society of Anesthesiologists Physical Status Classification System* |

P1 A normal healthy patient

P2 A patient with mild systemic disease

P3 A patient with severe systemic disease

P4 A patient with severe systemic disease that is a constant threat to life

P5 A moribund patient who is not expected to survive without the operation

P6 A declared brain-dead patient whose organs are being removed for donor purposes

From American Society of Anesthesiologists, 2003. Available at http://www.asahq.org/clinical/physicalstatus.htm.
Reprinted with permission of the American Society of Anesthesiologists, 520 North Northwest Highway, Park Ridge, IL 60068-2573.
*These definitions appear in each annual edition of the *American Society of Anesthesiologists Relative Value Guide*. There is no additional information that will help you further define these categories.

cardiac risk have been developed. These risk indices are reviewed in Chapter 15.

American Society of Anesthesiologists Physical Status Classification System

Of the various systems developed for perioperative assessment of medical status, the ASA Physical Status Classification is the most recognized system that provides a global impression of the clinical state of the patient. The ASA Physical Status Classification categorizes the patient according to preexisting diseases and conditions. Originally published in 1963, the ASA Physical Status Classification (ASA, 1963) has undergone only minimal revision in terminology. The current classification system is presented in Box 7-3. Each of the classes may be modified with the letter *E*, indicating emergency presentation and surgery.

Although the classification may provide an overall impression of the health of the patient, it is only one factor in the assessment of anesthetic and surgical risk. Surgical outcome also depends on other factors, including the level of surgical invasiveness (risk index for the surgical procedure), age of the patient, and emergency or elective nature of the operation (ASA Task Force on Preanesthesia Evaluation, 2002).

Preoperative Clearance Evaluation Form: Adult

This two-page form includes an abbreviated health history and physical examination report, suitable for primary care preoperative evaluation. Included on this form are the essential parameters of the preoperative examination, as noted in Box 7-1. Text block areas—most with detailed, cued documentation—are included for these parameters. The form contains a combination of narrative documentation space, check-off boxes, and lines for short answers and explanations of findings. Contained within the section under "Plan" are check-off boxes for provider-recommended preoperative laboratory and screening tests. The reader may use this form as printed or modify it to best suit individual practice by following instructions on the CD-ROM.

Preoperative Clearance Evaluation Form: Pediatric

This two-page form contains an abbreviated history and physical examination report for preoperative evaluation with a pediatric focus. Information regarding perinatal history, pediatric review of systems, and pediatric psychosocial information replaces the comorbid conditions review from the adult form. The reader may use this form as printed or modify it to best suit individual practice by following instructions on the CD-ROM.

COMMERCIAL DRIVER FITNESS EVALUATION

The U.S. Department of Transportation provides guidelines for commercial driver fitness evaluation through the Federal Motor Carrier Safety Administration (FMCSA). Under the FMCSA, the Commercial Driver's License Program, revised September 30, 2002, and mandated by the Motor Carrier Safety Improvement Act of 1999, is designed to enhance the safety of commercial motor vehicle operations on national highways by ensuring that only safe drivers operate commercial motor vehicles. The primary mission of the FMCSA is to reduce crashes, injuries, and fatalities involving large trucks and buses. Information published here is from the online resources cited within this section.

Of interest to primary care providers, a standardized medical screening protocol and report forms are available through the FMCSA. Documents include recommended physical qualifications for drivers, conference reports on specific medical conditions, instructions on determining a driver's physical qualification to operate a commercial motor vehicle, and forms for reporting results of examination and certification.

To meet regulatory agency requirements for United States licensure, commercial drivers are required to obtain a medical examination and certification of qualification. Documents included in this section provide the clinician with current forms and guidelines for conducting the examination and qualifying the driver. For further information and clarification regarding advisory criteria in certifying a driver for commercial license, clinicians may review online FMCSA reports on specific medical conditions as cited in Resources and References. The federal commercial driver fitness evaluation may be conducted and certified by a medical examiner with the following credentials: medical doctor, doctor of osteopathy, chiropractor, physician assistant, or advanced practice nurse.

Medical Examination Report for Commercial Driver Fitness Determination [649-F (6045)]

This three-page form is to be completed and signed by the medical examiner. The form has sections for the areas noted in Box 7-4. This report form is reprinted here and is also available online at http://www.fmcsa.dot.gov/ safetyprogs/spe_pdfs/Medical_Report.pdf.

Physical Qualifications for Drivers [49 CFR 391.41]

This one-page document, reprinted in this text, provides an overview of the driver's role and physical qualifications pursuant to Section 391.41 of the Federal Motor Carrier Safety Regulations (FMCSR). Unlike regulations that are codified and have a statutory base, the

| Box **7-4** | Content Areas of Medical Examination Report [Form 649-F (6045)] |

Driver's information
Health history
Vision, with applicable required standards
Hearing, with applicable required standards
Blood pressure/pulse rate, with qualifying standards
Laboratory and other test findings: Urinalysis is required
Physical examination, by body system
Certification status, determined by standards in "Physical Qualifications for Drivers" (49 CFR 391.41)

recommendations in this advisory are simply guidelines established to help the medical examiner determine a driver's medical qualifications. The medical examiner may, but is not required to, accept the recommendations. Section 390.3(d) of the FMCSR allows employers to have more stringent medical requirements. This document is also available as part of the online medical report at http://www.fmcsa.dot.gov/ safetyprogs/spe_pdfs/ Medical_Report.pdf.

Instructions to the Medical Examiner: Federal Motor Carrier Safety Regulations – Advisory Criteria

This five-page document provides specific information regarding physical qualification requirements and guidelines for making the qualification determination for commercial drivers. Clinicians are advised to read this document carefully so that they understand the criteria for qualification before they certify driver applicants. Specific criteria are documented for conditions listed in Table 7-2. If an applicant is found to have one or more of these conditions or deficits, the criteria should be reviewed to certify the driver accurately. Driver applicants who fail to meet certain specified criteria may be qualified subject to conditions of the Skill Performance Evaluation (SPE) Certification Program. The medical examiner instructions are also available as part of the online medical report at http://www.fmcsa.dot.gov/ safetyprogs/spe_pdfs/Medical_Report.pdf.

Medical Examiner's Certificate [650-FS-L2 6046] (1p)

The Medical Examiner's Certificate (650-FS-L2 6046) is completed by the medical examiner if he or she finds that the person examined is qualified to drive a commercial motor vehicle in accordance with Section 391.41 of the Federal Motor Carrier Safety Regulations. The form contains areas for qualifications and exceptions, as well as spaces for indicating the medical examiner's name, license or certificate number, and title. This certificate is also available as part of the online medical report at http://www.fmcsa. dot.gov/safetyprogs/spe_pdfs/Medical_Report.pdf.

Table 7-2 Federal Motor Carrier Safety Regulations: Medical Conditions and Advisory Criteria

Condition	Advisory Qualifying Criteria
Loss of Limb	Has no loss of a foot, leg, hand, or an arm or has been granted an SPE certificate pursuant to Section 391.49.
Limb Impairment	Has no impairment of: (i) A hand or finger that interferes with prehension or power grasping; or (ii) An arm, foot, or leg that interferes with the ability to perform normal tasks associated with operating a commercial motor vehicle; or (iii) Any other significant limb defect or limitation which interferes with the ability to perform normal tasks associated with operating a commercial motor vehicle; or (iv) Has been granted a SPE certificate pursuant to Section 391.49.
Diabetes	Has no established medical history or clinical diagnosis of diabetes mellitus currently requiring insulin for control.
Cardiovascular Condition	Has no current clinical diagnosis of myocardial infarction, angina pectoris, coronary insufficiency, thrombosis, or any other cardiovascular disease of a variety known to be accompanied by syncope, dyspnea, collapse, or congestive cardiac failure.
Respiratory Dysfunction	Has no established medical history or clinical diagnosis of a respiratory dysfunction likely to interfere with ability to control and drive a commercial motor vehicle safely.
Hypertension	Has no current clinical diagnosis of high blood pressure likely to interfere with ability to operate a commercial motor vehicle safely.
Rheumatic, Arthritic, Orthopedic, Muscular, Neuromuscular, or Vascular Disease	Has no established medical history or clinical diagnosis of rheumatic, arthritic, orthopedic, muscular, neuromuscular, or vascular disease that interferes with the ability to control and operate a commercial motor vehicle safely.
Epilepsy	Has no established medical history or clinical diagnosis of epilepsy or any other condition that is likely to cause loss of consciousness or any loss of ability to control a motor vehicle.
Mental Disorders	Has no mental, nervous, organic, or functional disease or psychiatric disorder likely to interfere with ability to drive a motor vehicle safely.
Vision	Has distant visual acuity of at least 20/40 (Snellen) in each eye with or without corrective lenses or visual acuity separately corrected to 20/40 (Snellen) or better with corrective lenses, distant binocular acuity of at least 20/40 (Snellen) in both eyes with or without corrective lenses, field of vision of at least 70 degrees in the horizontal meridian in each eye, and the ability to recognize the colors of traffic signals and devices showing standard red, green, and amber.
Hearing	First perceives a forced whispered voice in the better ear at not less than 5 feet with or without the use of a hearing aid, or, if tested by use of an audiometric device, does not have an average hearing loss in the better ear greater than 40 decibels at 500 Hz, 1000 Hz, and 2000 Hz with or without a hearing aid when the audiometric devices calibrated to the American National Standard [formerly ASA Standard] Z24.5—1951.
Drug Use	Does not use a controlled substance identified in 21 CFR 1308.ll. Schedule I, an amphetamine, a narcotic, or any other habit-forming drug. Exception: A driver may use such a substance or drug, if the substance or drug is prescribed by a licensed medical practitioner who is familiar with the driver's medical history and assigned duties and has advised the driver that the prescribed substance or drug will not adversely affect the driver's ability to safely operate a commercial motor vehicle.
Alcoholism	Has no current clinical diagnosis of alcoholism.

From Federal Motor Carrier Safety Regulations–Advisory Criteria. Available at http://www.fmcsa.dot.gov/safetyprogs/spe_pdfs/Medical_Report.pdf. SPE, Skill performance evaluation.

EVALUATION FOR ADJUSTMENT OF IMMIGRANT STATUS

In 2003 the United States government reorganized the former Immigration and Naturalization Service (INS) within the United States Department of Justice. The new agency is called *the United States Citizenship and Immigration Services (USCIS)* and resides within the Department of Homeland Security. Complete information pertaining to this new agency may be found online at http://www.uscis.gov/graphics/index.htm. Information included in this section is from the online resources cited in Resources and References.

Each candidate applying for an immigrant visa in the United States is required to have a physical examination and mental status assessment as part of the application process, which is officially reported with the use of designated forms from the USCIS. Candidates with mandatory examination requirements include refugees, U.S. aliens who apply for adjustment of their immigration status to that of permanent resident, and overseas applicants for immigrant visas. The purpose of the medical examination is to identify, for the Department of State and

Bureau of Citizenship and Immigration Services (BCIS), applicants with inadmissible health-related conditions. Medical examinations in the United States are performed by approximately 3000 physicians (called *civil surgeons*) who are designated by the BCIS.

The Centers for Disease Control and Prevention (CDC) National Center for Infectious Diseases, Division of Global Migration and Quarantine (formerly the Division of Quarantine) provides medical screening guidelines that outline in detail the scope of the required medical examination. Evaluation includes five components: past medical history, physical examination, chest radiograph (x-ray), laboratory tests, and immunization assessment. Results of the medical examination are generally valid for only 12 months.

The purpose of the migration health assessment is to determine whether medical conditions or mental disorders exist that would make the applicant inadmissible, have a need to be monitored after resettlement, or require long-term institutionalization or maintenance income to be provided by the U.S. government after resettlement. Institutionalization or incomes that will become a public charge are of particular concern. The CDC has the authority to develop the methods to identify health-related conditions that make applicants inadmissible and to develop methods to identify applicants who have medical conditions that have the potential to make them become public charges. *Medical grounds of inadmissibility* is a term used for denial of admission to the United States on the basis of health conditions that are of public health concern to the United States (Box 7-5). Waivers are available for applicants with inadmissible health-related conditions.

Medical Examination of Aliens Seeking Adjustment of Status (Form I-693, revised 4/25/02)

All aliens applying for adjustment of status in the United States must use Form I-693, Medical Examination of Aliens Seeking Adjustment of Status, to report the results of the medical exam to the USCIS. There is also a vaccination supplement form used to record the results of the vaccination assessment. If a person is applying for a visa at a U.S. consular post overseas, different forms, supplied by the consular officer, are used.

Form I-693, Medical Examination of Aliens Seeking Adjustment of Status, is reprinted here with instructions. It is available in its entirety, along with the Medical Clearance Requirements for Aliens Seeking Adjustment of Status, at http://www.uscis.gov/graphics/formsfee/forms/i-693.htm. The online set of forms repeats the same two pages four times. The destinations of each set of two pages are as follows:

Original and 1 copy to BCIS (in sealed envelope from the civil surgeon)
Copy to civil surgeon
Copy for applicant

The vaccination supplement that is to accompany Form I-693 is not included on the Internet posting; the civil surgeons receive this form directly from the CDC for attachment to Form I-693 for submission to the BCIS.

Immigrant applicants are advised to check the web page of their local immigration office under "Local Filing Procedures" to determine whether the local office wants Form I-693 at the time of filing the initial adjustment application (Form I-485) or at the time of interview.

Medical Clearance Requirements for Aliens Seeking Adjustment of Status

This list of medical clearance requirements is reprinted here as a point of reference for primary care clinicians. These requirements are available online as part of the Form I-693 document at http://www.uscis.gov/graphics/formsfee/forms/i-693.htm. Communicable diseases of public health significance, as defined in the Department of Health and Human Services (HHS) regulations, include nine infectious medical conditions listed in Box 7-6. If test results for a communicable disease are positive, a recommendation for a course of treatment should be made. For medical conditions that are not easily treatable, an applicant may obtain an adjustment of status by filing a

---

Box **7-5** **Health-Related Grounds for Inadmissibility or Ineligibility for Visas***

Presence of a communicable disease of public health significance
Failure to have received vaccination against vaccine-preventable diseases
A physical or mental disorder with associated harmful behavior
Drug abuse or drug addiction

From Centers for Disease and Control and Prevention, National Center for Infectious Disease, Division of Global Migration and Quarantine. *Medical Examinations*. Available at http://www.cdc.gov/ncidod/dq/health.htm.
*Developed in accordance with section 212(a)(1)(A) of the Immigration and Naturalization Service.

Box **7-6** **Communicable Diseases of Public Health Significance**

Severe acute respiratory syndrome (SARS)
Tuberculosis (TB)
Leprosy
Human immunodeficiency virus (HIV/AIDS)
Syphilis (infectious state)
Chancroid
Gonorrhea
Granuloma inguinale
Lymphogranuloma venereum

From United States Citizenship and Immigration Services. *Medical Examinations: medical grounds of inadmissibility*. Available at http://www.uscis.gov/graphics/Medical_Exam.htm.

waiver application. Specific requirements for the waiver process may be found online at http://www.uscis.gov/graphics/Medical_Exam.htm.

Resources and References

Online Resources

Preoperative Evaluation

Institute for Clinical Systems Improvement (ICSI): *Healthcare guideline: preoperative evaluation*, ed 6. Bloomington, Minn, September 2003, Institute for Clinical Systems Improvement. Website: http://www.icsi.org/.

This document in Adobe Acrobat format contains recommendations for preoperative evaluation from the Institute for Clinical Systems Improvement (ICSI). The ICSI is a collaboration of health care organizations based in Minnesota, with the objective of promoting health care quality and implementing the best clinical practices. An independent, nonprofit organization, ICSI provides health care quality improvement services to 43 medical organizations, representing more than 6000 physicians. The preoperative guidelines included at this site under "Healthcare Guidelines, September 2003" include a one-page preoperative form for adults and a similar one-page form for children younger than 15 years. Also included are two one-page preoperative questionnaires for adults and children.

Commercial Driver Fitness

United States Department of Transportation (USDOT) Federal Motor Carrier Safety Administration (FMCSA): The official government agency regulating motor carrier safety. Website: http://www.fmcsa.dot.gov/index.htm.

Fact Sheet-Commercial Driver's License (CDL): Information and regulations from the FMCSA regarding commercial driver licensing. Website: http://www.fmcsa.dot.gov/safetyprogs/CDLFactSheet.htm.

Commercial Driver's License Standards, Requirements and Penalties: This full text document in Adobe Acrobat format details federal regulatory information; commercial driver's license standards, requirements, and penalties; and state compliance regulations regarding the commercial driver's license. Website: http://www.fmcsa.dot.gov/pdfs/CDL%20Final%20Rule.pdf.

FMCSA Medical Reports: These include conference reports on insulin-dependent drivers; cardiovascular guidelines; and reports on diabetic, neurologic, pulmonary/respiratory, psychiatric, visual, and hearing disorders and are available in Adobe Acrobat format. Website: http://www.fmcsa.dot.gov/rulesregs/medreports.htm.

FMCSA 49 CFR Part 391: Physical Qualification of Drivers; Medical Examination; Certificate. This Adobe Acrobat–formatted document updates, simplifies, and clarifies the medical examination form and standards that are currently used to determine the physical qualification of commercial motor vehicle (CMV) drivers operating in interstate commerce. Website: http://www.fmcsa.dot.gov/rulesregs/fmcsr/final/100500.pdf.

Skill Performance Evaluation (SPE) Certification Regulations. Website: http://www.fmcsa.dot.gov/rulesregs/fmcsr/regs/391.49.htm

Medical Evaluation of Aliens in the United States

Medical screening guidelines. Website: http://www.cdc.gov/ncidod/dq/health.htm

Technical instructions for medical examination of aliens in the United States (June 1991, with changes of July 1992, including the Vaccination Requirements for Immigrant Visa applicants, revised in July 2003) to be used by the designated physicians (available in Adobe Acrobat format). Website: http://www.cdc.gov/ncidod/dq/civil.htm

Civil Surgeons Locator (list of current designated civil surgeons by area): Website: http://www.uscis.gov/graphics/surgeonportal.htm, or the National Customer Service Center: (800)-375-5283.

Form I-693, Medical Examination of Aliens Seeking Adjustment of Status and Medical Clearance Requirements for Aliens Seeking Adjustment of Status. Website: http://ww.uscis.gov/graphics/formsfee/forms/i-693.htm

References

American Society of Anesthesiologists: New classification of physical status, *Anesthesiology* 24:111, 1963.

American Society of Anesthesiologists Task Force on Preanesthesia Evaluation: Practice advisory for preanesthesia evaluation: a report by the American Society of Anesthesiologists Task Force on Preanesthesia Evaluation, *Anesthesiology* 96:485-496, 2002.

Eagle KA, Berger PB, Calkins H, et al: ACC/AHA guideline update for perioperative cardiovascular evaluation for noncardiac surgery–executive summary: a report of the American College of Cardiology/American Heart Association Task Force on Practice Guidelines (Committee to Update the 1996 Guidelines on Perioperative Cardiovascular Evaluation for Noncardiac Surgery), *J Am Coll Cardiol* 39:542-553, 2002. Available at http://www.acc.org/clinical/guidelines/perio/update/pdf/perio_update.pdf and http://www.americanheart.org/downloadable/heart/1013454973885perio_update.pdf.

Heffernan JJ, Witzburg RA, Smetana GW: Medical evaluation of the patient undergoing surgery. In Noble J, editor. *Textbook of primary care medicine*, ed 3, St Louis, 2001, Mosby.

Pasternak LR: Preoperative screening for ambulatory patients, *Anesthesiol Clin North Am* 21:229-242, vii, 2003.

Roizen MF, Foss JF, Fischer SP: Preoperative evaluation. In Miller RD, editor, *Anesthesia*, ed 5, Philadelphia, 2000, Churchill Livingstone.

Shulkin D, Ratko T, Matuszewski M: Model guidelines for the preoperative evaluation of patients undergoing elective surgery, *J Clin Outcomes Manage* 3:39-48, 1996.

Takata MN, Benumof JL, Mazzei W: The preoperative evaluation form: assessment of quality from one hundred thirty-eight institutions and recommendations for a high-quality form, *J Clin Anesth* 13:345-352, 2001.

Stepwise Approach to Preoperative Cardiac Assessment

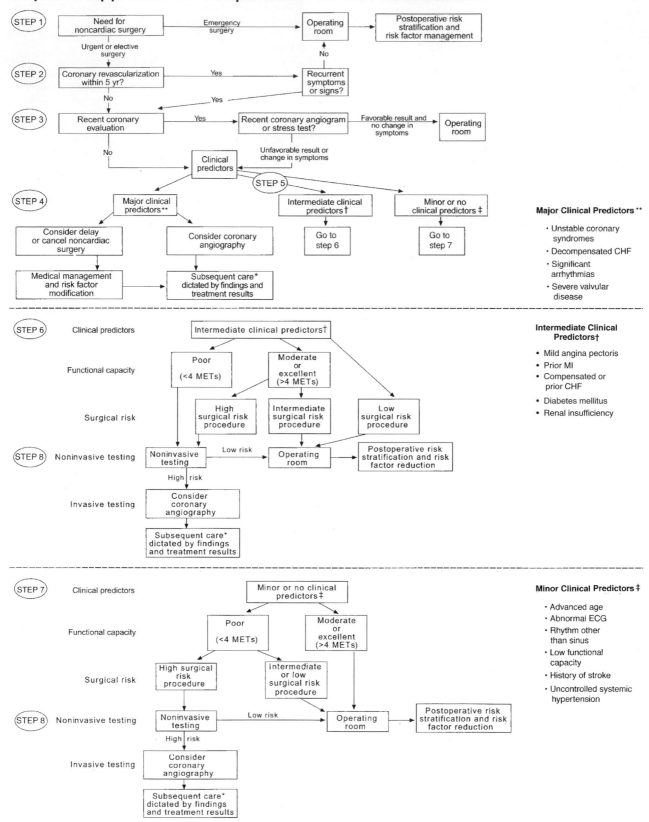

*Subsequent care may include cancellation or delay of surgery, coronary revascularization followed by noncardiac surgery, or intensified care. *CHF*, congestive heart failure; *ECG*, electrocardiogram; *MET*, metabolic equivalent; *MI*, myocardial infarction.

From ACC/AHA Guidelines for the Perioperative Cardiovascular Evaluation for Noncardiac Surgery, *J Am Coll Cardiol* 27:910-948, 1996. Copyright 2002 by the American College of Cardiology and the American Heart Asssociation, Inc. Reprinted with permission.

Preoperative Evaluation - Adult

Date of Visit: _____

Patient Name: _____

Medical Record #: _____

Date of Birth: _____ Age: _____ Gender: Male Female

Primary care provider:_____
Surgeon: _____
Diagnosis: _____
Planned procedure: _____
Date of surgery _____ Facility _____

Informant/Relationship: _____

Language _____ Interpreter present: ❏ Yes ❏ No

Reliability: ❏ Adequate ❏ Inadequate

Medical History

Cardiovascular ❏ Negative	Pulmonary ❏ Negative	Neurologic / Psych ❏ Negative	Hematology ❏ Negative
Exercise tolerance: _____ blocks _____ flights of stairs ❏ HTN ❏ Arrhythmia ❏ Angina ❏ Valve disease ❏ CAD ❏ History of MI (date ____) ❏ CHF ❏ CABG-PTCA (date ____) ❏ PVD ❏ Other: ❏ AAA	❏ Asthma ❏ Chronic Cough ❏ COPD ❏ Sputum ❏ Recent URI ❏ O₂ dependent ❏ Sleep Apnea ❏ Recent Pneum. ❏ Hx of TB ❏ Hx of PE ❏ Other:	❏ Seizures ❏ Numbness/Weakness ❏ Headaches ❏ Spinal Cord Injury ❏ Hx CVA/TIA ❏ Parkinsonism ❏ Elevated ICP ❏ Depression ❏ Dementia ❏ Other:	❏ Anemia ❏ Sickle Cell ❏ Hx of DVT ❏ Coagulopathy ❏ Thrombocytopenia ❏ Previous transfusions ❏ Other:

Renal ❏ Negative	GI ❏ Negative	Hepatic ❏ Negative	Endocrine ❏ Negative
❏ Chronic renal insufficiency ❏ Renal Failure ❏ Dialysis: Hemo • Peritoneal: ❏ Last transfused: _____ ❏ Other:	❏ GERD ❏ Hiatal hernia ❏ PUD ❏ S/P colectomy ❏ Vomiting • Diarrhea ❏ Dysphagia ❏ Other:	❏ History of hepatitis ❏ Jaundice ❏ Cirrhosis ❏ Other:	❏ Diabetes Mellitus: Age at onset: ___ ❏ Thyroid disorder: _____ ❏ Other:

Musculoskeletal ❏ Negative	Cancer ❏ Negative	Infectious Disease ❏ Negative	Comments:
❏ Back pain ❏ Musculodystrophy ❏ Arthritis: _____ ❏ Osteoporosis ❏ Other:	❏ Location: _____ ❏ Remission ❏ S/P chemo/radiation therapy ❏ Other:	❏ HIV ❏ MRSA ❏ Hepatitis B / C ❏ VRE ❏ Other:	

Allergies ❏ Negative	Medications (Rx and OTC) ❏ Negative	Previous Surgery ❏ Negative
❏ Eggs ❏ Medications: ❏ Latex ❏ IV Contrast Reactions:	(Name, dosage, frequency)	(Procedure/Date, Type Anesthesia, Complications)
Social Habits ❏ Negative Smoking: ❏ Yes: _____ ppd Quit date_____ ❏ No ETOH: ❏ Yes: Amount _____ ❏ No Drug Use: ❏ Yes: Describe _____ ❏ No Caffeine: ❏ Yes: cups/day _____ ❏ No		
Activity Level: ❏ Sedentary ❏ Moderate ❏ Strenuous		
Pregnant? ❏ No: LMP _____ ❏ Post-menopause ❏ Yes: gestational age _____ weeks		**Family History of Problems with Anesthesia:** ❏ No ❏ Yes: Describe:

Preoperative Evaluation - Adult - 2

Patient Name: _____

Medical Record #: _____

Date of Birth: _____

Physical Exam

Vitals						
Height	Weight	☐ Kg ☐ Lb		BMI:	☐ Thin ☐ Obese ☐ Average ☐ Mor. Obese	
BP		Pulse	☐ Regular ☐ Irregular	Resp Rate	Temperature	

N = normal A = abnormal (✔ appropriate box)	N	A
Airway: nares • dentition • oropharynx • trachea • neck ROM		
Pulmonary: excursion • palpation • percussion • auscultation		
Cardiac: rate • rhythm • S1 • S2 • murmur • extra sounds		
Neurologic : CNs • motor • sensory • cerebellar • DTR's • mental		
Regional Site:		
Other:		
Recent Laboratory Testing (dates) ☐ None ☐ See attached		

Document Abnormals / Comments:

Assessment and Plan

Problem List and Recommendations:

Recommended Laboratory Testing	
☐ CBC	☐ Serum / Urine HCG
☐ PT • INR • PTT • BT	☐ CXR
☐ Electrolytes	☐ Spirometry • ABG
☐ FBS	☐ EKG
☐ LFT's	☐ Cardiac stress test
☐ UA	☐ Coronary angiogram
Other:	

ASA Physical Classification Status: ☐ 1 ☐ 2 ☐ 3 ☐ 4 ☐ 5 ☐ E

Perioperative anticoagulation: ☐ per Surgery

Antibiotic prophylaxis: ☐ per Surgery

Advance Directive: ☐ None ☐ In office medical record ☐ With patient

Provider's Signature   **Date**
☐ Note dictated/written

Preoperative Evaluation - Pediatric

Date of Visit: _____

Patient Name: _____

Medical Record #: _____

Date of Birth: _____ Age: _____ Gender: Male Female

Primary care provider:_____

Surgeon: _____

Diagnosis: _____

Planned procedure: _____

Date of surgery _____ Facility _____

Informant/Relationship: _____

Language _____ Interpreter present: ❐ Yes ❐ No

Reliability: ❐ Adequate ❐ Inadequate

Medical History

Birth History ❐ Negative
❐ NSVD ❐ Cesarean section
❐ Term ❐ Pre-term: weight _____
❐ Complications: Apnea • Bradycardia •
Intubation • Bronchopulmonary dysplasia •
Retinopathy • Mechanical Ventilation
❐ Other:

Ear, Nose, Throat ❐ Negative
❐ URI ❐ Loose teeth
❐ Apnea ❐ Oral appliance
❐ Recent pharyngitis ❐ Braces
❐ Dysphagia ❐ Otitis media
❐ Blindness ❐ Deafness
❐ Other:

Cardiovascular ❐ Negative
❐ HTN ❐ Congenital abnormality
❐ Arrhythmia ❐ Murmur
❐ Cardiotoxic drugs
❐ Other:

Pulmonary ❐ Negative
❐ Asthma ❐ Bronchitis
❐ Recent URI ❐ Recent Pneumonia
❐ Hx of TB ❐ Chronic cough
❐ RSV ❐ Tracheostomy
❐ Other:

Neurologic ❐ Negative
❐ Seizures ❐ Weakness
❐ Headaches ❐ Myopathy
❐ Hydrocephalus ❐ Myelodysplasia
❐ Intraventricular hemorrhage
❐ Other:

GI • Hepatic ❐ Negative
❐ GERD ❐ Diarrhea
❐ Constipation ❐ Vomiting
❐ History of hepatitis ❐ Jaundice
❐ Other:

Hematology • CA ❐ Negative
❐ Anemia • Thalassemia ❐ Sickle Cell
❐ Bleeding disorder ❐ G6PD deficiency
❐ Leukemia ❐ Previous transfusions
❐ Other CA: _____
❐ S/P chemo/radiation therapy
❐ Other:

Endocrine ❐ Negative
❐ Diabetes Mellitus: Age at onset: ____
❐ Thyroid disorder: _____
❐ Adrenal disorder: _____
❐ Inborn error of metabolism (describe)
❐ Other:

Musculoskeletal ❐ Negative
❐ Scoliosis ❐ Musculodystrophy
❐ Hypotonia ❐ Fracture: _____
❐ Juvenile Arthritis: _____
❐ Other:

Genitourinary ❐ Negative
❐ UTI: (number) _____
❐ Renal disorder: _____
❐ Other:

Infectious Disease ❐ Negative
❐ HIV ❐ MRSA
❐ Hepatitis B / C ❐ VRE
❐ Other:

Comments:

Allergies ❐ Negative
❐ Eggs ❐ Medications:
❐ Latex
❐ IV Contrast
Reactions:

Substance Use ❐ Negative
Smoking: ❐ Yes: _____ ppd Quit date_____ ❐ No
ETOH: ❐ Yes: Amount _____ ❐ No
Drug Use: ❐ Yes: Describe_____ ❐ No
Caffeine: ❐ Yes: cups/day _____ ❐ No

Mental Health ❐ Negative
❐ ADHD ❐ Learning disability ❐ Depression
❐ Pervasive developmental disorder
❐ Other:

Pregnant? ❐ Prepubertal
❐ No: LMP _____
❐ Yes: gestational age _____ weeks

Medications (Rx and OTC) ❐ Negative
(Name, dosage, frequency)

Previous Surgery ❐ Negative
(Procedure/Date, Type Anesthesia, Complications)

Family History of Problems with Anesthesia:
❐ No ❐ Yes: Describe:

Preoperative Evaluation - Pediatric - 2

Patient Name: _____

Medical Record #: _____

Date of Birth: _____

Physical Exam

Vitals						
Height	Weight	☐ Kg ☐ Lb	BMI:	☐ Thin ☐ Obese		
				☐ Average ☐ Mor. Obese		
BP	Pulse	☐ Regular ☐ Irregular	Resp Rate	Temperature		

N = normal A = abnormal (✔ appropriate box)	N	A
Airway: nares • dentition • oropharynx • trachea • neck ROM		
Pulmonary: excursion • palpation • percussion • auscultation		
Cardiac: rate • rhythm • S1 • S2 • murmur • extra sounds		
Neurologic : CNs • motor • sensory • cerebellar • DTR's • mental		
Regional Site:		
Other:		
Recent Laboratory Testing (dates) ☐ **None** ☐ **See attached**		

Document Abnormals / Comments:

Assessment and Plan

Problem List and Recommendations:

Recommended Laboratory Testing	
☐ CBC	☐ Serum / Urine HCG
☐ PT • INR • PTT • BT	☐ CXR
☐ Electrolytes	☐ Spirometry • ABG
☐ FBS	☐ EKG
☐ LFT's	☐ Cardiac studies:
☐ UA	
Other:	

ASA Physical Classification Status: ☐ 1 ☐ 2 ☐ 3 ☐ 4 ☐ 5 ☐ E

Perioperative anticoagulation: ☐ **per Surgery**

Antibiotic prophylaxis: ☐ **per Surgery**

_____   _____
Provider's Signature   **Date**
☐ Note dictated/written

Medical Examination Report
For Commercial Driver Fitness Determination

649-F(6045)

1. DRIVER'S INFORMATION — Driver completes this section.

Driver's Name (Last, First, Middle)		Social Security No.			New certification Recertification Follow Up	Date of Exam

Address	City, State, Zip Code	Age	Birthdate M / D / Y	Sex M F	Driver License No.	License Class A □ C □ B □ D □ Other □	State of Issue

Work Tel: ( )
Home Tel: ( )

2. HEALTH HISTORY — Driver completes this section, but medical examiner is encouraged to discuss with driver.

Yes	No	
□	□	Any illness or injury in last 5 years?
□	□	Head/Brain injuries, disorders or illnesses
□	□	Seizures, epilepsy
□		□ medication
□	□	Eye disorders or impaired vision (except corrective lenses)
□	□	Ear disorders, loss of hearing or balance
□	□	Heart disease or heart attack; other cardiovascular condition
□		□ medication
□	□	Heart surgery (valve replacement/bypass, angioplasty, pacemaker)
□	□	High blood pressure □ medication
□	□	Muscular disease
□	□	Shortness of breath

Yes	No	
□	□	Lung disease, emphysema, asthma, chronic bronchitis
□	□	Kidney disease, dialysis
□	□	Liver disease
□	□	Digestive problems
□	□	Diabetes or elevated blood sugar controlled by:
	□	diet
	□	pills
	□	insulin
□	□	Nervous or psychiatric disorders, e.g., severe depression
□	□	Medication
□	□	Loss of or altered consciousness

Yes	No	
□	□	Fainting, dizziness
□	□	Sleep disorders, pauses in breathing while asleep, daytime sleepiness, loud snoring
□	□	Stroke or paralysis
□	□	Missing or impaired hand, arm, foot, leg, finger, toe
□	□	Spinal injury or disease
□	□	Chronic low back pain
□	□	Regular, frequent alcohol use
□	□	Narcotic or habit-forming drug use

For any YES answer, indicate onset date, diagnosis, treating physician's name and address, and any current limitation. List all medications (including over-the-counter medications) used regularly or recently.

_____

_____

_____

I certify that the above information is complete and true. I understand that inaccurate, false, or missing information may invalidate the examination and my Medical Examiner's Certificate.

_____   _____
Driver's Signature   Date

Medical Examiner's Comments on Health History (The medical examiner must review and discuss with the driver any "yes" answers and potential hazards of medications, including over-the-counter medications while driving.)

_____

_____

_____

TESTING (Medical Examiner completes Section 3 through 7)

3. VISION

Standard: At least 20/40 acuity (Snellen) in each eye with or without correction. At least 70° peripheral in horizontal meridian measured in each eye. The use of corrective lenses should be noted on the Medical Examiner's Certificate.

INSTRUCTIONS: *When other than the Snellen chart is used, give test results in Snellen-comparable values. In recording distance vision, use 20 feet as normal. Report visual acuity as a ratio with 20 as numerator and the smallest type read at 20 feet as denominator. If the applicant wears corrective lenses, these should be worn while visual acuity is being tested. If the driver habitually wears contact lenses or intends to do so while driving, sufficient evidence of good tolerance and adaptation to their use must be obvious. Monocular drivers are not qualified.*

Numerical readings must be provided.

ACUITY	UNCORRECTED	CORRECTED	HORIZONTAL FIELD OF VISION	
Right Eye	20/	20/	Right Eye	o
Left Eye	20/	20/	Left Eye	o
Both Eyes	20/	20/		o

Complete next line only if vision testing is done by an ophthalmologist or optometrist

Applicant can recognize and distinguish among traffic control signals and devices showing standard red, green, and amber colors? ☐ Yes ☐ No

Applicant meets visual acuity requirement only when wearing:
☐ Corrective Lenses
Monocular Vision: ☐ Yes ☐ No

Date of Examination   Name of Ophthalmologist or Optometrist (print)   Tel No.   License No./State of Issue   Signature

4. HEARING

Standard: a) Must first perceive forced whispered voice ≥ 5 ft, with or without hearing aid, or b) average hearing loss in better ear ≤ 40 dB ☐ Check if hearing aid used for tests. ☐ Check if hearing aid **required** to meet standard.

INSTRUCTIONS: *To convert audiometric test results from ISO to ANSI, -14 dB from ISO for 500 Hz, -10 dB for 1,000 Hz, -8.5 dB for 2,000 Hz. To average, add the readings for 3 frequencies tested and divide by 3.*

Numerical readings must be recorded.

a) Record distance from individual at which forced whispered voice can first be heard.

	Right Ear	Left Ear
	Feet	Feet
	Feet	Feet

b) If audiometer is used, record hearing loss in decibels. (acc. to ANSI Z24.5-1951)

	Right Ear			Left Ear		
	500 Hz	1000 Hz	2000 Hz	500 Hz	1000 Hz	2000 Hz
Average:				Average:		

5. BLOOD PRESSURE / PULSE RATE

Numerical readings must be recorded.

Blood Pressure	Systolic	Diastolic
Driver qualified if ≤160/90 on initial exam.		

Pulse Rate	☐ Regular	
	☐ Irregular	

GUIDELINES FOR BLOOD PRESSURE EVALUATION

On initial exam

Within 3 months

If 161-180 and/or 91-104, qualify 3 mos. only →

If >180 and/or 104, not qualified until reduced to <181/105. Then qualify for 3 mos. only.

If ≤160 and/or 90, qualify for 1 yr. Document Rx & control the 3rd month →

If ≤160 and/or 90, qualify for 6 mos. Document Rx & control the 3rd month →

Certify

Annually if acceptable BP is maintained

Biannually

Medical examiner should take at least 2 readings to confirm blood pressure.

6. LABORATORY AND OTHER TEST FINDINGS

Urinalysis is required: Protein, blood, or sugar in the urine may be an indication for further testing to rule out any underlying medical problem.

Other Testing *(Describe and record)*

URINE SPECIMEN	SP. GR.	PROTEIN	BLOOD	SUGAR

7. PHYSICAL EXAMINATION

Height: _____ (in.) Weight: _____ (lbs)

The presence of a certain condition may not necessarily disqualify a driver, particularly if the condition is controlled adequately, is not likely to worsen, or is readily amenable to treatment. Even if a condition does not disqualify a driver, the medical examiner may consider deferring the driver temporarily. Also, the driver should be advised to take the necessary steps to correct the condition as soon as possible particularly if the condition, if neglected, could result in more serious illness that might affect driving.

Check YES if there are any abnormalities. Check NO if the body system is normal. Discuss any YES answers in detail in the space below and indicate whether it would affect the driver's ability to operate a commercial motor vehicle safely. Enter applicable item number before each comment. If organic disease is present, note that it has been compensated for. See Instructions To The Medical Examiner for guidance.

BODY SYSTEM	CHECK FOR:	YES*	NO
1. General Appearance	Marked overweight, tremor, signs of alcoholism, problem drinking, or drug abuse.		
2. Eyes	Pupillary equality, reaction to light, accommodation, ocular motility, ocular muscle imbalance, extraocular movement, nystagmus, exophthalmos, strabismus uncorrected by corrective lenses, retinopathy, cataracts, aphakia, glaucoma, macular degeneration.		
3. Ears	Middle ear disease, occlusion of external canal, perforated eardrums.		
4. Mouth and Throat	Irremediable deformities likely to interfere with breathing or swallowing.		
5. Heart	Murmurs, extra sounds, enlarged heart, pacemaker.		
6. Lungs and chest, not including breast examination.	Abnormal chest wall expansion, abnormal respiratory rate, abnormal breath sounds including wheezes or alveolar rales, impaired respiratory function, dyspnea, cyanosis. Abnormal findings on physical exam may require further testing such as pulmonary tests and/or x-ray of chest.		

BODY SYSTEM	CHECK FOR:	YES*	NO
7. Abdomen and Viscera	Enlarged liver, enlarged spleen, masses, bruits, hernia, significant abdominal wall muscle weakness.		
8. Vascular system	Abnormal pulse and amplitude, carotid or arterial bruits, varicose veins.		
9. Genitourinary system	Hernias.		
10. Extremities - Limb impaired. Driver may be subject to SPE certificate if otherwise qualified.	Loss or impairment of leg, foot, toe, arm, hand, finger. Perceptible limp, deformities, atrophy, weakness, paralysis, clubbing, edema, hypotonia. Insufficient grasp and prehension in upper limb to maintain steering wheel grip. Insufficient mobility and strength in lower limb to operate pedals properly.		
11. Spine, other musculoskeletal	Previous surgery, deformities, limitation of motion, tenderness.		
12. Neurological	Impaired equilibrium, coordination or speech pattern; paresthesia, asymmetric deep tendon reflexes, sensory or positional abnormalities, abnormal patellar and Babinski's reflexes, ataxia.		

* COMMENTS: _____

Note certification status here. See Instructions to the Medical Examiner for guidance.

- ☐ Meets standards in 49 CFR 391.41; qualifies for 2-year certificate
- ☐ Does not meet standards
- ☐ Meets standards, but periodic evaluation required. _____ driver qualified only for:

Due to
- ☐ 3 months ☐ 1 year
- ☐ 6 months ☐ Other

- ☐ Temporarily disqualified due to (condition or medication): _____
  Return to medical examiner's office for follow-up on _____

- ☐ Wearing corrective lenses
- ☐ Wearing hearing aid
- ☐ Accompanied by a _____ waiver/exemption
- ☐ Skill Performance Evaluation (SPE) Certificate
- ☐ Driving within an exempt intracity zone.
- ☐ Qualified by operation of 49 CFR 391.64

Medical Examiner's Signature _____

Medical Examiner's Name (print) _____

Address _____

Telephone Number _____

If meets standards, complete a Medical Examiner's Certificate according to 49 CFR 391.43(h). (Driver must carry certificate when operating a commercial vehicle.)

49 CFR 391.41 Physical Qualifications for Drivers

THE DRIVER'S ROLE

Responsibilities, work schedules, physical and emotional demands, and lifestyles among commercial drivers vary by the type of driving that they do. Some of the main types of drivers include the following: turn around or short relay (drivers return to their home base each evening); long relay (drivers drive 8-10 hours and then have an 8-hour off-duty period), straight through haul (cross country drivers); and team drivers (drivers share the driving by alternating their 4-hour driving periods and 4-hour rest periods).

The following factors may be involved in a driver's performance of duties: abrupt schedule changes and rotating work schedules, which may result in irregular sleep patterns and a driver beginning a trip in a fatigued condition; long hours; extended time away from family and friends, which may result in lack of social support; tight pickup and delivery schedules, with irregularity in work, rest, and eating patterns, adverse road, weather and traffic conditions, which may cause delays and lead to hurriedly loading or unloading cargo in order to compensate for the lost time; and environmental conditions such as excessive vibration, noise, and extremes in temperature. Transporting passengers or hazardous materials may add to the demands on the commercial driver.

There may be duties in addition to the driving task for which a driver is responsible and needs to be fit. Some of these responsibilities are: coupling and uncoupling trailer(s) from the tractor, loading and unloading trailer(s) (sometimes a driver may lift a heavy load or unload as much as 50,000 lbs. of freight after sitting for a long period of time without any stretching period); inspecting the operating condition of tractor and trailer(s) before, during, and after delivery of cargo; lifting, installing, and removing heavy tire chains; and, lifting heavy tarpaulins to cover open top trailers. The above tasks demand agility, the ability to bend and stoop, the ability to maintain a crouching position to inspect the underside of the vehicle, frequent entering and exiting of the cab, and the ability to climb ladders on the tractor and/or trailer(s).

In addition, a driver must have the perceptual skills to monitor a sometimes complex driving situation, the judgment skills to make quick decisions, when necessary, and the manipulative skills to control an oversize steering wheel, shift gears using a manual transmission, and maneuver a vehicle in crowded areas.

§ 391.41 PHYSICAL QUALIFICATIONS FOR DRIVERS

(a) A person shall not drive a commercial motor vehicle unless he is physically qualified to do so and, except as provided in §391.67, has on his person the original, or a photographic copy, of a medical examiner's certificate that he is physically qualified to drive a commercial motor vehicle.

(b) A person is physically qualified to drive a motor vehicle if which person:

(1) Has no loss of a foot, a leg, a hand, or an arm, or has been granted a Skill Performance Evaluation (SPE) Certificate (formerly Limb Waiver Program) pursuant to §391.49.

(2) Has no impairment of: (i) A hand or finger which interferes with prehension or power grasping; or (ii) An arm, foot, or leg that interferes with the ability to perform normal tasks associated with operating a commercial motor vehicle; or any other significant limb defect or limitation which interferes with the ability to perform normal tasks associated with operating a commercial motor vehicle; or has been granted a SPE Certificate pursuant to §391.49.

(3) Has no established medical history or clinical diagnosis of diabetes mellitus currently requiring insulin for control;

(4) Has no current clinical diagnosis of myocardial infarction, angina pectoris, coronary insufficiency, thrombosis, or any other cardiovascular disease of a variety known to be accompanied by syncope, dyspnea, collapse, or congestive cardiac failure.

(5) Has no established medical history or clinical diagnosis of a respiratory dysfunction likely to interfere with his ability to control and drive a commercial motor vehicle safely.

(6) Has no current clinical diagnosis of high blood pressure likely to interfere with his ability to operate a commercial motor vehicle safely.

(7) Has no established medical history or clinical diagnosis of rheumatic, arthritic, orthopedic, muscular, neuromuscular, or vascular disease which interferes with his ability to control and operate a commercial motor vehicle safely.

(8) Has no established medical history or clinical diagnosis of epilepsy or any other condition which is likely to cause loss of consciousness or any loss of ability to control a commercial motor vehicle;

(9) Has no mental, nervous, organic, or functional disease or psychiatric disorder likely to interfere with his ability to drive a commercial motor vehicle safely;

(10) Has distant visual acuity of at least 20/40 (Snellen) in each eye without corrective lenses or visual acuity separately corrected to 20/40 (Snellen) or better with corrective lenses, distant binocular acuity of at least 20/40 (Snellen) in both eyes with or without corrective lenses, field of vision of at least 70 degrees in the horizontal meridian in each eye, and the ability to recognize the colors of traffic signals and devices showing standard red, green, and amber;

(11) First perceives a forced whispered voice in the better ear not less than 5 feet with or without the use of a hearing aid, or, if tested by use of an audiometric device, does not have an average hearing loss in the better ear greater than 40 decibels at 500 Hz, 1,000 Hz and 2,000 Hz with or without a hearing aid when the audiometric device is calibrated to American National Standard (formerly ASA Standard) Z24.5-1951;

(12) (i) Does not use a controlled substance identified in 21 CFR 1308.11 Schedule I, an amphetamine, a narcotic, or any other habit-forming drug. (ii) Exception: A driver may use such a substance or drug, if the substance or drug is prescribed by a licensed medical practitioner who: (A) Is familiar with the driver's medical history and assigned duties; and (B) Has advised the driver that the prescribed substance or drug will not adversely affect the driver's ability to safely operate a commercial motor vehicle; and

(13) Has no current clinical diagnosis of alcoholism.

INSTRUCTIONS TO THE MEDICAL EXAMINER

General Information

The purpose of this examination is to determine a driver's physical qualification to operate a commercial motor vehicle (CMV) in interstate commerce according to the requirements in 49 CFR 391.41-49. Therefore, the medical examiner must be knowledgeable of these requirements and guidelines developed by the Federal Motor Carrier Safety Administration (FMCSA) to assist the medical examiner in making the qualification determination. The medical examiner should be familiar with the driver's responsibilities and work environment and is referred to the section on the form, The Driver's Role.

In addition to reviewing the Health History section with the driver and conducting the physical examination, the medical examiner should discuss common prescriptions and over-the-counter medications relative to the side effects and hazards of these medications if used while driving. Educate driver to read warning labels on all medications. History of certain conditions may be cause for rejection, particularly if required by regulation, or may indicate the need for additional laboratory tests or more stringent examination, perhaps by a medical specialist. These decisions are usually made by the medical examiner in light of the driver's job responsibilities, work schedule, and potential for the condition to render the driver unsafe.

Medical conditions should be recorded even if they are not cause for denial, and they should be discussed with the driver to encourage appropriate remedial care. This advice is especially needed when a condition, if neglected, could develop into a serious illness that could affect driving.

If the medical examiner determines that the driver is fit to drive and is also able to perform nondriving responsibilities, and may be required, the medical examiner signs the medical certificate that the driver must carry with his/her license. The certificate must be dated. Under current regulations, the certificate is valid for two years, unless the driver has a medical condition that does not prohibit driving but does require more frequent monitoring. In such situations, the medical certificate should be issued for a shorter length of time. The physical examination should be done carefully and at least as completely as is indicated by the attached form. Contact the FMCSA at (202) 366-1790 for further information (a vision exemption, qualifying drivers under 49 CFR 391.64, etc.).

Interpretation of Medical Standards

Since the issuance of the regulations for physical qualifications of commercial drivers, the FMCSA has published recommendations called Advisory Criteria to help medical examiners in determining whether a driver meets the physical qualifications for commercial driving. These recommendations have been condensed to provide information to medical examiners that (1) is directly relevant to the physical examination and (2) is not already included in the medical examination form. The specific regulation is printed in italics and its reference by section is highlighted.

Federal Motor Carrier Safety Regulations
- Advisory Criteria -

Loss of Limb:
§ 391.41(b)(1)
A person is physically qualified to drive a commercial motor vehicle if that person:

Has no loss of a foot, leg, hand, or an arm, or has been granted a Skill Performance Evaluation (SPE) Certificate pursuant to Section 391.49.

Limb Impairment:
§ 391.41(b)(2)
A person is physically qualified to drive a commercial motor vehicle if that person:

Has no impairment of: (i) A hand or finger that interferes with prehension or power grasping; or (ii) An arm, foot, or leg that interferes with the ability to perform normal tasks associated with operating a commercial motor vehicle; or (iii) Any other significant limb defect or limitation that interferes with the ability to perform normal tasks associated with operating a commercial motor vehicle; or (iv) Has been granted a Skill Performance Evaluation Certificate pursuant to Section 391.49.

A person who suffers loss of a foot, leg, hand, or arm or whose limb impairment in any way interferes with the safe performance of normal tasks associated with operating a commercial motor vehicle is subject to the Skill Performance Evaluation (SPE) Certification Program pursuant to section 391.49, assuming the person is otherwise qualified.

With the advancement of technology, medical aids and equipment modifications have been developed to compensate for certain disabilities. The SPE Certification Program (formerly the Limb Waiver Program) was designed to allow persons with the loss of a foot or limb or with functional impairment to qualify under the Federal Motor Carrier Safety Regulations (FMCSRs) by use of prosthetic devices or equipment modifications that enable them to safely operate a commercial motor vehicle. Since there are no medical aids equivalent to the original body or limb, certain risks are still present, and thus restrictions may be included on individual SPE certificates when a State Director for the FMCSA determines they are necessary to be consistent with safety and public interest.

If the driver is found otherwise medically qualified (391.41(b)(3) through (13)), the medical examiner must check on the medical certificate that the driver is qualified only if accompanied by an SPE certificate. The driver and the employing motor carrier are subject to appropriate penalty if the driver operates a motor vehicle in interstate or foreign commerce without a current SPE certificate for his/her physical disability.

Diabetes
§ 391.41(b)(3)
A person is physically qualified to drive a commercial motor vehicle if that person:

Has no established medical history or clinical diagnosis of diabetes mellitus currently requiring insulin for control.

Diabetes mellitus is a disease that, on occasion, can result in a loss of consciousness or disorientation in time and space. Individuals who require insulin for control have conditions that can get out of control by the use of too much or too little insulin or by food intake not consistent with the insulin dosage. Incapacitation may occur from symptoms of hyperglycemic or hypoglycemic reactions (drowsiness, semiconsciousness, diabetic coma, or insulin shock).

The administration of insulin is, within itself, a complicated process requiring insulin, syringe, needle, alcohol sponge, and a sterile technique. Factors related to long-haul commercial motor vehicle operations, such as fatigue, lack of sleep, poor diet, emotional conditions, stress, and concomitant illness, compound the diabetic problem. Thus, because of these inherent dangers, the FMCSA has consistently held that a diabetic who uses insulin for control does not meet the minimum physical requirements of the FMCSRs.

Hypoglycemic drugs, taken orally, are sometimes prescribed for diabetic individuals to help stimulate natural body production of insulin. If the condition can be controlled by the use of oral medication and diet, then an individual may be qualified under the present rule.

(See Conference Report on Diabetic Disorders and Commercial Drivers and Insulin-Using Commercial Motor Vehicle Drivers at

http://www.fmcsa.dot.gov/rulesregs/medreports.htm)

Cardiovascular Condition
§ 391.41(b)(4)
A person is physically qualified to drive a commercial motor vehicle if that person:

Has no current clinical diagnosis of myocardial infarction, angina pectoris, coronary insufficiency, thrombosis, or any other cardiovascular disease of a variety known to be accompanied by syncope, dyspnea, collapse, or congestive cardiac failure. The term "has no current clinical diagnosis of" is specifically designed to encompass: "a clinical diagnosis of" (1) a current cardiovascular condition, or (2) a cardiovascular condition that has not fully stabilized regardless of the time limit. The term *"known to be accompanied by"* is defined to include: a clinical diagnosis of a cardiovascular disease (1) that is accompanied by symptoms of syncope, dyspnea, collapse, or congestive cardiac failure; and/or (2) that is likely to cause syncope, dyspnea, collapse, or congestive cardiac failure.

It is the intent of the FMCSRs to render unqualified a driver who has a current cardiovascular disease that is accompanied by and/or likely to cause symptoms of syncope, dyspnea, collapse, or congestive cardiac failure. However, the subjective decision of whether the nature and severity of an individual's condition will likely cause symptoms of cardiovascular insufficiency is on an individual basis and qualification rests with the medical examiner and the motor carrier. In those cases where there is an occurrence of cardiovascular insufficiency (myocardial infarction, thrombosis, etc.), it is suggested before a driver is certified that he or she have a normal resting and stress electrocardiogram (ECG), have no residual complications and no physical limitations, and be taking no medication likely to interfere with safe driving.

Coronary artery bypass surgery and pacemaker implantation are remedial procedures and thus, not unqualifying. Coumadin is a medical treatment which can improve the health and safety of the driver and should not, by its use, medically disqualify the commercial driver. The emphasis should be on the underlying medical condition(s) which require treatment and the general health of the driver. The FMCSA should be contacted at (202) 366-1790 for additional recommendations regarding the physical qualification of drivers on coumadin.
(See Conference on Cardiac Disorders and Commercial Drivers at http://www.fmcsa.dot.gov/rulesregs/medreports.htm)

Respiratory Dysfunction
§ 391.41(b)(5)

A person is physically qualified to drive a commercial motor vehicle if that person:
Has no established medical history or clinical diagnosis of a respiratory dysfunction likely to interfere with ability to control and drive a commercial motor vehicle safely.

Since a driver must be alert at all times, any change in his or her mental state is in direct conflict with highway safety. Even the slightest impairment in respiratory function under emergency conditions (when greater oxygen supply is necessary for performance) may be detrimental to safe driving.

There are many conditions that interfere with oxygen exchange and may result in incapacitation, including emphysema, chronic asthma, carcinoma, tuberculosis, chronic bronchitis, and sleep apnea. If the medical examiner detects a respiratory dysfunction that in any way is likely to interfere with the driver's ability to safely control and drive a commercial motor vehicle, the driver must be referred to a specialist for further evaluation and therapy. Anticoagulation therapy for deep vein thrombosis and/or pulmonary thromboembolism is not unqualifying once optimum dose is achieved, provided lower extremity venous examinations remain normal and the treating physician gives a favorable recommendation.

(See Conference on Pulmonary/Respiratory Disorders and Commercial Drivers at http://www.fmcsa.dot.gov/rulesregs/medreports.htm)

Hypertension
§ 391.41(b)(6)

A person is physically qualified to drive a commercial motor vehicle if that person:
Has no current clinical diagnosis of high blood pressure likely to interfere with ability to operate a commercial motor vehicle safely.

Hypertension alone is unlikely to cause sudden collapse; however, the likelihood increases when target organ damage, particularly cerebral vascular disease, is present. This regulatory criterion is based on FMCSA's Cardiac Conference recommendations, which used the report of the 1984 Joint National Committee on Detection, Evaluation, and Treatment of High Blood Pressure.

A blood pressure of 161-180 and/or 91-104 diastolic is considered mild hypertension, and the driver is not necessarily unqualified during evaluation and institution of treatment. The driver is given a 3-month period to reduce his or her blood pressure to less than or equal to 160/90; the certifying physician should state on the medical certificate that it is only valid for that 3-month period. If the driver is subsequently found qualified with a blood pressure less than or equal to 160/90, the certifying physician may issue a medical certificate for a 1-year period but should confirm blood pressure control in the third month of this 1-year period. The expiration date should be certified annually thereafter. The expiration date must be stated on the medical certificate.

A blood pressure of greater than 180 systolic and/or greater than 104 diastolic is considered moderate to severe. The driver may not be qualified, even temporarily, until his or her blood pressure has been reduced to less than 181/105. The examining physician may temporarily certify the individual once the individual's blood pressure is below 181 and/or 105. For blood pressure greater than 180 and/or 104, documentation of continued control should be made every 6 months. The individual should be certified biannually thereafter. The expiration date must be stated on the medical certificate. Commercial drivers who present for certification with normal blood pressures but are taking medication(s) for hypertension should be certified on the same basis as individuals who present with blood pressures in the mild or moderate to severe range. Annual recertification is recommended if the medical examiner is unable to establish the blood pressure at the time of diagnosis.

An elevated blood pressure finding should be confirmed by at least two subsequent measurements on different days. Inquiry should be made regarding smoking, cardiovascular disease in relatives, and immoderate use of alcohol. An electrocardiogram (ECG) and blood profile, including glucose, cholesterol, HDL cholesterol, creatinine, and potassium, should be done. An echocardiogram and chest x-ray are desirable in subjects with moderate or severe hypertension.

Since the presence of target damage increases the risk of sudden collapse, group 3 or 4 hypertensive retinopathy, left ventricular hypertrophy not otherwise explained (echocardiography or ECG by Estes criteria), evidence of severely reduced left ventricular function, or serum creatinine of greater than 2.5 warrants the driver being found unqualified to operate a commercial motor vehicle in interstate commerce.

Treatment includes nonpharmacologic and pharmacologic modalities, as well as counseling, to reduce other risk factors. Most antihypertensive medications also have side effects, the importance of which must be judged on an individual basis. Individuals must be alerted to the hazards of use of these medications while driving. Side effects of somnolence or syncope are particularly undesirable in commercial drivers.

A commercial driver who has normal blood pressure 3 or more months after a successful operation for pheochromocytoma, primary aldosteronism (unless bilateral adrenalectomy has been performed), renovascular disease, or unilateral renal parenchymal disease and who shows no evidence of target organ may be qualified. Hypertension that persists despite surgical intervention with no target organ disease should be evaluated and treated following the guidelines set forth above. (See Conference on Cardiac Disorders and Commercial Drivers at http://www.fmcsa.dot.gov/rulesregs/medreports.htm)

Rheumatic, Arthritic, Orthopedic, Muscular, Neuromuscular, or Vascular Disease
§ 391.41(b)(7)

A person is physically qualified to drive a commercial motor vehicle if that person:
Has no established medical history or clinical diagnosis of rheumatic, arthritic, orthopedic, muscular, neuromuscular, or vascular disease that interferes with ability to control and operate a commercial motor vehicle safely.

Certain diseases are known to have acute episodes of transient muscle weakness, poor muscular coordination (ataxia), abnormal sensations (paresthesia), decreased muscular tone (hypotonia), visual disturbances, and pain that may be suddenly incapacitating. With each recurring episode, these symptoms may become more pronounced and remain for longer periods. Other diseases have more insidious onsets and display symptoms of muscle wasting (atrophy), swelling, and paresthesia, which may not suddenly incapacitate a person but may restrict his/her movements and eventually interfere with the ability to safely operate a motor vehicle. In many instances these diseases are degenerative in nature or may result in deterioration of the involved area.

Once the individual has been diagnosed as having a rheumatic, arthritic, orthopedic, muscular, neuromuscular, or

vascular disease, then he/she has an established history of that disease. The physician, when examining an individual, should consider the following: (1) the nature and severity of the individual's condition (such as sensory loss or loss of strength); (2) the degree of limitation present (such as range of motion); (3) the likelihood of progressive limitation (not always present initially but may manifest itself over time); and (4) the likelihood of sudden incapacitation. If severe functional impairment exists, the driver does not qualify. In cases where more frequent monitoring is required, a certificate for a shorter time period may be issued.
(See Conference on Neurological Disorders and Commercial Drivers at
http://www.fmcsa.dot.gov/rulesregs/medreports.htm)

Epilepsy
§ 391.41(b)(8)
A person is physically qualified to drive a commercial motor vehicle if that person:

Has no established medical history or clinical diagnosis of epilepsy or any other condition that is likely to cause loss of consciousness or any loss of ability to control a motor vehicle.

Epilepsy is a chronic functional disease characterized by seizures or episodes that occur without warning, resulting in loss of voluntary control, which may lead to loss of consciousness and/or seizures. Therefore, the following drivers cannot be qualified: (I) a driver who has a medical history of epilepsy; (2) a driver who has a current clinical diagnosis of epilepsy; or (3) a driver who is taking antiseizure medication.

If an individual has had a sudden episode of a nonepileptic seizure or loss of consciousness of unknown cause that did not require antiseizure medication, the decision as to whether that person's condition will likely cause loss of consciousness or loss of ability to control a motor vehicle is made on an individual basis by the medical examiner in consultation with the treating physician. Before certification is considered, it is suggested that a 6-month waiting period elapse from the time of the episode. Following the waiting period, it is suggested that the individual have a complete neurological examination. If the results of the examination are negative and antiseizure medication is not required, then the driver may be qualified.

In those individual cases where a driver has a seizure or an episode of loss of consciousness that resulted from a known medical condition (e.g., drug reaction, high temperature, acute infectious disease, dehydration, or acute metabolic disturbance), certification should be deferred until the driver has fully recovered from that condition, has no existing residual complications, and is not taking antiseizure medication.
(See Conference on Neurological Disorders and Commercial Drivers at
http://www.fmcsa.dot.gov/rulesregs/medreports.htm)

Mental Disorders
§ 391.41(b)(9)
A person is physically qualified to drive a commercial motor vehicle if that person:

Has no mental, nervous, organic, or functional disease or psychiatric disorder likely to interfere with ability to drive a motor vehicle safely.

Emotional or adjustment problems contribute directly to an individual's level of memory, reasoning, attention, and judgment. These problems often underlie physical disorders. A variety of functional disorders can cause drowsiness, dizziness, confusion, weakness, or paralysis that may lead to incoordination, inattention, loss of functional control, and susceptibility to accidents while driving. Physical fatigue, headache, impaired coordination, recurring physical ailments, and chronic "nagging" pain may be present to such a degree that certification for commercial driving is inadvisable. Somatic and psychosomatic complaints should be thoroughly examined in determining an individual's overall fitness to drive. Disorders of a periodically incapacitating nature, even in the early stages of development, may warrant disqualification.

Many bus and truck drivers have documented that "nervous trouble" related to neurotic, personality, emotional, or adjustment problems is responsible for a significant fraction of their preventable accidents. The degree to which an individual is able to appreciate, evaluate, and adequately respond to environmental strain and emotional stress is critical when assessing an individual's mental alertness and flexibility to cope with the stresses of commercial motor vehicle driving.

On examination of the driver, it should be kept in mind that individuals who live under chronic emotional, upsets may have deeply ingrained maladaptive or erratic behavior patterns. Excessively antagonistic, instinctive, impulsive, openly aggressive, paranoid, or severely depressed behavior greatly interferes with the driver's ability to drive safely. Those individuals who are highly susceptible to frequent states of emotional instability (schizophrenia, affective psychoses, paranoia, anxiety, or depressive neuroses) may warrant disqualification. Careful consideration should be given to the side effects and interactions of medications in the overall qualification determination. See Psychiatric Conference Report for specific recommendations on the use of these medications and potential hazards for driving.
(See Conference on Psychiatric Disorders and Commercial Drivers at
http://www.fmcsa.dot.gov/rulesregs/medreports.htm)

Vision
§ 391.41(b)(10)
A person is physically qualified to drive a commercial motor vehicle if that person:

Has distant visual acuity of at least 20/40 (Snellen) in each eye with or without corrective lenses or visual acuity separately corrected to 20/40 (Snellen) or better with corrective lenses, distant binocular acuity of at least 20/40 (Snellen) in both eyes with or without corrective lenses, field of vision of at least 70 degrees in the horizontal meridian in each eye, and the ability to recognize the colors of traffic signals and devices showing standard red, green, and amber.

The term "ability to recognize the colors of" is interpreted to mean if a person can recognize and distinguish among traffic control signals and devices showing standard red, green, and amber, he or she meets the minimum standard, even though he or she may have some type of color perception deficiency. If certain color perception tests are administered (such as Ishihara, Pseudoisochromatic, Yarn) and doubtful findings are discovered, a controlled test using signal red, green and amber may be employed to determine the driver's ability to recognize these colors.

Contact lenses are permissible if there is sufficient evidence to indicate that the driver has good tolerance and is well adapted to their use. Use of a contact lens in one eye for distance visual acuity and another lens in the other eye for near vision is not acceptable, nor are telescopic lenses acceptable for the driving of commercial motor vehicles.

If an individual meets the criteria by the use of glasses or contact lenses, the following statement shall appear on the Medical Examiner's Certificate: "Qualified only if wearing corrective lenses."
(See Visual Disorders and Commercial Drivers at
http://www.fmcsa.dot.gov/rulesregs/medreports.htm)

Hearing
§ 391.41(b)(11)
A person is physically qualified to drive a commercial motor vehicle if that person:

First perceives a forced whispered voice in the better ear at not less than 5 feet with or without the use of a hearing aid, or, if tested by use of an audiometric device, does not have an average hearing loss in the better ear greater than 40 decibels at 500 Hz, 1,000 Hz, and 2,000 Hz with or without a hearing aid when the audiometric device is calibrated to American National Standard (formerly ASA Standard) Z24.5-1951.

Since the prescribed standard under the FMCSRs is the American Standards Association (ANSI), it may be necessary to convert the audiometric results from the ISO standard to the ANSI standard. Instructions are included on the Medical Examination report form.

If an individual meets the criteria by using a hearing aid, the driver must wear that hearing aid and have it in operation at all times while driving. Also, the driver must be in possession of a spare power source for the hearing aid.

For the whispered voice test, the individual should be stationed at least 5 feet from the examiner with the ear being tested turned toward the examiner. The other ear is covered. Using the breath that remains after a normal expiration, the examiner whispers words or random numbers such as 66, 18, 23, etc. The examiner should not use only sibilants (s-sounding test materials). The opposite ear should be tested in the same manner. If the individual fails the whispered voice test, the audiometric test should be administered.

If an individual meets the criteria by the use of a hearing aid, the following statement must appear on the Medical Examiner's Certificate "Qualified only when wearing a hearing aid."
(See Hearing Disorders and Commercial Motor Vehicle Drivers at:
http://www.fmcsa.dot.gov/rulesregs/medreports.htm)

Drug Use
§ 391.41(b)(12)
A person is physically qualified to drive a commercial motor vehicle if that person:
Does not use a controlled substance identified in 21 CFR 1308.II, Schedule I, an amphetamine, a narcotic, or any other habit-forming drug. Exception: A driver may use such a substance or drug, if the substance or drug is prescribed by a licensed medical practitioner who is familiar with the driver's medical history and assigned duties and has advised the driver that the prescribed substance or drug will not adversely affect the driver's ability to safely operate a commercial motor vehicle.

This exception does not apply to methadone. The intent of the medical certification process is to medically evaluate a driver to ensure that the driver has no medical condition that interferes with the safe performance of driving tasks on a public road. If a driver uses a Schedule I drug or other substance, an amphetamine, a narcotic, or any other habit-forming drug, it may be cause for the driver to be found medically unqualified. Motor carriers are encouraged to obtain a practitioner's written statement about the effects on transportation safety of the use of a particular drug.

A test for controlled substances is not required as part of this biennial certification process. The FMCSA or the driver's employer should be contacted directly for information on controlled substances and alcohol testing under Part 382 of the FMCSRs.

The term "uses" is designed to encompass instances of prohibited drug use determined by a physician through established medical means. This may or may not involve body fluid testing. If body fluid testing takes place, positive test results should be confirmed by a second test of greater specificity. The term "habit-forming" is intended to include any drug or medication generally recognized as capable of becoming habitual, which may impair the user's ability to operate a commercial motor vehicle safely.

The driver is medically unqualified for the duration of use of the prohibited drug(s) and until a second examination shows the driver is free from use of the prohibited drug(s). Recertification may involve a substance abuse evaluation, the successful completion of a drug rehabilitation program, and a negative drug test result. Additionally, given that the certification period is normally two years, the examiner has the option to certify for a period of less than 2 years if this examiner determines more frequent monitoring is required.
(See Conference on Neurological Disorders and Commercial Drivers and Conference on Psychiatric Disorders and Commercial Drivers at
http://www.fmcsa.dot.gov/rulesregs/medreports.htm)

Alcoholism
§ 391.41(b)(13)
A person is physically qualified to drive a commercial motor vehicle if that person:
Has no current clinical diagnosis of alcoholism.
The term "current clinical diagnosis of" is specifically designed to encompass a current alcoholic illness or those instances where the individual's physical condition has not fully stabilized, regardless of the time element. If an individual shows signs of having an alcohol-use problem, he or she should be referred to a specialist. After counseling and/or treatment, he or she may be considered for certification.

MEDICAL EXAMINER'S CERTIFICATE

I certify that I have examined _____ in accordance with the Federal Motor Carrier Safety Regulations (49 CFR 391.41-391.49) and with knowledge of the driving duties, I find this person is qualified; and, if applicable, only when:

☐ wearing corrective lenses

☐ wearing hearing aid

☐ accompanied by a _____ waiver/exemption

☐ driving within an exempt intracity zone (49 CFR 391.62)

☐ accompanied by a Skill Performance Evaluation Certificate (SPE)

☐ Qualified by operation of 49 CFR 391.64

The information I have provided regarding this physical examination is true and complete. A complete examination form with any attachment embodies my findings completely and correctly, and is on file in my office.

SIGNATURE OF MEDICAL EXAMINER	TELEPHONE	DATE

MEDICAL EXAMINER'S NAME (PRINT)	☐ MD ☐ DO ☐ Chiropractor ☐ Physician Assistant ☐ Advanced Practice Nurse

MEDICAL EXAMINER'S LICENSE OR CERTIFICATE NO. / ISSUING STATE

SIGNATURE OF DRIVER	DRIVER'S LICENSE NO.	STATE

ADDRESS OF DRIVER

MEDICAL CERTIFICATE EXPIRATION DATE

OMB No. 1115-0134

U.S. Department of Justice
Immigration and Naturalization Service

Medical Examination of Aliens
Seeking Adjustment of Status

Instructions to Alien Applying for Adjustment of Status

A medical examination is necessary as part of your application for adjustment of status. Please communicate immediately with one of the physicians on the attached list to arrange for your medical examination, which must be completed before your status can be adjusted. The purpose of the medical examination is to determine whether you have certain health conditions that may need further follow-up. The information requested is required in order for a proper evaluation to be made of your health status. The results of your examination will be provided to an Immigration officer and may be shared with health departments and other public health or cooperating medical authorities. All expenses in connection with this examination must be paid by you.

The examining physician may refer you to your personal physician or a local public health department and you must comply with some health follow-up or treatment recommendations for certain health conditions before your status will be adjusted.

This form should be presented to the examining physician. You must sign the form in the presence of the examining physician. *The law provides severe penalties for knowingly and willfully falsifying or concealing a material fact or using any false documents in connection with this medical examination. The medical examination must be completed in order for us to process your application.*

Medical Examination and Health Information

A medical examination is necessary as part of your application for adjustment of status. You should go for your medical examination as soon as possible. You will have to choose a doctor from a list you will be given. The list will have the names of doctors or clinics in your area that have been approved by the Immigration and Naturalization Service for this examination. You must pay for the examination. If you become a temporary legal resident and later apply to become a permanent resident, you may need to have another medical examination at that time.

The purpose of the medical examination is to find out whether you have certain health conditions that may need further follow-up. The doctor will examine you for certain physical and mental health conditions. You will have to take off your clothes. If you need more tests because of a condition found during your medical examination, the doctor may send you to your own doctor or to the local public health department. For some conditions, before you can become a temporary or permanent resident, you will have to show that you have followed the doctor's advice to get more tests or receive treatment.

If you have any records of immunizations (vaccinations), you should bring them to show to the doctor. This is especially important for preschool and school-age children. The doctor will tell you whether any more immunizations are needed and where you can get them (usually at your local public health department). It is important for your health that you follow the doctor's advice and get any immunizations.

One of the conditions you will be tested for is tuberculosis. If you are 15 years of age or older, you will be required to have a chest x-ray examination. **Exception:** If you are pregnant or applying for adjustment of status under the Immigration Reform and Control Act of 1986, you may choose to have either a chest x-ray or a tuberculin skin test. If you choose the skin test, you will have to return in 2 to 3 days to have it checked. If you do not have any reaction to the skin test, you will not need any more tests for tuberculosis. If you do have any reaction to the skin test, you will also need to have a chest x-ray examination. If the doctor thinks you are infected with tuberculosis, you may have to go to the local health department, and more tests may have to be done. The doctor will explain these to you.

If you are 14 years of age or younger, you will not need to have a test for tuberculosis, unless a member of your immediate family has chest x-ray findings that may be tuberculosis. If you are in this age group and you do have to be tested for tuberculosis, you may choose either the chest x-ray or the skin test.

You must also have a blood test for syphilis if you are 15 years of age or older.

You will also be tested to determine whether you have the human immunodeficiency virus (HIV) infection. This virus is the cause of AIDS. If you have this virus, it may damage your body's ability to fight off other diseases. The blood test you will take will tell whether you have been exposed to this virus.

Instructions to Physician Performing the Examination

Please medically examine for adjustment of status the individual presenting this form. The medical examination should be performed according to the U.S. Public Health Service "Guidelines for Medical Examination of Aliens in the United States" and Supplements, which have been provided to you separately.

If the applicant is free of medical defects listed in Section 212(a) of the Immigration and Nationality Act, endorse the form in the space provided. While in your presence, the applicant must also sign the form in the space provided. You should retain one copy for your files and return all other copies in a sealed envelope to the applicant for presentation at the immigration interview.

Form I-693 Instructions (Rev. 04/25/02) Y

If the applicant has a health condition that requires follow-up as specified in the "Guidelines for Medical Examination of Aliens in the United States" and Supplements, complete the referral information on the pink copy of the medical examination form, and advise the applicant that appropriate follow-up must be obtained before medical clearance can be granted. Retain the blue copy of the form for your files and return all other copies to the applicant in a sealed envelope. The applicant should return to you when the necessary follow-up has been completed for your final verification and signature. *Do not* sign the form until the applicant has met health follow-up requirements. All medical documents, including chest x-ray films if a chest x-ray examination was performed, should be returned to the applicant upon final medical clearance.

Instructions to Physician Providing Health Follow-Up

The individual presenting this form has been found to have a medical condition(s) requiring resolution before medical clearance for adjustment of status can be granted. Please evaluate the applicant for the condition(s) identified.

The requirements for clearance are outlined on the reverse of this page. When the individual has completed clearance requirements, please sign the form in the space provided and return the medical examination form to the applicant.

Privacy Act Notice

The authority for collection of the information requested on this form is contained in 8 U.S.C. 1182, 1183A, 1184(a), 1252, 1255, and 1258. The information will be used principally by the Immigration and Naturalization Service to whom it may be furnished to support an individual's application for adjustment of status under the Immigration and Nationality Act. Submission of the information is voluntary. It may also, as a matter of routine use, be disclosed to other federal, state, local, and foreign law enforcement and regulatory agencies. Failure to provide the necessary information may result in the denial of the applicant's request.

Paperwork Reduction Act Notice

An agency may not conduct or sponsor an information collection and a person is not required to respond to an information collection unless it displays a currently valid OMB control number. We try to create forms and instructions that are accurate, can be easily understood, and impose the least possible burden on you to provide us with information. Often this is difficult because some immigration laws are very complex. The estimated average time to complete and file this application is 90 minutes per application. If you have comments regarding the accuracy of this estimate or suggestions for making this form simpler, you may write to the Immigration and Naturalization Service, Regulations and Forms Services Division, 425 I Street, N.W., Suite 4034, Washington, DC 20536; OMB No. 1115-01234. *(Do not mail your completed application to this address.)*

OMB No. 1115-0134

U.S. Department of Justice
Immigration and Naturalization Service

Medical Examination of Aliens
Seeking Adjustment of Status

(Please type or print clearly)
I certify that on the date shown I examined:

1. Name (Last in CAPS)

_____
(First)   (Middle Initial)

2. Address (Street number and name)   (Apt. number)

_____
(City)   (State)   (Zip Code)

3. File number (A number)

4. Sex
☐ Male   ☐ Female

5. Date of birth (MM/DD/YYYY)

6. Country of birth

7. Date of examination (MM/DD/YYYY)

General Physical Examination: I examined specifically for evidence of the conditions listed below. My examination revealed:
☐ No apparent defect, disease, or disability.   ☐ The conditions listed below were found (check all boxes that apply).

Class A Conditions
☐ Chancroid   ☐ Hansen's disease, infectious   ☐ Mental defect   ☐ Psychopathic personality
☐ Chronic alcoholism ☐ HIV infection   ☐ Mental retardation   ☐ Sexual deviation
☐ Gonorrhea   ☐ Insanity   ☐ Narcotic drug addiction ☐ Syphilis, infectious
☐ Granuloma inguinale ☐ Lymphogranuloma venereum   ☐ Previous occurrence of one ☐ Tuberculosis active
                                                             or more attacks of insanity

Class B Conditions
☐ Hansen's disease, not infectious   ☐ Tuberculosis, not active   ☐ Other physical defect, disease, or disability (specify below).

Examination for Tuberculosis-Tuberculin Skin Test
☐ Reaction _____ mm   ☐ No Reaction   ☐ Not Done
Doctor's name (please print)   Date read

Examination for Tuberculosis-Chest X-Ray Report
☐ Abnormal   ☐ Normal   ☐ Not done
Doctor's name (please print)   Date read

Serologic Test for Syphilis
☐ Reactive Titer (confirmatory test performed)   ☐ Nonreactive
Test Type

Doctor's name (please print)   Date read

Serologic Test for HIV Antibody
☐ Positive (confirmed by Western blot)   ☐ Negative
Test Type

Doctor's name (please print)   Date read

Immunization Determination (DTP, OPV, MMR, Td-Refer to *PHS Guidelines* for recommendations.)

☐ Applicant is current for recommended age-specific immunizations.

☐ Applicant is not current for recommended age-specific immunizations and I have encouraged that appropriate immunizations be obtained.

REMARKS:

_____
_____
_____

Civil Surgeon Referral for Follow-Up of Medical Condition
☐ The alien named above has applied for adjustment of status. A medical examination conducted by me identified the conditions above, which require resolution before medical clearance is granted or for which the alien may seek medical advice. Please provide follow-up services or refer the alien to an appropriate health care provider. The actions necessary for medical clearance are detailed on the reverse of this form.

Follow-Up Information:
The alien named above has complied with the recommended health follow-up.

Doctor's name and address (please type or print clearly)   Doctor's signature   Date

Application Certification
I certify that I understand the purpose of the medical examination, I authorize the required tests to be completed, and the information on this form refers to me.

Signature   Date

Civil Surgeon Certification:
My examination showed the applicant to have met the medical examination and health follow-up requirements for adjustment of status.

Doctor's name and address (please type or print clearly)   Doctor's signature   Date

I-693

Medical Clearance Requirements
for Aliens Seeking Adjustment of Status

Medical Condition	Estimated Time For Clearance	Action Required
*Suspected Mental Conditions	5 - 30 Days	The applicant must provide to a civil surgeon a psychological or psychiatric evaluation from a specialist or medical facility for final classification and clearance.
Tuberculin Skin Test Reaction and Normal Chest X-Ray or Abnormal Chest X-Ray	Immediate	The applicant should be encouraged to seek further medical evaluation for possible preventive treatment.
Tuberculin Skin Test Reaction and Abnormal Chest X-Ray (Inactive/Class B)	10 - 30 Days	The applicant should be referred to a physician or local health department for further evaluation. Medical clearance may not be granted until the applicant returns to the civil surgeon with documentation of medical evaluation for tuberculosis.
Tuberculin Skin Test Reaction and Abnormal Chest X-Ray or Abnormal Chest X-Ray (Active or Suspected Active/Class A)	10 - 300 Days	The applicant should obtain an appointment with a physician or local health department. If treatment for active disease is started, it must be completed (usually 9 months) before medical clearance may be granted. At the completion of treatment, the applicant must present to the civil surgeon documentation of completion. If treatment is not started, the applicant must present to the civil surgeon documentation of medical evaluation for tuberculosis.
Hansen's Disease	30 - 210 Days	Obtain an evaluation from a specialist or Hansen's disease clinic. If the disease is indeterminate or tuberculoid, the applicant must present to the civil surgeon documentation of medical evaluation. It disease is lepromotous of borderline (dimorphous) and treatment is started, the applicant must complete at least 6 months of treatment and present documentation to the civil surgeon showing adequate supervision, treatment, and clinical response before medical clearance is granted.
**Venereal Diseases	1 - 30 Days	Obtain an appointment with a physician or local public health department. An applicant with a reactive serologic test for syphilis must provide to the civil surgeon documentation of evaluation for treatment. If any of the venereal diseases are infectious, the applicant must present to the civil surgeon documentation of completion of treatment.
Immunizations Incomplete	Immediate	Immunizations are not required, but the applicant should be encouraged to go to a physician or local health department for appropriate immunizations.
HIV Infection	Immediate	Post-test counseling is not required, but the applicant should be encouraged to seek appropriate post-test counseling.

*Mental retardation; insanity; previous attack of insanity; psychopathic personality, sexual deviation, or mental defect; narcotic drug addiction; and chronic alcoholism.

**Chancroid; gonorrhea; granuloma inguinale; lymphogranuloma venereum; and syphilis.

Form I-693 (Rev. 04/25/02) Page 2

PART TWO

Measurement Tools and Rating Scales

Introduction to Chapters 8 through 16

The goal of Part Two is to provide the reader with a concise compendium of health measurement tools for primary care clinical use. Thousands of health measurement instruments are scattered throughout the medical, social science, and nursing literature. Although several excellent texts that describe or reprint tools for a specialty subject area (such as psychiatry, health quality measurement, or geriatrics) are available, a compilation of tools covering a wide range of primary care topics does not exist. The purpose of this text is to fill this gap by gathering tools from many health-related areas that are of interest to primary care practitioners and placing them in one volume.

Contents of Part Two

Chapters 8 through 16 contain charts, scoring systems, checklists, and validated rating scales and measures in the areas of pediatrics and development, mental health, geriatrics, health quality, pain, wound evaluation, nutrition, social and spiritual well-being, and selected medical specialties. Assessment instruments were identified by the author from personal knowledge, consultation with other health care professionals and educators, review books of measures, and MEDLINE/CINAHL literature searches for measures within various disciplines. Of the many thousands available, the tools in this text were chosen on the basis of their prevalence of use in the medical and nursing literature, published validity and reliability, and potential usefulness in clinical practice. Several lesser known but excellent assessment measures are included to promote awareness among primary care clinicians of their existence and usefulness. All rating scales included in this section have been previously published, tested, and validated and are suitable for clinical use. Omitted from this text are pediatric health quality indices, scales measuring specific forms of impairment (such as orthopedic, rehabilitation, and disability assessment tools), and tools used primarily for research or psychiatric sampling studies. The reader is encouraged to consult other collections of rating scales[1-16] that pertain to his or her specialty interests.

Charts, checklists, and rating scales have been grouped into subject chapters that cover a broad topic. Within each chapter, tools are loosely ordered by subtopic, with more familiar tools listed first. The reader will note that there is considerable overlap between chapter topics, with a particular instrument often fitting into two or three chapter headings. Tools were placed in the topic chapter that is the most likely place the primary care clinician would look for that resource. For example, scales measuring mobility and falls were placed in Chapter 10: Geriatric Instruments, rather than in Chapter 15: System Specific Assessment Tools–Neurology, because the tools are most likely to be used with the geriatric population.

Box 1	What this text does:

- Provides a wide selection of rating scales and charts for clinical use in primary care
- Describes characteristics for each rating scale, chart, or screening tool
- Gives a summary of reliability and validation studies for each tool
- Lists references for each rating scale for further information
- Includes charts and scales in printable format on CD-ROM for personal use

Box 2	What this text does not do:

- Discuss development of rating scales or their use in research
- Provide detailed statistical information for reliability and validity studies
- Instruct the reader on fine points of implementing use of rating scales in the practice setting
- Recommend a particular scale over another within the same specialty

Box 3	Advantages and Disadvantages for Use of Rating Scales

ADVANTAGES:
- Screens for individuals who need treatment, monitoring, or other interventions
- Provides a reference for assessment as compared with the tested population
- Documents symptoms and individual perceptions regarding a particular condition
- Ensures a comprehensive assessment according to previously established criteria
- Provides validated documentation for referrals to specialists
- Provides documented justification for treatment plans to patients and insurance providers
- Allows systematic monitoring of patient progress with treatment

DISADVANTAGES:
- Cannot exclusively diagnose a condition
- Does not provide an individualized assessment
- Does not include a narrative, historical basis for symptoms
- May require training for administration and scoring techniques
- Requires additional time with the patient for administration, scoring, and interpretation
- May add additional costs to the practice for purchasing, scoring, or reprinting of the tool

Within subject chapters, each tool is reprinted if permission was obtained from the copyright holder of the tool. Permission was also requested to reprint each tool on an accompanying CD-ROM and was granted for most tools printed in their entirety. For those tools under restricted copyright protection or only available commercially, contact information for Internet download or purchase is provided.

Rating Scales and Measures

Rating scales and measures provide formal assessment of symptoms and perceptions, which are measured on a continuum. From individual responses, the assessment is scored and interpreted according to standardized results from research studies conducted in patient groups with similar symptoms or diagnoses.

Rating scales can be useful tools in clinical practice to identify individuals who would benefit from treatment or monitoring (Box 3). They assist in diagnosis of many medical conditions and provide more information about an individual's symptoms and response to illness. Formal assessments can assist in determining the level of care required and monitor the effects of treatment. By documenting patient responses with a standardized tool, clinicians provide support for administrative functions such as insurance and disability benefits, forensic evaluations, and third-party assessment of health care delivery. Rating scales may not be as useful if the patient has symptoms that indicate a straightforward diagnosis. However, for more complex presentations or conditions, a measurement tool can provide additional information that assists in making a diagnosis and planning treatment.

Each rating scale included or reviewed in this text is described with the following information:

- *Title:* The title of each scale, as given by the original author, is stated, along with any abbreviation used within published literature.
- *Author:* The original author(s) of the tool with the date of first publication is cited. If available, citations for primary author revisions or important modifications by other authors are also included.
- *Source:* If the tool is available on the Internet, the URL available at the time of publication of this

text is listed. If the measure is proprietary, contact information for purchase is provided.
- *Targeted Population:* The patient population for which the tool is designed is noted here.
- *Description of Tool:* The purpose of the tool, description of the content, and details of administration are discussed.
- *Scoring:* The method of scoring for the tool is described here, along with interpretation of scores, if available.
- *Accuracy:* Reliability and validity studies available for the tool are summarized; references are included for the reader who desires more details on psychometric properties. Information was obtained from published studies and reviews or meta-analyses, when available.
- *Administration Time:* Approximate administration times, as determined by the author of the instrument or other published studies, are stated. The method of administration is also cited.
- *References:* Citations for published studies describing the instrument and its accuracy characteristics are listed, along with further resources for information pertaining to the tool.

The information presented in this text regarding each instrument is by no means a thorough review of the tool's application, reliability, and validity; nor is it a recommendation for use. The intent is to provide the reader with preliminary information about the tool and access to the instrument itself. For further information regarding utility and appropriateness of an instrument, the reader is encouraged to consult one of the referenced articles or review texts cited for the tool.

Psychometric Properties of Rating Scales

Psychometric properties are those that describe the performance characteristics of a measurement instrument. Reliability and validity are the two primary psychometric properties of a measure and are defined in Box 4. Terms used to describe specific forms of reliability and validity are also briefly defined. The reader who wants a more in-depth explanation of how these properties are measured, used for rating scale development and research, and applied to clinical data may consult reference texts listed in *Resources and References* or any text on psychometrics and statistics.

Measures that have demonstrated good reliability and validity within a broader patient population and varying settings are more advantageous to the primary care practice than those that tested smaller groups in narrowly defined settings. For the purpose of assisting the reader in selection of a measure for clinical use, the known psychometric properties have been summarized for each scale that is reviewed. When examining the psychometric properties for any tool, the reader should keep in mind that published reliability data tend to overestimate the reliability that can be achieved in everyday clinical practice.[17] This is because research studies are generally conducted under optimal testing conditions and employ extensively trained raters to perform assessments.

Selection and Use of Rating Scales in the Primary Care Setting

Decisions for selection and use of the "best tool" are left to the reader. Choice of a rating scale for clinical use depends on the needs of the patient population, practice management style, availability of the tool, and use of the resultant score. Each scale has strengths and weaknesses and may be continually developed or revised. The clinician may examine and try different tools within a subject area to get a feel for their characteristics and ease of use. The reader should then choose one tool within a topic and use it consistently for appropriate patients. In doing so, the clinician will become more familiar with administration, scoring, typical results, and any idiosyncrasies for that tool.

When choosing a tool, the reader should consider the following:
- The characteristics of the patient population being tested
- Strength of evidence for reliability and validity of the instrument
- Ease of method of administration and scoring

| Box 4 | Psychometric Terms and Definitions[3, 4, 9, 11, 17-19] |

Reliability: The ability of an instrument to measure consistent and reproducible information across respondents and institutional settings. Reliability is expressed as a number between 0 and 1, with 0 indicating no reliability and 1 indicating perfect reliability.

Internal consistency: The measure of agreement among the individual components of a measure; the degree to which each of the items in a scale is measuring the same thing.

Interrater reliability: The extent of agreement between two or more raters evaluating the same or similar subjects and using the same information.

Test-retest reliability: The measure of agreement between evaluations of the same population on two separate occasions, provided the subjects' true condition remain stable in the time interval.

Validity: The degree to which the scale actually measures the underlying quality it is designed to measure.

Content validity: Assesses the extent to which the components of a scale sample all aspects of the relevant domain, that is, whether all items are relevant to the scale's objectives.

Face validity: Indicates whether the items appear to be assessing the qualities they claim to measure.

Criterion validity: Compares the scale with a gold standard (the criterion measure) or some other valid measure of the disorder under study. There are two types:

Concurrent validity: Correlation of the measure with the criterion measure within a similar time frame.

Predictive validity: The ability of the measure to predict future changes.

Construct validity: Assesses the validity of the items to assess the concept in question, with external validators other than gold standards, such as behavioral theories. Construct validity is divided into two types:

Convergent validity: Degree of correlation of the scale with related variables.

Discriminant validity: Degree that the scale does not correlate with dissimilar variables.

Positive predictive value: Probability in a given population that a positive test result corresponds to a true case.

Negative predictive value: Probability in a given population that a negative test result corresponds to a non-case.

Sensitivity: The ability of the measure to detect true cases.

Specificity: The ability of the measure to detect non-cases.

- Time and staff required to complete administration and scoring
- Cost of obtaining or printing the measure
- How the clinician will use the scores to guide treatment planning

In examining the benefits of using rating scales in clinical practice, the clinician needs to consider the costs of time and staff required for administration, as well as cost of the tool. These costs may be balanced by reimbursement for testing, although many insurance carriers will not cover rating scale evaluations. Use of rating scales may provide less tangible benefits such as clearer diagnostic implications and treatment guidance and may have some value for substantiating a diagnosis for third-party reimbursement for treatment. Testing also provides evidence for a particular diagnosis to patients or parents and supports the clinician's recommendation for treatment.

Incorporation of rating scale administration into the office setting can be done in a variety of ways. Self-administration measures are completed independently by the individual. A screening form can be filled out by patients or parents in the office waiting room just before they are seen by the practitioner. Some scales can be completed at home before or after an office visit and can be returned to the office for scoring. Provided that treatment rooms are available, patients may be instructed on form completion, then left alone to confidentially complete the screening while the clinician sees another patient. Measures may also be administered orally by a clinician or office personnel; the clinician should keep in mind that some scales require specific training in administration and should only be used by persons instructed in use of the measure.

After the patient completes the questionnaire, the form is scored and the clinician follows up with additional questions and evaluates the results. Results of a rating scale screening do not offer a concrete diagnosis but help provide support for a clinical diagnosis and identify concerns and may provide guidelines for management.

Permissions for Clinical Use and Content Disclaimers

Some of the tools reproduced in this text are within "public domain" and thus may be copied or used without restriction for personal, clinical, or noncommercial purposes at no charge. However, many of the tools are copyrighted and owned by the original author or other entity, requiring permission before use is allowed. Permissions contact information and any guidelines available for copyrighted tools are available in Appendix C.

All rating scales reviewed in this text are provided for the information and convenience of the reader and should not be used as the sole means for making clinical decisions pertaining to patient diagnosis, care, or management. Scores obtained from use of any rating scale should be compared with, and tempered by, personal clinical knowledge and judgment. Tools are intended only for the educational and personal use of health care professionals and students and are not intended for persons who have not received appropriate medical training. Use of rating scales and screening instruments are not intended to be used as a substitute for consulting a licensed health care professional.

Inclusion of an instrument in this text does not constitute an official endorsement or approval by the author or publisher. The reader is reminded that rating scales are developed from outcomes data through original research. Reliability and validity of rating scales used in private clinical practice may differ from results obtained in research studies that may reflect institutional bias or a particular patient population characteristic.

Resources and References

1. American Psychiatric Association. *Handbook of psychiatric measures.* Washington, DC, 2000, American Psychiatric Association.
2. Antony MM, Orsillo SM, Roemer L. *Practitioner's guide to empirically based measures of anxiety.* New York, 2001, Plenum.
3. Bowling A. *Measuring health: a review of quality of life measurement scales.* Philadelphia, 1997, Open University Press.
4. Bowling A. *Measuring disease,* ed 2. Philadelphia, 2001, Open University Press.
5. Burns A, Lawlor B, Craig S. *Assessment scales in old age psychiatry.* London, 1999, Martin Dunitz Ltd.
6. Corcoran K, Fischer J. *Measures for clinical practice: a sourcebook* (2 vols.), ed 3. New York, 2000, Free Press.
7. Jones RL. *Handbook of tests and measurements for black populations* (2 vols.). Hampton, VA, 1996, Cobb & Henry Publishers.
8. Maruish ME, editor. *Handbook of psychological assessment in primary care settings.* Mahwah, NJ, 2000, Lawrence Erlbaum Associates.
9. McDowell I, Newell C. *Measuring health: a guide to rating scales and questionnaires,* ed 2. New York, 1996, Oxford University Press.
10. Nezu AM, Ronan GF, Meadows EA, et al. *Practitioner's guide to empirically based measures of depression.* New York, 2000, Plenum.
11. Sajatovic M, Ramirez LF. *Rating scales in mental health.* Hudson, OH, 2001, Lexi-Comp Inc.
12. Salek S. *Compendium of quality of life instruments* (5 vols). Chichester, West Sussex, United Kingdom, 1998, Wiley.
13. Schutte NS, Malouff JM. *Sourcebook of adult assessment (applied clinical psychology).* New York, 1995, Plenum Press.
14. Stanhope M, Knollmueller RN. *Handbook of community-based and home health nursing practice.* St. Louis, 2000, Mosby.
15. Quanta Healthcare Solutions, Inc. *The Medical Algorithms Project.* Available at http://www.medal.org/ (The Medical Algorithms Project, developed by Quanta Healthcare Solutions, Inc, 2002, provides access to hundreds of tools and algorithms published for professional use.)
16. Turk DC, Melzack R, editors. *Handbook of pain assessment,* ed 2. New York, 2001, Guilford Press.
17. Blacker D, Endicott J. Psychometric properties: concepts of reliability and validity. In *Handbook of psychiatric measures.* Washington, DC, 2000, American Psychiatric Association.
18. Bowling A. *Research methods in health: investigating health and health services.* Philadelphia, 2002, Open University Press.
19. Streiner DL, Norman GR. *Health measurement scales: a practical guide to their development and use.* New York, 1989, Oxford University Press.

CHAPTER 8

Developmental and Pediatric Tools

Chapter Contents

ICON KEY: 📄 Tool Printed   ✐ Tool on CD-ROM   ∞ Customizable Tool   **i** Information and Resources Provided for Further Acquisition

Chapter Contents—cont'd

ICON KEY: 📄 Tool Printed   💿 Tool on CD-ROM   ∞ Customizable Tool   **i** Information and Resources Provided for Further Acquisition

Introduction and Contents

This chapter contains reference tools and charts for measuring growth and instruments applicable to pediatric primary care. Screening assessment tools encompassing developmental issues, behavioral disorders, and injury risk behaviors are included here.

A great many tools and instruments that evaluate the developmental and behavioral status of the child exist. Most of these useful and validated tools are now copyrighted and only available by purchase from the copyright owner. A summary of tools applicable to primary care is included here, with a short description of the tool and purchasing information. If the tool is available online, the reader is referred to this source for downloading. Online resources for useful pediatric practice information are also described and cited.

GROWTH EVALUATION TOOLS AND CHARTS

Maturational Assessment of Gestational Age (New Ballard Score)

Authors: Ballard JL et al., 1991.

Targeted Population: Neonates.

Description: The widely used New Ballard Maturational Score rates six measures of neuromuscular maturity and seven measures of physical maturity by assigning points of −1 to 5 for each measure. The New Ballard Maturational Score is an enhancement of the original Ballard Score, which was refined and expanded in 1991 (Ballard et al) with goals of greater accuracy and inclusion of extremely premature neonates. In 1999, Donovan et al assessed gestational age of extremely premature infants (<28 weeks) by comparing the New Ballard Score and accurate menstrual history. New Ballard Scores exceeded the gestational age by dates with wide variation. The authors suggest that clinicians should consider inaccuracies in gestational age as determined by the New Ballard Score when treating extremely premature infants, particularly in making decisions about whether to forego or administer intensive care. Small differences in gestational age for very premature infants can result in large differences in outcome and may even determine whether intensive care is given.

Scores: Points for each measure are summed; scores may range from −11 to 54. Scores are then correlated with gestational age by using a table.

Accuracy: Use of this scoring system was found to accurately estimate maturity to ± 2 weeks (correlation = .97). For infants less than 26 weeks of gestational age, examinations performed before 12 hours of postnatal age resulted in the greatest validity (97% to ± 2 weeks of gestational age by prenatal ultrasonography). Interrater reliability was reported to be excellent at 0.95.

Administration Time: ~5-10 minutes.

References

Ballard JL, Khoury JC, Wedig K, et al: New Ballard Score expanded to include extremely premature infants. *J Pediatr* 119: 417-423, 1991.

Donovan EF, Tyson JE, Ehrenkranz RA, et al: Inaccuracy of Ballard scores before 28 weeks' gestation. National Institute of Child Health and Human Development Neonatal Research Network. *J Pediatr* 135:147-152, 1999.

Centers for Disease Control and Prevention 2000 Growth Charts for the United States

- **Boys 0-36 months: Length for age/Weight for age**
- **Boys 0-36 months: Head circumference for age/ Weight for length**
- **Girls 0-36 months: Length for age/Weight for age**
- **Girls 0-36 months: Head circumference for age/ Weight for length**
- **Boys 2-20 years: Stature for age/Weight for age**
- **Boys 2-20 years: Body mass index for age**
- **Boys 2-20 years: Weight for stature**
- **Girls 2-20 years: Stature for age/Weight for age**
- **Girls 2-20 years: Body mass index for age**
- **Girls 2-20 years: Weight for stature**

Authors: Ogden CL et al, 2000; Centers for Disease Control and Prevention (CDC), 2000.

Source: Set 1 is reproduced in this text and includes CDC modifications through April 2001. Set 1 (most commonly used in the United States) and Set 2 (percentiles for specialized applications) are available online, in Adobe Acrobat, at *http://www.cdc.gov/growthcharts*. The charts may be downloaded and printed in color or black and white and in English, Spanish, or French. Other helpful resources regarding pediatric growth evaluation are included on this website.

Targeted Population: Children, birth to 20 years.

Description: The CDC presented a revised version of pediatric growth charts in 2000 (Ogden et al, 2000). These charts replaced the 1977 National Center for Health Statistics (NCHS) growth charts, which have been used widely in pediatric practice for routine monitoring of growth in infants, children, and adolescents. The 2000 CDC growth charts were developed from extensive analysis of data collected in a series of five surveys performed between 1963 and 1994.

The 2000 CDC growth charts consist of a set of curves for infants, birth to 36 months, including weight for age, recumbent length for age, head circumference for age, and weight for recumbent length. Also created is a set of curves for children and adolescents, 2 to 20 years of age, including weight for age, stature for age, and body mass index for age. Weight for stature charts were also created for children between 77 and 121 cm in stature; children of this stature are primarily 2 to 5 years of age.

The clinical pediatric growth charts were published in two sets. Set 1 has the outer limits of the curves at the 5th and 95th percentiles and is most commonly used in the United States. Set 2 has the outer limits of the curves at the 3rd and 97th percentiles for specialized applications, such as assessment of the growth of children with special health care requirements.

The following printing guidelines are recommended by the CDC National Center for Health Statistics:
- The recommended paper weight is 80#.
- Charts should be printed as two-sided copies, in the following combinations for each sex:
  - Infants, birth to 36 months:
    - Side 1: Length for age + Weight for age
    - Side 2: Head circumference for age + Weight for length
  - Children and adolescents, 2 to 20 years:
    - Side 1: Stature for age + Weight for age
    - Side 2: Body mass index for age *or* Weight for stature (age 2 to 5 years only)

Accuracy: The 2000 CDC growth charts represent a cross-section of children living in the United States between 1971 and 1994. They include breastfed infants on the basis of their distribution in the U.S. population. The national distribution of birth weights is better represented in the 2000 CDC growth charts than in the 1977 National Center for Health Statistics series. Disjunctions between length and stature present in the 1977 versions of the growth charts have been corrected with the 2000 releases.

References

Denniston CR: Assessing normal and abnormal patterns of growth. *Prim Care* 21:637-654, 1994.

Legler JD, Rose LC: Assessment of abnormal growth curves. *Am Fam Physician* 58:153-158, 1998.

Ogden CL, Kuczmarski RJ, Flegal KM, et al: Centers for Disease Control and Prevention 2000 Growth Charts for the United States: improvements to the 1977 National Center for Health Statistics version. *Pediatrics* 109:45-60, 2000.

Growth Charts for Children with Down Syndrome

- Weight: Birth-3 years, girls
- Weight: 2-18 years, girls
- Weight: Birth-3 years, boys
- Weight: 2-18 years, boys
- Length: Birth-3 years, girls
- Height: 2-18 years, girls
- Length: Birth-3 years, boys
- Height: 2-18 years, boys
- Head circumference: Birth-3 years, girls
- Head circumference: Birth-3 years, boys

Author: Greg Richards, 2001.

Source: The growth charts for children with Down syndrome are reprinted here and are also available online at *http://www.growthcharts.com.*

Targeted Population: Children with Down syndrome, birth to age 3 years.

Description: Growth charts for children with Down syndrome were created by Greg Richards, a computer software consultant. The author notes that deviations from a given percentile level commonly occur between 9 and 24 months in children with Down syndrome.

Accuracy: Height, length, and weight charts were adapted from information published by Cronk et al (1988). Head circumference charts were created from data published by Palmer et al (1992).

References

Cronk C, Crocker AC, Pueschel SM, et al: Growth charts for children with Down syndrome: 1 month to 18 years of age. *Pediatrics* 81:102-110, 1988.

Palmer CG, Cronk C, Pueschel SM, et al: Head circumference of children with Down syndrome (0-36 months) [published erratum appears in *Am J Med Genet* 1992;43:768]. *Am J Med Genet* 42: 61-67, 1992.

Other Specialized Growth Chart Resources

Some pediatric subpopulations may fall out of the ranges of the 2000 CDC growth charts on the basis of their medical condition or ethnicity. The resources that follow contain information regarding growth charts for these specialized populations. These specialized growth charts may be limited by small sample size, older data, lack of population diversity, absence of nutritional status of subjects included in data, inconsistent measuring techniques, or presence of secondary medical conditions.

The CDC Growth Charts for Children with Special Health Needs: This instructional tool describes some of the effects that special health care needs can have on growth and illustrates how the CDC growth charts can be used with children with special health care needs. Website: *http://depts.washington.edu/growth/cshcn/text/page1a.htm.*

Achondroplasia Growth Charts: This 1995 policy statement from the American Academy of Pediatrics (AAP) contains figures for male and female height, mean growth velocities, upper and lower segment lengths, and head circumference. American Academy of Pediatrics Committee on Genetics, 1995. Health supervision for children with achondroplasia. *Pediatrics* 95:443-451. Website: *http://aappolicy.aappublications.org/cgi/reprint/pediatrics;95/3/443.*

Cerebral Palsy Growth Charts: Charts include weight for age, length for age, and weight for length for males and females with quadriplegic cerebral palsy. In: Krick J, Murphy-Miller P, Zeger S et al: Pattern of growth in children with cerebral palsy. *J Am Diet Assoc* 96:680-685, 1996.

Noonan Syndrome Growth Curves: Height-for-age charts are available for males and females. In: Witt DR,

Keena BA, Hall JG, et al: Growth curves for height in Noonan syndrome. *Clin Genet* 30:150-153, 1986.

Prader-Willi Syndrome Growth Charts: Charts include height for age for males and females. In: Holm VA: Growth charts for Prader-Willi syndrome. In Greenswag LR, Alexander RC, eds. *Management of Prader-Willi syndrome,* ed 2. New York, 1995, Springer-Verlag.

Turner Syndrome Growth Chart: Available free of charge from the Turner Syndrome Society. Website: *http://www.turner-syndrome-us.org/store/publication.html*

Vietnamese and Asian Growth Charts: Growth charts for Vietnamese babies (weight, 0-36 months), Vietnamese children (weight, 0-60 months), and Southeast Asian girls (weight, 0-7 years) are available. A link to growth charts for Chinese boys and girls in Hong Kong (height and weight, ages 1 month to 18 years, boys and girls; head circumference, ages 0 months to 18 years, girls) is also included. *Website: http://www. adoptvietnam.org/adoption/growth-chart.htm.*

Williams Syndrome Growth Charts: Charts include stature for age and weight for age for males and females ages 0 to 20 years. In: Morris CA, Demsey SA, Leonard CO, et al: Natural history of Williams syndrome: physical characteristics. *J Pediatr* 113:318-326, 1988.

Tanner Stages of Development

Author: Tanner JM, 1962.

Targeted Population: Pubertal males and females.

Description: Tanner stages, or sexual maturity ratings, depict the typical sequence of pubertal changes in males and females. Stages of breast, pubic hair, and penile development are described and used to grade the sexual maturity of the pediatric patient. Progression through the Tanner stages varies widely depending on the nationality, ethnic group, and the individual child.

Scores: Development occurs in five stages based on size, shape, appearance, and relative changes. Tanner stage 1 represents preadolescence, stages 2 through 4 represent various levels within adolescence, and stage 5 represents adulthood. The recommended method of assigning a Tanner stage for females is to average the levels for genitalia and breasts. Tanner stage progression from stage 2 to stage 5 (adulthood) takes 4 years on average, varying by plus or minus 2 years.

References

Johns Hopkins Hospital, Nechyba C, Gunn VL: *The Harriet Lane handbook: a manual for pediatric house officers,* ed 16. St. Louis, 2002, Mosby.

Marshall WA, Tanner JM: Variations in pattern of pubertal changes in girls. *Arch Dis Child* 44:291-303, 1969.

Marshall WA, Tanner JM: Variations in the pattern of pubertal changes in boys. *Arch Dis Child* 45:13-23, 1970.

Tanner JM: *Growth at adolescence.* Oxford, 1962, Blackwell Scientific Publications.

OTHER PEDIATRIC SCREENING INSTRUMENTS

Apgar Newborn Scoring System

Authors: Apgar V, 1953.

Targeted Population: Neonates.

Description: The Apgar scoring system is used to assess infants immediately after birth to help identify those who require resuscitation. Cardiopulmonary and neurologic functions are assessed by using five indicators.

Scores: Scoring is done at 1 and 5 minutes after birth. Scores range from 1 to 10; the lower the score, the more profoundly the infant is affected. One-minute Apgar scores of 0 to 3 indicate the need for prompt resuscitation and subsequent close observation. A low initial score with no improvement in the 5-minute score is associated with neonatal problems including death.

Reference

Apgar V: A proposal for a new method of evaluation of the newborn infant. *Anesth Analg* 32:260-267, 1953.

Baby Check Scoring System

Authors: Morley et al, 1991a.

Source: The Baby Check Scoring System is reprinted here and is also available online at *http://www.medal.org/ch44.html.*

Targeted Population: Infants, 0-6 months of age.

Description: The Baby Check Scoring System is used for the evaluation of sick infants less than 6 months of age. The scoring system is particularly suited for use in developing countries or busy outpatient clinics and allows parents and professionals to more easily assess the severity of a baby's illness. It can help separate high-risk infants who need more intensive care from healthy or mildly affected ones. The Baby Check Scoring System consists of 19 questions concerning symptoms and signs during illness. These questions, when presented in combination, have been statistically identified to accurately grade the severity of the illness. The scoring system has been shown to be both specific and sensitive in predicting serious illness.

Scores: Each item is assigned predetermined points only if the symptom is definitely present. The Baby Check Score is a sum of points for symptoms, examination of the awake baby, and examination of the undressed infant. Scores range from 0 to 111 points. Scores are interpreted by Morley et al (1991a) as follows: 0 to 7, well or mildly ill; 8 to 12, unwell but not likely to be seriously ill at the moment; 13 to 19, moderately to severely ill; and ≥20, seriously ill.

Accuracy: The tool has been tested in Chinese infants in Taipei (Chen et al, 1997), infants presenting to a clinic in a West African village in Gambia, and infants presenting to a polyclinic in Oman (Morley et al, 1994); the tool has also been tested for parental use in inner

cities in the United States (Kai, 1994) and in other home environments (Morley et al, 1991b; Thomson et al, 1999).
Administration Time: ~ 5 minutes by clinician review of symptoms and clinical examination.

References

Chen CK, Chen SJ, Hwang B: Evaluation of the severity of illness in infants by the Baby Check Score. *Chung Hua I Hsueh Tsa Chih (Taipei)* [*Chinese Medical Journal*] 59:15-20, 1997.

Kai J: 'Baby Check' in the inner city—use and value to parents. *Fam Pract* 11:245-250, 1994.

Morley CJ, Rashiq H, Thomas IR, et al: Use of Baby Check to assess the severity of illness in babies attending a clinic in Gambia. *J Trop Pediatr* 40:144-148, 1994.

Morley CJ, Thornton AJ, Cole TJ, et al: Baby Check: a scoring system to grade the severity of acute systemic illness in babies under 6 months old. *Arch Dis Child* 66:100-105, 1991a.

Morley CJ, Thornton AJ, Green SJ, et al: Field trials of the Baby Check score card in general practice. *Arch Dis Child* 66:111-114, 1991b.

Thomson H, Ross S, Wilson PMJ, et al: Randomised controlled trial of effect of Baby Check on use of health services in first 6 months of life. *Br Med J* 318:1740-1744, 1999.

Diagnostic Criteria for Prader-Willi Syndrome   i

The Prader-Willi Syndrome Association includes a diagnostic criteria calculator for Prader-Willi syndrome. The scoring system is based on criteria identified by Holm et al (1993) and is available online at *http://www.pwsausa.org/syndrome/Diagnos.htm.*

Reference

Holm VA, Cassidy SB, Butler MG, et al: Prader-Willi syndrome: consensus diagnostic criteria. *Pediatrics* 91:398-402, 1993.

INJURY PREVENTION TOOLS

The Injury Behavior Checklist

Authors: Speltz ML et al, 1990.
Source: This widely used checklist is reprinted in this chapter and is also available online at *http://www.medal.org/ch44.html.*
Targeted Population: Children, aged 2 years through adolescence.
Description: The Injury Behavior Checklist can be used to identify children at high risk for physical injury. The tool consists of 24 items of high-risk behavior.
Scores: Each item is scored on a Likert-type 5-point scale ranging from 0 (not at all) to 4 (very often, more than once a week). Scores are summed and range from 0 to 96 points. Children with mean scores of 22 are considered to be at low risk for injury, those with mean scores of 24.4 are considered to be at moderate risk for injury, and those with mean scores of 33.7 are considered to be at high risk for injury (Speltz et al, 1990). The scores can separate the child with low to moderate risk of injury from the child with high risk for injury.

Accuracy: Speltz et al (1990) reported acceptable reliability and were able to significantly discriminate children with two or more injuries from those with one or none.
Administration Time: 5 minutes by parent report.

References

Potts R, Martinez IG, Dedmon A, et al: Brief report: cross-validation of the Injury Behavior Checklist in a school-age sample. *J Pediatr Psychol* 22:533-540, 1997.

Speltz ML, Gonzales N, Sulzbacher S, et al: Assessment of injury risk in children: a preliminary study of the Injury Behavior Checklist. *J Pediatr Psychol* 15:373-383, 1990.

The Injury Prevention Program (TIPP™)   i

Authors: American Academy of Pediatrics (AAP).
Source: TIPP™ materials and ordering information are available online at http://www.aap.org/family/tippmain.htm.
Targeted Population: Children, newborn through 12 years of age.
Description: The AAP developed The Injury Prevention Program (TIPP™), an educational program for parents of newborns and children through 12 years of age. The program goals are to help prevent common pediatric injuries through regular screening and counseling activities and to set policy on making pediatric injury prevention counseling a standard of care for pediatricians. TIPP™ safety counseling has been shown to be a cost-effective method of preventing childhood injuries. Through use of resources available from the AAP, clinicians may survey parents on safety issues and provide age-appropriate safety education materials. The surveys and informational notes are designed to be integrated into the well-child visit schedule. Surveys allow the provider to tailor the counseling to the educational needs of the parents. Injury prevention topics covered for parents of children 5 years old and younger include child safety seat and smoke detector use, crib safety, water safety, firearm safety, pedestrian safety, play equipment safety, fall prevention, burn prevention, choking and suffocation prevention, and poisoning prevention. Topics covered for parents of children ages 6 to 12 include fire safety, firearm hazards, bike safety, street safety, car safety, sports safety, and water safety.

References

American Academy of Pediatrics Committee on Injury and Poison Prevention: Office-based counseling for injury prevention. *Pediatrics* 94:566-567, 1994.

Miller TR, Galbraith M: Injury prevention counseling by pediatricians: a benefit-cost comparison. *Pediatrics* 96:1-4, 1995.

Framingham Safety Surveys   i

Authors: Bass J, Mehta KA. Developed 1976.
Source: The safety surveys are available for purchase from the American Academy of Pediatrics (AAP) at *http://www.aap.org/bst/showdetl.cfm?&DID=15&Product_ID=1292&CatID=138.* The survey for ages 1 to 4 (part 1)

is also available online at *http://www.medal.org/ch44.html.*

Targeted Population: Children, ages 0 to 12 years of age.

Description: The Framingham Safety Surveys were developed to help health care professionals evaluate the risk of injury to a child, to better target risk areas for counseling on childhood injury prevention. These surveys have been incorporated into the TIPP™ program, which is available through the AAP. There are five different surveys for age ranges 0 to 12 months, 1 to 4 years (part 1), 1 to 4 years (part 2), 5 to 9 years, and 10 to 12 years. The age-specific surveys demonstrate the changes in risk as a child develops.

Administration Time: 1 minute by parent report.

References

Bass JL, Christoffel KK, Widome M, et al: Childhood injury prevention counseling in primary care settings: a critical review of the literature. *Pediatrics* 92:544-550, 1993.

Bass JL, Mehta KA: Developmentally oriented safety surveys: reported parental and adolescent practices. *Clin Pediatr* 19:350-356, 1980.

Bass J, Mehta K, Ostrovsky M, et al: Educating parents about injury prevention. *Pediatr Clin North Am* 32:233-242, 1985.

Hansen K, Wong D, Young PC: Do the Framingham Safety Surveys improve injury prevention counseling during pediatric health supervision visits? *J Pediatr* 129:494-498, 1996.

DEVELOPMENTAL SCREENING TOOLS

The majority of tools in this section can only be obtained by purchase or are available online for downloading. A summary description of each tool and resource information are included in each review. Reprinted in this text is The CHAT (Checklist for Autism in Toddlers).

Pediatric professionals concur that developmental surveillance should be performed at regular intervals from infancy through school age and at any time thereafter if behavioral, learning, or social concerns are raised (AAP, 2001; Filipek, 2000; Glascoe, 2000). It is especially important to recognize delays in language skills early, because early intervention and diagnosis greatly improve outcomes (AAP, 2001). Periodic, regular screening will lead to detection of a delay at a subsequent screening in a child not identified by a single screening. Specific screening for autism should be performed for all children who fail routine developmental screening (Filipek, 2000).

There are many developmental screening instruments from which to choose. Selection of the instrument can be based on presence of good psychometric properties (sensitivity, specificity, validity, and reliability), ease of use, time for administration, and cost. Each screening tool has inherent advantages and disadvantages in these selection criteria. Clinicians must choose the tool that will best fit the needs of the practice, so that the tool will be used consistently.

There are two groups of instruments based on time of administration, parent report, and direct elicitation.

The parent-report instruments included in this chapter have good psychometric properties and require much less time from the clinician than tools requiring direct elicitation. A disadvantage of parent-report instruments is the possibility of parents reporting skills not observed by the clinician or overestimating the abilities of their child. Direct elicitation tools eliminate these risks but have their own disadvantage of lengthier administration time. Reimbursement issues also present a significant barrier to incorporation of formal developmental screening services (Dobrez et al, 2001). Screening services may not be reimbursed consistently among insurance panels; thus the time and staff costs required to conduct and evaluate the screenings will figure into the selection process for the instrument. Cost models, such as those created by Dobrez et al (2001), may be used to select the best screens for the practice patient population at an acceptable cost. Clinicians may also choose to conduct a cost-effective, parent-report screen for regular encounters, identifying children at risk for developmental or behavioral problems. These "at-risk" children may then be given another appointment for a full, direct-elicitation screening or referred to a specialist for further evaluation.

References

American Academy of Pediatrics Committee on Children with Disabilities, 2000–2001. Developmental surveillance and screening of infants and young children. *Pediatrics* 108:192-196. Available at http://www.aap.org/policy/re0062.html.

Dobrez D, Lo Sasso A, Holl J, et al: Estimating the cost of developmental and behavioral screening of preschool children in general pediatric practice. *Pediatrics* 108:913-922, 2001.

Glascoe FP: Early detection of developmental and behavioral problems. *Pediatr Rev* 21:272-279, 2000.

Glascoe FP, Shapiro HL: Pediatric development and behavior: developmental screening. Available at http://www.dbpeds.org/articles/detail.cfm?id=5.

Ages and Stages Questionnaires (ASQ™)　　　i

Authors: Bricker D, Squires J: *Ages and Stages Questionnaires (ASQ)*™, ed 2, 1997. Squires J, Bricker D, Twombly E: *Ages & Stages Questionnaires: Social-Emotional (ASQ:SE)*™.

Source: Paul H. Brookes, Publishing Co., Inc., PO Box 10624, Baltimore, MD 21285 (phone: 410-337-9580, fax: 410-337-8539, U.S. toll-free: 800-638-3775, e-mail: custserv@brookespublishing.com); available for purchase online at *http://www.brookespublishing.com/store/books/bricker-asq/index.htm.*

Targeted Population: 4 to 60 months.

Description:
- The ASQ™ screening system consists of 19 reproducible questionnaires to be completed at well-visit intervals between the ages of 4 and 60 months and a user's guide. Each questionnaire contains 30 items covering five areas of development and a general area for caregiver concerns.

The questionnaires are designed for both first-level screening and monitoring of development.

- The Ages and Stages Questionnaire: Social Emotional (ASQ:SE) works similarly to screen for emotional and behavioral problems and is available for children ages 6 to 60 months. The ASQ™ system includes color-coded, reproducible questionnaires, scoring sheets, and the ASQ™ User's Guide.

Scores: Responses are converted to a point value; values are summed and compared with established screening cutoff points.

Accuracy: The ASQ™ has high specificity (range, 76% to 91%) with variable sensitivity across age intervals (range, 70% to 90%) and also indicates high test-retest reliability, interobserver reliability, and internal consistency. ASQ™ is one of four tools recommended for developmental screening by the Academy of Neurology (Filipek et al, 2000).

Administration Time: ~15 minutes; parents may complete independently.

References

Bricker D, Squires, J: *Introduction to ASQ™*, ed 2. Baltimore, MD: Brookes Publishing Co. Available at http://www.brookespublishing.com/store/books/bricker-asq/asq-introduction.pdf.

Filipek PA, Accardo PJ, Ashwal S, et al: Practice parameter: screening and diagnosis of autism: report of the Quality Standards Subcommittee of the American Academy of Neurology and the Child Neurology Society. *Neurology* 55:468-479, 2000.

Squires J, Bricker D, Potter L: Revision of a parent-completed development screening tool: Ages and Stages Questionnaires. *J Pediatr Psychol* 22:313-328, 1997.

Child Development Inventories (CDI)   i

- Infant Development Inventory (IDI) (0-18 months)
- Child Development Review (CDR) (18-60 months)
- Child Development Inventory (CDI) (15-60 months)
- Child Development Chart (CDC) (3-60 months)

Author: Ireton H. Developed 1990.

Source: Behavior Science Systems Inc., Box 580274, Minneapolis, MN 55458 (phone: 612-998-4784, fax: 360-351-1374, or e-mail to heidi@childdevrev.com); more information is available online at *http://www.childdevrev.com/*. Samples of the IDI and CDR may be viewed online at First Signs: *http://www.firstsigns.org/pages/parent_resources/documents.html*.

Targeted Population: 3 to 60 months.

Description:

- The IDI and CDR are two separate parent survey screening tools recommended for initial developmental screening. The IDI, for infants ages 3 to 18 months, tracks developmental skills in five areas—social, self-help, gross motor, fine motor, and language—and includes monthly developmental milestones. The CDR replaces the Early Child Development Inventory (18 months-36 months)

and the Preschool Development Inventory (36-60 months), which are currently being retired. The CDR contains six questions for parents with a 26-item possible problem checklist. The screening tools include developmental charts for the first 5 years on the reverse side. These inventories can be completed independently by families or administered in the office setting.

- The CDI assessment tool may be used for further assessment after screening. This 300-item tool may be completed by parents at home and assesses the development of social, self-help, motor, language, letter, and number skills, and the presence of symptoms and behavior problems in children between the ages of 15 months and 5 years.

- The Child Development Chart, for ages 3 to 60 months, is a brief, one-page screener consisting of two charts: The Infant Development Chart, for birth through 21 months, and a First Five Years Development Chart. The charts cover five developmental areas and typical developmental milestones.

Scores: The IDI and CDR produce a single cutoff tied to 1.5 standard deviations. The CDI provides cutoffs for five developmental domains and illustrates both significantly advanced and delayed development.

Accuracy: Sensitivity in identifying children with difficulties is excellent (greater than 75% across studies) and specificity in correctly identifying normally developing children is good (70% across studies). The CDI series are one of four tool groups recommended for developmental screening by the Academy of Neurology (Filipek et al, 2000).

Administration Time: ~10 minutes for IDI and CDR; parents may complete all tools independently.

References

Filipek PA, Accardo PJ, Ashwal S, et al: Practice parameter: screening and diagnosis of autism: report of the Quality Standards Subcommittee of the American Academy of Neurology and the Child Neurology Society. *Neurology* 55:468-479, 2000.

Ireton H, Glascoe FP: Assessing children's development using parents' reports: The Child Development Inventory. *Clin Pediatr* 34:248-255, 1995.

Ireton, H, ed: *Child development inventories in education and health care*. Minneapolis, 1997, Behavior Science Systems, Inc.

Pediatric Development and Behavior: Child Development Inventories (formerly Minnesota Child Development Inventories). Available at: http://www.dbpeds.org/articles/dbtesting/cdi.html.

Parents' Evaluation of Developmental Status (PEDS)   i

Author: Glascoe FP, 1998.

Source: Ellsworth & Vandermeer Press, LLC, PO Box 68164, Nashville, TN 37206 (phone: 615-226-4460, fax: 615-227-0411, U.S. toll-free: 888-729-1697); available for purchase online at *http://www.pedstest.com/*.

Targeted Population: Birth to 8 years.

Description: This validated and standardized screening tool is designed to elicit parental concerns regarding development. The tool consists of 10 questions written at the fifth-grade level. It identifies when to screen further or refer for additional screening and when to counsel, reassure, or monitor development, behavior, and academic progress. Parents' Evaluation of Developmental Status (PEDS) can detect autism, pervasive developmental disorders, or other spectrum disabilities, and is one of four tools recommended for developmental screening by the Academy of Neurology (Filipek et al, 2000).

Scores: Total scores are graded as high, moderate, or low risk for developmental and behavioral/mental health problems.

Accuracy: Sensitivity ranges from 74% to 79% and specificity ranges from 70% to 80% across age levels.

Administration Time: ~2 minutes; parents may complete independently.

References

Filipek PA, Accardo PJ, Ashwal S, et al: Practice parameter: screening and diagnosis of autism: report of the Quality Standards Subcommittee of the American Academy of Neurology and the Child Neurology Society. *Neurology* 55: 468-479, 2000.

Glascoe F: *PEDS manual: collaborating with parents: using parent's evaluations of developmental status to detect and address developmental and behavioral problems.* Nashville, TN, 1998, Ellsworth and Vandermeer Press. Available at http://www.pedstest.com/test/ peds_manual.html

Pediatric Development and Behavior: Parent's Evaluations of Developmental Status (PEDS). Available at: http://www.dbpeds.org/articles/dbtesting/peds.html.

Battelle Developmental Inventory (BDI) Screening Test   i

Authors: Newborg J, Stock JR, Wnek L, 1984.

Source: Riverside Publishing, 425 Spring Lake Drive, Itasca, IL 60143 (phone: 630-467-7000, fax: 630-467-7192, U.S. toll-free: 800-767-8378); available for purchase online at *http://www.riverpub.com/products/clinical/ bdi/home.html.*

Targeted Population: 6 months to 8 years.

Description: The complete Battelle Developmental Inventory (BDI) is a comprehensive instrument used for screening, diagnosis, evaluation, and program development for children. The BDI Screening Test contains 96 items, selected from the complete BDI to represent the full scope and content of development. Items include a combination of direct elicitation, observation, and parental interview. Screening results can identify areas in need of in-depth evaluation with the complete BDI. A second edition of the BDI is scheduled for release in 2004, after standardization testing has been performed.

Scores: The BDI Screening Test yields cutoff scores and age equivalents.

Accuracy: Reliability and validity data for the BDI Screening Test were derived from the complete BDI. Independent testing showed sensitivity of 72% and specificities of 50% to 76% (Glascoe & Byrne, 1993;

McLean, et al, 1987). Interrater reliabilities for the complete BDI were in the .90 to .99 range.

Administration Time: 10 to 30 minutes for direct assessment, observation, and caregiver interview.

References

Berls AT, McEwen IR: Battelle Developmental Inventory. *Physical Therapy* 79:776-783, 1999.

Glascoe FP, Byrne KE: The usefulness of the Battelle Developmental Inventory Screening Test. *Clin Pediatrics* 32:273-280, 1993.

McLean M, McCormick K, Baird S, et al: Concurrent validity of the Battelle Developmental Inventory Screening Test. *Diagnostique* 13:10-20, 1987.

Newborg J, Stock JR, Wnek L, et al: *Battelle Developmental Inventory.* Itasca, IL, 1994, Riverside Publishing.

Bayley Infant Neurodevelopmental Screener® (BINS™)   i

Author: Aylward GP, 1995.

Source: The Psychological Corporation, 555 Academic Court, San Antonio, TX 78204 (phone: 800-228-0752); *http://www.psychcorp.com.*

Targeted Population: 3-24 months.

Description: The BINS™ comprises six item sets, one per 3- to 6-month age range, with each set including 11 to 13 directly elicited items selected from the *Bayley Scales of Infant Development®–Second Edition (BSID–II)*. Items assess neurologic function, neurodevelopmental skills, and developmental accomplishments. Forms, a carrying case of needed materials, and an instructional videotape are available.

Scores: Items are scored as optimal or nonoptimal. Items that are performed optimally by the infant are summed; score cutoffs result in low-, moderate-, or high-risk categories for each of the three domains.

Accuracy: A validation study with *BSID–II* shows 80% to 88% classification agreement for infants who are developmentally delayed. Test-retest reliability ranges from .71 to .84 across ages; interrater reliability ranges from .79 to .96; and internal consistency reliability ranges from .73 to .85.

Administration Time: ~5 to 10 minutes for directly elicited items.

Reference

Aylward GP, Verhulst SJ: Predictive utility of the Bayley Infant Neurodevelopmental Screener (BINS) risk status classifications: clinical interpretation and application. *Dev Med Child Neurol* 42:25-31, 2000.

Early Screening Inventory–Revised™ (ESI-R™)   i

Authors: Meisels SJ, Marsden DB, Wiske MS, Henderson LW, 1997.

Source: Pearson Early Learning, 330 East Liberty, Suite 3C, Ann Arbor, MI 48104 (phone: U.S. toll-free: 800-435-3085; email: mail@rebusinc.com); product and ordering information is available from *http://www. pearsonearlylearning.com/index3.html.*

Targeted Population: 3 to 6 years.

Description: The Early Screening Inventory–Revised (ESI-R™) was first published in 1993 and was re-standardized with new norms and cutoffs in 1997 . It is a brief, developmental screening tool divided into two sections: ESI-P for ages 3 to 4½ and ESI-K for ages 4½ to 6. Items cover visual motor/adaptive, language, cognitive, and gross motor skills through a combination of direct assessment and a parental questionnaire. This tool is designed to detect relative weaknesses in developmental skills to identify children who may need special educational services to perform successfully in school. A training package is available and it contains two demonstration videotapes, a trainer's manual, and a set of reproducible black-line masters.

Scores: Responses are compared with established screening cutoff points and grouped into "refer," "rescreen," and "satisfactory" categories within each age range.

Accuracy: Sensitivity is >.92, and specificity is .80 for both tests, indicating that the ESI-R™ is highly reliable and valid. Interrater reliability is >.97 for both tests, and test-retest stability is also high at .87.

Administration Time: ~15 to 20 minutes for directly elicited items and parent questionnaire.

References

Meisels SJ, Henderson LW, Liaw F, et al: New evidence for the effectiveness of the Early Screening Inventory. *Early Child Res Q* 8:327-346, 1993.

Meisels SJ, Marsden DB, Wiske MS, et al: *The Early Screening Inventory–Revised.* Ann Arbor, MI, 1997, Rebus Inc.

Brigance Screens   i

- Infant and Toddler Screen for children 0-23 months
- Early Preschool Screen for children 2 years 0 months to 2 years 8 months
- Preschool Screen for children 2 years 9 months to 4 years 8 months
- K & 1 Screen for children 4 years 9 months through the end of first grade.

Author: Brigance A. Developed 1979. Re-standardized in 1995 and 2001.

Source: Curriculum Associates, Inc. (1985) 153 Rangeway Road, PO Box 2001, North Billerica, MA 01862-090 (phone: 978-667-8000, fax: 978-667-5706/ 800-366-1158, U.S. toll-free: 800-225-0248); available for purchase online at *http://www.curriculumassociates.com/.*

Targeted Population: Birth to 4 years 9 months (end of first grade).

Descriptions:

- Infant and Toddler Screen: two forms, 0-11 months and 12-23 months. Accommodations are made for infants born prematurely (until age 2 years).
- Early Preschool Screens: two forms: 2 years and 2½ years.
- Preschool Screens: two forms: 3 years and 4 years.
- K & 1 Screens: three forms: kindergarten, first grade, end of first grade.

The Brigance Screens assess fine and gross motor skills, speech and language, school readiness, and general knowledge. The Infant and Toddler Screens also assess social-emotional and self-help skills. The K & 1 Screens additionally measure reading and math skills, identifying developmental problems and children who have academic talent or intellectual giftedness.

Available materials include the screening forms, instruction manual, instructional video, data charts, scoring software, and technical reports. Screening materials are available for the Infant and Toddler Screen.

Scores: Cutoff, age-equivalent, percentile, and quotient scores for motor, language, readiness, and general knowledge are calculated for all age levels except the Infant and Toddler level, which provides scores for nonverbal and communication. Overall cutoff scores are calculated for all age levels; cutoffs indicate potential giftedness and/or psychosocial risk. Growth indicator scores plot progress over time.

Accuracy: Sensitivity and specificity to giftedness and to developmental and academic problems range from 70% to 86% across ages. Internal consistency, test-retest, and interrater reliability range from 0.98 to 0.99 for both the Infant and Toddler Screens (Glascoe, 2002a, 2002b, 2002c). The Brigance Screens are one of four tool groups recommended for developmental screening by the Academy of Neurology (Filipek et al, 2000).

Administration Time: ~10 to 12 minutes for Infant and Toddler Screen by parent report; ~10 to 15 minutes for all others by direct elicitation and observation.

References

Filipek PA, Accardo PJ, Ashwal S, et al: Practice parameter: screening and diagnosis of autism: report of the Quality Standards Subcommittee of the American Academy of Neurology and the Child Neurology Society. *Neurology* 55:468-479, 2000.

Glascoe FP: The Brigance Infant and Toddler Screen: standardization and validation. *J Dev Behav Pediatr* 23:145-150, 2002a.

Glascoe, FP: *Technical report for the Brigance® Screens: infant & toddler, early preschool, preschool, and K & 1 screens.* North Billerica, MA, 2002b, Curriculum Associates, Inc. Available at http://www.casamples.com/downloads/screen_techreport.pdf

Glascoe, FP: *A validation study of the psychometric properties of the Brigance® Screens: infant & toddler, early preschool, preschool, and K & 1 screens.* North Billerica, MA, 2002c, Curriculum Associates, Inc. Available at http://www.casamples.com/downloads/validate-study.pdf

Denver Developmental Materials   i

- Denver II Developmental Screening Tool
- PDQII Developmental Tools

Authors: Frankenburg WK, Dodds JB, 1989.

Source: Denver Developmental Materials, Inc., PO Box 371075, Denver, CO, 80237 (phone: 303-355-4729, fax: 303-355-5622, U.S. toll-free: 800-419-4729); available for purchase online at *http://www.denverii.com/*

Targeted Population: 1 month to 6 years.

Descriptions:

- Denver II Developmental Screening Tool: The Denver II consists of 125 tasks, or items, which are arranged on the test form in four sectors to screen personal/social, fine motor/adaptive, language, and gross motor skills. Also included are five "test behavior" items for completion after administration of the test: typical, compliance, interest in surroundings, fearfulness, and attention span. Screening results are recorded repeatedly on the same Denver II form, marking developmental progress over time. The results are not diagnostic. The Denver II materials include test forms, a training manual, a test supply kit, and a technical manual. Administration time is ~ 20 minutes by direct elicitation.

- PDQII Developmental Tools: Four different age-related forms are available to be completed by the parent or caregiver. The PDQ-II consists of 91 questions from the Denver II; only a subset of questions are asked for each age group. The form may need to be read to parents and caregivers who are less educated. Administration time is ~10 minutes by parent report.

Scores:

- Denver-II: Individual, directly elicited items are scored as "advanced," "normal," "caution," or "delayed" on the basis of predetermined normal age ranges of success on that item. The number of items for which the child scores below the expected age range determines whether the child is classified as "within normal range," "suspect," or "delayed." Suspect scores are monitored by more frequent screening; delayed scores are referred for further assessment.
- PDQ-II: Scoring is based on the number of delays or cautions as defined for the Denver II. Children who have no delays or cautions are considered to be developing normally; children with one delay or two cautions are recommended for re-screening with the PDQ-II 1 month later. When delays are detected during re-screening or when two or more delays or three or more cautions are found during the first screening, the Denver II should be administered as soon as possible.

Accuracy: The Denver-II has sensitivity of 56% to 83%, depending on the scoring method used. Specificity ranges from 43% to 80%, again depending on the scoring method. Sensitivity and specificity data were standardized from a nondiverse population in Colorado, and validation studies have not been performed, drawing criticism of this tool from other developmental pediatric experts (Glascoe et al, 1992; Glascoe, 2002; Filipek et al, 2000). Denver-II has demonstrated good interrater and test-retest reliability (correlations .90 or higher for most tests). There is no direct reliability data for the PDQ-II screens.

Administration Time: See individual screening tool.

References

Filipek PA, Accardo PJ, Ashwal S, et al: Practice parameter: screening and diagnosis of autism: report of the Quality Standards Subcommittee of the American Academy of Neurology and the Child Neurology Society. *Neurology* 55:468-479, 2000.

Frankenburg WK: The Denver II: a major revision and restandardization of the Denver Developmental Screening Test. *Pediatrics* 89: 91-97, 1992.
Frankenburg WK: Developmental surveillance and screening of infants and young children. *Pediatrics* 109:144-145, 2002.
Glascoe FP: Two views of developmental testing. *Pediatrics* 109: 1181-1183; author reply 1181-1183, 2002.
Glascoe FP, Byrne KE, Chang B, et al: Accuracy of the Denver-II in developmental screening. *Pediatrics* 89:1221-1225, 1992.

CHAT (Checklist for Autism in Toddlers)

Authors: Baron-Cohen S et al, 1992.

Source: The CHAT is reprinted in this text. The checklist is also available online at several sources including the Autism 99 Information Centre (*http://trainland. tripod.com/gillian.htm*) and The Medical Algorithms Project (*http://www.medal.org/ch17.html*).

Targeted Population: 18 months.

Description: The CHAT is widely used to identify cases of autism and related pervasive developmental disorders and language and other developmental disorders. The CHAT combines parent responses to nine questions with a semistructured observation of five items by a health care provider. The CHAT was designed to be used with 18-month-old children; recent studies have indicated that it is also sensitive in the 18- to 24-month developmental range (Charman et al, 2002; Scambler et al, 2001).

Scores: Responses are "yes" or "no"; "no" responses (failures) are categorized as high, medium, or low risk of autism. Failure of all five key items on the CHAT (protodeclarative pointing [A7 + Biv], gaze monitoring [Bii] and pretend play [A5 + Biii]) both initially and on repeat administration suggest high risk for autism. Failure of the two key items relating to protodeclarative pointing (A7 + Biv), but passing of at least one of the other key items (A5, Bii, Biii) both initially and on repeat administration suggest medium risk for autism. It is emphasized that the CHAT is not a diagnostic instrument but can identify potential cases of autism spectrum disorders for a full diagnostic assessment (Baird et al, 2000).

Accuracy: The CHAT has been validated in large populations of children. The CHAT originally demonstrated sensitivity and specificity of 65% and 100%, respectively; Baird et al (2000) found the CHAT had a sensitivity of 38% and a specificity of 98% for identifying childhood autism. The CHAT may be less sensitive to milder symptoms of autism (Filipek et al, 2000); Scambler et al (2000) noted that the CHAT successfully discriminated 2-year-old children with autism from those with other developmental disorders (sensitivity of 85% in a group of children with developmental disabilities; specificity of 100%).

Administration Time: ~10 to 15 minutes for both parent responses and direct elicitation.

References

Baird G, Charman T, Baron-Cohen S, et al: A screening instrument for autism at 18 months of age: a 6-year follow-up study. *J Am Acad Child Adolesc Psychiatry* 39:694-702, 2000.

Baron-Cohen S, Allen J, Gillberg C: Can autism be detected at 18 months? The needle, the haystack, and the CHAT. *Br J Psychiatry* 161:839-843, 1992.

Baron-Cohen S, Cox A, Baird G, et al: Psychological markers of autism at 18 months of age in a large population. *Br J Psychiatry* 168:158-163, 1996.

Baron-Cohen S, Wheelwright S, Cox A, et al: Early identification of autism by the Checklist for Autism in Toddlers (CHAT). *J R Soc Med* 93: 521-525, 2000.

Charman T, Baron-Cohen S, Baird G, et al: Is 18 months too early for the CHAT? *J Am Acad Child Adolesc Psychiatry* 41(3):235-236, 2002.

Filipek PA, Accardo PJ, Ashwal S, et al: Practice parameter: screening and diagnosis of autism: report of the Quality Standards Subcommittee of the American Academy of Neurology and the Child Neurology Society. *Neurology* 55:468-479, 2000.

Scambler D, Rogers SJ, Wehner EA: Can the checklist for autism in toddlers differentiate young children with autism from those with developmental delays? *J Am Acad Child Adolesc Psychiatry* 40: 1457-1463, 2001.

Modified Checklist for Autism in Toddlers (M-CHAT)   i

Authors: Robins DL et al, 2001.

Source: The M-CHAT is available for downloading online at *http://www.firstsigns.org/pages/parent_resources/documents.html*.

Targeted Population: 18 months.

Description: The Modified Checklist for Autism in Toddlers (M-CHAT) is an expanded American version of the parental portion of the CHAT. A parent report questionnaire, the M-CHAT has a total of 23 items, which incorporate the nine original questions from the CHAT.

Scores: Responses are "yes" or "no"; when 2 or more *critical* items are failed ("no"), or when *any three* items are failed, the authors recommend more detailed evaluation or referral for developmental evaluation with a specialist.

Accuracy: Sensitivity, specificity, and validation studies are ongoing and results are anticipated in 2004.

Administration Time: ~5 to 10 minutes; parents complete independently.

Reference

Robins DL, Fein D, Barton ML, et al: The Modified Checklist for Autism in Toddlers: an initial study investigating the early detection of autism and pervasive developmental disorders. *J Autism Dev Disord* 31:131-144, 2001.

Pediatric Symptom Checklist (PSC)   i

Authors: Jellinek MS et al, 1988.

Source: The Pediatric Symptom Checklist (PSC) can be downloaded free of charge in English or Spanish at *http://psc.partners.org/*. This site is maintained by the authors of the PSC and contains a full discussion of technical aspects and references. A copy of the scoring criteria, with three factor subscales, is available free of charge at *http://www.pedstest.com/links/resources.html*.

Targeted Population: 4 to 18 years.

Description: A brief parent-completed psychosocial screening questionnaire, the PSC obtains parents' reports of children's behavioral/emotional problems on 35 items. The PSC is a screening instrument and not a diagnostic tool. It is designed to alert clinicians early to difficulties in functioning that may indicate current or potential psychosocial problems. This test is considered to be well validated and is accepted throughout the pediatric professional community.

Scores: The 35 items are rated as never, sometimes, or often present and scored 0, 1, and 2, respectively. Items that are left blank by parents are ignored (score = 0). If four or more items are left blank, the questionnaire is considered invalid. Item scores are summed; three subscale measures also screen for attention-deficit/hyperactivity disorder, depression and anxiety, and conduct disorder (Gardner et al, 1999). For children aged 6 through 16 years, the cutoff score is 28 or higher. For 4- and 5-year-old children, the PSC cutoff score is 24 or higher. A positive score on the PSC suggests the need for further evaluation by a qualified health or mental health professional.

Accuracy: The PSC has been extensively tested in various populations. A PSC cutoff score of 28 has a specificity of 0.68 and a sensitivity of 0.95 when compared with clinicians' ratings of children's psychosocial dysfunction (Jellinek et al, 1988). Strong internal consistency (.91) of PSC items and highly significant ($P < 0.0001$) correlations between individual PSC items and positive PSC screening scores have been demonstrated (Murphy et al, 1996). Test-retest reliability ranges from .84 to .91.

Administration Time: ~2 to 5 minutes; parents complete independently.

References

Gardner W, Murphy M, Childs G, et al: The PSC-17: a brief symptom checklist of psychosocial problem subscales: a report from PROS and ASPN. *Ambulatory Child Health* 5:225-236, 1999.

Jellinek MS, Murphy JM, Little M, et al: Use of the Pediatric Symptom Checklist to screen for psychosocial problems in pediatric primary care: a national feasibility study. *Arch Pediatr Adolesc Med* 153:254-260, 1999.

Jellinek MS, Murphy JM, Robinson J, et al: Pediatric Symptom Checklist: screening school-age children for psychosocial dysfunction. *J Pediatr* 112:201-209, 1988.

Murphy JM, Ichinose C, Hicks RC, et al: Utility of the Pediatric Symptom Checklist as a psychosocial screen to meet the federal Early and Periodic Screening, Diagnosis, and Treatment (EPSDT) standards: a pilot study. *J Pediatr* 129:864-869, 1996.

Pediatric Symptom Checklist. Available at http://www.psc.partners.org/

Family Psychosocial Screening   i

Authors: Kemper KJ, Kelleher KJ, 1996.

Source: The Family Psychosocial Screening can be freely downloaded through *http://www.pedstest.com/links/resources.html* or directly from *http://www.pedstest.com/links/files/fampsych.pdf*.

Targeted Population: Screens families for a range of psychosocial risk factors.

Description: A two-page form consists of questions identifying psychosocial risk factors associated with developmental and behavioral problems. These include items on parental history of physical abuse as a child, items on parental substance abuse, and items on parental depression. Other items include family health history, social support, family activities, home safety issues, and family demographics.

Scores: Positive responses to certain items are considered a positive screen; such items are clearly identified in the introduction to this measure available at the above website. Further questions, professional assistance, counseling, or referral to appropriate resources are warranted with a positive screen.

Accuracy: Reliability and validation data are not available.

Administration Time: ~15 minutes, less if completed independently.

Reference

Kemper KJ, Kelleher KJ: Family psychosocial screening: instruments and techniques. *Ambulatory Child Health* 4:325-339, 1996.

Safety Word Inventory and Literacy Screener (SWILS)   i

Authors: Glascoe FP, 2002.

Source: A copy of the Safety Word Inventory and Literacy Screener (SWILS) can be freely downloaded through *http://www.pedstest.com/links/resources.html* or directly from *http://www.pedstest.com/links/files/SWILS.pdf*.

Targeted Population: 6 to 14 years.

Description: The SWILS consists of 29 common safety words (e.g., *Walk, High Voltage, Poison*). Children are asked to read each word aloud. The number of correctly read words is compared with a cutoff score. Performance predicts skills in reading, math, and written language. Items were drawn from the Brigance Comprehensive Inventory of Basic Skills–Revised, a diagnostic inventory of academic skills, which itself includes a more in-depth screener of school dysfunction (available at *http://www.curriculumassociates.com*). The SWILS, with its emphasis on safety words, may also serve as a springboard to injury prevention counseling. A single longitudinal form remains in the medical record.

Scores: A single cutoff score indicates the need for a referral to a school psychologist or other professional. Cutoff scores increase with age.

Accuracy: Sensitivity of 78% (range, 73%-88%) and specificity of 84% (range, 77%-87%) to academic performance in the areas of reading, math, and written language have been documented. Interrater reliability coefficients were high and ranged from .64 to .98.

Administration Time: ~3 to 4 minutes to administer and score.

Reference

Glascoe FP: Safety words inventory and literacy screener: standardization and validation. *Clin Pediatr* 41:697-704, 2002.

LANGUAGE

Dyslexia Screening Tests   i

- Dyslexia Early Screening Test (DEST)
- Dyslexia Screening Test (DST)
- Dyslexia Adult Screening Test (DAST)

Authors: Nicolson RI, Fawcett AJ. 1996 (DEST and DST). 1998 (DAST).

Source: The Psychological Corporation, 555 Academic Court, San Antonio, TX 78204 (phone: 800-228-0752); available for purchase online at *http://www.psychcorp.com*.

Targeted Population: The Dyslexia Early Screening Test (DEST): 4 years 6 months to 6 years 5 months; The Dyslexia Screening Test (DST): 6 years 6 months to 16 years 6 months; The Dyslexia Adult Screening Test (DAST): adults aged 16 years 7 months to 75 years.

Description: The Dyslexia Screening Tests are designed as screening instruments for routine use in schools and in employment (Plake et al, 2003). Each test contains 10 to 11 subtests; IQ is not tested. The DAST includes a 5-minute, nonverbal memory test. The object of these tests is to identify children who are in need of further support. Available for purchase are the screening tests, instruction manual, score keys, record forms, and screening materials.

Scores: Through 10 to 11 subtests, a profile of strengths and weaknesses is provided. Subjects with "at risk" profiles are recommended for further tests.

Accuracy: The Dyslexia Screening Tests have been normed on more than 3000 children and adults in the United Kingdom. Reliability and validity data are not available.

Administration Time: ~30 minutes by direct elicitation.

References

Nicolson RI, Fawcett AJ: Dyslexia Screening Tests. Available at http://www.shef.ac.uk/psychology/research/lrg/dyslexia/dest.html.

Plake BS, Impara JC, Spies RA, eds: *The fifteenth mental measurements yearbook*. Lincoln, NE, 2003, Buros Institute of Mental Measurements.

ATTENTION-DEFICIT/HYPERACTIVITY DISORDER (ADHD) EVALUATION

National Initiative for Children's Healthcare Quality (NICHQ) ADHD Practitioners' Toolkit   i

Authors: NICHQ committee, sponsored by the American Academy of Pediatrics (AAP), 2000, 2001.

Source: Available as a PDF format zip file, the complete NICHQ ADHD Toolkit may be downloaded from *http://www.nichq.org/resources/toolkit/*. The Toolkit may also be ordered from the AAP at *http://www.aap.org/bst/showdetl.cfm?&DID=15&Product_ID=3787&CatID=132*.

Targeted Population: 6 to 12 years.

Description: The NICHQ ADHD Practitioners' Toolkit contains a set of practical tools and assessment scales for primary care practitioners to use in implementing the 2001 AAP guidelines for treating ADHD. Included in the Toolkit are the following forms and scales:

- Primary Care Initial Evaluation Form
- NICHQ Vanderbilt Assessment Scale–Parent Informant
- NICHQ Vanderbilt Assessment Scale–Teacher Informant
- NICHQ Vanderbilt Assessment Follow-up–Parent Informant
- NICHQ Vanderbilt Assessment Follow-up–Teacher Informant
- Scoring Instructions for NICHQ Vanderbilt Assessment Scales

Other valuable resources related to the management of ADHD, school issues, and reimbursement documentation are also included.

The NICHQ Vanderbilt Assessment Scales for parent and teacher evaluation are divided into symptom assessment and performance rating question sections, which screen the child for one of three subtypes of ADHD diagnosis: predominantly inattentive, predominantly hyperactive/impulsive, and combined inattentive/hyperactive. The assessment scales also screen for oppositional-defiant disorder, conduct disorder, and anxiety/depression.

Scores: Cutoff scores within subsets of questions, based on the *Diagnostic and Statistical Manual of Mental Disorders, Fourth Edition* (*DSM-IV*) criteria for the diagnosis of ADHD, are used to evaluate whether a child meets these criteria. It is recommended to use information from multiple sources in addition to the screening scales to diagnose ADHD (Brown et al, 2001).

Accuracy: Reliability and validity data are not available.

Administration Time: ~10-15 minutes by parent/teacher report.

References

American Academy of Pediatrics Committee on Quality Improvement and Subcommittee on Attention-Deficit/Hyperactivity Disorder: Clinical practice guideline: diagnosis and evaluation of the child with attention-deficit/hyperactivity disorder. *Pediatrics* 105:1158-1170, 2000.

American Academy of Pediatrics Subcommittee on Attention-Deficit/Hyperactivity Disorder and Committee on Quality Improvement: Clinical practice guideline: treatment of the school-aged child with attention-deficit/hyperactivity disorder. *Pediatrics* 108:1033-1044, 2001.

Brown RT, Freeman WS, Perrin JM, Stein MT, Amler RW, Feldman HM, Pierce K, Wolraich ML: Prevalence and assessment of attention-deficit/hyperactivity disorder in primary care settings. *Pediatrics* 107:E43, 2001.

Conners' Rating Scales-Revised (CSR-R)   i

Authors: Conners CK, 1997.

Source: Available for purchase at *http://www.widerange. com/conners.html*; The Psychological Corporation, 555 Academic Court, San Antonio, TX 78204 (phone: 800-228-0752); *http://www.psychcorp.com*.

Targeted Population: 6 to 17 years.

Description: The Conners' Rating Scales–Revised is a set of parent and teacher report measures for assessing attention-deficit/hyperactivity disorder (ADHD) in children and adolescents. The scales correspond to symptoms used in the *DSM-IV* as criteria for ADHD. Both reports have long and short forms. The parent long form (80 items) has the following subscales: oppositional, cognitive problems, hyperactive-impulsive, ADHD index, anxious/shy, perfectionism, social problems, psychosomatic, *DSM-IV* symptom subscales, and Conners' Global Index. The teacher report long form (59 items) includes the same subscales as the parent's form with the exception of the psychosomatic scale. The parent's short form (27 items) and teacher's short form (28 items) include the first four of the subscales. A self-assessment version for input directly from adolescents (an 87-item long form and a 27-item short form) is also offered. Available for purchase are a kit containing all rating scales, a user's manual, a technical manual, scoring, short and long forms for parent and teacher feedback, and a progress form for presenting assessment results to parents.

Scores: Scores based on the *DSM-IV* criteria for the diagnosis of ADHD identify children at risk for ADHD. It is recommended to use information from multiple sources in addition to the screening scales to diagnose ADHD (Brown et al, 2001).

Accuracy: Reliability and validity data are not available. Normative data for the revised forms come from a large sample of community-based North American children aged 3 to 17 years.

Administration Time: ~20-45 minutes for long forms; ~10-15 minutes for short forms; all forms by parent, teacher, or self-report.

References

Brown RT, Freeman WS, Perrin JM, et al: Prevalence and assessment of attention-deficit/hyperactivity disorder in primary care settings. *Pediatrics* 107:E43, 2001.

Conners CK: *Conners' rating scales–revised: instruments for use with children and adolescents.* New York, 1997, Multi-Systems, Inc.

Online Resources

The Pediatric Development and Behavior Homepage: *http:// www.dbpeds.org/*
This independent website was created to promote better care and outcomes for children and families affected by developmental, learning, and behavioral problems by providing access to clinically relevant information and educational material for physicians, fellows, resident physicians, and students. The site may also be of interest to psychologists, nurses, nurse practitioners, physician assistants, social workers, therapists, educators, and parents.

The Medical Algorithms Project: *http://www.medal.org/ch44.html*
The Medical Algorithms Project; developed by Quanta Healthcare Solutions, Inc, 2002, provides access to tools and algorithms published for professional use. Pediatric tools include assessment

of neonatal well-being and development, disorders in neonates, assessment of infants and small children, clinical evaluation of sick children, assessing pain in pediatric patients, fetal alcohol syndrome, injuries in children and adolescents, febrile seizures in children, effect of childhood illness on patients and family members, evaluation of feeding in infants, bedwetting, and puberty.

Harriet Lane Links: *http://derm.med.jhmi.edu/poi/*

The Harriet Lane Links (formerly Pediatric Points of Interest) provide an edited collection of pediatric resources (6071 links) on the World Wide Web. Maintained and edited at Johns Hopkins University, this site attempts to catalog, review, and score existing links to pediatric information on the Internet.

GeneralPediatrics.com: *http://www.generalpediatrics.com/*

This site is an award-winning pediatric digital library that identifies and organizes high-quality, authoritative general pediatric World Wide Web sites. Continuously updated information links are available and organized into the following subheadings: Case Studies and Patient Simulations, Continuing Medical Education Courses, Evidence Based Medicine Resources, Journals and News, Policy Statements and Clinical Practice Guidelines, Professional Societies, Internet Directories, Search Engines, and Handheld Computer Resources. GeneralPediatrics.com is curated and maintained by Donna M. D'Alessandro, MD, and is partially supported by a Robert Wood Johnson Foundation Generalist Faculty Scholar Grant.

MATURATIONAL ASSESSMENT OF GESTATIONAL AGE (New Ballard Score)

NAME _____ SEX _____

HOSPITAL NO. _____ BIRTH WEIGHT _____

RACE _____ LENGTH _____

DATE/TIME OF BIRTH _____ HEAD CIRC. _____

DATE/TIME OF EXAM _____ EXAMINER _____

AGE WHEN EXAMINED _____

APGAR SCORE: 1 MINUTE _____ 5 MINUTES _____ 10 MINUTES _____

NEUROMUSCULAR MATURITY

NEUROMUSCULAR MATURITY SIGN	SCORE							RECORD SCORE HERE
	-1	0	1	2	3	4	5	
POSTURE								
SQUARE WINDOW (Wrist)	>90°	90°	60°	45°	30°	0°		
ARM RECOIL		180°	140°-180°	110°-140°	90°-110°	<90°		
POPLITEAL ANGLE	180°	160°	140°	120°	100°	90°	<90°	
SCARF SIGN								
HEEL TO EAR								

TOTAL NEUROMUSCULAR MATURITY SCORE

PHYSICAL MATURITY

PHYSICAL MATURITY SIGN	SCORE							RECORD SCORE HERE
	-1	0	1	2	3	4	5	
SKIN	sticky friable transparent	gelatinous red translucent	smooth pink visible veins	superficial peeling &/or rash, few veins	cracking pale areas rare veins	parchment deep cracking no vessels	leathery cracked wrinkled	
LANUGO	none	sparse	abundant	thinning	bald areas	mostly bald		
PLANTAR SURFACE	heel-toe 40-50 mm: -1 <40 mm: -2	>50 mm no crease	faint red marks	anterior transverse crease only	creases ant. 2/3	creases over entire sole		
BREAST	imperceptible	barely perceptible	flat areola no bud	stippled areola 1-2 mm bud	raised areola 3-4 mm bud	full areola 5-10 mm bud		
EYE/EAR	lids fused loosely: -1 tightly: -2	lids open pinna flat stays folded	sl. curved pinna; soft; slow recoil	well-curved pinna; soft but ready recoil	formed & firm instant recoil	thick cartilage ear stiff		
GENITALS (Male)	scrotum flat, smooth	scrotum empty faint rugae	testes in upper canal rare rugae	testes descending few rugae	testes down good rugae	testes pendulous deep rugae		
GENITALS (Female)	clitoris prominent & labia flat	prominent clitoris & small labia minora	prominent clitoris & enlarging minora	majora & minora equally prominent	majora large minora small	majora cover clitoris & minora		

TOTAL PHYSICAL MATURITY SCORE

SCORE

Neuromuscular _____

Physical _____

Total _____

MATURITY RATING

score	weeks
-10	20
-5	22
0	24
5	26
10	28
15	30
20	32
25	34
30	36
35	38
40	40
45	42
50	44

GESTATIONAL AGE (weeks)

By dates _____

By ultrasound _____

By exam _____

From Ballard JL, Khoury JC, Wedig K, et al: New Ballard Score, expanded to include extremely premature infants. *J Pediatr* 119:417-423, 1991.

Birth to 36 months: Boys
Length-for-age & Weight-for-age percentiles

NAME _____

RECORD # _____

AGE (MONTHS)

Birth 3 6 9 12 15 18 21 24 27 30 33 36

LENGTH

95
90
75
50
25
10
5

LENGTH

WEIGHT

95
90
75
50
25
10
5

AGE (MONTHS)

12 15 18 21 24 27 30 33 36

		Mother's Stature _____	Gestational		
		Father's Stature _____	Age: _____ Weeks		Comment
Date	Age	Weight	Length	Head Circ.	
	Birth				

WEIGHT

Birth 3 6 9

Published May 30, 2000 (modified 4/20/01).
SOURCE: Developed by the National Center for Health Statistics in collaboration with
the National Center for Chronic Disease Prevention and Health Promotion (2000).
http://www.cdc.gov/growthcharts

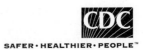

SAFER · HEALTHIER · PEOPLE™

212

Birth to 36 months: Boys
Head circumference-for-age &
Weight-for-length percentiles

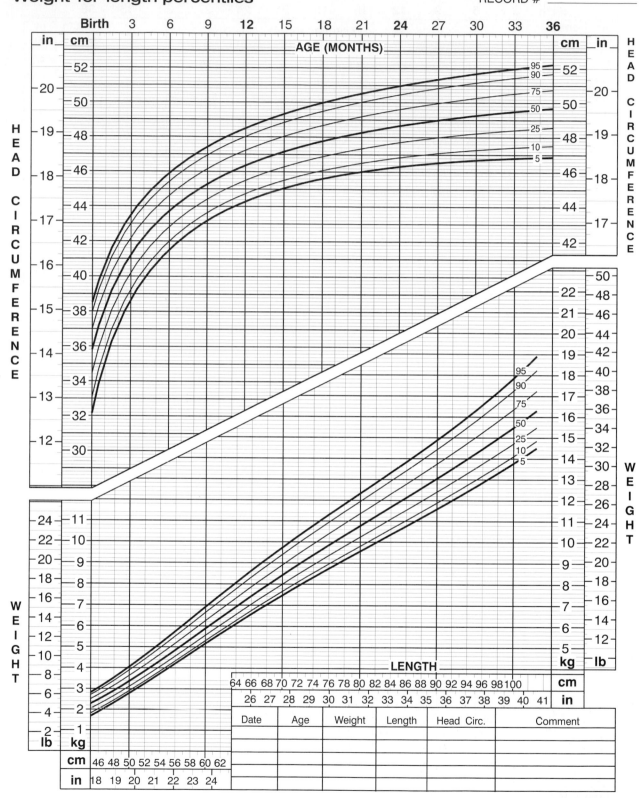

Published May 30, 2000 (modified 10/16/00).
SOURCE: Developed by the National Center for Health Statistics in collaboration with
the National Center for Chronic Disease Prevention and Health Promotion (2000).
http://www.cdc.gov/growthcharts

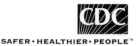

SAFER · HEALTHIER · PEOPLE™

Birth to 36 months: Girls
Length-for-age & Weight-for-age percentiles

NAME _____

RECORD # _____

AGE (MONTHS)

Birth 3 6 9 **12** 15 18 21 **24** 27 30 33 **36**

in cm

L
E
N
G
T
H

95
90
75
50
25
10
5

cm in

L
E
N
G
T
H

95
90
75
50
25
10
5

W
E
I
G
H
T

kg lb

AGE (MONTHS)

12 15 18 21 **24** 27 30 33 **36**

Mother's Stature _____			Gestational		
Father's Stature _____			Age: _____ Weeks		Comment
Date	Age	Weight	Length	Head Circ.	
	Birth				

W
E
I
G
H
T

lb kg

Birth 3 6 9

Published May 30, 2000 (modified 4/20/01).
SOURCE: Developed by the National Center for Health Statistics in collaboration with
the National Center for Chronic Disease Prevention and Health Promotion (2000).
http://www.cdc.gov/growthcharts

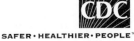

SAFER · HEALTHIER · PEOPLE™

Copyright © 2005 by Mosby, Inc.

214

Birth to 36 months: Girls
Head circumference-for-age &
Weight-for-length percentiles

NAME _____

RECORD # _____

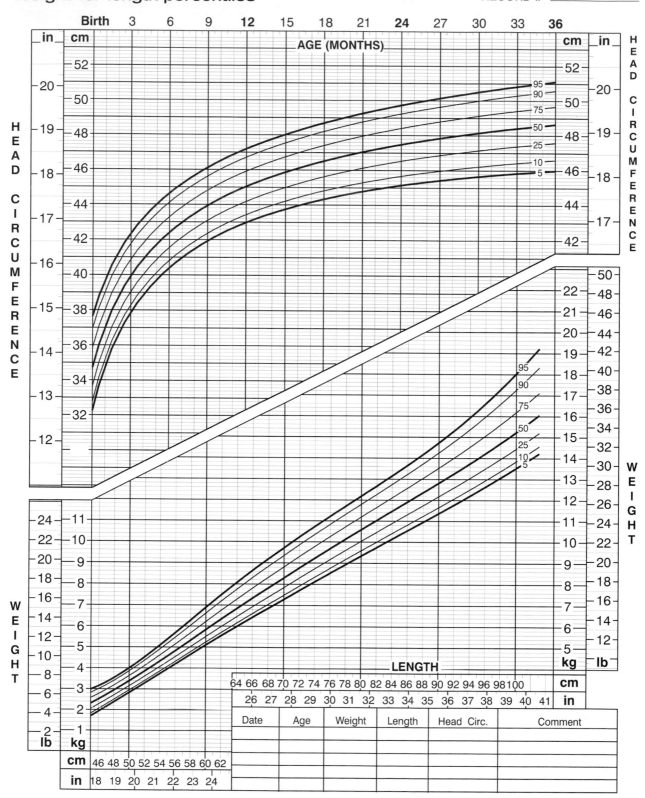

Published May 30, 2000 (modified 10/16/00).
SOURCE: Developed by the National Center for Health Statistics in collaboration with
the National Center for Chronic Disease Prevention and Health Promotion (2000).
http://www.cdc.gov/growthcharts

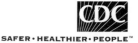

SAFER · HEALTHIER · PEOPLE™

2 to 20 years: Boys
Stature-for-age & Weight-for-age percentiles

NAME _____

RECORD # _____

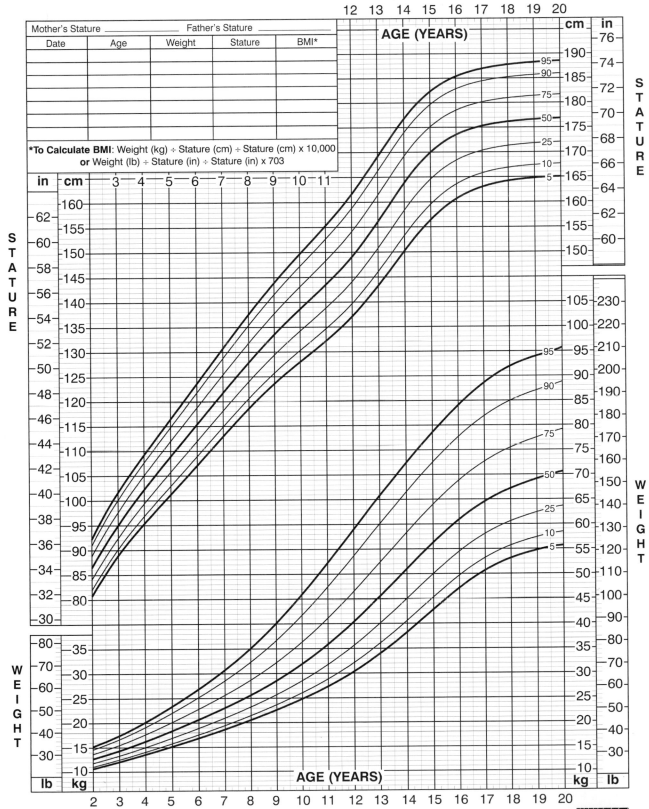

*To Calculate BMI: Weight (kg) ÷ Stature (cm) ÷ Stature (cm) x 10,000
or Weight (lb) ÷ Stature (in) ÷ Stature (in) x 703

Published May 30, 2000 (modified 11/21/00).
SOURCE: Developed by the National Center for Health Statistics in collaboration with
the National Center for Chronic Disease Prevention and Health Promotion (2000).
http://www.cdc.gov/growthcharts

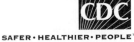

SAFER • HEALTHIER • PEOPLE™

2 to 20 years: Boys
Body mass index-for-age percentiles

NAME _____

RECORD # _____

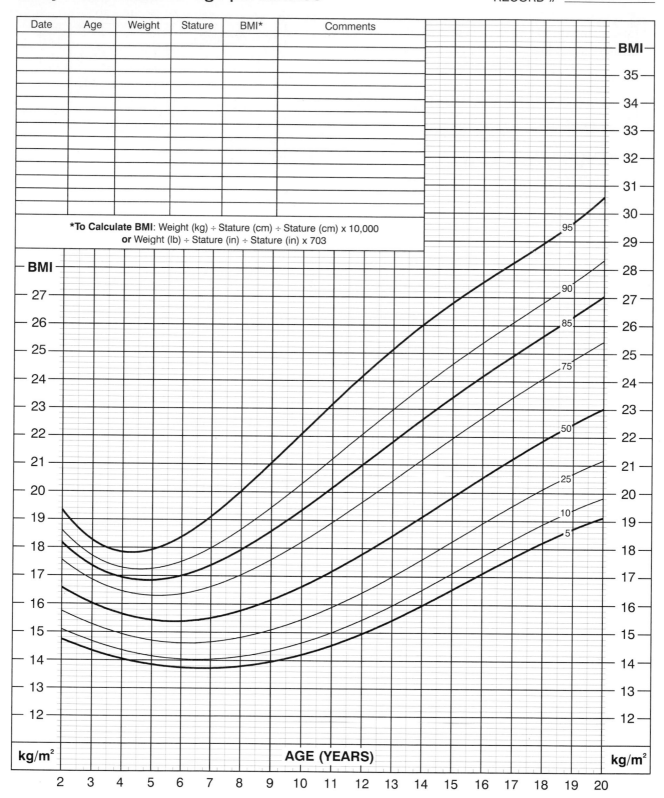

Date	Age	Weight	Stature	BMI*	Comments

*To Calculate BMI: Weight (kg) ÷ Stature (cm) ÷ Stature (cm) x 10,000
or Weight (lb) ÷ Stature (in) ÷ Stature (in) x 703

AGE (YEARS)

kg/m²

Published May 30, 2000 (modified 10/16/00).
SOURCE: Developed by the National Center for Health Statistics in collaboration with
the National Center for Chronic Disease Prevention and Health Promotion (2000).
http://www.cdc.gov/growthcharts

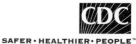

SAFER · HEALTHIER · PEOPLE™

Weight-for-stature percentiles: Boys

NAME _____

RECORD # _____

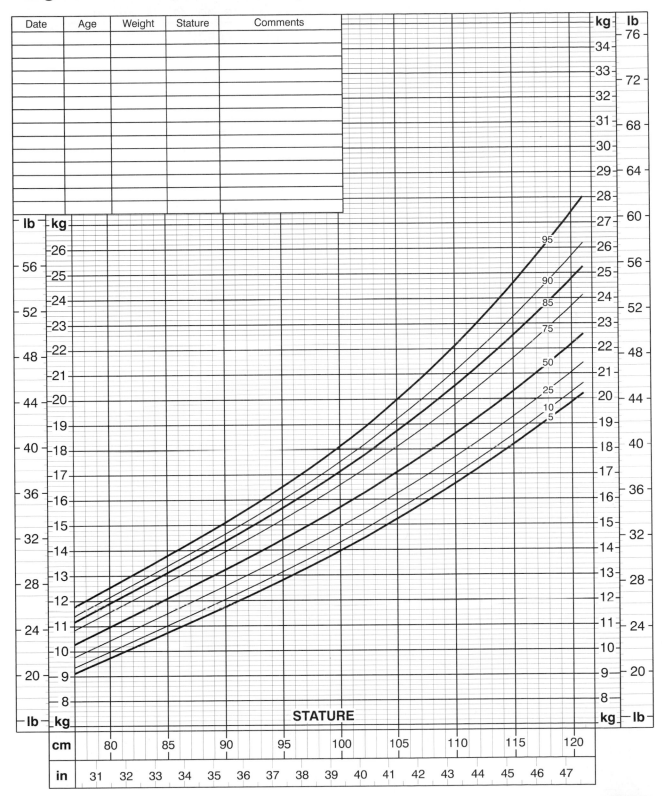

Published May 30, 2000 (modified 10/16/00).
SOURCE: Developed by the National Center for Health Statistics in collaboration with
the National Center for Chronic Disease Prevention and Health Promotion (2000).
http://www.cdc.gov/growthcharts

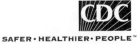

SAFER • HEALTHIER • PEOPLE™

2 to 20 years: Girls
Stature-for-age & Weight-for-age percentiles

NAME _____

RECORD # _____

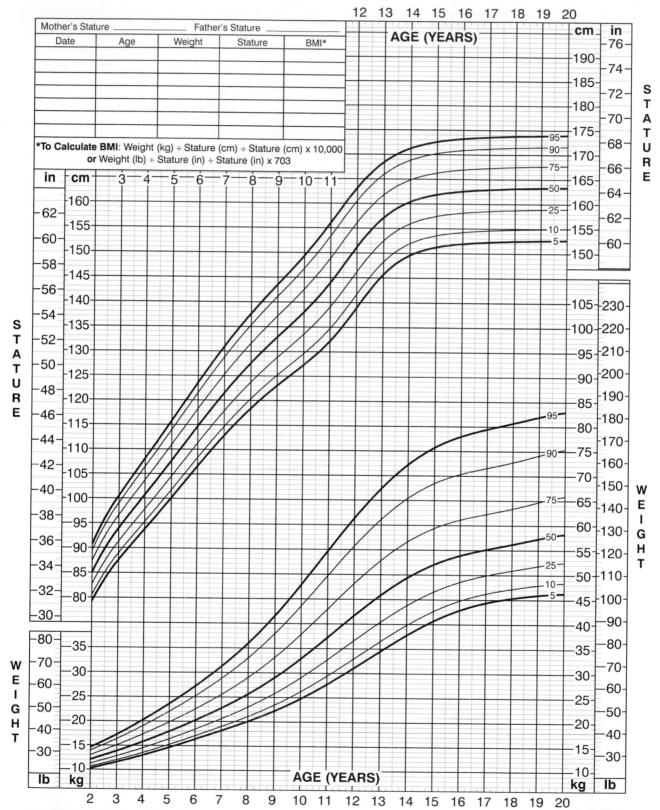

*To Calculate BMI: Weight (kg) ÷ Stature (cm) ÷ Stature (cm) x 10,000
or Weight (lb) ÷ Stature (in) ÷ Stature (in) x 703

Published May 30, 2000 (modified 11/21/00).
SOURCE: Developed by the National Center for Health Statistics in collaboration with
   the National Center for Chronic Disease Prevention and Health Promotion (2000).
   http://www.cdc.gov/growthcharts

SAFER • HEALTHIER • PEOPLE™

Copyright © 2005 by Mosby, Inc.

2 to 20 years: Girls
Body mass index-for-age percentiles

NAME _____

RECORD # _____

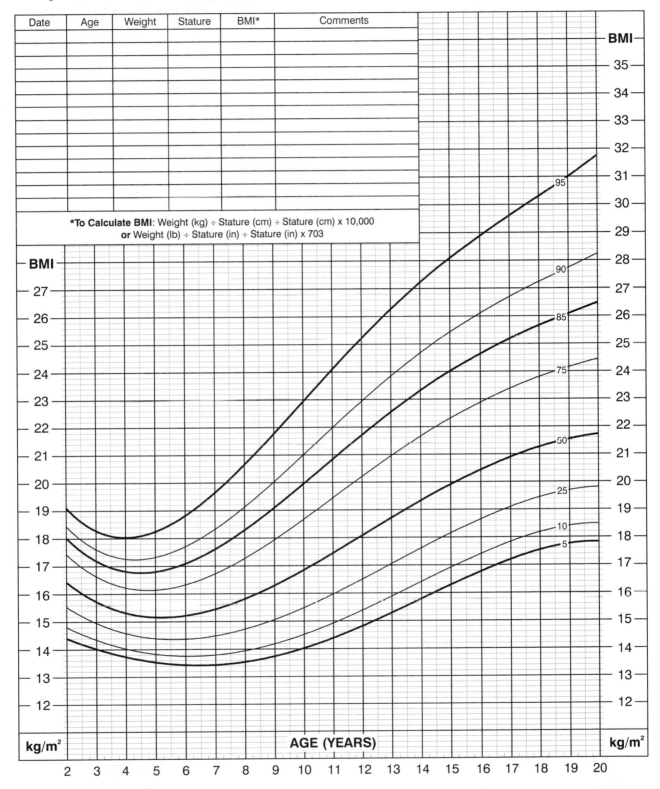

Date	Age	Weight	Stature	BMI*	Comments

*To Calculate BMI: Weight (kg) ÷ Stature (cm) ÷ Stature (cm) x 10,000
or Weight (lb) ÷ Stature (in) ÷ Stature (in) x 703

BMI

AGE (YEARS)

kg/m²

Published May 30, 2000 (modified 10/16/00).
SOURCE: Developed by the National Center for Health Statistics in collaboration with
the National Center for Chronic Disease Prevention and Health Promotion (2000).
http://www.cdc.gov/growthcharts

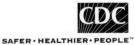

SAFER · HEALTHIER · PEOPLE™

Weight-for-stature percentiles: Girls

NAME _____

RECORD # _____

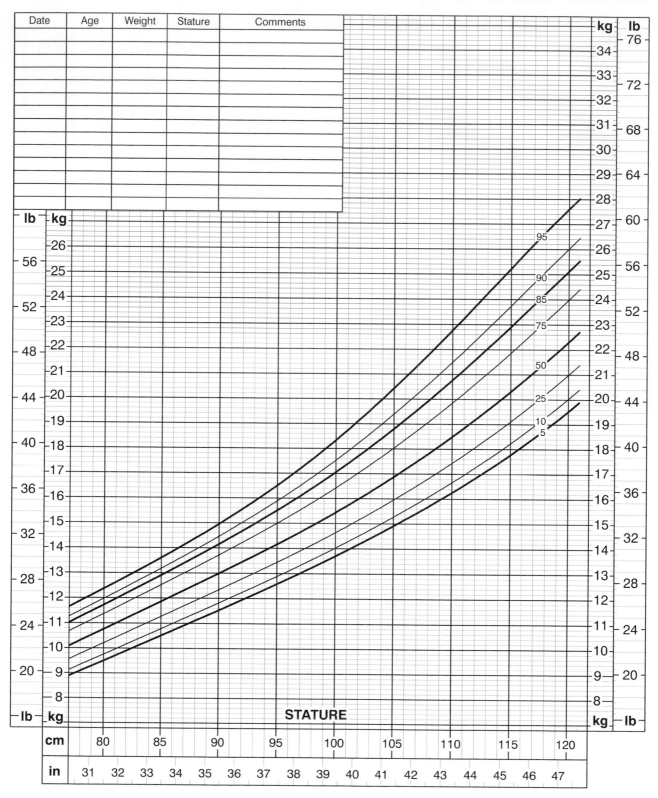

Date	Age	Weight	Stature	Comments

STATURE

Published May 30, 2000 (modified 10/16/00).

SOURCE: Developed by the National Center for Health Statistics in collaboration with
the National Center for Chronic Disease Prevention and Health Promotion (2000).
http://www.cdc.gov/growthcharts

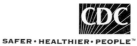

SAFER · HEALTHIER · PEOPLE™

Growth Chart for Girls with Down Syndrome (0-3 yrs)
WEIGHT

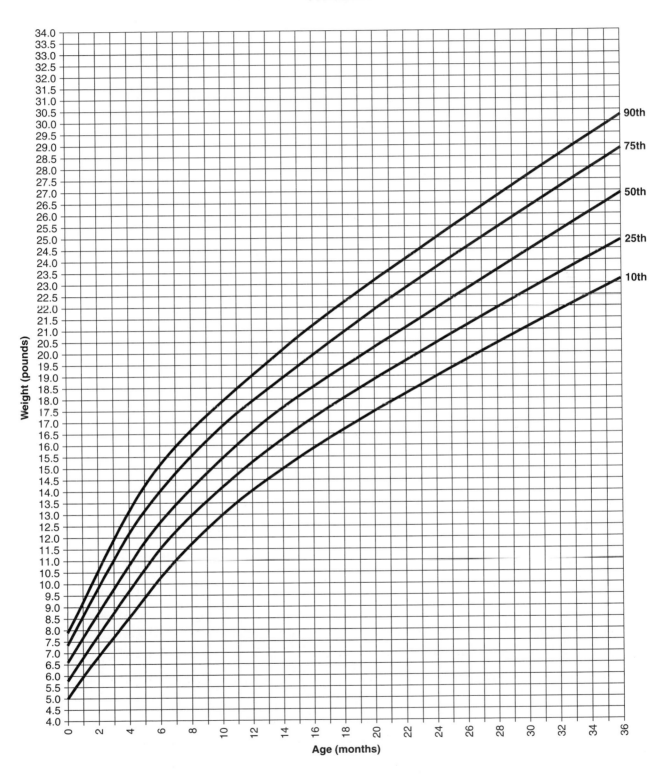

Weight (pounds)

Age (months)

90th
75th
50th
25th
10th

Growth Chart for Girls with Down Syndrome (2-18 yrs)
WEIGHT

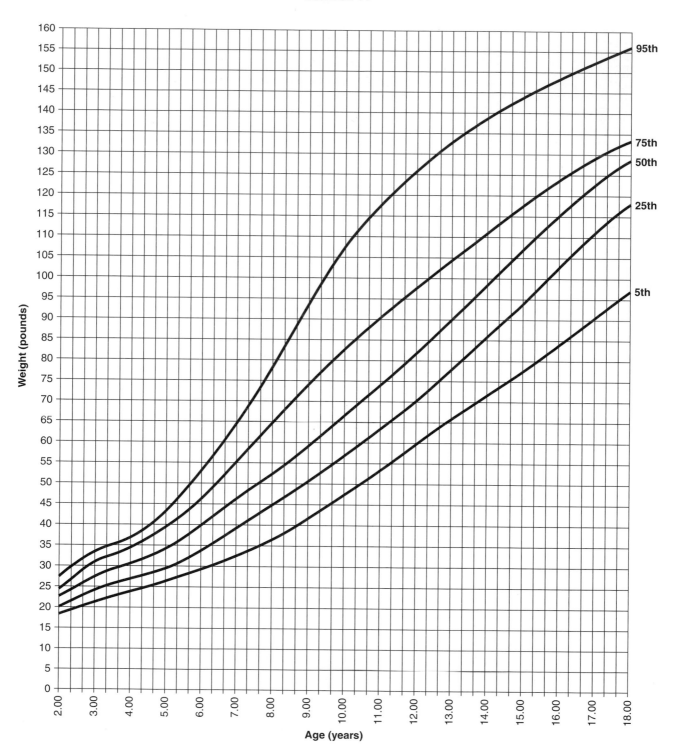

Growth Chart for Boys with Down Syndrome (0-3 yrs)
WEIGHT

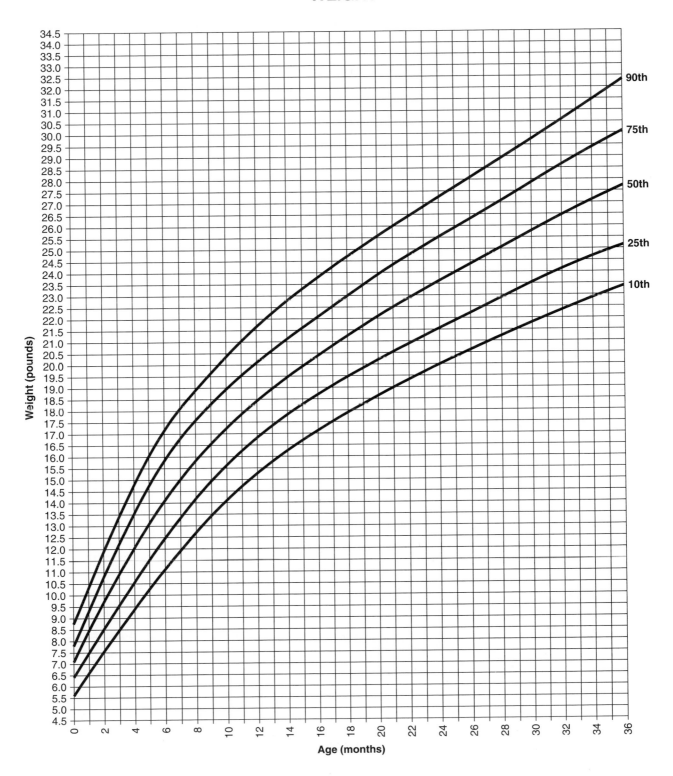

Growth Chart for Boys with Down Syndrome (2-18 yrs)
WEIGHT

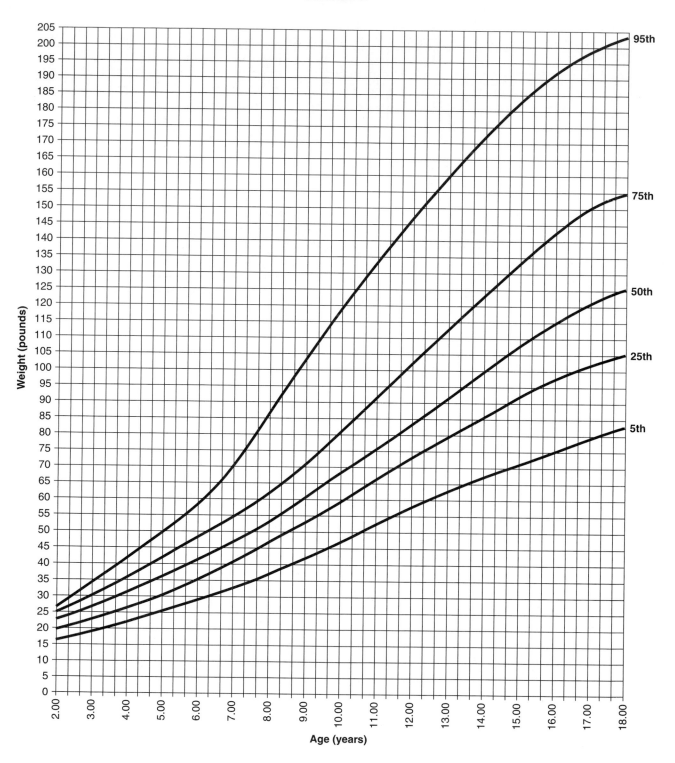

Weight (pounds) vs. Age (years)

Growth Chart for Girls with Down Syndrome (0-3 yrs)
LENGTH

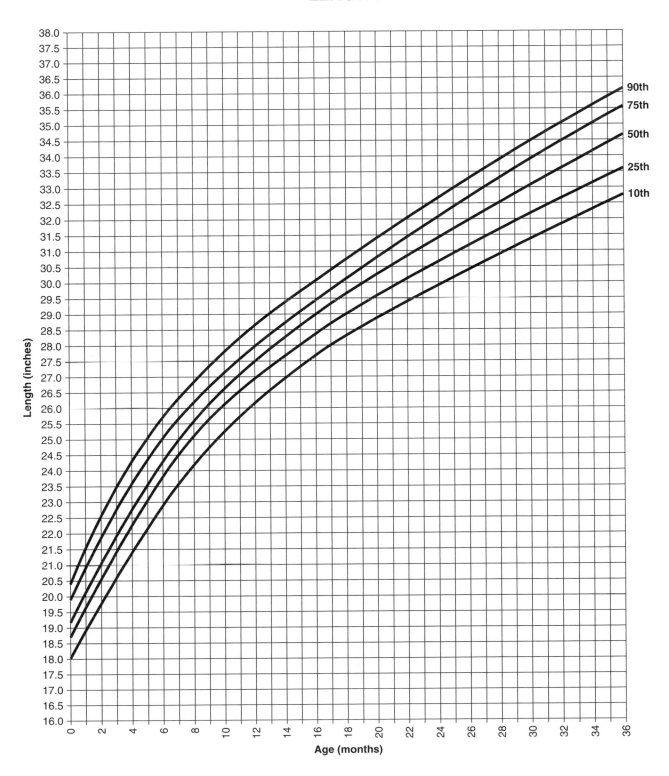

Growth Chart for Girls with Down Syndrome (2-18 yrs)
HEIGHT

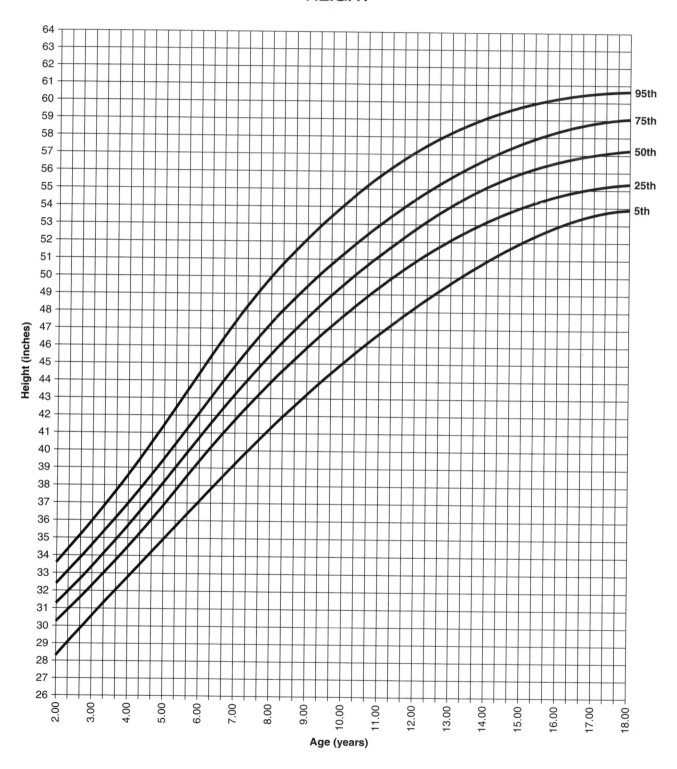

Growth Chart for Boys with Down Syndrome (0-3 yrs)
LENGTH

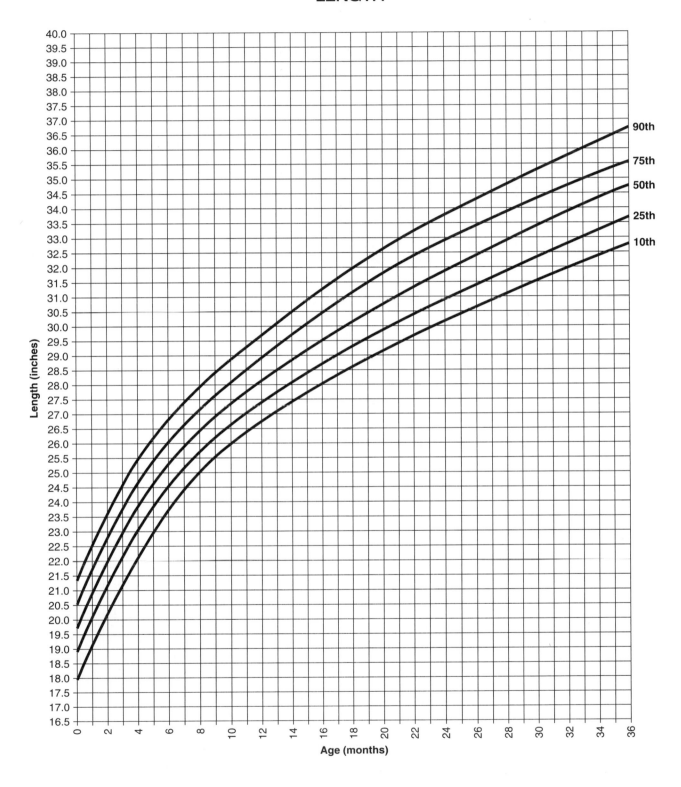

Growth Chart for Boys with Down Syndrome (2-18 yrs)
HEIGHT

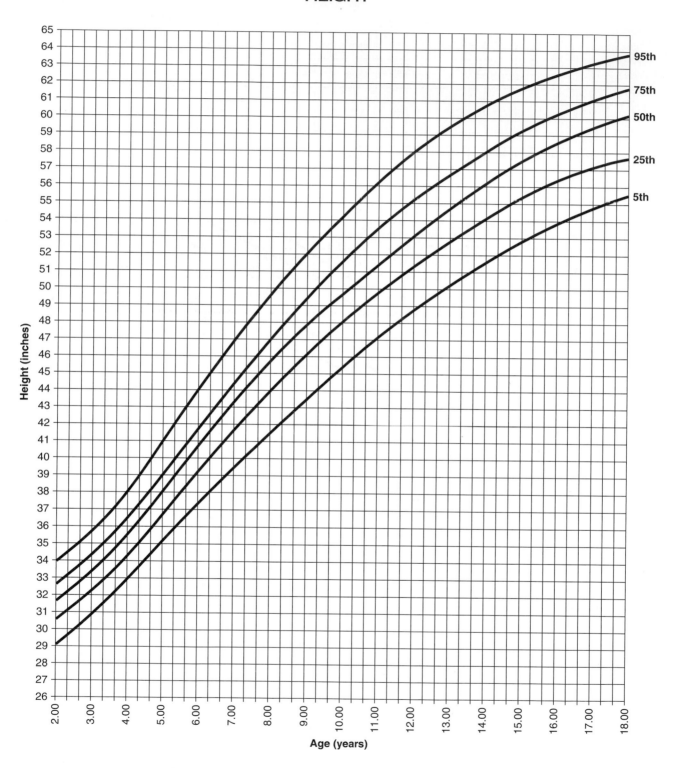

Head Circumference for Girls (0-3) w/Down Syndrome

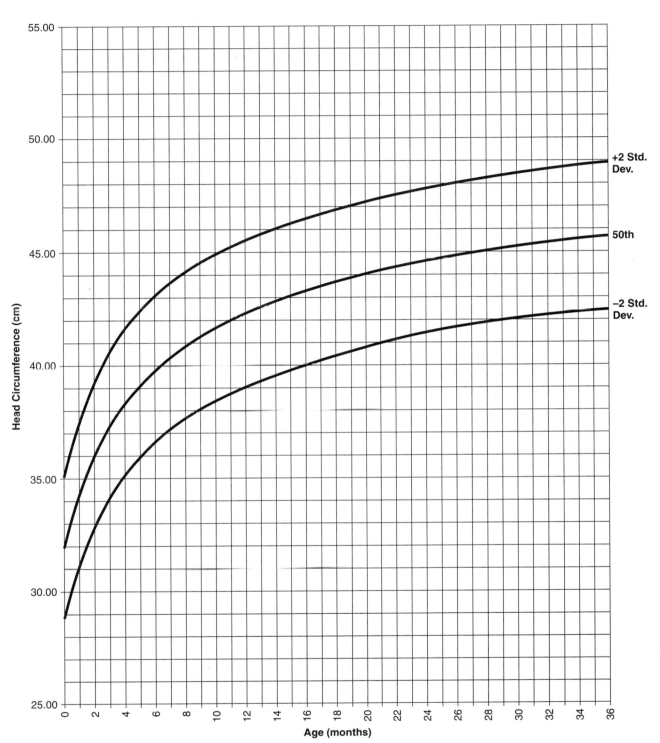

Reprinted with permission from Richards G: Growth charts for children with Down syndrome. Website: *http://www.growthcharts.com.*

Head Circumference for Boys (0-3) w/Down Syndrome

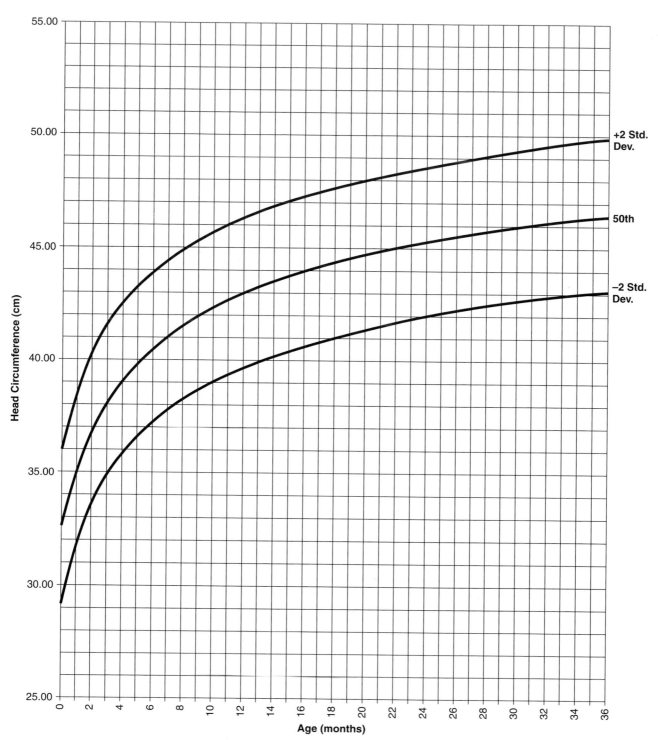

Reprinted with permission from Richards G: Growth charts for children with Down syndrome. Website: *http://www.growthcharts.com.*

Tanner Stages of Breast Development in Females

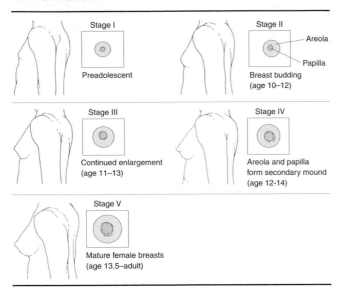

Tanner Stages of Pubic Hair Development in Females

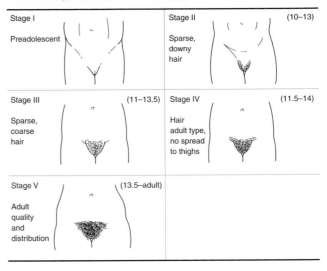

Pubic Hair Development in Males: Tanner Stages 1–5 with Age Range

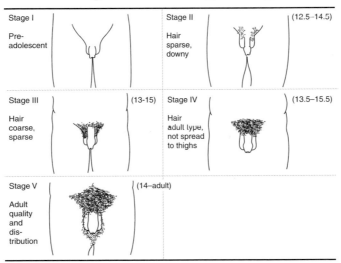

From Johns Hopkins Hospital, Nechyba C, Gunn VL: *The Harriet Lane handbook: a manual for pediatric house officers*, ed 16, St. Louis, 2002, Mosby. (Figures 5-1 to 5-3, Table 5-2: Tanner stages of development.)

Apgar Newborn Scoring System

Sign	0	1	2
Heart rate	Absent	Below 100	Over 100
Respiratory effort	Absent	Slow, irregular, shallow	Good, sustained crying, regular respirations
Muscle tone	Limp	Some flexion of extremities, some resistance to extension	Active motion, spontaneous flexion
Response to catheter in nostril (tested after oropharynx is clear)	No response	Grimace	Cough, sneeze, or cry
Color	Blue, pale	Body pink, extremities blue	Completely pink

Sixty seconds after the complete birth of the infant (disregarding the cord and placenta), the 5 objective signs above are evaluated, and each is given a score of 0, 1, or 2. A total score of 10 indicates an infant in the best possible condition. An infant with a score of 0-3 requires immediate resuscitation.

Modified from Apgar V: *Res Anesth Analg* 32:260-267, 1953.

Baby Check Scoring System

Date of Visit: _____

Patient Name: _____

Medical Record #: _____

Symptoms in the Past 24 Hours	Points
Has the baby vomited at least half the feed after each of the last 3 feeds?	4
Has the baby had any bile-stained (green) vomiting?	13
Has the baby taken less fluids than usual in the past 24 hours? If so, score the total amount of fluid taken as follows: • taken only slightly less than usual (more than two thirds of usual intake) • taken about half the usual amount (between one third and two thirds of the usual amount) • taken very little (< one third of usual intake) (NOTE: If baby is breastfed, ask the mother to estimate the amount taken. Fluids that have been vomited should still be scored.)	3 4 9
Has the baby passed less urine than usual?	3
Has there been any frank blood mixed with the baby's stools? (NOTE: Do not score for streaks.)	11
Has the baby been drowsy (less alert than usual) when awake? If so, score for the degree of drowsiness when awake as follows: • occasionally drowsy (but usually alert) • drowsy most of the time (occasionally alert) • drowsy all of the time (NOTE: Ensure that the mother is reporting drowsiness and not just irritability or increased sleeping.)	3 5 5
Has the baby had an unusual cry (sounds unusual to mother)?	2

Examination of the Awake Baby	Points
Is the baby's muscle tone reduced? (Compare tone and head control to normal for baby's age.)	4
Talk to the baby. Is the baby concentrating on you less than you would expect?	4
Is the baby wheezing on expiration? (NOTE: Do not score for snuffles or upper respiratory noises.)	3
Is the baby responding to what is going on less than you would expect?	5

Examination of the Undressed Baby	Points
Is there any indrawing (recession) of the lower ribs, sternum, or upper abdomen? If so, score as follows: • mild recession (slight indrawing just visible) • moderate recession (obvious indrawing clearly visible) • severe recession (deep indrawing)	4 15 15
Is the baby very pale or does the parent think that the baby has looked very pale in the past 24 hours?	3
Is the baby peripherally cyanosed?	3
Squeeze the baby's big toe firmly for two seconds to make it white. Release and observe color return for 3 seconds. Score if return is not complete within 3 seconds or if toe was completely white to start with.	3
Does the infant have an inguinal hernia? (NOTE: 60% of babies with inguinal hernia develop complications.)	13
Has the baby an obvious generalized truncal rash or a raw or weeping rash covering an area greater than 5 cm × 5 cm?	4
Is the baby's rectal temperature ≥ 38.3° C	4
Has the baby cried during the assessment (more than just a grizzle)?	3

Instructions:

(1) Score each item according to the exact wording of the question.

(2) Only score an item if it is definitely present.

(3) The baby can be re-scored at any time to assess changes in the severity of the illness.

Baby Check score = (points for symptoms) + (points for examination of the baby awake) + (points for examination of undressed infant)

Interpretation: • minimum score: 0 • maximum score: 111 points

Score	Group	Action
0-7	well or mildly ill	Infant unlikely to need medical care at the moment.
8-12	unwell but not likely to be seriously ill at the moment	Contact health care provider for advice. Monitor the child closely and reassess if condition worsens.
13-19	moderately to severely ill	Arrange to have child examined by a physician.
≥ 20	seriously ill	Take the infant to see a physician immediately.

Adapted from Morley CJ, Thornton AJ, Cole TJ, et al: Baby check: a scoring system to grade the severity of acute systemic illness in babies under 6 months old. *Arch Dis Child* 66:100-106, 1991.

The Injury Behavior Checklist

Date of Visit: _____

Patient Name: _____

Medical Record #: _____

The Injury Behavior Checklist can be used to identify children at high risk for physical injury. Please check the answer that best describes your child.

Behavior Checklist: How often does the child?	Not at all	Very seldom	Sometimes	Pretty often	Very often
(1) run out into the street	☐	☐	☐	☐	☐
(2) jump off furniture or other structures	☐	☐	☐	☐	☐
(3) jump down stairs	☐	☐	☐	☐	☐
(4) ride bike in unsafe areas	☐	☐	☐	☐	☐
(5) run or bump into things	☐	☐	☐	☐	☐
(6) fall down	☐	☐	☐	☐	☐
(7) play with fire	☐	☐	☐	☐	☐
(8) put finger or objects in electrical sockets or appliances	☐	☐	☐	☐	☐
(9) leave the house without permission	☐	☐	☐	☐	☐
(10) refuse to use car seat or stay seated in car	☐	☐	☐	☐	☐
(11) play with sharp objects	☐	☐	☐	☐	☐
(12) pull/push furniture or heavy objects over	☐	☐	☐	☐	☐
(13) fall out of windows or down stairways	☐	☐	☐	☐	☐
(14) put objects or nonfood items in mouth	☐	☐	☐	☐	☐
(15) get scratches, scrapes, or bruises during play	☐	☐	☐	☐	☐
(16) "take chances" on playground equipment	☐	☐	☐	☐	☐
(17) try to climb on top of furniture cabinets, etc.	☐	☐	☐	☐	☐
(18) stand on chairs	☐	☐	☐	☐	☐
(19) explore places that are off limits	☐	☐	☐	☐	☐
(20) get into dangerous substances	☐	☐	☐	☐	☐
(21) play carelessly or recklessly	☐	☐	☐	☐	☐
(22) come into contact with hot objects	☐	☐	☐	☐	☐
(23) behave carelessly in or around water hazards	☐	☐	☐	☐	☐
(24) tease and/or approach unfamiliar animals such as dogs	☐	☐	☐	☐	☐

SCORING

Frequency of Occurrence	Points
not at all	0
very seldom (once or twice)	1
sometimes (about once a month)	2
pretty often (about once a week)	3
very often (more than once a week)	4

Injury Behavior Checklist Score = the sum of points for all 24 questions

Interpretation:

Scores range from 0-96

Risk of Injury	Mean Score	Standard Deviation	Mean +/− 2 SD
low	22	10.5	1-41
moderate	24.4	9.7	5-43.8
high	33.7	13.4	6.8-60.5

Adapted from Speltz ML, Gonzales N, Sulzbacher S, et al: Assessment of injury risk in children: a preliminary study of the Injury Behavior Checklist. *J Pediatric Psychol* 15:373-383, 1990. Reprinted with permission of Oxford University Press.

The CHAT (Checklist for Autism in Toddlers)

Date of Visit: _____

Patient Name: _____

Medical Record #: _____

SECTION A: ASK PARENT

1. Does your child enjoy being swung, bounced on your knee, etc?	Yes	No
2. Does your child take an interest in other children?	Yes	No
3. Does your child like climbing on things, such as up stairs?	Yes	No
4. Does your child enjoy playing peek-a-boo/hide-and-seek?	Yes	No
5. Does your child ever PRETEND, for example, to make a cup of tea using a toy cup and teapot, or pretend other things?	Yes	No
6. Does your child ever use his/her index finger to point, to ASK for something?	Yes	No
7. Does your child ever use his/her index finger to point, to indicate INTEREST in something?	Yes	No
8. Can your child play properly with small toys (e.g., cars or blocks) without just mouthing, fiddling with, or dropping them?	Yes	No
9. Does your child ever bring objects over to you (parent) to SHOW you something?	Yes	No

SECTION B: GP OR HV OBSERVATION

i. During the appointment, has the child made eye contact with you?	Yes	No
ii. Get the child's attention, then point across the room at an interesting object and say "Oh look! There's a (name of toy)!" Watch child's face. Does the child look across to see what you are pointing at?	Yes	No*
iii. Get the child's attention, then give child a miniature toy cup and teapot and say "Can you make a cup of tea?" Does the child pretend to pour out tea, drink it, etc?	Yes	No**
iv. Say to the child "Where's the light?" or "Show me the light." Does the child POINT with his/her index finger at the light?	Yes	No***
v. Can the child build a tower of blocks? (If so, how many?) (No. of blocks _____)	Yes	No

* To record YES on this item, ensure the child has not simply looked at your hand, but has actually looked at the object you are pointing at.

** If you can elicit an example of pretending in some other game, score a YES on this item.

*** Repeat this with "Where's the teddy?" or some other unreachable item if child does not understand the word "light." To record YES on this item, the child must have looked up at your face around the time of pointing.

"No" Responses (Failures)	Risk of Autism
questions A5 and A7 AND observations Bii, Biii and Biv	high
question A7 AND observation Biv	medium
all other patterns	low

From Baron-Cohen S, et al: Can autism be detected at 18 months? The needle, the haystack, and the CHAT. *Br J Psychiatry* 161:839-843, 1992; and Baron-Cohen S, et al: Psychological markers of autism at 18 months of age in a large population. *Br J Psychiatry* 168:158–163, 1996.

Behavioral and Psychiatric Instruments

Chapter Contents

ICON KEY: ▤ Tool Printed   ⊘ Tool on CD-ROM   ∞ Customizable Tool   i Information and Resources Provided for Further Acquisition

Chapter Contents—cont'd

ICON KEY: 📖 Tool Printed   ✑ Tool on CD-ROM   ∞ Customizable Tool   i Information and Resources Provided for Further Acquisition

Introduction and Contents

Of all the health-related fields, behavioral medicine has produced the most extensively developed compilation of rating scales and measures. Most of these measures were developed for psychiatric research; however, many instruments are also suitable for clinical use. Although the majority of tools with a clinical application are used in specialty behavioral practices, a few are suitable for primary care screening for behavioral problems. This chapter focuses on the measures that are best suited for use in primary care practice or are so well known that they are included for educational purposes.

Scales deemed appropriate for primary care practice are brief, easy to use by clinicians and staff, cost-effective, accurate, acceptable to patients, and easy to read; and they may involve a self-report. The tools need to be easily integrated into the practice management structure to assist in the identification or monitoring of patients with behavioral health problems. Once a tool is implemented, a protocol that guides adequate treatment of the problem by the primary care clinician or ensures appropriate referral for further assessment and focused treatment services is recommended. Collaboration with mental health professionals in the community can facilitate a successful treatment outcome.

Measures in this chapter fall into two general categories: screening tools for *detection* of a problem and rating scales that measure the *severity* of a problem. Most of the screening measures are not considered to be diagnostic but indicate a potential problem in the screening subject area. A positive screen result should prompt the primary care clinician to seek further assessment by means of a diagnostic measure, a structured interview, or referral for such services. Rating scales that measure the severity of a problem are most often used in primary care to monitor a treatment course rather than to predict outcome.

Measures included in this chapter are grouped into sections under the general subject headings of General Psychiatric, Affective Disorders, Anxiety Disorders, Aggression and Domestic Violence, Suicidality, Substance Abuse Disorders, and Eating Disorders. The instruments were selected for their application to primary care clinical practice, professional recognition or popularity, psychometric integrity, and availability. Most of the tools are reprinted at the end of this chapter; proprietary measures are included in the reference list at the end of each section.

A recent mode of rating scale administration termed *interactive voice response* (*IVR*) has been introduced as a valid method of gathering measured information. The Hamilton Rating Scale for Depression (HRSD), the Hamilton Anxiety Rating Scale (HARS), and other psychiatric measures are available in this format. Kobak et al (1996, 1999) found that the Hamilton scales demonstrated good to excellent reliability and validity when administered by IVR and were highly correlated to the clinician-administered scales. The IVR format takes less administration time than the clinician-administered format, offering an advantage to busy clinicians. IVR for the Hamilton Rating Scales and other psychiatric measures is available at http://www.clinphone.com/HTS.asp.

Numerous resources for psychiatric assessment and treatment planning are available. Space precludes the inclusion of many rating scales that may be appropriate for primary care practice. Several extensive compendiums of psychiatric measures are referenced below; the reader is invited to explore these resources to obtain further information on behavioral and psychiatric rating scales.

As with other measures in Part II, the tools contained in this chapter have scoring mechanisms by which the screening results are assessed. For behavioral questionnaires and histories that do not contain a scoring system, please see Chapter 5.

References

American Psychiatric Association: Handbook of psychiatric measures. 2000, 852 pages.

Corcoran K, Fischer J: *Measures for clinical practice: a sourcebook*, ed 3. New York: 2000, Free Press.

Kobak KA, Greist JH, Jefferson JW, et al: Computer-administered clinical rating scales. A review. *Psychopharmacology* (Berl) 127:291-301, 1996.

Kobak KA, Greist JH, Jefferson JWE, et al: Computerized assessment of depression and anxiety over the telephone using interactive voice response. *MD Comput* 16:64-68, 1999.

Maruish ME, ed.: *Handbook of psychological assessment in primary care settings*. Mahwah, NJ: 2000, Lawrence Erlbaum Associates.

McDowell I, Newell C: *Measuring health: a guide to rating scales and questionnaires*, ed 2. New York: 1996, Oxford University Press.

Sajatovic M, Ramirez LF: *Rating scales in mental health*. Hudson, OH: 2001, Lexi-Comp Inc.

Varcarolis, EM: Psychiatric nursing clinical guide. Assessment tools and diagnosis. Philadelphia: 2000, WB Saunders Co.

GENERAL PSYCHIATRIC

General psychiatric measures are often long, cumbersome tools, best used in research protocols or psychiatric practice. General measures can provide a picture of overall mental health and assist in pinpointing problematic psychiatric areas. Although not used extensively in primary care practice, two measures deserve inclusion here for informational purposes. The Global Assessment of Functioning (GAF) Scale is often used for assessment of patients on admission to a psychiatric service. The GAF Scale or Global Assessment Scale (GAS) score may be noted in the medical record and serve as information for the primary care clinician by assessing the overall status of the patient. The Problem-Oriented Screening Instrument for Teenagers (POSIT) is a widely known adolescent screening tool and is often used in settings such as detention centers, schools, and rehabilitation units to assess adolescents for behavioral problems. The POSIT has been shown to have particular value in its use as a substance abuse screen.

Global Assessment of Functioning Scale (GAF); Global Assessment Scale (GAS)

Authors: GAF Scale: American Psychiatric Association, 2000a. GAS: Endicott J et al, 1976.

Source: The GAF Scale, reprinted in this text, comprises axis V of the *Diagnostic and Statistical Manual of Mental Disorders, Fourth Edition, Text Revision* (DSM-IV-TR) multiaxial system and is under copyright to the American Psychiatric Association. Permission to copy or reprint the GAF Scale should be obtained from the American Psychiatric Publishing, Inc., 1000 Wilson Blvd, Suite 1825, Arlington, VA 22209-3901; phone: 703-907-7322 or 800-368-5777; website: http://www.appi.org/permissions.cfx. The GAF Scale may also be viewed for academic purposes online at http://www.enabling.org/ia/sft/GAF.rtf and other sites.

The modified GAF Scale (Hall, 1995) may be viewed at http://www.dmh.missouri.gov/cps/outcomes/table1.pdf, and article information is available at http://www.dmh.missouri.gov/cps/outcomes/globalassess.pdf.

The Children's Global Assessment Scale (CGAS) (Shaffer et al, 1983) is available for viewing online at http://www.health.nsw.gov.au/policy/cmh/mhoat/ outcome_measures/CGASv1.pdf or http://www.southal-abama.edu/nursing/psynp/cgas.pdf.

Targeted Population: Adults.

Description: The GAS is a 100-point single-item rating scale for evaluating overall psychosocial functioning during a specified period on a continuum from psychologic or psychiatric sickness to health (Endicott et al, 1976). The scale provides a summary score that reflects the level of a patient's psychologic, social, and occupational functioning; impairment in functioning caused by physical (or environmental) limitations is not included in the rating. The GAF Scale is a derivative of the GAS and may be used to plan treatment, measure the impact of treatment, monitor a patient's change in level of functioning over time, evaluate quality of life, and predict outcome (American Psychiatric Association, 2000b). The GAF Scale is used for the current period (i.e., the level of functioning during the week before the evaluation). For inpatient care, ratings may be assessed at both admission and discharge as an outcomes measure.

Several modifications of the GAF Scale have been developed. A modified GAF Scale has more detailed criteria and a more structured scoring system than the original GAF Scale and was found to correlate well with the original GAF Scale (Hall, 1995). The modified GAF Scale was also found to have higher interrater reliability than the GAF. A self-report version of the GAF Scale was found to be valid and reliable by Bodlund et al (1994). The Children's Global Assessment Scale (CGAS) is an adaptation of the GAS for adults (Shaffer et al, 1983).

Scores: Instructions for using the GAF Scale appear in the *DSM-IV-TR. The Structured Clinical Interview for DSM-IV (SCID-CV) User's Guide* (First et al, 1995b) also provides detailed guidelines about making GAF Scale ratings.

The scale is completed by a clinician using information from any clinical source, such as patient records, clinical evaluation or interview, or a reliable informant. The scale values range from 1, which represents the hypothetically most impaired individual, to 100, the hypothetically healthiest individual. A rating point of 0 is also included in case information is inadequate. The scale is divided into 10 equal intervals, or deciles: 1 to 10, 11 to 20, and so on up to 91 to 100. Each 10-point interval is accompanied by a description, which defines that decile.

To make a rating, a clinician chooses the lowest decile that describes the patient's functioning during the past week. If a patient meets criteria for two or more levels, the clinician chooses the lowest level for rating. Within each decile, the clinician then chooses the single number that best describes the level of patient functioning, with lower numbers representing a lower level of functioning. To better select the specific scale point within the decile, the clinician examines descriptions of the two adjacent intervals to determine whether the subject is closer to one or the other and chooses point values that are closer to the matching adjacent interval description for the patient. If a patient seems to be equidistant from the two adjoining ranges, the clinician assigns a midrange point value.

Accuracy: The GAS and GAF Scale have been used in hundreds of studies to describe subject samples, to monitor changes in functioning over time, to assess treatment effects, to validate other measures, and to predict outcomes.

Reliability (intraclass correlation coefficients) on the GAS and the GAF Scale ranged from 0.61 to 0.91, indicating fair to excellent agreement, across several studies (American Psychiatric Association, 2000b). The GAF Scale discriminated significantly between patients who had a personality disorder (mean GAF score of 70) and those who did not (mean GAF score of 80) in a study of community subjects who were not receiving psychiatric treatment (First et al, 1995a). Endicott et al (1976) found that former inpatients in the community with a GAS rating below 40 had a higher probability of readmission to the hospital than did patients with higher GAS scores. The validity of the GAF Scale may depend on the quality of the information available to guide the clinical rating.

Administration Time: <2 minutes to assign a rating based on information from varying sources such as patient records, observation over time, or a comprehensive clinical interview. The scales may be used with minimal training.

References

American Psychiatric Association: *Diagnostic and statistical manual of mental disorders*, ed 4, text revision. Washington, DC, 2000a, American Psychiatric Publishing, Inc.

American Psychiatric Association: *Handbook of psychiatric measures.* Washington, DC, 2000b, American Psychiatric Association.

Bodlund O, Kullgren G, Ekselius L, et al: Axis V—Global Assessment of Functioning Scale: evaluation of a self-report version. *Acta Psychiatr Scand* 90:342-347, 1994.

Endicott J, Spitzer RL, Fleiss JL, et al: The Global Assessment Scale. A procedure for measuring overall severity of psychiatric disturbance. *Arch Gen Psychiatry* 33:766-771, 1976.

First MB, Spitzer RL, Gibbon M, et al: The Structured Clinical Interview for DSM-III-R Personality Disorders (SCID-II), II: multisite test-retest reliability study. *J Personal Disord* 9:92-104, 1995a.

First MB, Spitzer RL, Williams JBW, et al: *Structured clinical interview for DSM-IV (SCID-I) (user's guide and interview), research version.* New York, 1995b, Biometrics Research Department, New York Psychiatric Institute.

Hall RC: Global assessment of functioning. A modified scale. *Psychosomatics* 36:267-275, 1995.

Shaffer D, Gould MS, Brasic J, et al: A children's global assessment scale (CGAS). *Arch Gen Psychiatry* 40:1228-1231, 1983.

Problem Oriented Screening Instrument for Teenagers (POSIT)

Author: Rahdert E; National Institute on Drug Abuse, 1991.

Source: The Problem Oriented Screening Instrument for Teenagers (POSIT) is reprinted here and is available online at http://www.ncadi.samhsa.gov/govpubs/BKD234/241.aspx and other sites.

The POSIT has no copyright and may be ordered along with its scoring templates at no cost by contacting Adolescent Assessment-Referral System Manual (DHHS publication No. ADM 91-1735), National Clearinghouse for Alcohol and Drug Information, PO Box 2345, Rockville, MD 20847-2345; phone: 800-729-6686. For more information, please see http://www.niaaa.nih.gov/publications/posit.htm.

Targeted Population: Adolescents ages 12 to 19 years.

Description: The POSIT is a brief, general screening tool designed to identify problems in adolescents requiring subsequent in-depth assessment. It can also help determine a potential need for treatment. The self-report questionnaire assesses 10 functional areas: Substance Use/Abuse, Physical Health, Mental Health, Family Relationships, Peer Relationships, Educational Status, Vocational Status, Social Skills, Leisure and Recreation, and Aggressive Behavior/Delinquency. The POSIT contains 139 items with yes/no responses. The screen was developed by a panel of expert clinicians as part of a more extensive assessment and referral system for use with adolescents ages 12 to 19 years (Rahdert, 1991).

Scores: Two scoring systems are available: the original system presented in the Adolescent Assessment-Referral System (AARS) manual and a newer scoring system available from the National Institute on Drug Abuse (NIDA). The original scoring system includes "red flag" items and one expert-based cut-off score that indicates either a high or low risk for each of the 10 problem areas. The newer scoring system does not consider red flag items but includes two empirically based cut-off scores that indicate low, medium, or high risk for each of the 10 problem areas. In the newer system, the total raw score for each problem determines the level of risk for that area. Scores that are above the cut-off score for each functional area do not necessarily indicate the actual existence of a problem but are intended to identify functional areas in need of further evaluation (Rahdert, 1991). To obtain the scoring system, please consult the resource listed previously.

Accuracy: McLaney et al (1994) evaluated the reliability and validity of the POSIT, examining internal consistency, inter-correlation of subscales, convergent and divergent validity, and sensitivity and specificity of three POSIT subscales. The scales with acceptable levels of reliability are Substance Use/Abuse, Mental Health Status, Family Relations, and Aggressive Behavior/Delinquency. Results generally supported the validity of the POSIT under the kind of clinical conditions for which it is intended to be used. In reporting mixed findings on reliability and validity among the various subscales, the authors suggest that the POSIT be viewed as a screen for areas of potential problems that should be evaluated by means of additional diagnostic assessments.

Knight et al (2001) found evidence for the reliability of the POSIT in primary care medical settings, although they noted that some POSIT scales could likely be improved. Dembo et al (1996) described the POSIT as reliable in identifying potentially troubled youths on initial and second admissions to a juvenile assessment center. The POSIT Substance Use/Abuse subscale has been validated as an isolated measure for adolescent substance abuse (Knight et al, 2003; Latimer et al, 1997; Shrier et al, 2003). Data supporting the criterion validity of the POSIT Family Relationships subscale have been reported by Santisteban et al (1999). Extensive validity studies on the complete POSIT have not been documented.

Administration Time: 20-30 minutes by self-administration or interview. The POSIT requires no special training for administration.

References

Dembo R, Schmeidler J, Borden P, et al: Examination of the reliability of the Problem Oriented Screening Instrument for Teenagers (POSIT) among arrested youths entering a juvenile assessment center. *Subst Use Misuse* 31:785-824, 1996.

Gruenewald PJ, Klitzner M: Results of a preliminary POSIT analyses. In Rahdert E, ed. *The adolescent assessment/referral system manual.* Rockville, MD, 1991, National Institute on Drug Abuse. Website: http://www.niaaa.nih.gov/publications/posit.htm.

Knight JR, Goodman E, Pulerwitz T, et al: Reliability of the Problem Oriented Screening Instrument for Teenagers (POSIT) in adolescent medical practice. *J Adolesc Health* 29:125-130, 2001.

Knight JR, Sherritt L, Harris SK, et al: Validity of brief alcohol screening tests among adolescents: a comparison of the AUDIT, POSIT, CAGE, and CRAFFT. *Alcohol Clin Exp Res* 27:67-73, 2003.

Latimer WW, Winters KC, Stinchfield RD: Screening for drug abuse among adolescents in clinical and correctional settings using the Problem Oriented Screening Instrument for Teenagers. *Am J Drug Alcohol Abuse* 23:79-98, 1997.

Rahdert E, ed: *The adolescent assessment/referral system manual.* DHHS Pub. No. (ADM) 91-1735. Rockville, MD, 1991, National Institute on Drug Abuse.

Santisteban DA, Tejeda M, Dominicis C, et al: An efficient tool for screening for maladaptive family functioning in adolescent drug abusers: the Problem Oriented Screening Instrument for Teenagers. *Am J Drug Alcohol Abuse* 25:197-206, 1999.

McLaney MA, Del Boca FK, Babor T: A validation study of the Problem Oriented Screening Instrument for Teenagers (POSIT). *J Ment Health* 3:363-376, 1994.

Shrier LA, Harris SK, Kurland M, et al: Substance use problems and associated psychiatric symptoms among adolescents in primary care. *Pediatrics* 111(6 Pt 1):E699-E705, 2003.

AFFECTIVE DISORDERS

The U.S. Preventive Services Task Force (USPSTF) has issued depression screening recommendations that encourage primary care clinicians to routinely screen their adult patients for depression (USPSTF, 2002). Identification of patients with depression can be challenging in busy primary care settings; practice management protocols can ensure accurate diagnosis and effective treatment and follow-up so that patients benefit from screening.

Certain depression screening measures may be implemented during routine physical examinations and postnatal follow-up visits. Patients who score above the established cut-off level for the screening measure should be interviewed to assess for the depressive disorders criteria found in the *DSM-IV-TR* (American Psychiatric Association, 2000). If a patient is given a diagnosis of a depressive disorder, he or she may be treated within the primary care clinician's scope of practice or referred to a mental health specialist. Targeted screening in high-risk patients (those with chronic diseases, pain, undiagnosed somatic complaints, stressful environments, or social isolation) may also be implemented within a primary care practice.

The measures contained in this section include depression screening tools, which are used to detect symptoms consistent with a diagnosis of depression, and depression rating scales, which assess the severity of a preexisting diagnosis of depression. Targeted populations include adults, women receiving postpartum care, children, the elderly, and patients with dementia.

References

American Psychiatric Association: *Diagnostic and statistical manual of mental disorders*, ed 4, text revision. Washington, DC: 2000, American Psychiatric Publishing, Inc.

United States Preventive Services Task Force: Screening for depression: recommendations and rationale. *Ann Intern Med* 136:760-764, 2002.

Center for Epidemiologic Studies-Depression (CES-D) Scale and Center for Epidemiologic Studies–Depression Scale for Children (CES-DC)

Authors: Radloff LS, 1977; Weissman MM et al, 1980.

Source: The Center for Epidemiologic Studies-Depression (CES-D) Scale is reprinted here and is also available at multiple sites online including: http://www.mhhe.com/hper/health/personalhealth/labs/Stress/activ2-2.html. A revised version, the CES-DR (Eaton et al, 2004), has recently been published and is available online at: http://www.mdlogix.com. A pediatric version, CES-DC, is available for downloading at: http://www.brightfutures.org/mentalhealth/pdf/professionals/bridges/ces_dc.pdf.

Targeted Population: Adults (CES-D); children and adolescents (CES-DC) to screen for symptoms of depression.

Description: The CES-D is a 20-item scale developed by the Center for Epidemiological Studies at the National Institute of Mental Health in 1971 (Radloff, 1977). This measure was designed to assess the frequency and severity of symptoms related to depression. Items were chosen from existing depression scales and assess symptoms occurring in the past week. Responses to item statements are graded from 0 (rarely or none of the time) to 3 (most or all of the time). The CES-D is intended to be used as a screening tool to identify those at risk for depression and is one of the best known instruments for this purpose (McDowell & Newell, 1996).

The CES-DC is a similar scale, with items and responses phrased to be understandable by children.

Scores: Scores for each item in the CES-D and CES-DC are summed to obtain an overall score. Four questions (#4, 8, 12, 16) are worded positively and are reverse-scored. The overall scores range from 0 to 60. Higher scores indicate higher frequency of depressive symptoms. Several cutoff points indicative of depression have been suggested; a cut-off score of 16 for the CES-D is generally accepted as differentiating those with symptoms of depression from those without (Bowling, 2001; McDowell & Newell, 1996). Fendrich et al (1990) recommended a cutoff score of 15 as being suggestive of depressive symptoms in children for the CES-DC.

Accuracy: The CES-D has been used extensively in research studies, has shown good internal consistency in various populations, and has demonstrated fair test-retest reliability (Bowling, 2001; Radloff, 1977). Validity has been demonstrated in many studies; the scale shows the ability to discriminate between depressed patients and other populations, with high sensitivity in detecting depression in a variety of patient groups (McDowell & Newell, 1996). The CES-D compares favorably to other depression scales, including the Zung Scale and the Beck Depression Inventory (BDI).

The CES-DC was found to be reliable and valid in children, especially for girls and for children and adolescents aged 12-18 years (Fendrich et al, 1990). Faulstich et al (1986) reported mixed findings for reliability and validity in children, with better psychometric properties for adolescents.

Administration Time: 5-10 minutes by self-administration or interview.

References

Bowling A: *Measuring disease*, ed 2. Philadelphia, 2001, Open University Press. Pages 81-82.

Eaton WW, Muntaner C, Smith C, et al: Revision of the center for epidemiologic studies depression (CESD) scale. In: Maruish ME, editor. *The use of psychological testing for treatment planning and outcomes assessment*, ed 3. Mahwah, NJ, 2004, Lawrence Erlbaum Associates.

Faulstich ME, Carey MP, Ruggiero L, et al: Assessment of depression in childhood and adolescence: an evaluation of the Center for Epidemiological Studies Depression Scale for Children (CES-DC). *Am J Psychiatry* 143:1024-7, 1986.

Fendrich M, Weissman MM, Warner V: Screening for depressive disorder in children and adolescents: validating the Center for Epidemiologic Studies Depression Scale for Children. *American Journal of Epidemiology* 131:538-551, 1990.

McDowell I, Newell C: Measuring health: a guide to rating scales and questionnaires. ed 2, 1996 Oxford University Press. Pages 254-259.

Radloff LS: The CES-D scale: A self-report depression scale for research in the general population. *Appl Psychol Measure* 1:385-401, 1977.

Weissman MM, Orvaschel H, Padian N: Children's symptom and social functioning self-report scales: comparison of mothers' and children's reports. *J Nervous Mental Disorders* 168:736-740, 1980.

Hamilton Rating Scale for Depression (HRSD)

Author: Hamilton M, 1960.

Source: The original Hamilton Rating Scale for Depression (HRSD; also known as HAM-D) is reproduced here; this instrument is in the public domain and is available online in scoring form at the following websites: http://www.fpinfo.medicine.uiowa.edu/Docs/hamd.pdf and http://www.healthnet.umassmed.edu/mhealth/HAMD.pdf (21-item version) and http://www.strokecenter.org/trials/scales/hamilton.pdf (17-item version).

Targeted Population: Adults; also widely used with adolescents to measure the severity of depression.

Description: The HRSD was developed by Hamilton in 1960 and contains 21 items or themes assessing symptoms related to depression. A rating scale was published later (Hamilton, 1967), and further guidelines were published in 1986 (Hamilton, 1986). The survey is administered by a trained professional. Scores vary for each theme, depending on the presence or absence of a symptom (scores 0 to 2) or degree of symptom intensity (scores 0 to 4). Because of the length and depth of the interview process and the amount of training required to properly use the HRSD, this instrument may not be suitable for most primary care practices. It is presented here for reference because of its widespread recognition and place as the mainstay of depression rating scales.

Many alternate versions of the HRSD have been developed with corresponding guidelines, scoring, and psychometric studies. The HRSD has been widely used with adolescents (17-item and 14-item versions), despite limited data regarding its functioning (Myers & Winters, 2002). The HRSD is widely used in psychiatric research and clinical programs. In a thorough review of the literature on HRSD, McDowell and Newell (1996) concluded that the scale is suitable for determining the severity of depression in patients with depression but cannot be used to make a diagnosis of depression. They also advise thorough training in use of the instrument; the version used for testing should be reported.

Scores: A total score is obtained by summing the item responses and ranges from 0 to 52 for the 21-item instrument. Although Hamilton did not interpret scores with clinical diagnoses, the following interpretation is generally accepted (McDowell & Newell, 1996):

　　<7 = absence of depression
　　7 to 17 = mild depression
　　18 to 24 = moderate depression
　　≥25 = severe depression

Accuracy: Reliability and validity have been extensively tested, and the HRSD is consistently included as a criterion against which self-report scales are validated (McDowell & Newell, 1996). Overall, reliability reports are good for internal consistency with high inter-rater reliability. Although the HRSD's content validity has been criticized because the instrument favors somatic symptoms over cognitive and affective symptoms and mixes items that cover intensity of symptoms with items that measure presence of symptoms, the HRSD has been generally considered valid as a measure of severity of depression in patients given a diagnosis of a depressive disorder.

Administration Time: 30 minutes or more by semistructured interview, no specified questions; two raters are recommended, interviewers should be trained. Available as Interactive Voice Response (IVR) at http://www.clinphone.com/HTS.asp.

References

Hamilton M: A rating scale for depression. *J Neurol Neurosurg Psychiatry* 25:56-62, 1960.

Hamilton M: Development of a rating scale for primary depressive illness. *Br J Soc Clin Psychol* 6:278-296, 1967.

Hamilton M: The Hamilton Rating Scale for Depression. In Sartorious N, Ban T, eds. *Assessment of depression* (pp 143-152). Berlin, 1986, Springer-Verlag.

McDowell I, Newell C: *Measuring health: a guide to rating scales and questionnaires*, ed 2 (pp 269-276). Oxford, 1996, Oxford University Press.

Myers K, Winters NC: Ten-year review of rating scales. II: scales for internalizing disorders. *J Am Acad Child Adolesc Psychiatry* 41:634-659, 2002.

Warren WL: *Revised Hamilton Rating Scale for Depression (HRSD): manual*. Los Angeles, 1997, Western Psychological Services.

Montgomery-Åsberg Depression Rating Scale (MADRS)

Authors: Montgomery S, Åsberg M, 1979.

Source: Reprinted in this text; the Montgomery-Åsberg Depression Rating Scale (MADRS) is also available online at *http://www.medal.org/ch18.htm*.

Targeted Population: Adults with a diagnosis of depression.

Description: The MADRS was designed to detect changes in depressive illness (Montgomery & Åsberg, 1979). The scale contains 10 items describing psychic symptoms of depression; somatic and psychomotor symptoms are omitted. Items were selected for the MADRS from items most sensitive to change in depressive illness in Åsberg's Comprehensive Psychopathological Rating Scale (Åsberg et al, 1978). The items are rated according to findings obtained from a clinical interview; the rating reflects the measure of severity of a symptom. Ratings are graded from 0 to 6, with 0 representing a normal finding or absence of a symptom and 6 corresponding to the most severe degree of the symptom in question. Ratings numbered 0, 2, 4, and 6 for each item are defined with a phrase; whereas items 1, 3, and 5 represent intermediate steps between two defined phrases. Raters use responses elicited during the interview, as well as observations of the patient and interviews with other informants to choose the rating (McDowell & Newell, 1996).

Scores: A total score is obtained by summing the item ratings; the total score may range from 0 to 60. Interpretation of the total score has been suggested as 0 to 6, absence of symptoms; 7 to 19, mild depression; 20 to 34, moderate depression; and 35 to 60, severe depression (Snaith et al, 1986).

Accuracy: Reliability, including interrater reliability, has been reported to be adequate to good. Validity studies have confirmed the ability of the MADRS to differentiate severity levels of depression, and the scale compares favorably with the HRSD, the BDI, and other scales of this type (McDowell & Newell, 1996). The MADRS differs from the HRSD, BDI, and others in its omission of somatic symptoms.

Administration Time: 20-60 minutes by clinical interview.

References

Åsberg M, Montgomery SA, Perris C, et al: A comprehensive psychopathological rating scale. *Acta Psychiatr Scand Suppl* 271:5-27, 1978.

McDowell I, Newell C: *Measuring health: a guide to rating scales and questionnaires,* ed 2 (pp 276-281). Oxford, 1996, Oxford University Press.

Montgomery S, Åsberg M: A new depression scale designed to be sensitive to change. *Br J Psychiatry* 134:382-389, 1979.

Snaith RP, Harrop FM, Newby DA, et al: Grade scores of the Montgomery-Åsberg Depression and the Clinical Anxiety Scales. *Br J Psychiatry* 148:599-601, 1986.

Primary Care Evaluation of Mental Disorders: Patient Health Questionnaire 9-Item Depression Module (PRIME-MD PHQ-9)

Authors: Spitzer RL, et al, 1995, 1999.

Source: The Primary Care Evaluation of Mental Disorders: Patient Health Questionnaire 9-Item Depression Module (PRIME-MD PHQ-9) is reprinted here and is also available at http://www.neclinicians.org/pdf/depression/PrimeMDPATIENTQUESTIONNAIRE.pdf. A 16-item adaptation of the PRIME-MD PHQ is available online at http://www.montana.edu/wwwebm/Archives/PHQ.doc. The PRIME-MD is also available online in Greek, Italian, and Vietnamese at http://www.vtpu.org.au/resources/translated_instruments/prime_md/prime_md.html. Information about the PRIME-MD, provided by its sponsor, Pfizer, is available at http://www.zoloft.com/psd/healthmanagement/primemd.pdf.

Targeted Population: Adults.

Description: The PRIME-MD PHQ was developed for primary care providers to use as a screen for minor psychiatric disorders (Spitzer et al, 1995, 1999). The full-length questionnaire consists of a brief, self-report somatic symptom questionnaire and a series of interview questions on mood disorder, anxiety disorder, psychosomatic disorder, eating disorder, alcohol abuse, stress and specific questions for women on menstruation, pregnancy and childbirth. The PRIME-MD PHQ-9-item depression module (PHQ-9) is the subset of mood disorder questions, which use each of the *DSM-IV-TR* (American Psychiatric Association, 2000) criteria for diagnosis of depression. An additional question has the patient rate the level of interference in work, home life, or relationships caused by any of the problems listed. The reported good validity and brevity of this screening tool make it popular for use in primary care practices.

Scores: Answers are scored as the frequency of the symptom, ranging from 0 (not at all) to 3 (nearly every day). Item scores are summed for a total score. PHQ-9 scores of 5, 10, 15, and 20 represent mild, moderate, moderately severe, and severe depression, respectively, with similar results found for primary care and obstetrics-gynecology samples (Kroenke et al, 2001).

Accuracy: Kroenke et al (2001), in a prospective study, found good reliability and validity for the PHQ-9 as a measure of depression severity. PHQ-9 scores ≥10 had a sensitivity of 88% and a specificity of 88% for major depression. Spitzer et al (1999) noted that it took approximately 3 minutes for physicians to review the questionnaire and that most of the physicians agreed with the PRIME-MD PHQ-9 result.

Administration Time: 1-2 minutes by self-administration.

References

American Psychiatric Association: *Diagnostic and statistical manual of mental disorders,* ed 4, text revision. Washington, DC, 2000, American Psychiatric Publishing, Inc.

Kroenke K, Spitzer RL, Williams JB: The PHQ-9: validity of a brief depression severity measure. *J Gen Intern Med* 16:606-613, 2001.

Spitzer RL, Kroenke K, Linzer M, et al: Health-related quality of life in primary care patients with mental disorders. Results from the PRIME-MD 1000 Study. *JAMA* 274:1511-1517, 1995.

Spitzer RL, Kroenke K, Williams JB: Validation and utility of a self-report version of PRIME-MD: the PHQ primary care study. *JAMA* 282:1737-1744, 1999.

Zung Self-Rating Depression Scale (SDS)

Author: Zung WWK, 1965.

Source: The Zung Self-Rating Depression Scale (SDS) is reprinted here and is also available online at many sites, including http://www.fpinfo.medicine.uiowa.edu/calculat.htm, http://www.healthnet.umassmed.edu/mhealth/mhscales.cfm, and http://www.medal.org/ch18.htm.

Targeted Population: Adults.

Description: The Zung SDS contains 20 items, which consist of 10 positively worded and 10 negatively worded phrases describing symptoms of depression. The patient chooses the frequency at which the symptoms have been present over the past week: none or a little of the time, some of the time, a good part of the time, and most or all of the time (scored 1 to 4, respectively; positively phrased items are reverse-scored).

Scores: The point values for the responses are summed to obtain a raw score ranging from 20 to 80. The raw score of 50 or above is associated with depression. Most often, the raw score is converted to a 100-point scale called the *SDS Index* as follows:

SDS Index = (Raw Score/80 total points) × 100 or
SDS Index = Raw Score × 1.25

Interpretation of the SDS Index is as follows:
<50: Normal
50-59: Mild depression
60-69: Moderate to marked major depression
>70: Severe or extreme major depression

Accuracy: Other than good internal consistency, there is little evidence of reliability for Zung's SDS (Bowling, 2001). The validity of the scale has been extensively studied with mixed results. The SDS has failed to distinguish among inpatients with severe depression, outpatients with moderate depression, and patients with mild depression seen in general practice (Carroll et al, 1973). Many other studies also indicated mixed results in sensitivity and correlation with other instruments (McDowell & Newell, 1996). Zung's SDS is a historically important scale and is widely used; however, for accuracy in screening, other depression instruments should be considered.

Administration Time: 5-10 minutes by self-administration.

References

Bowling A: *Measuring disease*, ed 2. Philadelphia, 2001, Open University Press, pp. 91-92.

Carroll BJ, Fielding JM, Blashki TG: Depression rating scales: a critical review. *Arch Gen Psychiatry* 28:361-366, 1973.

McDowell I, Newell C: *Measuring health: a guide to rating scales and questionnaires*, ed 2 (pp 249-254). Oxford, 1996, Oxford University Press.

Zung WWK: A self-rating depression scale. *Arch Gen Psychiatry* 12: 63-70, 1965.

Zung WW, Richards CB, Short MJ: Self-rating depression scale in an outpatient clinic. Further validation of the SDS. *Arch Gen Psychiatry* 13:508-515, 1965.

Edinburgh Postnatal Depression Scale (EPDS)

Authors: Cox JL et al, 1987.

Source: The Edinburgh Postnatal Depression Scale (EPDS) is reprinted here and is also available online at http://www.fpinfo.medicine.uiowa.edu/Docs/epds_scale.pdf.

Targeted Population: Women receiving postpartum care.

Description: The EPDS, developed at the University of Edinburgh in Scotland, is a 10-item self-rating scale for depression in women who have recently been pregnant. Symptoms occurring during the previous 7 days are assessed and rated according to frequency on a 4-point Likert-type scale. The EPDS is considered by many to be a valuable and efficient tool for the identification of patients who are at risk for postpartum depression (Gold, 2002; Epperson, 1999).

Scores: Responses are scored 0, 1, 2, and 3 according to the increased severity of symptoms. Items 3 and 5 through 10 are reverse-scored. Item scores are summed for a total score ranging from 0 to 30. Higher scores are indicative of more severe depressive symptoms. A score of 12 or greater or an affirmative answer to question 10, the presence of suicidal thoughts, raises concern and indicates a need for more thorough evaluation (Cox et al, 1987).

Accuracy: Cox et al (1987) found satisfactory sensitivity and specificity in the original development of the EPDS, as well as sensitivity to change in the severity of depression over time. More recently, studies have indicated that the incidence of detection of postpartum depression with the EPDS was significantly higher than the incidence of spontaneous detection during routine clinical evaluation (Evins et al, 2000; Fergerson et al, 2002). Fergerson et al (2002) also noted that a failed attempt at breastfeeding was associated with an increased risk of a score of ≥10 on the EPDS. The EPDS has been noted to be useful in screening for postpartum depression in various populations (Cox et al, 1996; Morris-Rush et al, 2003; Murray & Carothers, 1990), has correlated well with physician-rated scales for detecting depression (Thompson et al, 1998), and has been validated by many other studies worldwide.

Administration Time: 5 minutes by self-administration.

References

Cox JL, Chapman G, Murray D, et al: Validation of the Edinburgh Postnatal Depression Scale (EPDS) in postnatal women. *J Affect Disord* 39:185-189, 1996.

Cox JL, Holden JM, Sagovsky R: Detection of postnatal depression: development of the 10-item Edinburgh Postnatal Depression Scale. *Br J Psychiatry* 150:782-786, 1987.

Epperson CN: Postpartum major depression: detection and treatment. *Am Fam Physician* 59:2247-2254, 2259-2260, 1999.

Evins GG, Theofrastous JP, Galvin SL: Postpartum depression: a comparison of screening and routine clinical evaluation. *Am J Obstet Gynecol* 182:1080-1082, 2000.

Fergerson SS, Jamieson DJ, Lindsay M: Diagnosing postpartum depression: can we do better? *Am J Obstet Gynecol* 186:899-902, 2002.

Gold LH. Postpartum disorders in primary care: diagnosis and treatment. *Prim Care* 29:27-41, vi, 2002.

Morris-Rush JK, Freda MC, Bernstein PS: Screening for postpartum depression in an inner-city population. *Am J Obstet Gynecol* 188:1217-1219, 2003.

Murray L, Carothers AD: The validation of the Edinburgh Postnatal Depression Scale on a community sample. *Br J Psychiatry* 157: 288-290, 1990.

Thompson WM, Harris B, Lazarus J, et al: A comparison of the performance of rating scales used in the diagnosis of postnatal depression. *Acta Psychiatr Scand* 98:224-227, 1998.

Geriatric Depression Scale (GDS)

Authors: Yesavage JA et al, 1983.

Source: The Geriatric Depression Scale (GDS) is in the public domain and may be used freely for patient assessment. The GDS is reprinted in this text and is also available at multiple sites online including http://www.aafp.org/afp/monograph/200102/GDS.doc and http://www.acsu.buffalo.edu/~drstall/gds.txt.

Online testing and scoring are available at http://www.psychologynet.org/geriatric.html.

The 15-item GDS-short form and the GDS in more than 24 languages are available at http://www.stanford.edu/~yesavage/GDS.html.

Targeted Population: Older adults.

Description: The GDS is a self-rating screening test for depression in the elderly. This scale was specifically developed for use in geriatric patients and thus contains fewer somatic items. The test consists of 30 questions, which are answered with yes/no responses. A 15-item short form of the GDS was created for brevity to reduce fatigue and lack of focus (Sheikh & Yesavage, 1986). A 5-item version was created from the 15-item version (Hoyl et al, 1999).

Scores: One point is assigned for each depressive answer, with total scores ranging from 0 to 30 for the GDS. Scores of 0 to 10 are considered normal; scores of 11 to 20 indicate mild depression; and scores of 21 to 30 indicate moderate to severe depression (Brink et al, 1982; Yesavage et al, 1983). For the 15-item GDS, scores of 0 to 4 are considered normal, 5 to 9 indicate mild depression, and 10 to 15 indicate moderate to severe depression (Alden et al, 1989). In the 5-item GDS, a score of 2 or higher indicates possible depression (Hoyl et al, 1999).

Accuracy: The GDS has been well studied; reliability is good, with high sensitivity and specificity reported in a wide range of elderly populations without cognitive impairment (McDowell & Newell, 1996). Among the cognitively impaired, however, validity is not maintained (Burke et al, 1989; Kafonek et al, 1989; McDowell & Newell, 1996). The 15-item version of the GDS is highly correlated with reliability and validity for the 30-item GDS (Burke et al, 1991; Lesher & Berryhill, 1994). The 5-item GDS has been shown to be as effective as the 15-item GDS for depression screening (Hoyl et al, 1999).

Administration Time: GDS: 8-10 minutes; 15-item GDS: 5-7 minutes; 5-item GDS: 1-2 minutes; all by self-administration or interview.

References

Alden D, Austin C, Sturgeon R: A correlation between the Geriatric Depression Scale long and short forms. *J Gerontol* 44:P124-P125, 1989.

Brink TL, Yesavage JA, Lum O, et al: Screening tests for geriatric depression. *Clinical Gerontol* 1:37-44, 1982.

Burke WJ, Houston MJ, Boust SJ, et al: Use of the Geriatric Depression Scale in dementia of the Alzheimer's type. *J Am Geriatr Soc* 37: 856-860, 1989.

Burke WJ, Roccaforte WH, Wengel SP: The short form of the Geriatric Depression Scale: a comparison with the 30-item form. *J Geriatr Psychiatry Neurol* 4:173-178, 1991.

Hoyl MT, Alessi CA, Harker JO, et al: Development and testing of a five-item version of the Geriatric Depression Scale. *J Am Geriatr Soc* 47:873-878, 1999.

Kafonek S, Ettinger WH, Roca R, et al: Instruments for screening for depression and dementia in a long-term care facility. *J Am Geriatr Soc* 37:29-34, 1989.

Lesher EL, Berryhill JS: Validation of the Geriatric Depression Scale–Short Form among inpatients. *J Clin Psychol* 50:256-260, 1994.

McDowell I, Newell C: *Measuring health: a guide to rating scales and questionnaires*, ed 2 (pp 259-262). Oxford, 1996, Oxford University Press.

Sheikh JI, Yesavage JA: Geriatric Depression Scale (GDS): recent evidence and development of a shorter version. In Brink TL, editor: *Clinical gerontology: a guide to assessment and intervention* (pp.165-172). New York, 1986, The Haworth Press.

Yesavage JA, Brink TL, Rose TL, et al: Development and validation of a geriatric depression screening scale: a preliminary report. *J Psychiatr Res* 17:37-49, 1983.

Cornell Scale for Depression in Dementia (CSDD)

Authors: Alexopoulos GS et al, 1988.

Targeted Population: Older adults with cognitive impairment.

Description: The Cornell Scale for Depression in Dementia (CSDD) is a 19-item clinician-administered instrument that uses information from interviews with both the patient and a caregiver to screen for depression in the cognitively impaired adult (Alexopoulos et al, 1988a). Items are grouped into categories of mood-related signs, behavioral disturbance, physical signs, cyclic functions, and ideational disturbance. Each item is rated on the basis of behavior occurring the week before the interview.

Scores: Each item is scored on a scale of 0 to 2: 0 = absence of sign, 1 = mild or intermittent, and 2 = severe. Interviewers may also rate the sign as "a" (unable to evaluate). The total score ranges from 0 to 38, with higher scores indicating a greater need for further evaluation. A cut-off score of 8 or higher suggests significant depressive symptoms (Alexopoulos et al, 1988a).

Accuracy: The CSDD has demonstrated high reliability, including interrater reliability, internal consistency, and sensitivity (Alexopoulos et al, 1988a, 1988b; Harwood et al, 1998; Kurlowicz et al, 2002). The CSDD has been validated in patients with and without dementia (Alexopoulos et al, 1988b); in frail, institutionalized older adults with high rates of dementia, medical illness, and functional disability (Kurlowicz et al, 2002); and in samples of Anglo and Hispanic patients (Ownby et al, 2001). When the Hamilton Depression Scale was compared with the CSDD, both demonstrated statistically significant discriminating ability for major depression in patients with mild to moderate, probable Alzheimer's disease (Vida et al, 1994).

Administration Time: 10 minutes with the patient, 20 minutes with the caregiver by interview.

References

Alexopoulos GS, Abrams RC, Young RC, et al: Cornell Scale for Depression in Dementia. *Biol Psychiatry* 23:271-284, 1988a.

Alexopoulos GS, Abrams RC, Young RC, et al: Use of the Cornell scale in nondemented patients. *J Am Geriatr Soc* 36:230-236, 1988b.

Harwood DG, Ownby RL, Barker WW, et al: The factor structure of the Cornell Scale for Depression in Dementia among probable Alzheimer's disease patients. *Am J Geriatr Psychiatry* 6:212-220, 1998.

Kurlowicz LH, Evans LK, Strumpf NE, et al: A psychometric evaluation of the Cornell Scale for Depression in Dementia in a frail, nursing home population. *Am J Geriatr Psychiatry* 10:600-608, 2002.

Ownby RL, Harwood DG, Acevedo A, et al: Factor structure of the Cornell Scale for Depression in Dementia for Anglo and Hispanic patients with dementia. *Am J Geriatr Psychiatry* 9:217-224, 2001.

Vida S, Des Rosiers P, Carrier L, et al: Depression in Alzheimer's disease: receiver operating characteristic analysis of the Cornell Scale for Depression in Dementia and the Hamilton Depression Scale. *J Geriatr Psychiatry Neurol* 7:159-162, 1994.

Other Measures:

Beck Depression Inventories: BDI, BDI-II, BDI-FastScreen for Medical Patients

Authors: BDI: Beck AT et al, 1961; revised, 1978; BDI-II: Beck AT et al, 1996; BDI-FastScreen (BDI-FS): Beck AT et al, 2000.

Source: The BDI-II and BDI-FS are copyrighted by the Psychological Corporation, 19500 Bulverde Rd,

San Antonio, TX 78259; phone: 800-872-1726; website: http://www.PsychCorp.com. The tools may be purchased online at http://www.marketplace.psychcorp.com. Kits include a manual and record forms and are available in English and Spanish.

Targeted Population: Ages 13 through 80 years.

Description: The BDI-II consists of 21 items to assess the intensity of depression. Each inventory is not a diagnostic screening, but a measure of severity of depression, and is used to monitor treatment progress. Each item is a list of four statements arranged in increasing severity about a particular symptom of depression. The BDI-II symptoms were modified from the original BDI to align with *DSM-IV* criteria (American Psychiatric Association, 2000). Symptoms are assessed over the preceding 2 weeks.

The BDI-FS (also known as the *BDI–Primary Care*) consists of seven items drawn from the BDI-II. The BDI-FS may be used for screening for clinical depression at the time of routine medical examinations (Scheinthal et al, 2001; Steer et al, 1999).

The BDI and BDI-II are well known and have been used extensively with adults. They are also the depression rating scales most often used with adolescents, drawing criticism only for the lack of items relevant to school and lack of corresponding parent or teacher rating forms (Myers & Winters, 2002).

Scores: BDI-II: Each item is rated on a 4-point scale, from 0 to 3, with the total score being a sum of the item ratings. Total scores range from 0 to 63. Suggested interpretation of scores for patients with a diagnosis of major depression are as follows: 0 to 13, minimal; 14 to 19, moderate; 29 to 63, severe (Beck et al, 1996). BDI-FS: Items are scored as in the BDI-II; a cut-off score of 4 identifies patients who were and were not given a diagnosis of depression (Scheinthal et al, 2001; Steer et al, 1999).

Accuracy: The BDI and BDI-II have been extensively tested and are considered to be standards by which other similar instruments are measured. Reliabilities for the BDI and BDI-II are high, including internal consistency and test-retest reliability (Arnau et al, 2001; McDowell & Newell, 1996). Sensitivity and specificity are good to excellent, and the BDI and BDI-II correlate well with other depression rating scales including the Hamilton Scale, the Zung Scale and the Geriatric Depression Scale (McDowell & Newell, 1996; Myers & Winters, 2002). Likewise, the reliability and validity studies for the BDI–Primary Care revealed high internal consistency; good concurrent validity; and lack of association with age, gender, ethnicity, or medical disorder (Beck et al, 1997; Steer et al, 1999; Winter et al, 1999). The corresponding BDI-FS also demonstrates good to excellent reliability and validity (Beck et al, 2000; Scheinthal et al, 2001).

Administration Time: BDI-II: 5 to 10 minutes; BDI-FS: 1 to 2 minutes; both by self-administration or interview.

References

American Psychiatric Association: *Diagnostic and statistical manual of mental disorders*, ed 4, text revision. Washington, DC, 2002, American Psychiatric Association.

Arnau RC, Meagher MW, Norris MP, et al: Psychometric evaluation of the Beck Depression Inventory-II with primary care medical patients. *Health Psychol* 20:112-119, 2001.

Beck AT, Brown GK, Steer RA: Psychometric characteristics of the Scale for Suicide Ideation with psychiatric outpatients. *Behav Res Ther* 35:1039-1046, 1997.

Beck AT, Steer RA, Brown GK: *Manual for the Beck Depression Inventory-II*. San Antonio, TX, 1996, Psychological Corporation.

Beck AT, Steer RA, Brown GK: *BDI-II, Beck depression inventory—FastScreen for medical patients: manual*. San Antonio, TX, 2000, Psychological Corporation.

Beck AT, Ward CH, et al: An inventory for measuring depression. *Arch Gen Psychiatry* 4:561-571, 1961.

McDowell I, Newell C: *Measuring health: a guide to rating scales and questionnaires*, ed 2 (pp 242-249). Oxford, 1996, Oxford University Press.

Myers K, Winters NC: Ten-year review of rating scales. II: scales for internalizing disorders. *J Am Acad Child Adolesc Psychiatry* 41: 634-659, 2002.

Scheinthal SM, Steer RA, Giffin L, et al: Evaluating geriatric medical outpatients with the Beck Depression Inventory-FastScreen for medical patients. *Aging Ment Health* 5:143-148, 2001.

Steer RA, Cavalieri TA, Leonard DM, et al: Use of the Beck Depression Inventory for Primary Care to screen for major depression disorders. *Gen Hosp Psychiatry* 21:106-111, 1999.

Winter LB, Steer RA, Jones-Hicks L, et al: Screening for major depression disorders in adolescent medical outpatients with the Beck Depression Inventory for Primary Care. *J Adolesc Health* 24:389-394, 1999.

Reynolds Child Depression Scale (RCDS) and Reynolds Adolescent Depression Scale–2nd Edition (RADS-2)   i

Author: Reynolds WM, 1987, 1989.

Source: The Reynolds Child Depression Scale (RCDS) and Reynolds Adolescent Depression Scale–2nd Edition (RADS-2) are proprietary and may be ordered from Psychological Assessment Resources, Inc. (PAR) at http://www.parinc.com/product.cfm?ProductID= 187 (RCDS) or http://www.parinc.com/product.cfm? ProductID=188 (RADS-2). For information contact: Psychological Assessment Resources, Inc. (PAR), 16204 N. Florida Ave, Lutz, FL 33549; phone: 800-331-8378 (orders), 813-968-3003 (all other calls); fax: 800-727-9329 (orders), 813-968-2598 (all other faxes); website: http://www.parinc.com/. Products include test manuals, summary/profile forms, hand-scorable test booklets, answer sheets, and a scoring key.

Targeted Population: Ages 8 to 13 years (RCDS). Ages 11-20 years (RADS-2).

Description: The RCDS and the RADS-2 are two related scales that screen for depressive symptoms in children on the basis of symptoms occurring over the past 2 weeks. For each instrument, 30 items are rated on a 4-point scale. Items are based on *DSM-III* diagnostic criteria for depression. The recently revised RADS-2 includes four subscales that evaluate four dimensions of depression: Dysphoric Mood, Anhedonia/Negative Affect, Negative Self-Evaluation, and Somatic Complaints. **Scores:** Item scores provide an indication of the clinical severity of a youth's depressive symptoms (normal, mild, moderate, or severe). A total score representing the over-all severity of depressive symptoms is calculated. For the RADS-2, standard (T) scores and a clinical cut-off score are provided in a summary/profile form. The cut-off score discriminates between adolescents with major depressive disorder and an age- and gender-matched control group. **Accuracy:** The Reynolds scales have been standardized with thousands of youths, providing normative data. In an extensive review, Myers and Winters (2002) cite numer-ous studies that suggest that the RADS is applicable to diverse samples and may distinguish depression from dis-tress. The RCDS has been studied with school children and mentally retarded teenagers and functions almost as well as the RADS. Solid psychometric properties have been established with reports of good to excellent reliabil-ity and validity (Myers and Winters, 2002; Reynolds and Graves, 1989; Reynolds and Mazza, 1998). The RADS also correlates well with other depression measures (Reynolds and Mazza, 1998). Limiting factors include test-ing and use with predominantly school-based samples. **Administration Time:** 5-10 minutes for administration; <20 minutes to complete and score. May be administered to individuals or in groups. Items are read aloud to assist students in grades 3 and 4.

References

Myers K, Winters NC: Ten-year review of rating scales. II: scales for internalizing disorders. *J Am Acad Child Adolesc Psychiatry* 41: 634-659, 2002.
Reynolds WM: *Reynolds Adolescent Depression Scale (RADS)*. Odessa, FL, 1987, Psychological Assessment Resources.
Reynolds WM: *Reynolds Child Depression Scale (RCDS)*. Odessa, FL, 1989, Psychological Assessment Resources.
Reynolds WM, Graves A: Reliability of children's reports of depressive symptomatology. *J Abnorm Child Psychol* 17:647-655, 1989.
Reynolds WM, Mazza JJ: Reliability and validity of the Reynolds Adolescent Depression Scale with young adolescents. *J Sch Psychol* 36:353-376, 1998.

ANXIETY DISORDERS

Anxiety rating scales may measure presence of symptoms of generalized anxiety disorder or symptoms specific to focused constructs such as social phobia or obsessive-compulsive disorder (OCD). Overall screening measures of anxiety reviewed here include the Zung Self-Rating Anxiety Scale and Beck Anxiety Inventory. The Hamilton Anxiety Rating Scale (HARS) measures the severity of symptoms that occur in diagnosed anxiety disorders. The Yale-Brown Obsessive-Compulsive Scale (Y-BOCS) assesses severity of OCD symptoms. The cor-responding screening test can detect symptoms consistent with a diagnosis of OCD. Also included in this section

are a social anxiety scale and the well-recognized Recent Life Changes Questionnaire.

Hamilton Anxiety Rating Scale (HARS)

Author: Hamilton M, 1959.
Targeted Population: Adults and adolescents.
Description: Designed to evaluate changes in symptoms over time, the Hamilton Anxiety Rating Scale (HARS, also known as HAM-A) (Hamilton, 1959) is a semistruc-tured scale consisting of 14 items that characterize anxiety. These are anxious mood, tension, fears, insomnia, intel-lectual (cognitive) symptoms, depressed mood, somatic (muscular) symptoms, somatic (sensory) symptoms, car-diovascular symptoms, respiratory symptoms, gastroin-testinal symptoms, genitourinary symptoms, autonomic symptoms, and behavior at interview. Each of the items has a list of component signs that define the item's characteristics.
Scores: Each item, with its cluster of signs, is rated on a 5-point scale, ranging from 0 (not present) to 4 (severe). No other guidelines for scoring were offered by Hamilton (1959). The item scores are summed for a total score, which ranges from 0 to 56; higher scores indicate increased anxiety.
Accuracy: In a limited number of adult studies, the reli-ability and the concurrent validity of the HARS was noted to be sufficient (American Psychiatric Association, 2000; Maier et al, 1988). A single study in which the HARS was administered to adolescents revealed good overall internal reliability, comparable to that found for adults, and good construct validity (Clark and Donovan, 1994). Despite the lack of reliability and validity studies, the HARS has been used consistently in clinical trials and pharmaceutical studies to rate changes in anxiety levels after interventions. Although often used as a base-line screening tool, the HARS is not recommended as a screening or diagnostic instrument but is recommended for monitoring changes in anxiety during treatment and in pharmacotherapy studies of anxiety (American Psychiatric Association, 2000).
Administration Time: Approximately 15 to 30 minutes by clinician interview. Available as Interactive Voice Response (IVR) at http://www.clinphone.com/HTS.asp.

References

American Psychiatric Association: *Handbook of psychiatric measures*. Washington, DC, 2000b, American Psychiatric Association.
Clark DB, Donovan JE: Reliability and validity of the Hamilton Anxiety Rating Scale in an adolescent sample. *J Am Acad Child Adolesc Psychiatry* 33:354-360, 1994.
Hamilton M: The assessment of anxiety states by rating. *Br J Med Psychol* 32:50–55, 1959.
Maier W, Buller R, Philipp M, et al: The Hamilton Anxiety Scale: reli-ability, validity and sensitivity to change in anxiety and depressive disorders. *J Affect Disord* 14:61-68, 1988.
Varcarolis EM: *Psychiatric nursing clinical guide. Assessment tools and diagnosis* (pp 142-143). Philadelphia, 2000, W. B. Saunders.

Zung Self-Rating Anxiety Scale (SAS)

Author: Zung WWK, 1971.

Source: The Zung Self-Rating Anxiety Scale (SAS) is reprinted here and is available online at http://www.healthnet.umassmed.edu/mhealth/mhscales.cfm

Targeted Population: Adults.

Description: The Zung SAS contains 20 items, consisting of 5 positively worded and 15 negatively worded phrases describing symptoms of anxiety. The patient chooses the frequency at which the symptoms have been present over the past week: none or a little of the time, some of the time, good part of the time, most or all of the time (scored 1 to 4, respectively; positively phrased items are reverse-scored).

Scores: The point values for the responses are summed to obtain a raw score ranging from 20 to 80. When the SAS was administered to family practice patients, Zung (1986) found that a cut-off score of 50 resulted in 20% of the patients diagnosed with clinically significant anxiety. An index for the SAS may be calculated by converting the raw score to a 100-point scale called *the SAS Index* as follows (Zung, 1971):

$$\text{SAS Index} = (\text{Raw Score}/80 \text{ total points}) \times 100 \text{ or}$$
$$\text{SAS Index} = \text{Raw Score} \times 1.25$$

Interpretation of the SAS Index is not readily available.

Accuracy: Zung (1971) found good reliability and validity in his initial report. Little information on the reliability and validity of the SAS is available; however, the scale has been used extensively as a screening tool for anxiety. The SAS is often used as a measure of anxiety during and after treatment for such.

Administration Time: 5-10 minutes by self-administration.

References

Zung WWK: A rating instrument for anxiety disorders. *Psychosomatics* 12:371-379, 1971.

Zung WW: Prevalence of clinically significant anxiety in a family practice setting. *Am J Psychiatry* 143:1471-1472, 1986.

Yale-Brown Obsessive Compulsive Scale (Y-BOCS), Florida Obsessive Compulsive Inventory (FOCI) and Children's Yale-Brown Obsessive Compulsive Scale (CY-BOCS)

Authors: Goodman WK, et al, 1989a.

Source: The Y-BOCS is reprinted here and is also available online at: http://healthnet.umassmed.edu/mhealth/mhscales.cfm. For more information about Obsessive Compulsive Disorder and screening, please see: http://www.ufocd.org/

The self-report form of the Y-BOCS, known as the Florida Obsessive Compulsive Inventory (FOCI), is reprinted here and is also is available online at: http://www.ocfoundation.org/ocf1070a.htm. This screening test may be more suitable for primary care clinical use. Permission is required to use this screening tool in clinical practice and may be obtained by contacting: Wayne K. Goodman, M.D., care of Beverly Hollingsworth, University of Florida, College of Medicine, Department of Psychiatry, PO Box 100256, Gainesville, Florida 32610-0256, phone: (352) 392-3681; fax: (352) 392-9887.

A children's version, the Children's Yale-Brown Obsessive Compulsive Scale (CY-BOCS), a developmental modification of the Y-BOCS, is also available and has become the standard assessment for OCD in children (Goodman, 1991; Leckman, 1997; Scahill et al, 1997; Myers & Winters, 2002). The obsessive and compulsive checklists for the CY-BOC may be found online at: http://www.bipolarchild.com/survey/ybocs.html.

Targeted Population: Adults.

Description: The Y-BOCS is a 10-item instrument, containing two 5-item subscales, obsession and compulsion. Each item assesses the severity of obsessions or compulsions, rated on a 5-item Likert-type scale from 0 (no symptoms) to 4 (extreme symptoms). Items are rated by hours per day spent, interference from, distress from, resistance to, and control over obsessions and compulsions. The Y-BOCS Symptom Checklist allows the clinician to ask the patient about specific obsessions and compulsions, both past and present. The indicated responses form the basis of a target symptoms list.

Scores: Scores for the individual 10 items are summed to yield a total severity score and separate obsession and compulsion subscale scores. Total scores indicate the range of severity: 0 to 7 = subclinical, 8 to 15 = mild, 16 to 23 = moderate, 24 to 31 = severe, and 32 to 40 = extreme.

Accuracy: The Y-BOCS has demonstrated excellent reliability, including interrater reliability for the total score and each of the 10 individual item scores. A high degree of internal consistency and good test-retest reliability were also demonstrated (Goodman et al, 1989a). Validity for assessment of OCD symptom severity has also been demonstrated, and the Y-BOCS has been used as an outcomes measure with good sensitivity to changes noted with treatment (Goodman et al, 1989b; Kim et al, 1990, 1992; Woody et al, 1995).

Administration Time: 5-10 minutes by interview or self-administration for Y-BOCS and Symptom Checklist. Available as Interactive Voice Response (IVR) at http://www.clinphone.com/HTS.asp.

References

Goodman WK: *Children's Yale-Brown Obsessive Compulsive Scale (CY-BOCS).* New Haven, CT, 1991, Clinical Neuroscience Research Unit, Connecticut Mental Health Center.

Goodman WK, Price LH, Rasmussen SA, et al: The Yale-Brown Obsessive Compulsive Scale. I. Development, use, and reliability. *Arch Gen Psychiatry* 46:1006-1011, 1989a.

Goodman WK, Price LH, Rasmussen SA, et al: The Yale-Brown Obsessive Compulsive Scale. II. Validity. *Arch Gen Psychiatry* 46:1012-1016, 1989b.

Kim SW, Dysken MW, Kuskowski M: The Yale-Brown Obsessive-Compulsive Scale: a reliability and validity study. *Psychiatry Res* 34:99-106, 1990.

Kim SW, Dysken MW, Kuskowski M: The Symptom Checklist-90: obsessive-compulsive subscale: a reliability and validity study. *Psychiatry Res* 41:37–44, 1992.

Myers K, Winters NC: Ten-year review of rating scales. II: scales for internalizing disorders. *J Am Acad Child Adolesc Psychiatry* 41: 634-659, 2002.

Scahill L, Riddle MA, McSwiggin-Hardin M, et al: Children's Yale-Brown Obsessive Compulsive Scale: reliability and validity. *J Am Acad Child Adolesc Psychiatry* 36:844-852, 1997.

Woody SR, Steketee GS, Chambless DL: Reliability and validity of the Yale-Brown Obsessive-Compulsive Scale. *Behav Res Ther* 33:597-605, 1995.

Liebowitz Social Anxiety Scale (LSAS)

Author: Liebowitz MR, 1987.

Source: The Liebowitz Social Anxiety Scale (LSAS) is reprinted here and is also available online at http://www.healthnet.umassmed.edu/mhealth/mhscales.cfm. A child and adolescent version is also available from Carrie L. Masia, PhD, NYU Child Study Center, 550 First Ave, New York, NY 10016; website: carrie.masia@med.nyu.edu.

Targeted Population: Adults.

Description: The LSAS evaluates both anxiety and avoidance in a broad range of social situations that are difficult for individuals with social phobia. The LSAS contains 24 items, 13 concerning performance anxiety (P) and 11 concerning social situations (S). Each item is rated separately for fear (0 to 3 = none, mild, moderate, severe) and avoidance behavior (0 to 3 = never, occasionally, often, usually).

Scores: Scores are summed to form four subscale scores (performance fear, performance avoidance, social fear, and social avoidance) and an overall social anxiety severity rating. Scores from 50 to 65 suggest moderate social phobia; 65 to 80, marked; 80 to 95, severe; and greater than 95, extremely severe social phobia (Raj & Sheehan, 2001).

Accuracy: The LSAS has demonstrated good internal consistency and convergent validity (Heimberg et al, 1999; Horner et al, 1996). The LSAS was not originally intended for use as a self-report measure; however, recent studies have shown it to be reliable and valid when used as such (Baker et al, 2001; Fresco et al, 2001).

Administration Time: 15 minutes by clinician interview; 2 to 5 minutes by self-report. Available as Interactive Voice Response (IVR) at http://www.clinphone.com/HTS.asp.

References

Baker SL, Heinrichs N, Kim HJ, et al: The Liebowitz Social Anxiety Scale as a self-report instrument: a preliminary psychometric analysis. *Behav Res Ther* 40:701-715, 2002.

Fresco DM, Coles ME, Heimberg RG, et al: The Liebowitz Social Anxiety Scale: a comparison of the psychometric properties of self-report and clinician-administered formats. *Psychol Med* 31: 1025-1035, 2001.

Heimberg RG, Horner KJ, Juster HR, et al: Psychometric properties of Liebowitz Social Phobia Scale. *Psychol Med* 29:199-212, 1999.

Horner KJ, Juster HR, Brown EJ, et al: *Psychometric properties of the Liebowitz Social Anxiety Scale* [poster]. Presented at the 16th Annual Meeting of the Anxiety Disorders Association of America. Orlando, Fla. March 28-31, 1996.

Liebowitz MR: Social phobia. *Mod Probl Pharmacopsychiatry* 22:141-173, 1987.

Masia CL, Hoffman SG, Klein RG, et al: The Liebowitz Social Anxiety Scale for Children and Adolescents (LSAS-CA). New York, 1999, NYU Child Study Center.

Raj BA, Sheehan DV: Social anxiety disorder. *Med Clin North Am* 85:711-733, 2001.

Recent Life Changes Questionnaire (RLCQ)

Author: Rahe RH, 1967; revised 1978, 1995.

Source: The Recent Life Changes Questionnaire (RLCQ) and 1995 Life Change Units table are reprinted here. For more information about the RLCQ, the author may be contacted atv Richard H. Rahe, MD, Health Assessment Programs, Inc., 638 St. Lawrence Ave, Reno, NV 89509-1440; office phone: 775-348-8584; e-mail: rahe@equinox.unr.edu.

Targeted Population: Adults and older adolescents with a minimum of a tenth-grade reading level.

Description: The RLCQ contains 74 items representing life events, which result in changes to accustomed patterns. The current RLCQ is a tool that evolved through several rescalings from an original 43-item measurement of life change events in family, personal, work, and financial domains (Holmes and Rahe, 1967). To complete the questionnaire, the respondent selects events that have occurred in the past 2 years; the period may be divided into four consecutive 6-month intervals. Multiple occurrences of some events during the recall period can also be recorded.

In their original work, Holmes and Rahe (1967) assigned a rank order for life change events with a corresponding mean life change value. This original scale has been modified several times to reflect ongoing research conducted by Rahe and others (Miller & Rahe, 1997; Rahe, 1978, 1990; Rahe et al, 1980). Additional events were added to the original scale, and item value scores were adjusted to reflect the life change magnitude appropriate for the current population. The authors suggest that this measure can be used for applications in behavioral medicine in which life stressors are a concern and as part of routine assessment to ensure that no life circumstances will be overlooked. When this measure is used as a basis for further history taking, recognition of life events that have led to adjustment difficulties and increased use of coping behaviors may be identified.

Scores: Several methods of scoring the RLCQ exist. Basic scoring is a simple item count of the number of events indicated (range, 0 to 74). For a more thorough rating, the positive responses on the RLCQ over the past 6 months are noted. Point values are assigned from the 1995 Life Change Units table (Miller & Rahe, 1997). The total points are summed; the total is rated for illness risk as follows: 0 to 125 is low; 126 to 200 is moderate; 201 to 300 is elevated; and over 300 is high. Argument through the years has been concerned with whether the sum of Life Change Units or the simple item count is more accurate as a measure of environmental stress. Studies have shown both methods of scoring to be equally reliable, which has led Rahe and others to suggest that a simple item count may be the most valid estimate of environmental stress.

Accuracy: The RLCQ has demonstrated good test-retest reliability. To demonstrate validity, Rahe's extensive body of work, including the research studies cited here, related Life Change Units and item counts from the scale to measures of physical and psychological health. Statistically significant correlations have been noted with measures of general psychologic distress, hospitalization, medical resource use, report of physical health symptoms, depression, myocardial infarction, control of diabetes, onset of narcolepsy, mortality after spinal cord injury, risk of suicide, medical compliance, and rehabilitation after surgery (American Psychiatric Association, 2000; Rahe, 1979, 1988; Rahe et al, 1967). Concurrent validity has been difficult to establish because the RCLQ was the first, fully developed life event checklist, and as such, correlates highly with later measures.

Administration Time: 10 to 15 minutes by self-administration.

References

American Psychiatric Association: *Handbook of psychiatric measures.* Washington, DC, 2000, American Psychiatric Association.

Holmes TH, Rahe RH: The Social Readjustment Rating Scale. *J Psychosom Res* 11:213-218, 1967.

Miller MA, Rahe RH: Life changes scaling for the 1990s. *J Psychosom Res* 43:279-292, 1997.

Rahe RH: Multi-cultural correlations of life change scaling. America, Japan, Denmark and Sweden. *J Psychosom Res* 13:191-195, 1969.

Rahe RH: Epidemiological studies of life change and illness. *Int J Psychiatry Med* 6:133-146, 1975.

Rahe RH: Life change measurement clarification. *Psychosom Med* 40:95-98, 1978.

Rahe RH: Life change events and mental illness: an overview. *J Human Stress* 5:2-10, 1979.

Rahe RH: Anxiety and physical illness. *J Clin Psychiatry* 49(Suppl): 26-29, 1988.

Rahe RH: Life change, stress responsivity, and captivity research. *Psychosom Med* 52:373-396, 1990.

Rahe RH, McKean JD Jr, Arthur RJ: A longitudinal study of life-change and illness patterns. *J Psychosom Res* 10:355-366, 1967.

Rahe RH, Ryman DH, Ward HW: Simplified scaling for life change events. *J Human Stress* 6:22-27, 1980.

Other Measures:

Beck Anxiety Inventory (BAI)   i

Authors: Beck et al, 1988.

Source: The Beck Anxiety Inventory (BAI) is copyrighted by the Psychological Corporation, 19500 Bulverde Rd, San Antonio, TX 78259; phone: 800-872-1726; website: http://www.PsychCorp.com. The tools may be purchased online at http://www.marketplace.psychcorp.com. Kits include a manual and record forms and are available in English and Spanish.

Targeted Population: Adults, ages 17 through 80 years.

Description: The BAI is a 21-item self-report questionnaire. Items include subjective, somatic, and panic-related symptoms of anxiety. Fourteen items denote physiologic symptoms, and seven items denote subjective perceptions such as fears. Each item is rated on a 4-point Likert-type scale, ranging from 0 (not at all) to 3 (severely/I could barely stand it). Items are rated on the basis of experiences from the past week, including the current day.

Scores: Items are summed for a total score, which ranges from 0 to 63. Score interpretation varies, depending on the authors. Beck and Steer (1993) interpreted the BAI score as follows: 0-7, minimal anxiety; 8-15, mild anxiety; 16-25, moderate anxiety; and 26-63, severe anxiety. Ferguson (2000) recommends caution in applying an interpretive standard to the BAI score, because a patient's demographics may not match those of the normative group, and the interpretation of a total score does not necessarily correspond to a diagnosis of anxiety disorder.

Accuracy: The BAI has demonstrated excellent internal consistency (Beck et al, 1988; Cox et al, 1996; Creamer et al, 1995; Kabacoff et al, 1997; Osman et al, 1997) and good test-retest reliability (Creamer et al, 1995; Fydrich et al, 1992). The BAI is especially noted for convergent and discriminant validity, in that the items correlate with other anxiety inventories but do not correlate with items from depression inventories (Beck et al, 1988; Creamer et al, 1995; Fydrich et al, 1992). Studies indicate that the instrument is more sensitive to panic or physiologic symptoms than to cognitive or behavioral symptoms of anxiety such as worry or avoidance behavior (Cox et al, 1996; Creamer et al, 1995; de Beurs et al, 1997; Fydrich et al, 1992; Kabacoff et al, 1997). In summary, the BAI is a reliable screening tool for detection of many anxiety disorders but may be less sensitive to detection of anxiety disorders not involving physiologic symptoms, such as phobias.

Administration Time: 5 to 10 minutes by self-administration or interview.

References

Beck AT, Steer RA, Ranieri WF: Scale for suicide ideation: psychometric properties of a self-report version. *J Clin Psychol* 44:499-505, 1988.

Beck AT, Steer RA: *The Beck Anxiety Inventory manual.* San Antonio, TX, 1993, Psychological Corporation.

Cox BJ, Cohen E, Direnfeld DM, et al: Does the Beck Anxiety Inventory measure anything beyond panic attack symptoms? *Behav Res Ther* 34:949-954, 1996.

Creamer M, Foran J, Bell R: The Beck Anxiety Inventory in a non-clinical sample. *Behav Res Ther* 33:477-485, 1995.

de Beurs E, Wilson KA, Chambless DL, et al: Convergent and divergent validity of the Beck Anxiety Inventory for patients with panic disorder and agoraphobia. *Depress Anxiety* 6:140-146, 1997.

Ferguson RJ: Using the Beck Anxiety Inventory in primary care. In Maruish ME, ed. *Handbook of psychological assessment in primary care settings* (pp. 509-535). Mahwah, NJ, 2000, Lawrence Erlbaum Associates.

Fydrich T, Dowdall D, Chambless DL: Reliability and validity of the Beck Anxiety Inventory. *J Anxiety Disord* 6:55-61, 1992.

Kabacoff RI, Segal DL, Hersen M, et al: Psychometric properties and diagnostic utility of the Beck Anxiety Inventory and State-Trait Anxiety Inventory with older adult psychiatric outpatients. *J Anxiety Disord* 11:33-47, 1997.

Osman A, Kopper BA, Barrios FX, et al: The Beck Anxiety Inventory: reexamination of factor structure and psychometric properties. *J Clin Psychol* 53:7-14, 1997.

AGGRESSION AND DOMESTIC VIOLENCE

A great number of screening tools and questionnaires have been developed for the assessment of aggression and domestic violence. Many of these tools consist of guidelines for directed questioning; these tools and resources are included in Chapter 5. This chapter includes two tools that quantifiably measure the level or presence of aggressive or violent behavior, the Overt Aggression Scale–Modified (OAS-M) and the Rating Scale for Aggressive Behavior in the Elderly (RAGE). These tools may assist primary care clinicians in evaluating the response to treatment interventions.

Routine screening for domestic violence has become a standard of care for primary care practice. Older measures of partner violence, including the Index of Spouse Abuse (Hudson & McIntosh, 1981) and the Conflict Tactics Scale (Strauss, 1979), were designed to measure the severity of abuse. Both tools are lengthy, which discourages their use in primary care practice. Included in this chapter is HITS, a domestic violence screening tool that combines four scored questions with an acronym to prompt easy recall in primary care settings.

References

Hudson WW, McIntosh S: The index of spouse abuse: two quantifiable dimensions. *J Marriage Fam* 43:873-888, 1981.

Straus MA: Measuring intrafamily conflict and violence: the Conflict Tactics Scales. *J Marriage Fam* 41:75-88, 1979.

Overt Aggression Scale–Modified (OAS-M)

Authors: Coccaro EF et al, 1991.

Source: The Overt Aggression Scale–Modified (OAS-M) is reprinted in this text. Copyright is held by Emil Coccaro, MD.

Targeted Population: School-age children and adults.

Description: The Overt Aggression Scale–Modified (Coccaro et al, 1991) is a 25-item tool designed to assess aggressive or violent behavior in outpatients. A modification of the original Overt Aggression Scale (Yudofsky et al, 1986), the OAS-M is divided into three domains. The first domain, Aggression, assesses four subscales: Verbal Aggression, Aggression Against Objects, Aggression Against Others, and Auto (self) Aggression. The second domain, Irritability, measures two subscales: Global Irritability and Subjective Irritability. The third domain, Suicidality, measures three subscales: Suicidal Tendencies (Ideation and Behavior), Intent of Attempt, and Lethality of Attempt.

Scores: Two methods are used in scoring the OAS-M. For the Aggression domain, each of the four subscales lists six behaviors with assigned point values of 0 to 5. All behaviors within each subscale that have occurred in the past week are noted; the points within each subscale are summed, then multiplied by the "weighted score" assigned to that subscale. The sum of these subscale scores results in a "Total Aggression Score." For the Irritability and Suicidality domains, a Likert-type scale is used to grade the level of intensity or intent for each of the subscales. Points are summed for the two Irritability subscales to produce a "Total Irritability Score." For the Suicidality domain, the second and third subscales are scored only if the first subscale (Suicidal Tendencies) is scored at 4 or higher. The sum of these three subscales forms the "Total Suicidality Score."

Scores range from 0 to 10 for the Irritability domain and 0 to 16 for the Suicidality domain. Because the Aggression domain uses a weighted score format, the total score may range from 0 to 135. Cut-off scores and norms are not available. Higher scores imply increased aggressive behavior.

Accuracy: Although data on the reliability and validity of the OAS-M are limited, it has demonstrated high interrater reliability (Endicott et al, 2002). The OAS-M authors found only moderate test-retest reliability, attributed to sample characteristics (Coccaro et al, 1991). The OAS-M Irritability and Aggression domains correlated well, but the Suicidality domain has not been tested. The OAS-M has been successfully used to monitor changes in aggressive behavior during various treatment protocols (Armenteros & Lewis, 2002; Donovan et al, 2000; Kavoussi & Coccaro, 1998; Mischoulon et al, 2002).

Administration Time: ~20-30 minutes by clinician interview.

References

Armenteros JL, Lewis JE: Citalopram treatment for impulsive aggression in children and adolescents: an open pilot study. *J Am Acad Child Adolesc Psychiatry* 41:522-529, 2002.

Coccaro EF, Harvey PD, Kupsaw-Lawrence E, et al: Development of neuropharmacologically based behavioral assessments of impulsive aggressive behavior. *J Neuropsychiatry Clin Neurosci* 3:S44-S51, 1991.

Coccaro EF, Kavoussi RJ: Fluoxetine and impulsive aggressive behavior in personality disordered subjects. *Arch Gen Psychiatry* 54:1081-1088, 1997.

Donovan SJ, Stewart JW, Nunes EV, et al: Divalproex treatment for youth with explosive temper and mood lability: a double-blind, placebo-controlled crossover design. *Am J Psychiatry* 157:818-820, 2000.

Endicott J, Tracy K, Burt D, et al: A novel approach to assess inter-rater reliability in the use of the Overt Aggression Scale-Modified. *Psychiatry Res* 112:153-159, 2002.

Kafantaris V, Lee DO, Magee H, et al: Assessment of children with the overt aggression scale. *J Neuropsychiatry Clin Neurosci* 8:186-193, 1996.

Kavoussi RJ, Coccaro EF: Divalproex sodium for impulsive aggressive behavior in patients with personality disorder. *J Clin Psychiatry* 59:676-680, 1998.

Mischoulon D, Dougherty DD, Bottonari KA, et al: An open pilot study of nefazodone in depression with anger attacks: relationship between clinical response and receptor binding. *Psychiatry Res* 116:151-161, 2002.

Yudofsky SC, Silver JM, Jackson W, et al: The Overt Aggression Scale for the objective rating of verbal and physical aggression. *Am J Psychol* 143:35-39, 1986.

Rating Scale for Aggressive Behavior in the Elderly (RAGE)

Authors: Patel V, and Hope RA, 1992.

Source: The Rating Scale for Aggressive Behavior in the Elderly (RAGE) is reprinted here and is also available online at http://www.medafile.com/zyweb/Default.htm.

Targeted Population: Older adults.

Description: The RAGE consists of 21 items designed to detect aggressive behavior in the elderly. Nineteen items consist of specific examples of aggressive behavior. One item notes any measures taken by staff to control aggressive behavior, and the last item asks for an overall assessment of the degree of aggressive behavior. All items assess behavior occurring over the past 3 days. Responses assess the frequency of behavior on a 4-point Likert-type scale, ranging from 0 (never) to 3 (more than once every day in the past 3 days). The authors recommend a brief training period for those using the RAGE in clinical practice. The training should outline the scale and emphasize the need for objectivity in assessment. Additionally recommended is use of a checklist to monitor behaviors for 3 days before completion of the scale.

Scores: The point values assigned to each response for the 21 items are summed to produce a total score, which may range from 0 to 63. Higher scores indicate greater frequency of aggressive behavior. A cut-off score was not provided by the authors; the scale may be used to monitor changes in aggressive behavior over time.

Accuracy: Reliability, including interrater and test-retest reliability and sensitivity, was tested by the authors. Interrater reliability was found to be significantly higher when staff kept a checklist in addition to completing the RAGE. Test-retest correlations were high, and sensitivity was also good, with changes in test scores corresponding to behavioral changes as observed by an independent rater. The RAGE was externally validated by comparing the scale with results of direct observation.

Administration Time: <5 minutes by clinician observation.

Reference

Patel V, Hope RA: A rating scale for aggressive behaviour in the elderly—the RAGE. *Psychol Med* 22:211-221, 1992.

HITS–Safety Questionnaire

Authors: Sherin KM et al, 1998.

Source: This questionnaire is reprinted in this text as a safety questionnaire.

Targeted Population: Adults.

Description: This four-item questionnaire for domestic violence screening uses the mnemonic *HITS* to promote recall of the instrument items. HITS stands for **H**urt, **I**nsult, **T**hreaten, or **S**cream. The patient responds to each question on a 5-point Likert-type scale with responses ranging from "never" to "frequently."

Scores: Each response is assigned a point value from 1 (never) to 5 (frequently). Responses to the four items are summed to produce a total score, which may range from 4 to 20. The authors suggest a cut-off score of 10 to differentiate abuse victims from nonvictims.

Accuracy: The HITS scale correlated well with verbal and physical aggression items of the Conflict Tactics Scale (CTS), showing good internal consistency and concurrent validity with the CTS verbal and physical aggression items (Sherin et al, 1998). The authors found that a cut-off score of 10.5 on the HITS accurately classified 91% of patients and 96% of abuse victims. The reliable differentiation of patients seen in a family practice office from abuse victim respondents demonstrated good construct validity.

Administration Time: <1 minute by self-report or interview.

Reference

Sherin KM, Sinacore JM, Li XQ, et al: HITS: a short domestic violence screening tool for use in a family practice setting. *Fam Med* 30:5085-12, 1998.

SUICIDALITY

Suicidal behavior is multidimensional, with complex factors contributing to the overall risk of a future suicide attempt. Many scales that seek to weigh and integrate the many parameters affecting suicidal behavior exist, but the evaluation of suicide risk ultimately rests on the impression of the clinician. Suicide screening tools often focus on previous attempts or intent to commit suicide, with various supportive items such as demographic information, level of social support, and coexisting mental health disorders.

Suicidality proceeds from ideation to attempt to completion. Because the goal of a suicide scale is to prevent completion, the sensitivity of the scale must be high so as not to miss a potential suicide. The risk of a high sensitivity scale is in overidentification of potential attempts. Because of the need for brevity and accuracy in primary care screening, the two suicidality scales reprinted here comprise basic, simple questions focusing on history and intent. Also reviewed are four popular proprietary instruments that may be of interest to practices with a mental health focus.

Modified SAD PERSONS Scale

Authors: Hockberger RS, and Rothstein RJ, 1988.

Targeted Population: Adults.

Description: Hockberger and Rothstein (1988) modified the SAD PERSONS Scale originally developed by

Patterson et al (1983). There are 10 factors to assess according to the acronym SAD PERSONS: **S**ex; **A**ge; **D**epression or hopelessness; **P**revious attempts or psychiatric care; **E**xcessive alcohol or drug use; **R**ational thinking loss; **S**eparated, divorced, or widowed; **O**rganized or serious attempt; **N**o social support; and **S**tated future intent. Each item is assigned 0 to 2 points, depending on the response.

Scores: The total score is the sum of points for all 10 parameters. Total scores range from 0 to 14; the higher the score, the greater is the risk of suicide. The authors suggest interpretation guidelines for total scores as follows: 0 to 5, questionable outpatient treatment; 6 to 8, emergency psychiatric consultation; 9 to 14, psychiatric hospitalization.

Accuracy: The modified SAD PERSONS scale was created because of the inability of the authors to validate the predictive ability of the original SAD PERSONS scale (Patterson et al, 1983) for determining the need for hospitalization of patients who have expressed suicidal ideation or behavior. Four of the original criteria were found to correlate with the need for hospitalization in patients expressing suicidal ideation and were weighted for scoring. The addition of weighted scoring greatly improved the sensitivity and specificity in identifying the need for hospitalization, which was confirmed by follow-up study of mortality rates over 6 to 12 months. The authors recommend this tool as a rapid screening measurement for nonpsychiatrists to obtain the objective information necessary to make an initial assessment of suicidality.

Administration Time: 1 to 2 minutes by clinician assessment.

References

Hockberger RS, Rothstein RJ: Assessment of suicide potential by nonpsychiatrists using the SAD PERSONS score. *J Emerg Med* 6:99-107, 1988.

Patterson WM, Dohn HH, Bird J, et al: Evaluation of suicidal patients: the SAD PERSONS scale. *Psychosomatics* 24:343-345, 348-349, 1983.

4-Item Risk of Suicide Questionnaire (RSQ-4)

Authors: Horowitz LM et al, 2001.

Source: A copy of the questionaire can be obtained by contacting the author, Lisa Horowitz; PhD, phone: 617-355-7447; fax 617-232-9562; e-mail: lisa.horowitz@tch.harvard.edu.

Targeted Population: Children and adolescents.

Description: The four items in the 4-Item Risk of Suicide Questionnaire (RSQ-4) were selected from a 14-item tool termed *the Risk of Suicide Questionnaire (RSQ)*, which was developed by Horowitz et al (2001). The four questions assess major factors in suicide risk: present and past thoughts of suicide, prior self-destructive behavior, and current stressors.

Scores: Each item is assigned a "yes" or "no" response. A positive response to any of the questions is considered a positive screen and alerts the clinician to possible imminent suicidal behavior.

Accuracy: By examining responses to the 14-item RSQ and the 30-item Suicide Ideation Questionnaire (SIQ) (Reynolds, 1987), Horowitz et al (2001), on the basis of statistical extrapolation, selected four items that produced the best sensitivity (0.98), specificity (0.37), and negative predictive value (0.97) for detection of suicidal behavior. Addition of the other 10 questions from the RSQ to these four did not significantly improve the accuracy of identifying suicidal patients. Limitations to use of this tool, stemming from its development, include the original small sample size, the homogenous patient sample population (patients with psychiatric problems in an urban pediatric teaching hospital), the use of the SIQ (which measures suicidal ideation, not behavior) as the comparison standard, and a tendency to identify children who are at relatively low risk of being suicidal. The authors recommend further study in larger, more diverse populations.

Administration Time: 1 to 2 minutes.

References

Horowitz LM, Wang PS, Koocher GP, et al: Detecting suicide risk in a pediatric emergency department: development of a brief screening tool. *Pediatrics* 107:1133-1137, 2001.

Reynolds WM: *Suicide Ideation Questionnaire.* Odessa, FL, 1987, Psychological Assessment Resources.

Other Measures:
Beck Scale for Suicidal Ideation (BSS) i

Authors: Beck AT, and Steer RA, 1991.

Source: The Beck Scale for Suicidal Ideation (BSS) is copyrighted by the Psychological Corporation, 19500 Bulverde Rd, San Antonio, TX 78259; phone: 800-872-1726; website: http://www.psychcorp.com. The tool may be purchased online at http://www.marketplace.psychcorp.com. Kits include a manual and record forms and are available in English and Spanish.

Targeted Population: Adults.

Description: The BSS includes 21 test items. The first five screening items may be used as a brief screen for patients not known to be suicidal. The 21 items are divided into three parts: active suicidal desire, suicidal ideation, and previous suicide attempts and intent. Items measure behavior occurring in the past week. The first 19 items contain three options graded according to the intensity of the suicidality and rated on a 3-point scale, ranging from 0 to 2. The last two items assess the number of previous suicide attempts and the seriousness of the intent to die associated with the last attempt.

Scores: The sum of the 19-item scores provides a total score with a range of 0 to 38. Higher scores indicate increased risk of suicide. If the respondent reports any active or passive desire to commit suicide, then an additional 14 items are administered. The authors recommend that the responses to individual items be examined over time for changes in suicide risk. Individual item responses may also initiate clinician-directed discussion of suicidal impulses and interventions for such.

Accuracy: Internal consistency, test-retest stability, and concurrent validity of this measure have been well-established for the BSS (Beck et al, 1988, 1991, 1997; Cochrane-Brink et al, 2000; Steer et al, 1993b). The BSI is moderately correlated with the Beck Depression Inventory Suicide Item, the BDI, and the Beck Hopelessness Scale (Beck et al, 1988, 1993; Steer et al, 1993a).

Administration Time: 5 to 10 minutes by self-administration or interview.

References

Beck AT, Brown GK, Steer RA: Psychometric characteristics of the Scale for Suicide Ideation with psychiatric outpatients. *Behav Res Ther* 35:1039-1046, 1997.

Beck AT, Steer RA: *Beck Scale for Suicide Ideation: manual.* San Antonio, TX, 1991, Psychological Corporation.

Beck AT, Steer RA, Beck JS, et al: Hopelessness, depression, suicidal ideation, and clinical diagnosis of depression. *Suicide Life Threat Behav* 23:139-145, 1993.

Beck AT, Steer RA, Ranieri WF: Scale for suicide ideation: psychometric properties of a self-report version. *J Clin Psychol* 44:499-505, 1988.

Cochrane-Brink KA, Lofchy JS, et al: Clinical rating scales in suicide risk assessment. *Gen Hosp Psychiatry* 22:445-451, 2000.

Steer RA, Rissmiller DJ, Ranieri WF, et al: Hopelessness, depression, suicidal ideation, and clinical diagnosis of depression. *Behav Res Ther* 31:229-236, 1993a.

Steer RA, Rissmiller DB, Ranieri WF, et al: Dimensions of suicidal ideation in psychiatric inpatients. *Behav Res Ther* 31:229-236, 1993b.

Beck Hopelessness Scale (BHS)   i

Authors: Beck AT, and Steer RA, 1988.

Source: The Beck Hopelessness Scale (BHS) is copyrighted by the Psychological Corporation, 19500 Bulverde Rd, San Antonio, TX 78259; phone: 800-872-1726; website: http://www.psychcorp.com. The tool may be purchased online at http://www.marketplace.psychcorp.com. Kits include a manual, record forms, and scoring key and are available in English and Spanish.

Targeted Population: Adults ages 17 through 80 years.

Description: The BHS contains 20 true or false items with pessimistic or optimistic statements. It is intended to be an indirect measure of suicidality.

Scores: Patients may endorse a pessimistic statement or deny an optimistic statement for a positive item score. Item scores are summed for a total score. A cut-off score of 9 on the BHS appears to be predictive of eventual suicide (Beck & Weishaar, 1990).

Accuracy: Hopelessness has been established as a suicide risk factor, as supported by results of prospective studies of inpatients and outpatients. Hopelessness was found to be 1.3 times more important than depression in explaining suicidal ideation (Beck et al, 1993).

Administration Time: 5 to 10 minutes by self-administration or interview.

References

Beck AT, Weishaar ME: Suicide risk assessment and prediction. *Crisis* 11:22-30, 1990.

Beck AT, Steer RA: *Manual for the Beck Hopelessness Scale.* San Antonio, TX, 1988, Psychological Corporation.

Beck AT, Steer RA, Beck JS, et al: Hopelessness, depression, suicidal ideation, and clinical diagnosis of depression. *Suicide Life Threat Behav* 23:139-145, 1993.

Suicide Probability Scale (SPS)   i

Authors: Cull JG, Gill WW, 1988.

Source: The Suicide Probability Scale (SPS) is copyrighted by Western Psychological Services, 12031 Wilshire Blvd, Los Angeles, CA 90025-1251; phone: 800-648-8857; fax: 310-478-7838; website: http://www.wpspublish.com/Inetpub4/index.htm. The tool may be purchased online at https://www-secure.earthlink.net/www.wpspublish.com/Inetpub4/catalog/W-172.htm. Kits include a manual, test forms, and profile forms.

Targeted Population: Adults and adolescents ages 13 and older.

Description: The SPS contains 36 items that describe particular feelings and behaviors. Each statement is rated on how often it applies to the respondent with the use of a 4-point Likert-type scale (never, rarely, usually, or always). The SPS is intended for use as a screening tool in a variety of outpatient and inpatient settings to identify adults and adolescents at risk for suicide attempts. It is also used as a continuous, systematic monitoring tool for psychiatric outpatients at risk for suicide.

Scores: Three summary scores are produced: a total weighted score, a T-score, and a probability score, which provide an overall indication of suicide risk. For more detailed interpretation, there are also four subscales: Hopelessness, Suicide Ideation, Negative Self-Evaluation, and Hostility. Cut-off norms are provided for interpretation for healthy subjects, psychiatric patients, and lethal suicide attempters.

Accuracy: The SPS was standardized in 1982 by Cull and Gill (1988) in a large sample population that included nonpsychiatric and psychiatric patients, as well as previous suicide attempters. Reliability, including internal consistency and test-retest reliability, was reported as good to excellent. In a review of available studies of the SPS as used with adolescents, Winters et al (2002) noted that reliability and validity were generally good. They cautioned, however, that adult normative data should not be applied to youths, as evidenced by higher scores obtained for adolescents in some studies.

Administration Time: 5 to 10 minutes by self-report or group administration.

References

Cull JG, Gill WW: *Suicide Probability Scale (SPS) manual.* Los Angeles, 1982, Western Psychological Services.

Winters NC, Myers K, Proud L: Ten-year review of rating scales. III: scales assessing suicidality, cognitive style, and self-esteem. *J Am Acad Child Adolesc Psychiatry* 41:1150-1181, 2002.

Suicidal Ideation Questionnaire (SIQ)   i

Author: Reynolds WM, 1987.

Source: The Suicidal Ideation Questionnaire (SIQ) and Suicidal Ideation Questionnaire-Junior (SIQ-JR) are copyrighted by Sigma Assessment Systems, Inc., PO Box 610984, Port Huron, MI 48061-0984; phone: 800-265-1285: fax: 800-361-9411; website: http://www.sigmaassessmentsystems.com/siq.htm. The tool may be purchased online at http://www.sigmaassessmentsystems.com/psiq.htm. Kits include a manual, test forms, and scoring templates.

Targeted Population: SIQ: Adolescents in grades 10 to 12. SIQ-JR: Adolescents in grades 7 to 9.

Description: The SIQ is a 30-item screening tool for adolescents in grades 10 to 12. A 15-item version, the SIQ-JR, is available for adolescents in grades 7 to 9. Both forms use a 7-point scale to assess the intensity and frequency of suicidal ideation during the past month.

Accuracy: Internal consistency, reliability, and validity have been demonstrated through content, construct, and clinical studies (Reynolds, 1987). In a review of adolescent studies, Winters et al (2002) reported good standardization and psychometric properties in diverse populations and noted that the SIQ and SIQ-JR are among the best suicidality scales for adolescents.

Administration Time: 5 to 10 minutes by self-administration or group administration.

References

Reynolds WM: *Suicidal Ideation Questionnaire (SIQ): professional manual.* Odessa, FL, 1987, Psychological Assessment Resources.

Winters NC, Myers K, Proud L: Ten-year review of rating scales. III: scales assessing suicidality, cognitive style, and self-esteem. *J Am Acad Child Adolesc Psychiatry* 41:1150-1181, 2002.

SUBSTANCE ABUSE DISORDERS

Screening for substance abuse has become a primary care issue, because patients with substance abuse problems often first turn to their primary care providers for assistance. The primary care clinician is also the first professional to see the at-risk, nondependent substance abuser in everyday practice. The ability to implement a screening protocol to identify these at-risk persons requires knowledge and skills in the area of behavioral health care. Knowledge of and familiarity with diagnostic screening tools for substance abuse are essential for implementation of a substance abuse protocol.

Extensive resources and screening tools for alcohol and substance abuse have been developed. The following resources cite online information of interest to the primary care clinician. Included in this chapter are the most well-known and frequently used screening tools for alcohol and drug abuse detection, including screens for adults, pregnant women, and adolescents. The brevity of these tools allows for easy incorporation into routine practice.

Resources: Substance Abuse Disorders

National Institute on Alcohol Abuse and Alcoholism (NIAAA): This online resource contains information and access to numerous resources, publications an databases pertaining to alcohol abuse. http://www.niaaa.nih.gov.

Project Cork: This resource provides authoritative information on substance abuse for clinicians, health care providers, human service personnel, and policy makers. Project Cork includes a database with more than 51,000 items on substance abuse, screening tools for substance abuse, newsletters for clinician use, and resources including a list of organizations, links to websites on substance abuse, and other publications. Additionally, a substance use history and physical examination, an adolescent interview guide, summary charts for drugs of abuse, and *DSM-IV* diagnostic criteria for substance abuse are available. Website: http://www.projectcork.org/

Treatment Improvement Exchange–Treatment Improvement Protocols (TIPs): This site is a resource sponsored by the Division of State and Community Assistance of the Center for Substance Abuse Treatment (CSAT), which provides information exchange between CSAT staff and state and local alcohol and substance abuse agencies. The best practice guidelines for the treatment of substance abuse are contained in 38 TIP documents, which draw on the experience and knowledge of clinical, research, and administrative experts in fields such as primary care, mental health, and social services. Website: http://www.treatment.org/Externals/tips.html

World Health Organization: Substance/Alcohol Dependence: This online resource includes World Health Organization (WHO) documents in electronic format on alcohol and substance use, abuse, and public health issues. Website: http://www.who.int/health_topics/en/

CAGE Questionnaire

Author: Ewing JA, 1984.

Source: The CAGE Questionnaire is reprinted here and is also available online at numerous sites including http://www.projectcork.org/clinical_tools/index.html. CAGE is copyrighted by the American Psychiatric Association; no permission is required for clinical use.

Targeted Population: Adults.

Description: The CAGE Questionnaire is a very brief, questionnaire consisting of four questions with "yes" or "no" answers for detection of alcoholism. CAGE is an acronym for the question topics: C = cut down, A = annoyed, G = guilt, E = eye opener. First validated in 1974 (Mayfield et al) and formally reported in 1984, the CAGE has been used clinically since the 1970s.

Scores: Items are assigned 1 point for a "yes" response and 0 points for a "no" response. A score of 1 or more raises a high index of suspicion and warrants further evaluation. Mayfield et al (1974) proposed a cut-off score of 2 as the criterion for a positive screen.

Accuracy: The CAGE Questionnaire has been used and tested extensively in many populations. It is considered to be a reliable method of screening for alcohol abuse in adults. In a systematic review of 38 studies in primary care, Fiellin et al (2000) noted that the CAGE questions proved to be superior for detecting alcohol abuse and dependence, with sensitivities ranging from 43% to 94% and specificities ranging from 70% to 97%. The CAGE Questionnaire is not recommended for use among adolescents because of significantly lower sensitivities in this population (Knight et al, 2003).

Administration Time: <1 minute by self-administration or interview.

Reference

Ewing JA: Detecting alcoholism. The CAGE questionnaire. *JAMA* 252:1905-1907, 1984.

Fiellin DA, Reid C, O'Connor PG: Screening for alcohol problems in primary care: a systematic review. *Arch Gen Psychiatry* 160: 1977-1989, 2000.

Knight JR, Sherritt L, Harris SK, et al: Validity of brief alcohol screening tests among adolescents: a comparison of the AUDIT, POSIT, CAGE, and CRAFFT. *Alcohol Clin Exp Res* 27:67-73, 2003.

Mayfield D, McLeod G, Hall P: The CAGE questionnaire: validation of a new alcoholism instrument. *Am J Psychiatry* 131:1121-1123, 1974.

T-ACE Questionnaire

Authors: Sokol RJ et al, 1989.

Targeted Population: Pregnant women.

Description: The T-ACE Questionnaire is a 4-item screen for alcoholism in pregnant women. Modeled after the CAGE Questionnaire, the T-ACE Questionnaire is an acronym for the following question topics: T = **t**olerance, A = **a**nnoyed, C = **c**ut down, E = **e**ye opener. The leading question focuses on the number of drinks it takes to make the patient feel "high." In the process of obtaining quantity and frequency data, potential at-risk prenatal drinking may be identified.

Scores: For the first question, the patient is considered tolerant if it takes more than two drinks to make her feel "high." Positive item responses are scored as 2 points for T and 1 each for A, C, or E. A total score of greater than or equal to 2 is considered a positive screen.

Accuracy: Sokol et al (1989) correctly identified 69% of the at-risk drinkers using the T-ACE Questionnaire with a positive predictive value of 23%. Russell et al (1996) found improved sensitivity for the T-ACE Questionnaire when it was administered with the MAST and the CAGE Questionnaire.

Administration Time: <1 minute by self-administration or interview.

References

Russell M, Martier SS, Sokol RJ, et al: Detecting risk drinking during pregnancy: a comparison of four screening questionnaires. *Am J Public Health* 86:1435-1439, 1996.

Sokol RJ, Martier SS, Ager JW: The T-ACE questions: practical prenatal detection of risk-drinking. *Am J Obstet Gynecol* 160:863-868, 1989.

Michigan Alcoholism Screening Test (MAST)

Author: Selzer ML, 1971.

Source: The Michigan Alcoholism Screening Test (MAST) is in the public domain and is reprinted here. The MAST and its derivatives may also be found at numerous online sites, including http://www.projectcork. org/clinical_tools/index.html (MAST and Brief-MAST), http://www.ncadi.samhsa.gov/govpubs/BKD250/26o. aspx#TIP26.FIG4-4 (MAST-G), and http://www.ncadi. samhsa.gov/govpubs/BKD234/24l.aspx (MAST, SMAST, and MAST-G).

Targeted Population: Adults.

Description: The MAST is a 24-item screening tool for alcoholism. Several derivations of the MAST are available. These include a 10-item Brief-MAST (Pokorny et al, 1972), a 13-item Short MAST (SMAST) (Selzer et al, 1975), a 9-item modified version called the *Malmo modification* (Mm-MAST) (Kristenson and Trell, 1982), a 24-item geriatric version (MAST-G) (Blow et al, 1992), and a 10-item Short MAST-Geriatric Version (SMAST-G) (Blow et al, 1998).

MAST items encompass a range of alcohol-related problems, such as perceptions of alcohol use, life consequences of drinking behavior, physical effects related to alcohol use, and drinking habits. The items included in the MAST and derivative tools are not directly linked to standard diagnostic criteria for alcohol use in *DSM-IV*.

Scores: The 24 questions for the MAST have yes/no responses and are weight-assigned 1, 2, or 5 points for positive responses; negative answers receive no points. Four items (1, 4, 6, and 7) are reverse-scored. A total score, ranging from 0 to 53, is obtained from the sum of the item scores.

The original citation rates a score of 5 as diagnostic of alcoholism; Ross et al (1990) reported an optimum cut-off score of 12/13, for detecting *DSM-III* alcohol dependence.

Accuracy: The MAST and its variants have been studied extensively since they were originally published. Reliability and validity have been reported as excellent (Blow et al, 1992; Hedlund and Vieweg, 1984; Ross et al, 1990; Selzer, 1971).

Administration Time: 5 to 15 minutes by self-administration or interview.

References

Blow FC, Gillespie BW, Barry KL, et al: Brief screening for alcohol problems in elderly populations using the Short Michigan Alcoholism Screening Test–Geriatric Version (SMAST-G). *Alcoholism Clin Exp Res* 22(Suppl):131A, 1998.

Blow FC, Brower KJ, Schulenberg JE, et al: The Michigan Alcoholism Screening Test–Geriatric Version (MAST-G): a new elderly-specific screening instrument. *Alcoholism Clin Exp Res* 16:372, 1992.

Hedlund JL, Vieweg BW: The Michigan Alcoholism Screening Test (MAST): a comprehensive review. *J Operational Psychiatry* 15:55-64, 1984.

Kristenson H, Trell E: Indicators of alcohol consumption: comparisons between a questionnaire (Mm-MAST), interviews and serum gamma-glutamyl transferase (GGT) in a health survey of middle-aged males. *Br J Addict* 77:297-304, 1982.

Pokorny AD, Miller BA, Kaplan HB: The brief MAST: a shortened version of the Michigan Alcohol Screening Test. *Am J Psychiatry* 129:342-345, 1972.

Ross HE, Gavin DR, Skinner HA: Diagnostic validity of the MAST and the Alcohol Dependence Scale in the assessment of DSM-III alcohol disorders. *J Stud Alcohol* 51:506-513, 1990.

Selzer ML: The Michigan Alcoholism Screening Test: the quest for a new diagnostic instrument. *Am J Psychiatry* 127:1653-1658, 1971.

Selzer ML, Vinokur A, van Roojen L: A self-administered Michigan Alcoholism Screening Test (SMAST). *J Stud Alcohol* 36:117-126, 1975.

Alcohol Use Disorders Identification Test (AUDIT)

Authors: World Health Organization: Babor TF et al, 1992, 2001.

Source: The Alcohol Use Disorders Identification Test (AUDIT) is reprinted here and is available at multiple locations online, including http://www.niaaa.nih.gov/publications/insaudit.htm, http://www.projectcork.org/clinical_tools/index.html, and http://www.ncadi.samhsa.gov/govpubs/BKD234/24l.aspx. The AUDIT is copyrighted but may be reproduced without permission.

Targeted Population: Adults and adolescents.

Description: The AUDIT is a two-part screening instrument that measures alcohol consumption and related harm. Developed over several years by the World Health Organization, the core questionnaire contains 10 items that measure amount and frequency of alcohol consumption, dependent drinking behaviors, and problems related to alcohol use during the past year. In addition to the questionnaire, the AUDIT program includes an optional clinical screening procedure consisting of two interview items, a brief physical examination, and a laboratory test. The optional screening, to be performed by a health care clinician, is useful in cases in which a patient is resistant, uncooperative, or unable to respond or if denial is likely or suspected. Guidelines for use of the AUDIT and corresponding recommendations for monitoring alcohol use and resultant harm are available from the World Health Organization (Babor et al, 2001; World Health Organization, 2000).

Scores: The 10 multiple-choice questions are scored by using a 5-point Likert-type scale with answers ranging from "never" or "no" (0 points) to the highest frequency of behavior (4 points). The total score is the sum of all item points and ranges from 0 to 40. A score ≥8 indicates a strong likelihood of hazardous or harmful alcohol use. A cut-off score of 10 will provide greater specificity but at the expense of sensitivity (Babor et al, 2001). For subscale items, a high score on the quantity and frequency items (1-3) indicates hazardous alcohol use, a high score on the second three items (4-6) implies alcohol dependence, and a high score on the last four items (7-10) suggests harmful use (Babor et al, 1992). Babor et al (2001) further recommend that scores between 8 and 15 are most appropriate for simple advice focused on the reduction of hazardous drinking, scores between 16 and 19 suggest brief counseling and continued monitoring, and scores of ≥20 warrant further diagnostic evaluation for alcohol dependence.

Accuracy: The AUDIT has a respected history of excellent reliability and validity (Babor et al, 2001). In a review of primary care studies on screening methods for alcohol problems conducted from 1966 through 1998, Fiellin et al (2000) reported that the AUDIT was the most effective measure for identifying subjects with at-risk, hazardous, or harmful drinking; sensitivities ranged from 51% to 97% and specificities ranged from 78% to 96%.

They noted that the CAGE questions were superior for detecting alcohol abuse and dependence and that the AUDIT and CAGE instruments consistently performed better than other screening methods. Two other meta-analyses of the AUDIT core questionnaire have been completed. Allen et al (1997) reported high sensitivities and specificities for the AUDIT, with correlations associated with other self-report alcohol screening tests, biochemical measures of drinking, and more distal indicators of problematic drinking. On review of studies performed on the AUDIT through 2001, Reinert et al (2002) found that the AUDIT demonstrated sensitivities and specificities, test-retest reliability, and internal consistency comparable, and typically superior, to those of other self-report screening measures.

Use of the AUDIT for screening of adolescents (ages 14-18 years) was examined by Knight et al (2003). In this prospective study, optimal cut points associated for problem alcohol use, sensitivities, and specificities were examined for the AUDIT, POSIT, CAGE, and CRAFFT measures. The AUDIT, POSIT, and CRAFFT demonstrated acceptable sensitivity for identifying alcohol problems or disorders in the adolescent age group.

Administration Time: ~2 to 4 minutes by self-administration or clinician interview.

References

Allen JP, Litten RZ, Fertig JB, et al: A review of research on the Alcohol Use Disorders Identification Test (AUDIT). *Alcoholism Clin Exp Res* 21:613-619, 1997.

Babor TF, de la Fuente JR, Saunders J, et al: *AUDIT, The Alcohol Use Disorders Identification Test: guidelines for use in primary health care.* Geneva, 1992, World Health Organization.

Babor TF, Higgins-Biddle JC, Saunders JB, et al: *The Alcohol Use Disorders Identification Test: guidelines for use in primary care,* ed 2. Geneva, 2001, World Health Organization, Department of Mental Health and Substance Dependence. Available at http://www.who.int/substance_abuse/publications/alcohol/en/

Fiellin DA, Reid C, O'Connor PG: Screening for alcohol problems in primary care: a systematic review. *Arch Gen Psychiatry* 160:1977-1989, 2000.

Knight JR, Sherritt L, Harris SK, et al: Validity of brief alcohol screening tests among adolescents: a comparison of the AUDIT, POSIT, CAGE, and CRAFFT. *Alcohol Clin Exp Res* 27:67-73, 2003.

Reinert DF, Allen JP: The Alcohol Use Disorders Identification Test (AUDIT): a review of recent research. *Alcohol Clin Exp Res* 26:272-279, 2002.

World Health Organization: Department of Mental Health and Substance Dependence, Noncommunicable Diseases and Mental Health Cluster. *International guide for monitoring alcohol consumption and related harm.* Geneva, 2000, World Health Organization. Available at http://www.who.int/substance_abuse/publications/alcohol/en/

Drug Abuse Screening Test (DAST)

Author: Skinner HA, 1982.

Source: The Drug Abuse Screening Test (DAST) is reprinted here and available online at http://www.projectcork.org/clinical_tools/index.html, http://www.psycounseling.com/screening_tests.htm (DAST-28), http://www.kc.vanderbilt.edu/addiction/dast.html, and http://www.eibdata.emcdda.org/Treatment/Needs/tdast.shtml (DAST-20).

The DAST-20 forms may also be ordered from Centre for Addiction and Mental Health, 33 Russell St, Toronto, Ontario, Canada M5S 2S1; phone: 800-661-1111 or 416-595-6059; website: http://www.camh.net/publications/index.html.

Targeted Population: Adults (DAST) and adolescents (DAST-A).

Description: The DAST is a screening tool used to identify individuals who are abusing psychoactive drugs and to measure the problem severity. Items screen for self-recognition of a drug problem, serious social consequences of drug use, help seeking for drug abuse, illegal drug-related activities, and inability to control drug use. Frequency and duration of drug use and specific drugs abused are not identified. The original DAST (Skinner, 1982) contains 28 items with yes/no responses. Variants include a 20-item DAST (brief-DAST or DAST-20), a 10-item DAST (DAST-10), and the Drug Abuse Screening Test for Adolescents (DAST-A) (Martino et al, 2000). The DAST-20 contains question numbers 1 to 5, 8 to 10, 12, 14 to 18, 21 to 25, and 27 from the DAST-28. The DAST-10 contains question numbers 1, 3, 5, 8 to 10, 15, 21, 23, and 24 from the DAST-28. The term *DAST* is often used in the literature for both the 28-item and 20-item versions.

Scores: Each "yes" response is scored 1 point; each "no" response is scored 0. Item numbers 4, 5, and 7 on the DAST-28 are reverse-scored. The item points are summed to provide a total score. The DAST-28 yields an overall score ranging from 0 to 28. A cut-off score of 5 or more on the DAST-28 indicates a probable drug use disorder. A range of valid clinical DAST cut-off scores from 5/6 through 10/11 was identified as valid in discriminating patients according to *DSM-III* substance abuse diagnostic criteria (Staley & el-Guebaly, 1990; Gavin et al, 1989). DAST-A scores of greater than 6 were found to differentiate adolescent psychiatric inpatients with and without drug-related disorders (Martino et al, 2000).

Accuracy: Skinner (1982) noted nearly perfect correlation between the DAST-28 and the DAST-20. Internal consistency is excellent; high sensitivity and specificity for detecting drug use disorders has confirmed the validity of the DAST (Gavin et al, 1989; Skinner, 1982; Staley & el-Guebaly, 1990). High face validity for all items, however, provides no protection from false reporting. DAST scores have also been shown to be significantly correlated with frequency of drug use in the past 12 months for a host of drugs (Skinner, 1982). The DAST items do not specify a time frame; because the DAST does not distinguish between current and past drug-related diagnoses, it has not been used as an outcome measure.

Administration Time: 5 minutes by self-administration.

References

Gavin DR, Ross HE, Skinner HA: Diagnostic validity of the Drug Abuse Screening Test in the assessment of DSM-III drug disorders. *Br J Addict* 84:301-307, 1989.

Skinner HA: The drug abuse screening test. *Addict Behav* 7:363-371, 1982.

Staley D, el-Guebaly N: Psychometric properties of the Drug Abuse Screening Test in a psychiatric patient population. *Addict Behav* 15:257-264, 1990.

Martino S, Grilo CM, Fehon DC: Development of the drug abuse screening test for adolescents (DAST-A). *Addict Behav* 25:57-70, 2000.

CRAFFT

Authors: Knight JR et al, 1999.

Source: The CRAFFT is reprinted in this text and is also available online at http://www.projectcork.org/clinical_tools/index.html. The CRAFFT may be used clinically without permission.

Targeted Population: Adolescents.

Description: The CRAFFT is a 6-item screening test for substance use and abuse in adolescents. CRAFFT is a mnemonic, with each of the letters based on a key word in each of the six questions of the screening tool: **C**ar, **R**elax, **A**lone, **F**orget, **F**amily/Friends, **T**rouble. The CRAFFT was designed to be brief, developmentally appropriate, to include both alcohol and other drugs in the screening, and to elicit yes/no responses.

Scores: Each of the six items is given 1 point for a "yes" response and 0 points for a "no" response. The item points are summed for a total score; a cut-off score of 2 or more suggests that the adolescent has a serious problem with alcohol abuse and is indicative of a need for long-term treatment (Knight et al, 1999).

Accuracy: The CRAFFT individual items were derived from three preexisting screening tools: the RAFFT (Riggs & Alario, 1989), the POSIT (Gruenewald & Klitzner, 1991) and the Drug and Alcohol Problem (DAP) Quickscreen (Klitzner et al, 1987). The six items were selected for high internal consistency, sensitivity, and specificity rates. When grouped as a 6-item screen, the model maintained internal consistency. In a comparison study for criterion validity among the AUDIT, POSIT, CRAFFT, and CAGE, Knight et al (2003) noted that the AUDIT, POSIT, and CRAFFT had acceptable sensitivity for identifying alcohol problems or disorders in adolescents. In this study, the optimal cut-off point associated with problem use was 1 for CRAFFT. Knight et al (1999) have recommended further validation study of the CRAFFT but note that this tool has the potential to quickly assist clinicians in identifying youth who need referral to substance abuse treatment programs.

Administration Time: 1 to 2 minutes by clinician interview.

References

Gruenewald PJ, Klitzner M: Results of a preliminary POSIT analyses. In Rahdert E, ed. *The adolescent assessment/referral system manual.* Rockville, MD, 1991, National Institute on Drug Abuse. Website: http://www.niaaa.nih.gov/publications/posit.htm.

Klitzner M, Schwartz RH, Gruenewald P, et al: Screening for risk factors for adolescent alcohol and drug use. *Am J Dis Child* 141:45-49, 1987.

Knight JR, Shrier LA, Bravender TD, et al: A new brief screen for adolescent substance abuse. *Arch Pediatr Adolesc Med* 153:591-596, 1999.

Knight JR, Sherritt L, Harris SK, et al: Validity of brief alcohol screening tests among adolescents: a comparison of the AUDIT, POSIT, CAGE, and CRAFFT. *Alcohol Clin Exp Res* 27:67-73, 2003.

Riggs SR, Alario A: Adolescent substance use instructor's guide. In Dube C, Goldstein M, Lewis D, et al, eds. *Project ADEPT curriculum for primary care physician training* (pp 1-57). Providence, RI, 1989, Brown University.

EATING DISORDERS

Eating disorders are common in the general population and particularly affect young women. The primary eating disorder diagnoses, according to *DSM-IV*, are anorexia nervosa, bulimia nervosa, and binge eating disorder. Primary care providers, the source of first contact for most patients, are in the unique position of being able to detect and manage an eating disorder before physical complications arise. Although many eating disorder screening tools comprise a long, structured interview format best served by a mental health professional, several brief screening tools have been proposed in recent years. Two brief questionnaires are included in this chapter. Although psychometric studies are lacking for these measures, their brevity and focus make them appropriate for primary care practice. A third instrument, the Eating Attitudes Test (26-item), measures a range of behaviors and attitudes characteristic of disordered eating. Information on the more comprehensive, proprietary Eating Disorders Inventory is also included.

SCOFF Questionnaire

Authors: Morgan JF et al, 1999.

Targeted Population: Adults and adolescents, with women as the primary focus group.

Description: The SCOFF Questionnaire, developed in England, consists of five questions designed to assess the presence of core features of anorexia nervosa and bulimia nervosa. SCOFF is a mnemonic, with each of the letters based on a key word in each of the six questions of the screening tool: **S**ick, **C**ontrol, **O**ne, **F**at, and **F**ood. The SCOFF was designed to be brief, memorable for primary care clinicians, and to elicit yes/no responses. Of note, the third question "Have you recently lost more than **O**ne stone in a 3-month period?" includes the British weight and measures term *stone*; this is the equivalent of 14 pounds in American weights and measures.

Scores: The number of "yes" responses is totaled; two or more "yes" responses are associated with the potential for an eating disorder.

Accuracy: Morgan et al (1999) developed the SCOFF questionnaire by studying women with diagnoses of eating disorders and a control group of women without eating disorders. A cut-off score of 2 or more "yes" responses provided

100% sensitivity for anorexia and bulimia; specificity was 87.5% for control subjects. In a more recent study of a non-clinical college population, sensitivity of the SCOFF was reported at 78%, with a specificity of 88% for a cut-off score of ≥2 (Cotton et al, 2003). Cotton et al (2003) suggested that the original psychometrics noted for the SCOFF were due to the extreme differences in the two groups included in the original study and that the SCOFF is less helpful in a primary care population. Both studies suggest that further validation of the SCOFF in larger populations is needed.

Administration Time: <1 minute by self-administration or interview.

References

Cotton M, Ball C, Robinson P: Four simple questions can help screen for eating disorders. *J Gen Intern Med* 18:53-56, 2003.

Morgan JF, Reid F, Lacey H: The SCOFF questionnaire: assessment of a new screening tool for eating disorders. *BMJ* 319:1467-1468, 1999.

Eating Disorder Screen for Primary Care (ESP)

Authors: Cotton M et al, 2003.

Targeted Population: Adults and adolescents, with women as the primary focus group.

Description: The Eating Disorder Screen for Primary Care (ESP) contains four screening questions derived from other eating disorder inventories. Each question has a yes/no response choice.

Scores: The first of the four items is given 1 point for a "no" response and 0 points for a "yes" response. The remaining three items are scored 1 point for a "yes" response and 0 points for a "no" response. The item points are summed for a total score; a score of ≥2 indicates a potential eating disorder and should prompt a more detailed assessment (Cotton et al, 2003).

Accuracy: In the development of the ESP, the authors compared answers given to the ESP and SCOFF Questionnaire (Morgan et al, 1999) with results from the standardized Questionnaire for Eating Disorder Diagnoses (Q-EDD) (Mintz et al, 1997). Each component of the ESP and SCOFF was compared with the Q-EDD by using sensitivity, specificity, and likelihood ratios. From this analysis, the questions on the ESP and SCOFF that were most likely to detect or rule out an eating disorder were determined. Use of a cut-off score of ≥2 maximized the sensitivity to 100% for the ESP, although the specificity was 71%. The authors recommend further study for this screen, with improvement in consecutive recruitment of subjects; they also recommend applying the measure to populations with a lower prevalence of eating disorders and using a larger population (Cotton et al, 2003).

Administration Time: <1 minute by self-administration or interview.

References

Cotton M, Ball C, Robinson P: Four simple questions can help screen for eating disorders. *J Gen Intern Med* 18:53-56, 2003.

Mintz LB, O'Halloran MS, Mulholland AM: Questionnaire for eating disorder diagnoses: reliability and validity of operationalizing DSM-IV criteria into a self-report format. *J Couns Psychol* 44:63-79, 1997.

Morgan JF, Reid F, Lacey H: The SCOFF questionnaire: assessment of a new screening tool for eating disorders. *BMJ* 319:1467-1468, 1999.

Eating Attitudes Test (EAT-26)

Authors: Garner DM et al, 1982.

Source: The Eating Attitudes Test (EAT-26) is reprinted here and may also be found online at http://www. eatingdisorderinfo.org/EAT-26.pdf and http://www. healthyplace.com/Communities/Eating_Disorders/ concernedcounseling/eat/.

The EAT-26 is also available in the text by Garner (1997).

Targeted Population: Adults and adolescents.

Description: The EAT-26 measures a range of behaviors and attitudes characteristic of disordered eating. The 26 items focus on dieting habits, preoccupation with food, and perceptions regarding food and control. Three subscales have been proposed: dieting, bulimia and food preoccupation, and oral control. The EAT-26 is an abbreviated version of the original 40-item Eating Attitudes Test (Garner and Garfinkel, 1979). Now widely used as a standardized measure of eating disorder symptoms, the EAT-26 is not, in itself, diagnostic. The tool is recommended for screening for eating disorder symptoms; patients who score at or above a cut-off point are then referred for a more definitive diagnostic interview.

Scores: The 26 items are scored on a 6-point Likert-type scale based on frequency of experience (never, rarely, sometimes, often, usually, always). Responses for item numbers 1 to 25 are weighted from 0 to 3, with a score of 3 assigned to "always," a score of 2 for "usually," a score of 1 for "often," and a score of 0 assigned to the last three responses. Item number 26 is reverse-scored in that "never" is scored 3, "rarely" is scored 2, and "sometimes" is scored 1 point. Item scores are summed for a total score; a total score of ≥20 identifies individuals likely to have an eating disorder, including anorexia nervosa and bulimia nervosa. Subscale items are calculated by adding the item scores for that particular subscale; norms are not available. Subscale:

Dieting: 1, 6, 7, 10, 11,12,14,16, 17, 22, 23, 24, 25
Bulimia and food preoccupation: 3, 4, 9, 18, 21, 26
Oral control: 2, 5, 8, 13, 15, 19, 20

Accuracy: Garner et al (1982) described psychometric and clinical correlates of the EAT-26 and original EAT-40 in patients with eating disorders and a control group. Both screens were highly correlated; no differences were found between patients with bulimia and those with anorexia nervosa in the total EAT-26 and EAT-40 scores. The authors concluded that the EAT-26 is a reliable, valid, and economical instrument that may be useful as an objective measure of the symptoms of anorexia nervosa. In a later study of a nonclinical group, the EAT-26 was found to be reliable; the factor structure was different from that obtained in clinical groups and was significantly

correlated with body image, weight, and diet (Koslowsky et al, 1992).

Administration Time: 2-5 minutes by self-administration.

References

Garner DM: Psychoeducational principles in treatment. In Garner DM, Garfinkel PE, eds. *Handbook of treatment for eating disorders.* New York, 1997, Guilford Press.

Garner DM, Garfinkel PE: The Eating Attitudes Test: an index of the symptoms of anorexia nervosa. *Psychol Med* 9:273-279, 1979.

Garner DM, Olmsted MP, Bohr Y, et al: The eating attitudes test: psychometric features and clinical correlates. *Psychol Med* 12: 871-878, 1982.

Koslowsky M, Scheinberg Z, Bleich A, et al: The factor structure and criterion validity of the short form of the Eating Attitudes Test. *J Pers Assess* 58:27-35, 1992.

Other Measures:

Eating Disorders Inventory–Second Edition (EDI-2)   **i**

Authors: Garner DM, 1991; Garner DM et al, 1983 ; and Garner DM, Olmstead MP, 1984.

Source: The Eating Disorders Inventory–Second Edition (EDI-2) is copyrighted and available from Psychological Assessment Resources, Inc. (PAR), 16204 N Florida Ave, Lutz, FL 33549; phone: 800-331-8378 or 813-968-3003; fax: 800-727-9329. The tool may be purchased online at http://www.parinc.com/product.cfm?ProductID=201. Kits include a manual, item booklets, answer sheets, profile forms, and symptom checklists. A computer version is available. More information may be found at http://www.river-centre.org/OrderEDI-2.html.

Targeted Population: Adults and adolescents, ages 12 and older.

Description: The EDI-2 is a standardized measure of symptoms associated with anorexia nervosa, bulimia nervosa, and other eating disorders (Garner, 1991). The EDI-2 contains 64 original items plus 27 additional items for a total of 91 items. Items are divided into 11 subscales: Ineffectiveness, Perfection, Interpersonal Distrust, Interoceptive Awareness, Maturity Fears, Asceticism, Impulse Regulation, Social Insecurity, Drive for Thinness, Bulimia, and Body Dissatisfaction. The items are presented in a 6-point Likert-type scale format (always, usually, often, sometimes, rarely, or never) and measure a range of psychologic symptoms that are relevant to the development and maintenance of eating disorders. A 4-page symptom checklist that documents information regarding the frequency and severity of symptoms relevant to the diagnosis of an eating disorder is also available.

The EDI-2 does not yield a specific diagnosis of an eating disorder. It is used as a screening instrument to identify eating disorders in nonpatient and patient populations.

Scores: A two-part answer sheet provides item scoring without the use of scoring keys. Subscale scores are obtained by adding all item scores for each subscale; these are plotted on profile forms. Norms are also provided for patients with bulimia and anorexia nervosa, patients with bulimia nervosa, high school boys and girls, and male and female college students.

Accuracy: The original EDI is considered a standard in assessment of eating disorders and has been cited in hundreds of research and clinical articles. The EDI-2 has demonstrated strong reliability and validity in college students and adults. Evidence of good psychometric performance for the EDI-2 was noted for adolescents by McCarthy et al (2002) and for women with binge eating disorder by Tasca et al (2003). Bizeul et al (2001) reported that a high EDI total score and high scores on subscales for perfectionism and interpersonal distrust could predict a long-term severe outcome in anorexia nervosa, supporting use of this measure as a long-term outcome predictor.

Administration Time: 20 minutes by self-administration.

References

Bizeul C, Sadowsky N, Rigaud D: The prognostic value of initial EDI scores in anorexia nervosa patients: a prospective follow-up study of 5-10 years. Eating Disorder Inventory. *Eur Psychiatry* 16:232-238, 2001.

Garner DM: *Eating Disorder Inventory. Professional manual.* Los Angeles, 1991, Western Psychological Services.

Garner DM, Olmstead MP: *Manual of Eating Disorder Inventory (EDI).* Odessa, FL, 1984, Psychological Assessment Resources, Inc.

Garner DM, Olmstead MP, Polivy J: Development and validation of a multidimensional eating disorder inventory for anorexia nervosa and bulimia. *Int J Eat Disord* 2:15-34, 1983.

McCarthy DM, Simmons JR, Smith GT, et al: Reliability, stability, and factor structure of the Bulimia Test-Revised and Eating Disorder Inventory-2 scales in adolescence. *Assessment* 9:382-389, 2002.

Tasca GA, Illing V, Lybanon-Daigle V, et al: Psychometric properties of the eating disorders inventory-2 among women seeking treatment for binge eating disorder. *Assessment* 10:228-236, 2003.

Global Assessment of Functioning (GAF) Scale

Consider psychological, social, and occupational functioning on a hypothetical continuum of mental health–mental illness. Do not include impairment in functioning due to physical (or environmental) limitations. NOTE: Use intermediate codes when appropriate, e.g., 45, 68, 72.

Code

Code	
100 | 91	Superior functioning in a wide range of activities, life's problems never seem to get out of hand, is sought out by others because of his or her many positive qualities. No symptoms.
90 | 81	Absent or minimal symptoms (e.g., mild anxiety before an examination), good functioning in all areas, interested and involved in a wide range of activities, socially effective, generally satisfied with life, no more than everyday problems or concerns (e.g., an occasional argument with family members).
80 | 71	If symptoms are present, they are transient and expected reactions to psychosocial stressors (e.g., difficulty concentrating after family argument); no more than slight impairment in social, occupational, or school functioning (e.g., temporarily behind in schoolwork).
70 | 61	Some mild symptoms (e.g., depressed mood and mild insomnia) OR some difficulty in social, occupational, or school functioning (e.g., occasional truancy, or theft within the household), but generally functioning pretty well, has some meaningful interpersonal relationships.
60 | 51	Moderate symptoms (e.g., flat affect and circumstantial speech, occasional panic attacks) OR moderate difficulty in social, occupational, or school functioning (e.g., few friends, conflicts with peers or co-workers).
50 | 41	Serious symptoms (e.g., suicidal ideation, severe obsessional rituals, frequent shoplifting) OR any serious impairment in social, occupational, or school functioning (e.g., no friends, unable to keep a job.)
40 | 31	Some impairment in reality testing or communication (e.g., speech is at times illogical, obscure, or irrelevant) OR major impairment in several areas, such as work or school, family relations, judgment, thinking, or mood (e.g., depressed man avoids friends, neglects family, and is unable to work; child frequently beats up younger children, is defiant at home, and is failing at school).
30 | 21	Behavior is considerably influenced by delusions or hallucinations OR serious impairment in communication or judgment (e.g., sometimes incoherent, acts grossly inappropriately, suicidal preoccupation) OR inability to function in almost all areas (e.g., stays in bed all day; no job, home, or friends).
20 | 11	Some danger of hurting self or others (e.g., suicide attempts without clear expectation of death; frequently violent; manic excitement) OR occasionally fails to maintain minimal personal hygiene (e.g., smears feces) OR gross impairment in communication (e.g., largely incoherent or mute).
10 | 1	Persistent danger of severely hurting self or others (e.g., recurrent violence) OR persistent inability to maintain minimal personal hygiene OR serious suicidal act with clear expectation of death.
0	Inadequate information.

Problem Oriented Screening Instrument for Teenagers (POSIT)

Name: _____

Date: _____

The purpose of these questions is to help us choose the best ways to help you. So, please try to answer the questions honestly.

Please answer all of the questions. If a question does not fit you exactly, pick the answer that is mostly true.

You may see the same or similar questions more than once. Please just answer each question as it comes up.

Please put an "X" through your answer.

If you do not understand a word, please ask for help.

You may begin.

1. Do you have so much energy you don't know what to do with it?	Yes	No
2. Do you brag?	Yes	No
3. Do you get into trouble because you use drugs or alcohol at school?	Yes	No
4. Do your friends get bored at parties when there is no alcohol served?	Yes	No
5. Is it hard for you to ask for help from others?	Yes	No
6. Has there been adult supervision at the parties you have gone to recently?	Yes	No
7. Do your parents or guardians argue a lot?	Yes	No
8. Do you usually think about how your actions will affect others?	Yes	No
9. Have you recently either lost or gained more than 10 pounds?	Yes	No
10. Have you ever had sex with someone who shot up drugs?	Yes	No
11. Do you often feel tired?	Yes	No
12. Have you had trouble with stomach pain or nausea?	Yes	No
13. Do you get easily frightened?	Yes	No
14. Have any of your best friends dated regularly during the past year?	Yes	No
15. Have you dated regularly in the past year?	Yes	No
16. Do you have a skill, craft, trade, or work experience?	Yes	No
17. Are most of your friends older than you are?	Yes	No
18. Do you have less energy than you think you should?	Yes	No
19. Do you get frustrated easily?	Yes	No
20. Do you threaten to hurt people?	Yes	No
21. Do you feel alone most of the time?	Yes	No
22. Do you sleep either too much or too little?	Yes	No
23. Do you swear or use dirty language?	Yes	No
24. Are you a good listener?	Yes	No
25. Do your parents or guardians approve of your friends?	Yes	No

26. Have you lied to anyone in the past week?	Yes	No
27. Do your parents or guardians refuse to talk with you when they are mad at you?	Yes	No
28. Do you rush into things without thinking about what could happen?	Yes	No
29. Did you have a paying job last summer?	Yes	No
30. Is your free time spent just hanging out with friends?	Yes	No
31. Have you accidentally hurt yourself or someone else while high on alcohol or drugs?	Yes	No
32. Have you had any accidents or injuries that still bother you?	Yes	No
33. Are you a good speller?	Yes	No
34. Do you have friends who damage or destroy things on purpose?	Yes	No
35. Have the whites of your eyes ever turned yellow?	Yes	No
36. Do your parents or guardians usually know where you are and what you are doing?	Yes	No
37. Do you miss out on activities because you spend too much money on drugs or alcohol?	Yes	No
38. Do people pick on you because of the way you look?	Yes	No
39. Do you know how to get a job if you want one?	Yes	No
40. Do your parents or guardians and you do lots of things together?	Yes	No
41. Do you get A's and B's in some classes and fail others?	Yes	No
42. Do you feel nervous most of the time?	Yes	No
43. Have you stolen things?	Yes	No
44. Have you ever been told you are hyperactive?	Yes	No
45. Do you ever feel you are addicted to alcohol or drugs?	Yes	No
46. Are you a good reader?	Yes	No
47. Do you have a hobby you are really interested in?	Yes	No
48. Do you plan to get a diploma (or already have one)?	Yes	No
49. Have you been frequently absent or late for work?	Yes	No
50. Do you feel people are against you?	Yes	No
51. Do you participate in team sports that have regular practices?	Yes	No
52. Have you ever read a book cover to cover for your own enjoyment?	Yes	No
53. Do you have chores that you must regularly do at home?	Yes	No
54. Do your friends bring drugs to parties?	Yes	No
55. Do you get into fights a lot?	Yes	No
56. Do you have a hot temper?	Yes	No
57. Do your parents or guardians pay attention when you talk with them?	Yes	No
58. Have you started using more and more drugs or alcohol to get the effect you want?	Yes	No

59. Do your parents or guardians have rules about what you can and cannot do?	Yes	No
60. Do people tell you that you are careless?	Yes	No
61. Are you stubborn?	Yes	No
62. Do any of your best friends go out on school nights without permission from their parents or guardians?	Yes	No
63. Have you ever had or do you now have a job?	Yes	No
64. Do you have trouble getting your mind off things?	Yes	No
65. Have you ever threatened anyone with a weapon?	Yes	No
66. Do you have a way to get to a job?	Yes	No
67. Do you ever leave a party because there is no alcohol or drugs?	Yes	No
68. Do your parents or guardians know what you really think or feel?	Yes	No
69. Do you often act on the spur of the moment?	Yes	No
70. Do you usually exercise for a half hour or more at least once a week?	Yes	No
71. Do you have a constant desire for alcohol or drugs?	Yes	No
72. Is it easy to learn new things?	Yes	No
73. Do you have trouble with your breathing or with coughing?	Yes	No
74. Do people your own age like and respect you?	Yes	No
75. Does your mind wander a lot?	Yes	No
76. Do you hear things no one else around you hears?	Yes	No
77. Do you have trouble concentrating?	Yes	No
78. Do you have a valid driver's license?	Yes	No
79. Have you ever had a paying job that lasted at least one month?	Yes	No
80. Do you and your parents or guardians have frequent arguments that involve yelling and screaming?	Yes	No
81. Have you had a car accident while high on alcohol or drugs?	Yes	No
82. Do you forget things you did while drinking or using drugs?	Yes	No
83. During the past month have you driven a car while you were drunk or high?	Yes	No
84. Are you louder than other kids?	Yes	No
85. Are most of your friends younger than you are?	Yes	No
86. Have you ever intentionally damaged someone else's property?	Yes	No
87. Have you ever stopped working at a job because you just didn't care?	Yes	No
88. Do your parents or guardians like talking with you and being with you?	Yes	No
89. Have you ever spent the night away from home when your parents didn't know where you were?	Yes	No

90.	Have any of your best friends participated in team sports that require regular practices?	Yes	No
91.	Are you suspicious of other people?	Yes	No
92.	Are you already too busy with school and other adult supervised activities to be interested in a job?	Yes	No
93.	Have you cut school at least 5 days in the past year?	Yes	No
94.	Are you usually pleased with how well you do in activities with your friends?	Yes	No
95.	Does alcohol or drug use cause your moods to change quickly, like from happy to sad or vice versa?	Yes	No
96.	Do you feel sad most of the time?	Yes	No
97.	Do you miss school or arrive late for school because of your alcohol or drug use?	Yes	No
98.	Is it important to you now to get or keep a satisfactory job?	Yes	No
99.	Do your family or friends ever tell you that you should cut down on your drinking or drug use?	Yes	No
100.	Do you have serious arguments with friends or family members because or your drinking or drug use?	Yes	No
101.	Do you tease others a lot?	Yes	No
102.	Do you have trouble sleeping?	Yes	No
103.	Do you have trouble with written work?	Yes	No
104.	Does your alcohol or drug use ever make you do something you would not normally do—like breaking rules, missing curfew, breaking the law, or having sex with someone?	Yes	No
105.	Do you feel you lose control and get into fights?	Yes	No
106.	Have you ever been fired from a job?	Yes	No
107.	During the past month, have you skipped school?	Yes	No
108.	Do you have trouble getting along with any of your friends because of your alcohol or drug use?	Yes	No
109.	Do you have a hard time following directions?	Yes	No
110.	Are you good at talking your way out of trouble?	Yes	No
111.	Do you have friends who have hit or threatened to hit someone without any real reason?	Yes	No
112.	Do you ever feel you can't control your alcohol or drug use?	Yes	No
113.	Do you have a good memory?	Yes	No
114.	Do your parents or guardians have a pretty good idea of your interests?	Yes	No
115.	Do your parents or guardians usually agree about how to handle you?	Yes	No
116.	Do you have a hard time planning and organizing?	Yes	No
117.	Do you have trouble with math?	Yes	No

118. Do your friends cut school a lot?	Yes	No
119. Do you worry a lot?	Yes	No
120. Do you find it difficult to complete class projects or work tasks?	Yes	No
121. Does school sometimes make you feel stupid?	Yes	No
122. Are you able to make friends easily in a new group?	Yes	No
123. Do you often feel like you want to cry?	Yes	No
124. Are you afraid to be around people?	Yes	No
125. Do you have friends who have stolen things?	Yes	No
126. Do you want to be a member of any organized group, team, or club?	Yes	No
127. Does one of your parents or guardians have a steady job?	Yes	No
128. Do you think it's a bad idea to trust other people?	Yes	No
129. Do you enjoy doing things with people your own age?	Yes	No
130. Do you feel you study longer than your classmates and still get poorer grades?	Yes	No
131. Have you ever failed a grade in school?	Yes	No
132. Do you go out for fun on school nights without your parents' or guardians' permission?	Yes	No
133. Is school hard for you?	Yes	No
134. Do you have an idea about the type of job or career that you want to have?	Yes	No
135. On a typical day, do you watch more than two hours of TV?	Yes	No
136. Are you restless and can't sit still?	Yes	No
137. Do you have trouble finding the right words to express what you are thinking?	Yes	No
138. Do you scream a lot?	Yes	No
139. Have you ever had sexual intercourse without using a condom?	Yes	No

POSIT: Problem Oriented Screening Instrument for Teenagers. From Rahdert E, ed: *The adolescent assessment/referral system manual.* DHHS pub. no. (ADM) 91-1735. Rockville, MD, 1991, National Institute on Drug Abuse.

Center for Epidemiologic Studies–Depression (CES-D) Scale

Name: _____

Date: _____

As I read the following statements, please tell me how often you felt or behaved this way.

IN THE LAST WEEK. Did you feel this way:

    0 = Rarely or none of the time (i.e., less than 1 day)?
    1 = Some or a little of the time (i.e., 1-2 days)?
    2 = Occasionally or a moderate amount of time (i.e., 3-4 days)?
    3 = Most or all of the time (i.e., 5-7 days)?
    — = No response

	Rarely	Some of of the time	Occasionally	Most of the time	No response
1. I was bothered by things that usually don't bother me	0	1	2	3	—
2. I did not feel like eating; my appetite was poor	0	1	2	3	—
3. I felt that I could not shake off the blues even with help from my family and friends	0	1	2	3	—
*4. I felt that I was just as good as other people	3	2	1	0	—
5. I had trouble keeping my mind on what I was doing	0	1	2	3	—
6. I felt depressed	0	1	2	3	—
7. I felt that everything I did was an effort	0	1	2	3	—
*8. I felt hopeful about the future	3	2	1	0	—
9. I thought my life had been a failure	0	1	2	3	—
10. I felt fearful	0	1	2	3	—
11. My sleep was restless	0	1	2	3	—
*12. I was happy	3	2	1	0	—
13. I talked less than usual	0	1	2	3	—
14. I felt lonely	0	1	2	3	—
15. People were unfriendly	0	1	2	3	—
*16. I enjoyed life	3	2	1	0	—
17. I had crying spells	0	1	2	3	—
18. I felt sad	0	1	2	3	—
19. I felt people disliked me	0	1	2	3	—
20. I could not get going	0	1	2	3	—

*Items are reverse-scored.

From Radloff LS: the CES-D Scale: a self-report depression scale for research in the general population, *Appl Psychol Measure* 2:385-401, 1977.

HAMILTON RATING SCALE FOR DEPRESSION (HRSD)

Name: _____

Date: _____

The total Hamilton Rating Scale for Depression (HRSD) provides an indication of depression and, over time, provides a valuable guide to progress.

Classification of symptoms which may be difficult to obtain can be scored as: 0 - absent; 1 - doubtful or trivial; 2 - present. Classification of symptoms where more detail can be obtained can be expanded to: 0 - absent; 1 - mild; 2 - moderate; 3 - severe; 4 - incapacitating. In general, the higher the total score, the more severe the depression.

HRSD score level of depression: 10-13 mild; 14-17 mild to moderate; >17 moderate to severe.

HRSD Rating Scale Symptoms	Pre-treatment Date: _____	1st follow up Date: _____	2nd follow up Date: _____
1. Depressed mood	0 1 2 3 4	0 1 2 3 4	0 1 2 3 4
2. Guilt feelings	0 1 2 3 4	0 1 2 3 4	0 1 2 3 4
3. Suicide	0 1 2 3 4	0 1 2 3 4	0 1 2 3 4
4. Insomnia - early	0 1 2	0 1 2	0 1 2
5. Insomnia - middle	0 1 2	0 1 2	0 1 2
6. Insomnia - late	0 1 2	0 1 2	0 1 2
7. Work and activities	0 1 2 3 4	0 1 2 3 4	0 1 2 3 4
8. Retardation - psychomotor	0 1 2 3 4	0 1 2 3 4	0 1 2 3 4
9. Agitation	0 1 2 3 4	0 1 2 3 4	0 1 2 3 4
10. Anxiety - psychological	0 1 2 3 4	0 1 2 3 4	0 1 2 3 4
11. Anxiety - somatic	0 1 2 3 4	0 1 2 3 4	0 1 2 3 4
12. Somatic symptoms GI	0 1 2	0 1 2	0 1 2
13. Somatic symptoms - General	0 1 2	0 1 2	0 1 2
14. Sexual dysfunction - menstrual disturbance	0 1 2	0 1 2	0 1 2
15. Hypochondrias	0 1 2 3 4	0 1 2 3 4	0 1 2 3 4
16. Weight loss - by history	0 1 2	0 1 2	0 1 2
- by scales	0 1 2	0 1 2	0 1 2
17. Insight	0 1 2	0 1 2	0 1 2

TOTAL SCORE: _____   _____   _____

Adapted from Hamilton Rating Scale for Depression (HRSD). From Hamilton M: A rating scale for depression, *J Neurol Neurosurg Psychiatry* 25:56-62, 1960.

Montgomery-Åsberg Depression Rating Scale (MADRS)

Name: _____

Date: _____

Responses: from 0 (normal) to 6 (severe depression); statements are provided for 0, 2, 4 and 6; 1, 3 and 5 are scored as in-between values.

(1) APPARENT SADNESS:

despondency, gloom, and despair that is more than just ordinary transient low spirits

Response	Points
no sadness	0
looks dispirited but does brighten up without difficulty	2
appears sad and unhappy most of the time	4
looks miserable all the time; extremely despondent	6

(2) REPORTED SADNESS:

reports of depressed mood regardless of whether it is reflected in appearance. This includes low spirits, despondency, or the feeling of being beyond help and without hope. Rate according to intensity, duration, and the extent to which the mood is reported to be influenced by events.

Response	Points
occasional sadness in keeping with the circumstances	0
sad or low but brightens up without difficulty	2
pervasive feelings of sadness or gloominess. The mood is still influenced by external circumstances.	4
continuous or unvarying sadness, misery, or despondency	6

(3) INNER TENSION:

feelings of ill-defined discomfort, edginess, inner turmoil, or mental tension mounting to panic, dread, or anguish. Rate according to intensity, frequency, duration, and the extent of reassurance called for.

Response	Points
placid with only fleeting inner tension	0
occasional feelings of edginess and ill-defined discomfort	2
continuous feelings of inner tension or intermittent panic that the patient can only master with some difficulty	4
unrelenting dread or anguish; overwhelming panic	6

(4) REDUCED SLEEP:

reduced duration or depth of sleep compared with the subject's own normal pattern when well

Response	Points
sleeps as usual	0
slight difficulty dropping off to sleep; slightly reduced, light, or fitful sleep	2
sleep reduced or broken by at least 2 hours	4
less than 2-3 hours of sleep	6

(5) REDUCED APPETITE:

loss of appetite compared with when well. There may be a loss of desire for food or the need to force oneself to eat.

Response	Points
normal or increased appetite	0
slightly reduced appetite	2
no appetite and food is tasteless	4
needs persuasion to eat at all	6

(6) CONCENTRATION DIFFICULTIES:

difficulties in collecting one's thoughts, mounting to an incapacitating lack of concentration. This is rated according to the intensity, frequency, and degree of incapacity produced.

Response	Points
no difficulties in concentrating	0
occasional difficulties in collecting one's thoughts	2
difficulties in concentrating and sustaining thought, which reduces the ability to read or hold a conversation	4
unable to read or converse without great difficulty	6

(7) LASSITUDE:

difficulty in getting started; slowness in initiating and performing everyday activities

Response	Points
hardly any difficulty in getting started; no sluggishness	0
difficulties in starting activities	2
difficulties in starting simple routine activities, which are carried out with effort	4
complete lassitude; unable to do anything without help	6

(8) INABILITY TO FEEL:

reduced interest in surroundings or in activities that normally give pleasure. The ability to react with adequate emotion to circumstances is reduced.

Response	Points
normal interest in surroundings and other people	0
reduced ability to enjoy usual interests	2
loss of interest in surroundings; loss of feelings for friends and acquaintances	4
emotionally paralyzed; unable to feel anger, grief, or pleasure; complete or even painful failure to feel for close relatives and friends	6

(9) PESSIMISTIC THOUGHTS:

feelings of guilt, inferiority, self-reproach, sinfulness, remorse, or ruin

Response	Points
none	0
fluctuating ideas of failure, self-reproach, or self-depreciation	2
persistent self-accusation or definite but still rational ideas of guilt or sin; increasingly pessimistic about the future	4
delusions of ruin, remorse, or unredeemable sin; self-accusations that are absurd and unshakable	6

(10) SUICIDAL THOUGHTS:

feeling that life is not worth living and/or that a natural death would be welcome; presence of suicidal thoughts and the making of preparations for suicide.

Response	Points
enjoys life or takes it as it comes	0
weary of life; only fleeting suicidal thoughts	2
probably better off dead; suicidal thoughts common and suicide is considered as a possible solution but without specific plans or intentions	4
explicit plans for suicide when there is an opportunity; active preparations for suicide	6

Total Score _____

Interpretation (Snaith et al, 1986): 0 to 6: absence of symptoms, 7-19: mild depression, 20-34: moderate depression, and 35-60: severe depression.

From Montgomery S, Åsberg M: A new depression scale designed to be sensitive to change, *Br J Psychiatry* 134:382-389, 1979.

Primary Care Evaluation of Mental Disorders:
Patient Health Questionnaire 9-Item Depression Module (PRIME-MD PHQ-9)

Name: _____

Date: _____

1. Over the **LAST TWO WEEKS,** how often have you been bothered by any of the following problems?

	Not at all 0	Several days 1	More than half the days 2	Nearly every day 3
a. Little interest or pleasure in doing things				
b. Feeling down, depressed, or hopeless				
c. Trouble falling/staying asleep, sleeping too much				
d. Feeling tired or having little energy				
e. Poor appetite or overeating				
f. Feeling bad about yourself - or that you are a failure or have let yourself or your family down				
g. Trouble concentrating on things, such as reading the newspaper or watching television				
h. Moving or speaking so slowly that other people could have noticed. Or the opposite - being so fidgety or restless that you have been moving around a lot more than usual				
i. Thoughts that you would be better off dead or of hurting yourself in some way				

2. If you checked off **ANY** problem on this questionnaire so far, how difficult have these problems made it for you to do your work, take care of things at home, or get along with other people?

Not difficult at all	Somewhat difficult	Very difficult	Extremely difficult

Total Score: _____

Primary Care Evaluation of Mental Disorders: Patient Health Questionnaire 9-Item Depression Module (PRIME-MD PHQ-9). Developed by Drs. Robert L. Spitzer, Janet B.W. Williams, and Kurt Kroenke with an educational grant from Pfizer, Inc. For research information, contact Dr. Spitzer at rls8@columbia.edu. The names PRIME-MD and PRIME-MD TODAY are trademarks of Pfizer, Inc.

Zung Self-Rating Depression Scale (SDS)

Name: _____

Date: _____

Please read each statement and decide how much of the time the statement describes how you have been feeling during the past several days.

Circle the appropriate number for each statement	None or a little of the time	Some of the time	Good part of the time	Most or all of the time
1. I feel down-hearted, blue, and sad	1	2	3	4
2. Morning is when I feel the best	4	3	2	1
3. I have crying spells or feel like crying	1	2	3	4
4. I have trouble sleeping through the night	1	2	3	4
5. I eat as much as I used to	4	3	2	1
6. I enjoy looking at, talking to, and being with attractive women/men	4	3	2	1
7. I notice that I am losing weight	1	2	3	4
8. I have trouble with constipation	1	2	3	4
9. My heart beats faster than usual	1	2	3	4
10. I get tired for no reason	1	2	3	4
11. My mind is as clear as it used to be	4	3	2	1
12. I find it easy to do the things I used to do	4	3	2	1
13. I am restless and can't keep still	1	2	3	4
14. I feel hopeful about the future	4	3	2	1
15. I am more irritable than usual	1	2	3	4
16. I find it easy to make decisions	4	3	2	1
17. I feel that I am useful and needed	4	3	2	1
18. My life is pretty full	4	3	2	1
19. I feel that others would be better off if I were dead	1	2	3	4
20. I still enjoy the things I used to do	4	3	2	1

Scoring: Add the numbers for a Total Raw Score.

Convert to an Index: Raw Score × 1.25

Index Score Interpretation: <50: normal; 50-59: mild depression; 60-69: moderate to marked depression; >70: severe or extreme depression.

From Zung WK: A self-rating depression scale, *Arch Gen Psychiatry* 12:63, 1965. Copyright 1965 by the American Medical Association. All rights reserved.

Edinburgh Postnatal Depression Scale (EPDS)

Name:_____   Address: _____

Your Date of Birth: _____   _____

Baby's Age: _____   Phone: _____

As you have recently had a baby, we would like to know how you are feeling. Please **check** the answer that comes closest to how you have felt **in the past 7 days,** not just how you feel today.

In the past 7 days:

1. I have been able to laugh and see the funny side of things
   - ☐ As much as I always could
   - ☐ Not quite so much now
   - ☐ Definitely not so much now
   - ☐ Not at all

2. I have looked forward with enjoyment to things
   - ☐ As much as I ever did
   - ☐ Rather less than I used to
   - ☐ Definitely less than I used to
   - ☐ Hardly at all

*3. I have blamed myself unnecessarily when things went wrong
   - ☐ Yes, most of the time
   - ☐ Yes, some of the time
   - ☐ Not very often
   - ☐ No, never

4. I have been anxious or worried for no good reason
   - ☐ No, not at all
   - ☐ Hardly ever
   - ☐ Yes, sometimes
   - ☐ Yes, very often

*5. I have felt scared or panicky for no very good reason
   - ☐ Yes, quite a lot
   - ☐ Yes, sometimes
   - ☐ No, not much
   - ☐ No, not at all

*6. Things have been getting on top of me
   - ☐ Yes, most of the time I haven't been able to cope at all
   - ☐ Yes, sometimes I haven't been coping as well as usual
   - ☐ No, most of the time I have coped quite well
   - ☐ No, I have been coping as well as ever

*7. I have been so unhappy that I have had difficulty sleeping
   - ☐ Yes, most of the time
   - ☐ Yes, sometimes
   - ☐ Not very often
   - ☐ No, not at all

*8. I have felt sad or miserable
   - ☐ Yes, most of the time
   - ☐ Yes, quite often
   - ☐ Not very often
   - ☐ No, not at all

*9. I have been so unhappy that I have been crying
   - ☐ Yes, most of the time
   - ☐ Yes, quite often
   - ☐ Only occasionally
   - ☐ No, never

*10. The thought of harming myself has occurred to me
   - ☐ Yes, quite often
   - ☐ Sometimes
   - ☐ Hardly ever
   - ☐ Never

Scoring: 0, 1, 2, 3, based on severity; * items are reverse-scored.

From Cox JL, Holden JM, Sagovsky R: Detection of postnatal depression: development of the 10-item Edinburgh Postnatal Depression Scale, *Br J Psychiatry* 150:782-786, 1987. Copyright 1987 The Royal College of Psychiatrists.

Geriatric Depression Scale (GDS)

Name: _____

Date: _____

Circle the best answer for how you felt over the past week.

1.	*Are you basically satisfied with your life?	Yes	No
2.	Have you dropped many of your activities and interests?.	Yes	No
3.	Do you feel that your life is empty?.	Yes	No
4.	Do you often get bored?	Yes	No
5.	*Are you hopeful about the future?.	Yes	No
6.	Are you bothered by thoughts you can't get out of your head?.	Yes	No
7.	*Are you in good spirits most of the time?	Yes	No
8.	Are you afraid something bad is going to happen to you?	Yes	No
9.	*Do you feel happy most of the time?.	Yes	No
10.	Do you often feel helpless?.	Yes	No
11.	Do you often get restless and fidgety?	Yes	No
12.	Do you prefer to stay at home, rather than going out and doing new things?.	Yes	No
13.	Do you frequently worry about the future?	Yes	No
14.	Do you feel you have more problems with memory than most?	Yes	No
15.	*Do you think it is wonderful to be alive now?.	Yes	No
16.	Do you often feel downhearted and blue?	Yes	No
17.	Do you feel pretty worthless the way you are now?	Yes	No
18.	Do you worry a lot about the past?.	Yes	No
19.	*Do you find life very exciting?	Yes	No
20.	Is it hard for you to get started on new projects?.	Yes	No
21.	*Do you feel full of energy?.	Yes	No
22.	Do you feel that your situation is hopeless?	Yes	No
23.	Do you think that most people are better off than you are?	Yes	No
24.	Do you frequently get upset over little things?	Yes	No
25.	Do you frequently feel like crying?	Yes	No
26.	Do you have trouble concentrating?	Yes	No
27.	*Do you enjoy getting up in the morning?.	Yes	No
28.	Do you prefer to avoid social gatherings?.	Yes	No
29.	*Is it easy for you to make decisions?.	Yes	No
30.	*Is your mind as clear as it used to be?	Yes	No

Scoring: Assign one point for each 'yes' answer: 2, 3, 4, 6, 8, 10, 11, 12, 13, 14, 16, 17, 18, 20, 22, 23, 24, 25, 26, 28
  *Assign one point for each 'no' answer: 1, 5, 7, 9, 15, 19, 21, 27, 29, 30

Score: _____ Completed by: _____ Date: _____

Normal: 0 to 10; Mildly depressed: 11 to 20; Very depressed: 21 to 30

Adapted from Yesavage JA, Brink TL: Development and a validation of a geriatric depression screening scale: a preliminary report, *J Psychiatr Res* 17(1):37-49, 1983.

Cornell Scale for Depression in Dementia (CSDD)

Name: _____

Date: _____

Scoring (based on symptoms/signs occurring during the week prior to testing):
a = unable to evaluate; 0 = absent; 1 = mild or intermittent; 2 = severe.

Location: ☐ Nursing Home Resident   ☐ Outpatient   ☐ Inpatient

A. MOOD-RELATED SIGNS

1.	ANXIETY	a	0	1	2
	anxious expression, ruminations, worrying				
2.	SADNESS	a	0	1	2
	sad expression, sad voice, tearfulness				
3.	LACK OF REACTIVITY TO PLEASANT EVENTS	a	0	1	2
4.	IRRITABILITY	a	0	1	2
	easily annoyed, short tempered				

B. BEHAVIORAL DISTURBANCES

5.	AGITATION	a	0	1	2
	restlessness, handwringing, hairpulling				
6.	RETARDATION	a	0	1	2
	slow movements, slow speech, slow reactions				
7.	MULTIPLE PHYSICAL COMPLAINTS	a	0	1	2
	(score 0 if gastrointestinal symptoms only)				
8.	LOSS OF INTEREST	a	0	1	2
	less involved in usual activities (score only if change occurred acutely-in less than 1 month)				

C. PHYSICAL SIGNS

9.	APPETITE LOSS	a	0	1	2
	eating less than usual				
10.	WEIGHT LOSS	a	0	1	2
	(score 2 if greater than 5 lb in one month)				
11.	LACK OF ENERGY	a	0	1	2
	fatigues easily, unable to sustain activities (score only if change occurred acutely—in less than 1 month)				

D. CYCLIC FUNCTIONS

12.	DIURNAL VARIATION ON MOOD	a	0	1	2
	symptoms worse in the morning				
13.	DIFFICULTY FALLING ASLEEP	a	0	1	2
	later than usual for this person				
14.	MULTIPLE AWAKENINGS DURING SLEEP	a	0	1	2
15.	EARLY MORNING AWAKENING	a	0	1	2
	earlier than usual for this person				

E. IDEATIONAL DISTURBANCES

16.	SUICIDE	a	0	1	2
	feels life is not worth living, has suicidal wishes, or makes suicidal attempt				
17.	POOR SELF-ESTEEM	a	0	1	2
	self-blame, self-deprecation, feelings of failure				
18.	PESSIMISM	a	0	1	2
	anticipation of the worst				
19.	MOOD-CONGRUENT DELUSIONS	a	0	1	2
	delusions of poverty, illness, or loss				

Score: _____

Total score ≥ 8 suggests significant depressive symptoms.

Reprinted with permission from Alexopoulos GS, Agrams RC, Young RC, et al: Cornell Scale for depression dementia, *Biol Psychiatry* 23(3): 271-284, 1988. Copyright 1988 The Society of Biological Psychiatry.

Hamilton Anxiety Rating Scale (HARS)

Name: _____

Rater: _____

Date: _____

The Hamilton Anxiety Scale (HARS, HAM-A) consists of 14 items, each defined by a series of symptoms. Each item is rated on a 5-point scale: 0-absent; 1-mild; 2-moderate; 3-severe; 4-incapacitating. Higher scores indicate increased anxiety.

SYMPTOMS

1. Anxious Mood   0 1 2 3 4
   - worries
   - anticipates worst

2. Tension   0 1 2 3 4
   - startles
   - cries easily
   - restless
   - trembling

3. Fears   0 1 2 3 4
   - fear of the dark
   - fear of strangers
   - fear of being alone
   - fear of animal

4. Insomnia   0 1 2 3 4
   - difficulty falling asleep or staying asleep
   - difficulty with nightmares

5. Intellectual   0 1 2 3 4
   - poor concentration
   - memory impairment

6. Depressed Mood   0 1 2 3 4
   - decreased interest in activities
   - anhedonia
   - insomnia

7. Somatic complaints–Muscular   0 1 2 3 4
   - muscle aches or pains
   - bruxism

8. Somatic complaints–Sensory   0 1 2 3 4
   - tinnitus
   - blurred vision

9. Cardiovascular Symptoms   0 1 2 3 4
   - tachycardia
   - palpitations
   - chest pain
   - sensation of feeling faint

10. Respiratory Symptoms   0 1 2 3 4
    - chest pressure
    - choking sensation
    - shortness of breath

11. Gastrointestinal Symptoms   0 1 2 3 4
    - dysphagia
    - nausea or vomiting
    - constipation
    - weight loss

12. Genitourinary Symptoms   0 1 2 3 4
    - urinary frequency or urgency
    - dysmenorrhea
    - impotence

13. Autonomic Symptoms   0 1 2 3 4
    - dry mouth
    - flushing
    - pallor
    - sweating

14. Behavior at Interview   0 1 2 3 4
    - fidgets
    - tremor
    - paces

TOTAL SCORE: _____

Adapted from Hamilton M: The assessment of anxiety states by rating, *Brit J Med Psychol* 32:50-55, 1959. Copyright 1959 The British Psychological Society. Reprinted with permission.

Zung Self-Rating Anxiety Scale (SAS)

Name: _____

Date: _____

Listed below are 20 statements. Please read each one carefully and decide how much of the statement describes how you have been feeling **during the past week.** Circle the appropriate number for each statement.

Statement	None or a little of the time	Some of the time	A good part of the time	Most or all of the time
1. I feel more nervous and anxious than usual.	1	2	3	4
2. I feel afraid for no reason at all.	1	2	3	4
3. I get upset easily or feel panicky.	1	2	3	4
4. I feel like I'm falling apart and going to pieces.	1	2	3	4
5. I feel that everything is all right and nothing bad will happen.	4	3	2	1
6. My arms and legs shake and tremble.	1	2	3	4
7. I am bothered by headaches, neck and back pains.	1	2	3	4
8. I feel weak and get tired easily.	1	2	3	4
9. I feel calm and can sit still easily.	4	3	2	1
10. I can feel my heart beating fast.	1	2	3	4
11. I am bothered by dizzy spells.	1	2	3	4
12. I have fainting spells or feel like it.	1	2	3	4
13. I can breathe in and out easily.	4	3	2	1
14. I get feelings of numbness and tingling in my fingers, toes.	1	2	3	4
15. I am bothered by stomach aches or indigestion.	1	2	3	4
16. I have to empty my bladder often.	1	2	3	4
17. My hands are usually warm and dry.	4	3	2	1
18. My face gets hot and blushes.	1	2	3	4
19. I fall asleep easily and get a good night's rest.				
20. I have nightmares.	1	2	3	4

Total (Raw) Score: _____

Scoring: SAS Index = Raw Score × 1.25

From Zung WK: A rating instrument for anxiety disorder, *Psychosomatics* 12:371-379, 1971. Copyright 1971 The American Psychiatric Association. Reprinted with permission.

Yale-Brown Obsessive Compulsive Scale (Y-BOCS)

Name: _____

Date: _____

Note: Scores should reflect the composite effect of all the patient's obsessive compulsive symptoms. Rate the average occurrence of each item during the prior week up to and including the time of interview.

Obsession Rate Scale (circle appropriate score)

Item	Range of Severity				
1. Time Spent on Obsessions	0 hr/day	0-1 hr/day	1-3 hr/day	3-8 hr/day	>8 hr/day
Score:	0	1	2	3	4
2. Interference From Obsessions	None	Mild	Definite but manageable	Substantial impairment	Incapacitating
Score:	0	1	2	3	4
3. Distress From Obsessions	None	Little	Moderate but manageable	Severe	Near constant, disabling
Score:	0	1	2	3	4
4. Resistance to Obsessions	Always resists	Much resistance	Some resistance	Often yields	Completely yields
Score:	0	1	2	3	4
5. Control Over Obsessions	Complete control	Much control	Some control	Little control	No control
Score:	0	1	2	3	4

Obsession subtotal (add items 1-5) _____

Compulsion Rating Scale (circle appropriate score)

Item	Range of Severity				
6. Time Spent on Compulsions	0 hr/day	0-1 hr/day	1-3 hr/day	3-8 hr/day	>8 hr/day
Score:	0	1	2	3	4
7. Interference From Compulsions	None	Mild	Definite but manageable	Substantial impairment	Incapacitating
Score:	0	1	2	3	4
8. Distress From Compulsions	None	Mild	Moderate but manageable	Severe	Near constant, disabling
Score:	0	1	2	3	4
9. Resistance to Compulsions	Always resists	Much resistance	Some resistance	Often yields	Completely yields
Score:	0	1	2	3	4
10. Control Over Compulsions	Complete control	Much control	Some control	Little control	No control
Score:	0	1	2	3	4

Compulsion subtotal (add items 6-10) _____

Y-BOCS total (add items 1-10) _____

Total Y-BOCS score range of severity for patients who have both obsessions and compulsions:

0-7 Subclinical   8-15 Mild   16-23 Moderate   24-31 Severe   32-40 Extreme

COMMENTS: _____

_____

_____

Y-BOCS Symptom Checklist

Date of Visit: _____

Patient Name: _____

Instructions: Generate a *Target Symptoms List* from the Y-BOCS Symptom Checklist by asking the patient about specific obsessions and compulsions. Check all that apply. Distinguish between current and past symptoms. Mark principal symptoms with a "p". These will form the basis of the *Target Symptoms List*. Items marked "*" may or may not be OCD phenomena.

Current	Past	
		AGGRESSIVE OBSESSIONS
___	___	Fear might harm self
___	___	Fear might harm others
___	___	Violent or horrific images
___	___	Fear of blurting out obscenities or insults
___	___	Fear of doing something else embarrassing*
___	___	Fear will act on unwanted impulses (e.g., to stab friend)
___	___	Fear will steal things
___	___	Fear will harm others because not careful enough (e.g., hit/run motor vehicle accident)
___	___	Fear will be responsible for something terrible happening (e.g., fire, burglary)
___	___	Other:
		CONTAMINATION OBSESSIONS
___	___	Concerns or disgust w/ with bodily waste or secretions (e.g., urine, feces, saliva)
___	___	Concern with dirt or germs
___	___	Excessive concern with environmental contaminants (e.g., asbestos, radiation, toxic waste)
___	___	Excessive concern with household items (e.g., cleansers, solvents)
___	___	Excessive concern with animals (e.g., insects)
___	___	Bothered by sticky substances or residues
___	___	Concerned will get ill because of contaminant
___	___	Concerned will get others ill by spreading contaminant (Aggressive)
___	___	No concern with consequences of contamination other than how it might feel
		SEXUAL OBSESSIONS
___	___	Forbidden or perverse sexual thoughts, images, or impulses
___	___	Content involves children or incest
___	___	Content involves homosexuality*
___	___	Sexual behavior towards others (Aggressive)*
___	___	Other:

HOARDING/SAVING OBSESSIONS
(distinguished from hobbies and concern with objects of monetary or senti-mental value)

___	___	
		RELIGIOUS OBSESSIONS (Scrupulosity)
___	___	Concerned with sacrilege and blasphemy
___	___	Excess concern with right/wrong, morality
___	___	Other:

OBSESSION WITH NEED FOR SYMMETRY OR EXACTNESS

___	___	Accompanied by magical thinking (e.g., concerned that another will have accident unless things are in the right place)
___	___	Not accompanied by magical thinking
		MISCELLANEOUS OBSESSIONS
___	___	Need to know or remember
___	___	Fear of saying certain things
___	___	Fear of not saying just the right thing
___	___	Fear of losing things
___	___	Intrusive (nonviolent) images
___	___	Intrusive nonsense sounds, words, or music
___	___	Bothered by certain sounds/noises*
___	___	Lucky/unlucky numbers
___	___	Colors with special significance
___	___	Superstitious fears
___	___	Other:

Current	Past	
		SOMATIC OBSESSIONS
___	___	Concern with illness or disease*
___	___	Excessive concern with body part or aspect of appearance (e.g., dysmorphophobia)*
___	___	Other:
		CLEANING/WASHING COMPULSIONS
___	___	Excessive or ritualized handwashing
___	___	Excessive or ritualized showering, bathing, toothbrushing, grooming, or toilet routine that involves cleaning of household items or other inanimate objects
___	___	Other measures to prevent or remove contact with contaminants
___	___	Other:
		CHECKING COMPULSIONS
___	___	Checking locks, stove, appliances, etc.
___	___	Checking that did not/will not harm others
___	___	Checking that did not/will not harm self
___	___	Checking that nothing terrible did/will happen
___	___	Checking that did not make mistake
___	___	Checking tied to somatic obsessions
___	___	Other:
		REPEATING RITUALS
___	___	Rereading or rewriting
___	___	Need to repeat routine activities (e.g., jog, in/out door, up/down from chair)
___	___	Other:
		COUNTING COMPULSIONS
___	___	
		ORDERING/ARRANGING COMPULSIONS
___	___	
		HOARDING/COLLECTING COMPULSIONS

(distinguish from hobbies and concern with objects of monetary or senti-mental value [e.g., carefully reads junk mail, piles up old newspapers, sorts through garbage, collects useless objects])

___	___	
		MISCELLANEOUS COMPULSIONS
___	___	Mental rituals (other than checking/counting)
___	___	Excessive list making
___	___	Need to tell, ask, or confess
___	___	Need to touch, tap, or rub*
___	___	Rituals involving blinking or staring*
___	___	Measures (not checking) to prevent harm to self, harm to others, terrible consequences
___	___	Ritualized eating behaviors*
___	___	Superstitious behaviors
___	___	Trichotillomania*
___	___	Other self-damaging or self-mutilating behaviors*
___	___	Other:

Adapted from Goodman WK et al: The Yale-Brown Obsessive Compulsive Scale, *Arch Gen Psychiatry* 46:1006-1011, 1989.

Florida Obsessive-Compulsive Inventory (FOCI)

Name: _____

Date: _____

People who have Obsessive Compulsive Disorder (OCD) experience recurrent, unpleasant thoughts (obsessions) and feel driven to perform certain acts over and over again (compulsions). Although sufferers usually recognize that the obsessions and compulsions are senseless or excessive, the symptoms of OCD often prove difficult to control without proper treatment. Obsessions and compulsions are not pleasurable; on the contrary, they are a source of distress. The following questions are designed to help people determine if they have symptoms of OCD and could benefit from professional help.

Part A. Please circle YES or NO based on your experiences in the past month.

Have you been bothered by unpleasant thoughts or images that repeatedly enter your mind, such as:

1. concerns with contamination (dirt, germs, chemicals, radiation) or acquiring a serious illness such as AIDS?	YES	NO
2. overconcern with keeping objects (clothing, groceries, tools) in perfect order or arranged exactly?	YES	NO
3. images of death or other horrible events?	YES	NO
4. personally unacceptable religious or sexual thoughts?	YES	NO

Have you worried a lot about terrible things happening, such as:

5. fire, burglary, or flooding the house?	YES	NO
6. accidentally hitting a pedestrian with your car or letting it roll down the hill?	YES	NO
7. spreading an illness (giving someone AIDS)?	YES	NO
8. losing something valuable?	YES	NO
9. harm coming to a loved one because you weren't careful enough?	YES	NO

Have you worried about acting on an unwanted and senseless urge or impulse, such as:

10. physically harming a loved one, pushing a stranger in front of a bus, steering your car into oncoming traffic; inappropriate sexual contact; or poisoning dinner guests?	YES	NO

Have you felt driven to perform certain acts over and over again, such as:

11. excessive or ritualized washing, cleaning, or grooming?	YES	NO
12. checking light switches, water faucets, the stove, door locks, or emergency brake?	YES	NO
13. counting; arranging; evening-up behaviors (making sure socks are at same height)?	YES	NO
14. collecting useless objects or inspecting the garbage before it is thrown out?	YES	NO
15. repeating certain actions (in/out of chair, going through doorway, re-lighting cigarette) a certain number of times or until it feels *just right*?	YES	NO
16. need to touch objects or people?	YES	NO
17. unnecessary re-reading or re-writing; re-opening envelopes before they are mailed?	YES	NO
18. examining your body for signs of illness?	YES	NO
19. avoiding colors ("red" means blood), numbers ("13" is unlucky), or names (those that start with "D" signify death) that are associated with dreaded events or unpleasant thoughts?	YES	NO
20. needing to "confess" or repeatedly asking for reassurance that you said or did something correctly?	YES	NO

If you answered YES to 2 or more of the above questions, please continue with Part B on the next page.

Part B. The following questions refer to the repeated thoughts, images, urges, or behaviors identified in Part A. Consider your experience during the past 30 days when selecting an answer. Circle the most appropriate number from 0 to 4.

	0	1	2	3	4
On average, how much *time* is occupied by these thoughts or behaviors each day?	None	Mild (less than 1 hour)	Moderate (1 to 3 hours)	Severe (3 to 8 hours)	Extreme (more than 8 hours)
How much *distress* do they cause you?	None	Mild	Moderate	Severe	Extreme (disabling)
How hard is it for you to *control* them?	Complete control	Much control	Moderate control	Little control	No control
How much do they cause you to *avoid* doing anything, going any place, or being with anyone?	No avoidance	Occasional avoidance	Moderate avoidance	Frequent and extensive	Extreme (housebound)
How much do they *interfere* with school, work, or your social or family life?	None	Slight interference	Definitely interferes with functioning	Much interference	Extreme (disabling)

Sum on Part B (Add items 1 to 5): _____

Scoring: If you answered YES to 2 or more of questions in Part A *and* scored 5 or more on Part B, you may wish to contact your physician, a mental health professional, or a patient advocacy group (such as the Obsessive Compulsive Foundation, Inc.) to obtain more information on OCD and its treatment. Remember, a high score on this questionnaire does not necessarily mean you have OCD—only an evaluation by an experienced clinician can make this determination.

Liebowitz Social Anxiety Scale (LSAS)

Name: _____

Date: _____

Fear or Anxiety:
0 = None
1 = Mild
2 = Moderate
3 = Severe

Avoidance:
0 = Never (0%)
1 = Occasionally (1%-33%)
2 = Often (33%-67%)
3 = Usually (67%-100%)

	Fear or Anxiety	Avoidance	
1. Telephoning in public (P)			1.
2. Participating in small groups (P)			2.
3. Eating in public places (P)			3.
4. Drinking with others in public places (P)			4.
5. Talking to people in authority (S)			5.
6. Acting, performing, or giving a talk in front of an audience (P)			6.
7. Going to a party (S)			7.
8. Working while being observed (P)			8.
9. Writing while being observed (P)			9.
10. Calling someone you don't know very well (S)			10.
11. Talking with people you don't know very well (S)			11.
12. Meeting strangers (S)			12.
13. Urinating in a public restroom (P)			13.
14. Entering a room when others are already seated (P)			14.
15. Being the center of attention (S)			15.
16. Speaking up at a meeting (P)			16.
17. Taking a test (P)			17.
18. Expressing a disagreement or disapproval to people you don't know very well (S)			18.
19. Looking people you don't know very well in the eyes (S)			19.
20. Giving a report to a group (P)			20.
21. Trying to pick up someone (P)			21.
22. Returning goods to a store (S)			22.
23. Giving a party (S)			23.
24. Resisting a high-pressure salesperson (S)			24.

Scores: Total (0-144) _____   Subscores (0-72):   Performance Fear _____   Performance Avoidance _____
Social Fear _____   Social Avoidance _____

P: performance anxiety
S: social situations

From Liebowitz MR: Social phobia, *Mod Probl Pharmacopsychiatry* 22:141-173, 1987, with permission S. Karger AG.

Recent Life Changes Questionnaire (RLCQ)

Name: _____

Date: _____

To answer the questions below, mark in one or more of the ovals to the right of each question. If the event in question happened to you within the past two years, indicate when it occurred by marking in the appropriate column: 0-6 months ago, 7-12 months ago, etc. If you experienced an event more than once over the past two years, mark all appropriate ovals. If the event did not occur over the last two years (or never occurred), leave all ovals empty.

Within the time periods listed, have you experienced:

	19-24 mo. ago	13-18 mo. ago	7-12 mo. ago	0-6 mo. ago
Health				
an illness or injury which:				
kept you in bed a week or more, or sent you to the hospital?	y	y	y	y
was less serious than above?	y	y	y	y
major dental work?	y	y	y	y
a major change in eating habits?	y	y	y	y
a major change in sleeping habits?	y	y	y	y
a major change in your usual type and/or amount of recreation?	y	y	y	y
Work				
a change to a new type of work?	y	y	y	y
a change in your work hours or conditions?	y	y	y	y
a change in your responsibilities at work:				
more responsibilities?	y	y	y	y
less responsibilities?	y	y	y	y
promotion?	y	y	y	y
demotion?	y	y	y	y
transfer?	y	y	y	y
troubles at work:				
with your boss?	y	y	y	y
with co-workers?	y	y	y	y
with persons under your supervision?	y	y	y	y
other work troubles?	y	y	y	y
a major business readjustment?	y	y	y	y
a retirement?	y	y	y	y
a loss of job:				
laid off work?	y	y	y	y
fired from work?	y	y	y	y
a correspondence course to help you in your work?	y	y	y	y
Home and Family				
a major change in your living conditions (home improvements or a decline in your home or neighborhood)?	y	y	y	y
a change in residence:				
move within the same town or city?	y	y	y	y
move to a different town, city, or state?	y	y	y	y
a change in family "get togethers"?	y	y	y	y
a major change in the health or behavior of a family member (illness, accidents, drug or disciplinary problems, etc.)?	y	y	y	y
marriage?	y	y	y	y
a pregnancy?	y	y	y	y
a miscarriage or an abortion?	y	y	y	y
a gain of a new family member:				
birth of a child?	y	y	y	y
adoption of a child?	y	y	y	y
a relative moving in with you?	y	y	y	y

	19-24 mo. ago	13-18 mo. ago	7-12 mo. ago	0-6 mo. ago
Home and Family—cont'd				
a spouse beginning or ending work outside the home?	y	y	y	y
a child leaving home:				
to attend college?	y	y	y	y
due to marriage?	y	y	y	y
for other reasons?	y	y	y	y
a change in arguments with your spouse?	y	y	y	y
in-law problems?	y	y	y	y
a change in the marital status of your parents:				
divorce?	y	y	y	y
remarriage?	y	y	y	y
a separation from your spouse:				
due to work?	y	y	y	y
marital problems?	y	y	y	y
a divorce?	y	y	y	y
the birth of a grandchild?	y	y	y	y
the death of a spouse?	y	y	y	y
the death of another family member:				
child?	y	y	y	y
brother or sister?	y	y	y	y
parent?	y	y	y	y
Personal and Social				
a change in personal habits (your dress, friends, life-style, etc.)?	y	y	y	y
beginning or ending school or college?	y	y	y	y
a change of school or college?	y	y	y	y
a change in political beliefs?	y	y	y	y
a change in religious beliefs?	y	y	y	y
a change in social activities (clubs, movies, visiting, etc.)?	y	y	y	y
a vacation?	y	y	y	y
a new, close, personal relationship?	y	y	y	y
an engagement to marry?	y	y	y	y
girlfriend or boyfriend problems?	y	y	y	y
sexual difficulties?	y	y	y	y
a "falling out" of a close personal relationship?	y	y	y	y
an accident?	y	y	y	y
a minor violation of the law (traffic ticket, etc.)?	y	y	y	y
being held in jail (DUI, felony, etc.)?	y	y	y	y
the death of a close friend?	y	y	y	y
a major decision regarding your immediate future?	y	y	y	y
a major personal achievement?	y	y	y	y
Financial				
a major change in finances:				
increased income?	y	y	y	y
decreased income?	y	y	y	y
investment and/or credit difficulties?	y	y	y	y
a loss or damage of personal property?	y	y	y	y
a moderate purchase (such as an automobile)?	y	y	y	y
a major purchase (such as a home)?	y	y	y	y
a foreclosure of a mortgage or loan?	y	y	y	y

From Miller RA, Rahe RH: Life Changes Scaling for the 1990's, *J Psychosomat Res* 43(3):279-292, 1997. Reprinted with permission from Richard H. Rahe, MD, President, Health Assessment Programs Inc., 5209 Boulevard Extension Road, SE, Olympia, WA 98501. http://www.DrRichardRahe.com.

1995 Life Change Units
to be used with the Recent Life Changes Questionnaire

Health	LCU
An injury or illness which:	
kept you in bed a week or more, or in the hospital	74
was less serious than described above	44
Major dental work	26
Major change in eating habits	27
Major change in sleeping habits	26
Major change in usual type and/or amount of recreation	28

Work	
Change to a new type of work	51
Change in work hours and conditions	35
Change in responsibilities at work:	
more responsibilities	29
fewer responsibilities	21
promotion	31
demotion	42
transfer	32
Troubles at work:	
with your boss	29
with co-workers	35
with persons under your supervision	35
other work troubles	28
Major business adjustment	60
Retirement	52
Loss of job:	
laid off from work	68
fired from work	79
Correspondence course	18

Home and Family	
Major change in living conditions	42
Change in residence:	
move within the same town or city	25
move to a different town, city, or state	47
Change in family get-togethers	25
Major change in health or behavior of family member	55
Marriage	50
Pregnancy	67
Miscarriage or abortion	65
Gain of a new family member:	
birth of a child	66
adoption of a child	65
a relative moving in with you	59
Spouse beginning or ending work outside the home	46
Child leaving home:	
to attend college	41
due to marriage	41
for other reasons	45

Home and Family—cont'd	LCU
Change in arguments with spouse	50
In-law problems	38
Change in the marital status of your parents:	
divorce	59
remarriage	50
Separation from spouse:	
due to work	53
due to marital problems	76
Divorce	96
Birth of grandchild	43
Death of spouse	119
Death of other family member:	
child	123
brother or sister	102
parent	100

Personal and Social	
Change in personal habits	26
Beginning or ending school or college	38
Change of school or college	35
Change in political beliefs	24
Change in religious beliefs	29
Change in social activities	27
Vacation	24
New, close, personal relationship	37
Engagement to marry	45
Girlfriend or boyfriend problems	39
Sexual difficulties	44
"Falling out" of a close personal relationship	47
An accident	48
Minor violation of the law	20
Being held in jail	75
Death of a close friend	70
Major decision regarding the immediate future	51
Major personal achievement	36

Financial	
Major change in finances:	
increased income	38
decreased income	60
investment and/or credit difficulties	56
Loss or damage of personal property	43
Moderate purchase	20
Major purchase	37
Foreclosure on a mortgage or loan	58

Evaluation

Over a period of 6 months, the Recent Life Change (LCU) totals are rated as follows for illness risk: 0-125 is low; 126-200 is moderate; 201-300 is elevated; and over 300 is high.

Adapted from Rahe R: Psychosocial stressors and adjustment disorder: Van Gogh's life chart illustrates stress and disease, *J Clin Psychiatry* 51(11, suppl 1):15, 1990. Physicians Postgraduate Press. Reprinted with permission.

Overt Aggression Scale—Modified for Outpatients (OAS-M)

Patient Name: _____

Date: _____

Rater I: _____

Rater II: _____

FREQUENCY (PAST WEEK)

1. **Verbal Assault:**

   Assessment of verbal outbursts or threats made at spouse, boy/girl friend, close friends, strangers.

   0 = No events.

   1 = Snapped or yelled at someone. _____

   2 = Cursed at or personally insulted someone. _____

   3 = Engaged in a verbal argument with someone. _____

   4 = Verbally threatened to hit someone pt knows well. _____

   5 = Verbally threatened to hit a stranger. _____

   TOTAL WEIGHTED SCORE = _____ × 1 = _____

2. **Assault Against Objects:**

   Assessments of intentional physical attacks against one's own property, another's property, or animals.

   0 = No events.

   1 = Slammed door, kicked chair, threw clothes, in anger. _____

   2 = Broke something in anger. _____

   3 = Broke several things in anger. _____

   4 = Set a fire, vandalism, damaged another's property. _____

   5 = Injured or tortured a pet or other living thing. _____

   TOTAL WEIGHTED SCORE = _____ × 2 = _____

3. **Assault Against Others:**

   Assessment of intentional physical attacks against other people.

   0 = No events.

   1 = Makes threatening gestures. _____

   2 = Assault resulting in no physical harm to another. _____

   3 = Assault resulting in some physical harm to another. _____

   4 = Assault resulting in serious physical injury to another. _____

   5 = Assault requiring medical attention. _____

   TOTAL WEIGHTED SCORE = _____ × 3 = _____

4. **Assault Against Self:**

   Assessment of intentional physical attacks against self, whether or not attacks are suicidal in purpose.

   0 = No events.

   1 = Hit, bit, scratched self. _____

   2 = Head banging or hitting fists against wall. _____

   3 = Cut, bruised, burned self but only superficially. _____

   4 = Cut, bruised, burned self deeply or seriously. _____

   5 = Broke teeth, bone, skull. _____

   TOTAL WEIGHTED SCORE = _____ × 3 = _____

FREQUENCY (PAST WEEK)

5. Global Subjective Irritability:

   Intensity and duration of externally
   directed feelings of irritability/anger/
   resentment/annoyance expressed
   overtly or not.

   0 = Not at all: not clinically significant.

   1 = Slight: doubtful clinical significance.   _____
   2 = Mild: more than called for but only occasional
       and never intense.   _____
   3 = Moderate: often aware of feeling angry or
       occasionally very angry.   _____
   4 = Marked: aware of feeling angry most of the
       time or often very angry.   _____
   5 = Extreme: almost constantly aware of
       feeling very angry.   _____

6. Global Overt Irritability:

   Overt irritability or anger NOT
   associated with mania or psychosis.

   0 = Not at all: only subjectively felt.

   1 = Slight: occasional snappiness of doubtful
       clinical significance.   _____
   2 = Mild: argumentative/quick to express
       annoyance.   _____
   3 = Moderate: often shouts/loses temper.   _____
   4 = Severe: throws/breaks things,
       occasionally assaultive.   _____
   5 = Extreme: repeatedly violent against
       things or persons.   _____

7. Suicidal Tendencies:
   Thoughts of death or suicide.

   0 = None at all.

   1 = Slight: occasional thoughts of his or her
       death (w/o suicidal thoughts).   _____
   2 = Mild: frequent thoughts of being better
       off dead/occasional thoughts of
       suicide (w/o plan).   _____
   3 = Moderate: often thinks of suicide or has
       thoughts of specific method.   _____
   4 = Severe: frequent suicidal thoughts, mentally
       rehearsed plan, has made a suicidal gesture.   _____
   5 = Extreme: made preparations for a serious
       suicidal attempt.   _____
   6 = Very extreme: suicidal attempt with definite
       intent to die or potential for death/serious
       medical consequences.   _____

If question 7 = 4, 5, or 6 (i.e. Extreme -Very Extreme), rate questions 7a & 7b below

---

7a. Suicide: Intent of Attempt:

0 = Obviously no intent, purely a manipulative gesture.

Seriousness of suicidal intent to kill self as judged by overall circumstances including likelihood of being rescued, precautions against discovery, action to gain help during or after attempt, degree of planning and the apparent purpose of attempt.

1 = Not sure or only minimal intent.   _____

2 = Definite but very ambivalent.   _____

3 = Serious.   _____

4 = Very Serious.   _____

5 = Extreme (every expectation of death).   _____

7b. Suicide: Medical Lethality:

0 = No danger: No effects, held pills in hand.

Actual medical threat to life or physical condition following the most serious gesture or suicide attempt.

1 = Minimal: scratch on the wrist.   _____

2 = Mild: 10 aspirins, mild gastritis.   _____

3 = Moderate: 10 Seconols, briefly unconscious.   _____

4 = Severe: cut throat.   _____

5 = Extreme: respiratory arrest or prolonged coma.   _____

OAS-M TOTAL SCORES

AGGRESSION (Q. 1-4) = _____

IRRITABILITY (Q. 5-6) = _____

SUICIDALITY (Q. 7-7b) = _____

SCORING OF THE OAS-M

Weight the scores for each "item" within a "question" appropriately and then add the scores for the items together. The sum score for the question should then be multiplied by the total weight for that particular Question: i.e., × 1 for Question 1, × 2 for Question 2, and × 3 for Questions 3 and 4.

Add up the total weighted scores for Questions 1, 2, 3, and 4. This is the "Aggression" score. Enter it on the appropriate line on the last page of the form. Add up the scores for Questions 5 and 6. This is the "Irritability" score. Enter it on the appropriate line on the last page of the form.

Question 7 is the "Suicidality" Question. Be sure and answer questions 7a and 7b only if the subject scored 4 or higher on Question 7. Add up the scores for 7, 7a, and 7b. Enter this score on the appropriate line on the last page of the form. Further information on the OAS-M is available from the authors.

Rating Scale for Aggressive Behavior in the Elderly (RAGE)

Name: _____

Date: _____

Has the patient in the past 3 days . . .

	0	1	2	3
1. Been demanding or argumentative?	0	1	2	3
2. Shouted, yelled, or screamed?	0	1	2	3
3. Sworn or used abusive language?	0	1	2	3
4. Disobeyed ward rules, e.g. deliberately passed urine outside the commode?	0	1	2	3
5. Been uncooperative or resisted help, e.g. whilst being given a bath or medication?	0	1	2	3
6. Been generally in a bad mood, irritable or quick to fly off the handle?	0	1	2	3
7. Been critical, sarcastic or derogatory, e.g. saying someone is stupid or incompetent?	0	1	2	3
8. Been inpatient or got angry if something does not suit him/her?	0	1	2	3
9. Threatened to harm or made statements to scare others?	0	1	2	3
10. Indulged in antisocial acts, e.g. deliberately stealing food or tripping someone?	0	1	2	3
11. Pushed or shoved others?	0	1	2	3
12. Destroyed property or thrown things around angrily, e.g. towels, medicines?	0	1	2	3
13. Been angry with him/herself?	0	1	2	3
14. Attempted to kick anyone?	0	1	2	3
15. Attempted to hit others?	0	1	2	3
16. Attempted to bite, scratch, spit at, or pinch others?	0	1	2	3
17. Used an object (such as a towel or a walking stick) to lash out or hurt someone?	0	1	2	3

In the past 3 days, has the patient inflicted any injury . . .

	0	1	2	3
18. On him/herself?	0	1	2	3
19. On others?	0	1	2	3

19. On others?
   0 no
   1 mild e.g. a scratch
   2 moderate e.g. a bruise
   3 severe e.g. a fracture

20. Has the patient in the past 3 days been required to be placed under sedation or in isolation or in physical restraints, in order to control his/her aggressiveness?
   0 no; 1 yes

21. Taking all factors into consideration, do you consider the patient's behavior in the last 3 days to have been aggressive?
   0 not at all
   1 mildly
   2 moderately
   3 severely

Total score:

Any additional comments:

Rating on frequency basis over last 3 days
0 = Never
1 = At least once in past 3 days
2 = At least once every day in past 3 days
3 = More than once every day in past 3 days

From Patel V, Hope RA: A rating scale for aggressive behaviour in the elderly—the RAGE, *Psychol Med* 22:211-212, 1992. Reprinted with permission of Cambridge University Press.

HITS Safety Questionnaire

Name: _____

Date: _____

Please check the box that best describes your experiences with your partner. Your answers will help us work together to ensure your personal safety.

	Never (1)	Rarely (2)	Sometimes (3)	Fairly Often (4)	Frequently (5)
How often does your partner physically **hurt** you?					
How often does your partner **insult** you or talk down to you?					
How often does your partner **threaten** you with harm?					
How often does your partner **scream** or curse at you?					

Scoring
Sum all responses; a score >10 suggests increased risk.

From Sherin KM, Sinacore JM, Li XQ, et al: HITS: a short domestic violence screening tool for use in a family practice setting, *Fam Med* 30(7):508-512, 1998. Reprinted with permission from the Society of Teachers of Family Medicine, www.stfm.org.

Modified "SAD PERSONS" Scale

Factor	Points assigned
Sex (male)	1
Age (<19 or >45)	1
Depression or hopelessness	2
Previous attempts or psychiatric care	1
Excessive alcohol or drug use	1
Rational thinking loss	2
Separated, divorced, or widowed	1
Organized or serious attempt	2
No social supports	1
Stated future intent	2

Scoring: 0-5 points: questionable outpatient treatment;
6-8 points: emergency psychiatric treatment/evaluation;
9-14 points: psychiatric hospitalization.

From Hockberger RS, Rothstein RJ: Assessment of suicide potential by nonpsychiatrists using the SAD PERSONS score, *J Emer Med* 6(2):99-107, 1988.

4-Item Risk of Suicide Questionnaire (RSQ-4)

1. Are you here because you tried to hurt yourself?   Yes   No

2. In the past week, have you been having thoughts about   Yes   No
   killing yourself?

3. Have you ever tried to hurt yourself in the past *other*   Yes   No
   than this time?

4. Has something stressful happened to you in the   Yes   No
   past few weeks?

From Horowitz LM, Wang PS, Koocher GP, et al: Detecting suicide risk in a pediatric emergency department: development of a brief screening tool, *Pediatrics* 107(5):1133-1137, 2001.

CAGE Questionnaire

		Yes	No
1. Have you ever felt you should	**C**ut down on your drinking?	1	—
2. Have people	**A**nnoyed you by criticizing your drinking?	1	—
3. Have you ever felt bad or	**G**uilty about your drinking?	1	—
4. Have you had an	**E**ye opener first thing in the morning to steady nerves or get rid of a hangover?	1	—

Score: _____

T-ACE Questionnaire

1. How many drinks does it **T**ake to make you feel high?   _____

2. Have people **A**nnoyed you by criticizing your drinking? Yes No

3. Have you ever felt you ought to **C**ut down on your drinking? Yes No

4. Have you ever had an **E**ye-opener drink first thing in the Yes No
morning to steady your nerves or get rid of a hangover?

SCORING: Positive item responses are scored as 2 points for "T"
and 1 each for A, C, or E. Total score >2 is a positive screen.

Score: _____

From Sokol RJ, Martier SS, Ager JW: The T-ACE questions: practical prenatal detection of risk drinking, *Am J Obstet Gynecol* 160:863, 1989.

Michigan Alcoholism Screening Test (MAST)

Name: _____

Date: _____

Score: _____

			Yes	No
*1.	(2)	Do you feel you are a normal drinker? (By normal we mean you drink less than or as much as most other people)	☐	☐
2.	(2)	Have you ever awakened the morning after some drinking the night before and found that you could not remember part of the evening?	☐	☐
3.	(1)	Does your wife, husband, a parent, or other near relative ever worry or complain about your drinking?	☐	☐
*4.	(2)	Can you stop drinking without a struggle after one or two drinks?	☐	☐
5.	(1)	Do you ever feel guilty about your drinking?	☐	☐
*6.	(2)	Do friends or relatives think you are a normal drinker?	☐	☐
*7.	(2)	Are you able to stop drinking when you want to?	☐	☐
8.	(5)	Have you ever attended a meeting of Alcoholics Anonymous (AA)?	☐	☐
9.	(1)	Have you gotten into physical fights when drinking?	☐	☐
10.	(2)	Has your drinking ever created problems between you and your wife, husband, a parent, or other relative?	☐	☐
11.	(2)	Has your wife, husband or other family member ever gone to anyone for help about your drinking?	☐	☐
12.	(2)	Have you ever lost friends because of your drinking?	☐	☐
13.	(2)	Have you ever gotten into trouble at work or school because of drinking?	☐	☐
14.	(2)	Have you ever lost a job because of drinking?	☐	☐
15.	(2)	Have you ever neglected your obligations, your family, or your work for two or more days in a row because you were drinking?	☐	☐
16.	(1)	Do you drink before noon fairly often?	☐	☐
17.	(2)	Have you ever been told you have liver trouble? Cirrhosis?	☐	☐
18.	(2)	After heavy drinking have you ever had Delirium Tremens (DTs) or severe shaking or heard voices or seen things that really weren't there?**	☐	☐
19.	(5)	Have you ever gone to anyone for help about your drinking?	☐	☐
20.	(5)	Have you ever been in a hospital because of drinking?	☐	☐
21.	(2)	Have you ever been a patient in a psychiatric hospital or on a psychiatric ward of a general hospital where drinking was part of the problem that resulted in hospitalization?	☐	☐
22.	(2)	Have you ever been seen at a psychiatric or mental health clinic or gone to any doctor, social worker, or clergyman for help with any emotional problem where drinking was part of the problem?	☐	☐
23.	(2)	***Have you ever been arrested for drunk driving, driving while intoxicated, or driving under the influence of alcoholic beverages? If YES, how many times? _____	☐	☐
24.	(2)	Have you ever been arrested, or taken into custody, even for a few hours, because of other drunk behavior? If YES, how many times? _____	☐	☐

*Negative responses are alcoholic responses.
**5 points for each Delirium Tremens.
***2 points for each arrest.

From Selzer ML: The Michigan Alcoholism Screening Test: the quest for a new diagnostic instrument, *Am J Psychiatry* 127:1653-1658, 1971.

Alcohol Use Disorders Identification Test (AUDIT)

Name: _____

Date: _____

PATIENT: Because alcohol use can affect your health and can interfere with certain medications and treatments, it is important that we ask some questions about your use of alcohol. Your answers will remain confidential so please be honest.

Place an X in one box that best describes your answer to each question.

Questions	0	1	2	3	4	
1. How often do you have a drink containing alcohol?	Never	Monthly or less	2-4 times a month	2-3 times a week	4 or more times a week	
2. How many drinks containing alcohol do you have on a typical day when you are drinking?	1 or 2	3 or 4	5 or 6	7 to 9	10 or more	
3. How often do you have six or more drinks on one occasion?	Never	Less than monthly	Monthly	Weekly	Daily or almost daily	
4. How often during the last year have you found that you were not able to stop drinking once you had started?	Never	Less than monthly	Monthly	Weekly	Daily or almost daily	
5. How often during the last year have you failed to do what was normally expected of you because of drinking?	Never	Less than monthly	Monthly	Weekly	Daily or almost daily	
6. How often during the last year have you needed a first drink in the morning to get yourself going after a heavy drinking session?	Never	Less than monthly	Monthly	Weekly	Daily or almost daily	
7. How often during the last year have you had a feeling of guilt or remorse after drinking?	Never	Less than monthly	Monthly	Weekly	Daily or almost daily	
8. How often during the last year have you been unable to remember what happened the night before because of your drinking?	Never	Less than monthly	Monthly	Weekly	Daily or almost daily	
9. Have you or someone else been injured because of your drinking?	No		Yes, but not in the last year		Yes, during the last year	
10. Has a relative, friend, doctor, or other health care worker been concerned about your drinking or suggested you cut down?	No		Yes, but not in the last year		Yes, during the last year	
					TOTAL	

From Babor TF, de la Fuente JR, Saunders J, et al: AUDIT—the Alcohol Use Identification Test: guidelines for use in primary health care, Geneva, 1992, World Health Organization.

Drug Abuse Screening Test (DAST)

Name: _____

Date: _____

Score: _____

1.	Have you used drugs other than those required for medical reasons?	Yes	No
2.	Have you abused prescription drugs?	Yes	No
3.	Do you abuse more than one drug at a time?	Yes	No
*4.	Can you get through the week without using drugs (other than those required for medical reasons)?	Yes	No
*5.	Are you always able to stop using drugs when you want to?	Yes	No
6.	Do you abuse drugs on a continuous basis?	Yes	No
*7.	Do you try to limit your drug use to certain situations?	Yes	No
8.	Have you had "blackouts" or "flashbacks" as a result of drug use?	Yes	No
9.	Do you ever feel bad about your drug abuse?	Yes	No
10.	Does your spouse (or parents) ever complain about your involvement with drugs?	Yes	No
11.	Do your friends or relatives know or suspect you abuse drugs?	Yes	No
12.	Has drug abuse ever created problems between you and your spouse?	Yes	No
13.	Has any family member ever sought help for problems related to your drug use?	Yes	No
14.	Have you ever lost friends because of your use of drugs?	Yes	No
15.	Have you ever neglected your family or missed work because of your use of drugs?	Yes	No
16.	Have you ever been in trouble at work because of drug abuse?	Yes	No
17.	Have you ever lost a job because of drug abuse?	Yes	No
18.	Have you gotten into fights when under the influence of drugs?	Yes	No
19.	Have you ever been arrested because of unusual behavior while under the influence of drugs?	Yes	No
20.	Have you ever been arrested for driving while under the influence of drugs?	Yes	No
21.	Have you engaged in illegal activities to obtain drugs?	Yes	No
22.	Have you ever been arrested for possession of illegal drugs?	Yes	No
23.	Have you ever experienced withdrawal symptoms as a result of heavy drug intake?	Yes	No
24.	Have you had medical problems as a result of your drug use (e.g., memory loss, hepatitis, convulsions, or bleeding)?	Yes	No
25.	Have you ever gone to anyone for help for a drug problem?	Yes	No
26.	Have you ever been in a hospital for medical problems related to your drug use?	Yes	No
27.	Have you ever been involved in a treatment program specifically related to drug use?	Yes	No
28.	Have you been treated as an outpatient for problems related to drug abuse?	Yes	No

Total Score: _____

('Yes' = 1 point; * reverse-scored)

From Skinner HA: Drug Abuse Screening Test (DAST), 1982. Copyright 1982 Elsevier Science.

CRAFFT

Name: _____

Date: _____

Score: _____

	Yes	**No**
1. Have you ever ridden in a <u>CAR</u> driven by someone (including yourself) who was "high" or had been using alcohol or drugs?	☐	☐
2. Do you ever use alcohol or drugs to <u>RELAX</u>, feel better about yourself, or fit in?	☐	☐
3. Do you ever use alcohol/drugs while you are by yourself, <u>ALONE</u>?	☐	☐
4. Do you ever <u>FORGET</u> things you did while using alcohol or drugs?	☐	☐
5. Do your family or <u>FRIENDS</u> ever tell you that you should cut down on your drinking or drug use?	☐	☐
6. Have you ever gotten into <u>TROUBLE</u> while you were using alcohol or drugs?	☐	☐

Scoring: Two or more positive items indicate the need for further assessment.

From Knight JR, Shrier LA, Bravender TD, et al: A new brief screening for adolescent substance abuse, *Arch Pediatr Adolesc Med* 153:591-596, 1999. Copyright 1999 American Medical Association. All rights reserved.

SCOFF QUESTIONNAIRE

Please check the appropriate box in answering these questions:

	Yes	No
Do you make yourself **S**ick because you feel uncomfortably full?	☐	☐
Do you worry you have lost **C**ontrol over how much you eat?	☐	☐
Have you recently lost more than 14 p**O**unds in a 3 month period?	☐	☐
Do you believe yourself to be **F**at when others say you are too thin?	☐	☐
Would you say that **F**ood dominates your life?	☐	☐

Scoring: One point for every "yes" answer; ≥2 indicates a positive screen.

From Morgan JF, Reid F, Lacey H: The SCOFF questionnaire: Assessment of a new screening tool for eating disorders, *BMJ* 319:1467-1468, 1999. Reprinted with permission.

ESP Questionnaire

Please check the appropriate box in answering these questions:

	Yes	No
Are you satisfied with your eating patterns?*	☐	☐
Do you ever eat in secret?	☐	☐
Does your weight affect the way you feel about yourself?	☐	☐
Do you currently suffer with or have you ever suffered in the past with an eating disorder?	☐	☐

Scoring: One point for every "yes" answer, * the first item is reverse-scored; ≥2 indicates a positive screen.

From Cotton M, Ball C, Robinson P: Four simple questions can help screen for eating disorders, *J Gen Intern Med* 18:53-56, 2003.

Eating Attitudes Test (EAT-26)

Name: _____

Date: _____

Height _____
Current Weight _____
Highest Weight (excluding pregnancy) _____
Lowest Adult Weight _____
Do you participate in athletics at any of the following level:
- ☐ Intramural
- ☐ Inter-Collegiate
- ☐ Recreational
- ☐ High School teams

	Always	Usually	Often	Sometimes	Rarely	Never	Score
1. Am terrified about being overweight	☐	☐	☐	☐	☐	☐	_____
2. Avoid eating when I am hungry	☐	☐	☐	☐	☐	☐	_____
3. Find myself preoccupied with food	☐	☐	☐	☐	☐	☐	_____
4. Have gone on eating binges where I feel that I may not be able to stop	☐	☐	☐	☐	☐	☐	_____
5. Cut my food into small pieces	☐	☐	☐	☐	☐	☐	_____
6. Aware of the calorie content of foods that I eat	☐	☐	☐	☐	☐	☐	_____
7. Particularly avoid foods with a high carbohydrate content (e.g., bread, rice, potatoes, etc.)	☐	☐	☐	☐	☐	☐	_____
8. Feel that others would prefer if I ate more	☐	☐	☐	☐	☐	☐	_____
9. Vomit after I have eaten	☐	☐	☐	☐	☐	☐	_____
10. Feel extremely guilty after eating	☐	☐	☐	☐	☐	☐	_____
11. Am preoccupied with a desire to be thinner	☐	☐	☐	☐	☐	☐	_____
12. Think about burning up calories when I exercise	☐	☐	☐	☐	☐	☐	_____
13. Other people think that I am too thin	☐	☐	☐	☐	☐	☐	_____
14. Am preoccupied with the thought of having fat on my body	☐	☐	☐	☐	☐	☐	_____
15. Take longer than others to eat my meals	☐	☐	☐	☐	☐	☐	_____
16. Avoid foods with sugar in them	☐	☐	☐	☐	☐	☐	_____
17. Eat diet foods	☐	☐	☐	☐	☐	☐	_____
18. Feel that food controls my life	☐	☐	☐	☐	☐	☐	_____
19. Display self-control around food	☐	☐	☐	☐	☐	☐	_____
20. Feel that others pressure me to eat	☐	☐	☐	☐	☐	☐	_____
21. Give too much time and thought to food	☐	☐	☐	☐	☐	☐	_____
22. Feel uncomfortable after eating sweets	☐	☐	☐	☐	☐	☐	_____
23. Engage in dieting behavior	☐	☐	☐	☐	☐	☐	_____
24. Like my stomach to be empty	☐	☐	☐	☐	☐	☐	_____
25. Enjoy trying new rich foods	☐	☐	☐	☐	☐	☐	_____
26. Have the impulse to vomit after meals	☐	☐	☐	☐	☐	☐	_____

TOTAL SCORE _____

Eating Attitudes Test (EAT-26) - 2

Please respond to each of the following questions:

1. Have you gone on eating binges where you feel that you may not be able to stop? (Eating much more than most people would eat under the same circumstances)

   No ☐   Yes ☐   How many times in the last 6 months? _____

2. Have you ever made yourself sick (vomited) to control your weight or shape?

   No ☐   Yes ☐   How many times in the last 6 months? _____

3. Have you ever used laxatives, diet pills or diuretics (water pills) to control your weight or shape?

   No ☐   Yes ☐   How many times in the last 6 months? _____

4. Have you ever been treated for an eating disorder?

   No ☐   Yes ☐   When? _____

5. Have you recently thought of or attempted suicide?

   No ☐   Yes ☐   When? _____

SCORING THE EATING ATTITUDES TEST

For all items **except #25,** each of the responses receives the following value:

          Always = 3
          Usually = 2
          Often = 1
          Sometimes = 0
          Rarely = 0
          Never = 0

For **item #25,** the responses receive these values:

          Always = 0
          Usually = 0
          Often = 0
          Sometimes = 1
          Rarely = 2
          Never = 3

→ After scoring each item, add the scores for a total. If your score is over **20,** we recommend that you discuss your responses with a counselor (take your responses to the EAT with you to your first appointment).

→ If you responded yes to any of the five YES/NO items on the bottom of the EAT, we also suggest that you discuss your responses with a counselor.

From Garner DM, Olmsted MP, Bohr Y, et al: The eating attitudes test: psychometric features and clinical correlates, *Psychol Med* 12(4):871-878, 1982. Reprinted with permission Cambridge University Press.

CHAPTER 10

Geriatric Assessment Tools

Chapter Contents

ICON KEY: 📄 Tool Printed   ⊘ Tool on CD-ROM   ∞ Customizable Tool   **i** Information and Resources Provided for Further Acquisition

Chapter Contents—cont'd

ICON KEY: 📄 Tool Printed   ✐ Tool on CD-ROM   ∞ Customizable Tool   **i** Information and Resources Provided for Further Acquisition

Introduction and Contents

Geriatric assessment is multidimensional, involving physical health, mental health, functioning, and evaluation of social circumstances. Numerous instruments have been developed to assist the clinician in assessing these domains. Instruments in this chapter focus on assessment of functioning, extent of risks, and cognitive impairment. Other measures pertinent for the older adult may be found in Chapter 9 (depression, anxiety, substance abuse), Chapter 11 (health status, more functional indices), Chapter 12 (pain assessment), Chapter 13 (wound evaluation), Chapter 14 (nutrition), Chapter 15 (system specific measures), and Chapter 16 (social and spiritual instruments).

It is important to appreciate the complexity of geriatric assessment as one begins to use validated measures in daily practice. These tools can be incorporated into routine office evaluation of older patients, and efficient protocols can be created for administration during waiting periods or before office appointments. Ancillary staff may be trained in administering many of these instruments. However, once the tools have been incorporated, it is essential to not lose sight of the potential complications of assessment and misdiagnosis in the elderly. In the fast-paced environment of primary care practice, these tools must be viewed only as support for clinical diagnosis; other factors that may influence test outcomes should be kept in mind. Decreased visual acuity, hearing deficits, baseline educational level, and social situations must be taken into consideration when the results of these tests are interpreted. A test score should never replace sound clinical judgment.

Finally, it is impossible to include or review all of the tools available in this area. Tools were selected for inclusion, as throughout this text, for demonstrated reliability and validity, popularity, and/or availability. Many other measures exist, and the reader is invited to explore the online and print resources cited in the list at the end of the chapter.

FUNCTIONAL ABILITY MEASURES

The functional health measures included here include the long-standing Instrumental Activities of Daily Living (IADL) Scale (Lawton & Brody, 1969), the Brief IADL Measure developed from the Older Americans Resources and Services (OARS) program at Duke University (Fillenbaum, 1985), and the more recent Structured Assessment of Independent Living Skills (SAILS) (Mahurin et al, 1991). The Hearing Handicap Inventory for the Elderly–Screening Version (HHIE-S) (Ventry & Weinstein, 1983) is included here, for lack of a better place, because hearing disability affects function. Additional measures, such as the Katz Index of Activities of Daily Living and the Barthel Index, may be found in Chapter 11. Impairments identified by these scales should alert the clinician to develop a plan to support the continuation of independent living.

Functional ability scales may be limited by their reliance on subjective self-reporting. More objective measures assess specific functions by focused demonstration and evaluation of a physical or cognitive activity. These measures are included in the next two sections of this chapter.

Instrumental Activities of Daily Living Scale (IADL)

Authors: Lawton MP, Brody EM, 1969.
Source: This tool is reprinted here and is also available online at http://www.upstate.edu/geriatric_education/library/lawton.pdf.
Targeted Population: Older adults.
Description: The Instrumental Activities of Daily Living (IADL) Scale is frequently used to evaluate functional ability of the older adult. Eight categories of activities are used to determine the patient's level of functioning in the community: ability to use the telephone, shopping, food preparation, housekeeping, laundry, mode of transportation, responsibility for own medications, and ability to handle finances. Three to five items are presented for each category; the evaluator chooses the category item that best indicates the level of functioning for the patient.
Scores: Each category item is assigned a score value of 0 or 1. The highest possible score for each category is 1, and the lowest possible score is 0. Category scores are summed for an overall score as follows:

7-8 = high level independence
5-6 = moderate level independence

3-4 = moderate level dependence

1-2 = dependence

Although the overall score gives a general assessment of the level of independence, category scores provide more specific identification of strengths and limitations to guide therapeutic interventions.

Administration Time: 5 minutes by proxy administration.

References

Lawton MP, Brody EM: Assessment of older people: self-maintaining and instrumental activities of daily living. *Gerontologist* 9:179-186, 1969.

Stanhope M, Knollmueller RN: *Handbook of community-based and home health nursing practice.* St. Louis, 2000, Mosby, pp. 146-148.

Structured Assessment of Independent Living Skills (SAILS)

Authors: Mahurin RK et al, 1991.

Targeted Population: Older adults with dementia.

Description: This tool offers a thorough assessment of independent living skills through observation of skill activity. SAILS assesses 10 areas (subscales) of everyday functioning: fine motor skills, gross motor skills, dressing, eating, expressive language, receptive language, time and orientation, money-related skills, instrumental activities, and social interaction. Each subscale contains five items, which are rated for ability on a 4-point scale.

Scores: Each of the five items within each subscale is graded from 0 to 3, with higher numbers indicating increased functional ability. The SAILS scores are divided into a motor score (fine motor skills, gross motor skills, dressing, eating) and a cognitive score (expressive language, receptive language, time and orientation, money-related skills). Instrumental activities and social interaction are rated separately. Motor and cognitive scores range from 0 to 60; instrumental activities and social interaction scores range from 0 to 15. The grand total score ranges from 0 to 150. Higher scores indicate more independent functional abilities.

Accuracy: The authors reported preliminary reliability and validity data for 18 patients with Alzheimer's disease and 18 control subjects. Test-retest reliability and interrater reliability were good. High correlations were noted between SAILS scores and visuospatial abilities, attention, and visual memory. Verbal memory, degree of depression, and praxis were not significantly correlated with SAILS scores.

Administration Time: Approximately 60 minutes by proxy administration and observation.

Reference

Mahurin RK, DeBettignies BH, Pirozzolo FJ: Structured assessment of independent living skills: preliminary report of a performance measure of functional abilities in dementia. *J Gerontol* 46:58-66, 1991.

Five-Item Instrumental Activities of Daily Living Screening (Brief IADL)

Author: Fillenbaum, GG, 1985.

Targeted Population: Older adults.

Description: The Five-Item Instrumental Activities of Daily Living Screening (Brief IADL) was developed from the OARS Multidimensional Functional Assessment Questionnaire. Five instrumental activities of daily living items were identified by factor analyses that most accurately identify adults who need help in performing essential independent living activities. The five items assess the ability to travel, shop, prepare meals, perform housework, and manage finances.

Scores: Each of the five items is scored as 1 (able to complete item without help), 0 (requires some help with item), or not answered. The total score ranges from 0 to 5, with a higher score indicating more independent functioning. Answers to the individual items provide rapid assessment of functional needs and enable targeted interventions for maintenance of functional independence.

Accuracy: The author noted both discriminant and predictive validity in the original development of this scale. All items substantially correlated with the concurrent mental and physical health functioning and the number of in-home services received. Because the items in this measure are statistically derived from the reliable and valid OARS Multidimensional Functional Assessment Questionnaire, this tool may be used as a rapid and meaningful screen for quick identification of those elderly who need help and/or fuller assessment.

Administration Time: 1-5 minutes by interview.

References

Fillenbaum GG: Screening the elderly: a brief instrumental activities of daily living measure. *J Am Geriatr Soc* 33:698-706, 1985.

Fillenbaum GG, Smyer MA: The development, validity and reliability of the OARS multidimensional functional assessment questionnaire: disability and pain scales. *J Gerontol* 36:428-433, 1981.

Hearing Handicap Inventory for the Elderly–Screening Version (HHIE-S)

Authors: Ventry IM, Weinstein BE, 1983.

Targeted Population: Older adults.

Description: Hearing impairment is defined as physical hearing loss that can be measured by audiometry (Ventry & Weinstein, 1983). Hearing handicap is a complex concept based on the perceived disadvantages caused by the hearing loss; hearing handicap cannot be measured by audiometry. The HHIE-S is a self-administered, 10-item questionnaire that quantifies the perceived emotional and social effects associated with impaired hearing. The 10 questions include five social/situational items and five emotional response items that assess the impact of hearing loss on respondents' lives. The patient selects an answer to each item: yes (4 points), sometimes (2 points), or no (0 points). The HHIE-S may be used to quickly identify older adults with a hearing handicap for further evaluation. The authors recommend that the HHIE-S be used in combination with a pure-tone audiometry screen for comprehensive assessment of hearing handicap and hearing impairment.

Scores: Total scores on the HHIE-S range from 0 to 40 and are interpreted as follows:

0-8 = no self-perceived handicap
10-22 = mild to moderate handicap
24-40 = significant handicap

Patients with scores >10 may be referred to an audiologist for further evaluation. Scores ≥18 suggest the need for amplification.

When pure-tone audiometry is also used for screening, patients should be referred to an audiologist if they are unable to hear a 40-dB tone in either ear at a frequency of either 1000 or 2000 Hz (Weinstein, 1994).

Accuracy: Items in the HHIE-S were selected from the 25-item clinical version (HHIE) (Ventry & Weinstein, 1982). Items were selected to ensure comparable reliability to the long form. Overall accuracy of the HHIE-S is 75%, with excellent specificity. In combination with pure-tone audiometry, the overall accuracy increases to 83% (Lichtenstein et al, 1988).

Administration Time: <2 minutes by self-administration.

References

Lichtenstein MJ, Bess FH, Logan SA: Validation of screening tools for identifying hearing-impaired elderly in primary care. *JAMA* 259:2875-2878, 1988.

Ventry I, Weinstein B: The Hearing Handicap Inventory for the Elderly. *Ear Hearing* 3:128-135, 1982.

Ventry IM, Weinstein BE: Identification of elderly people with hearing problems. *Am Speech-Language-Hearing Assoc* 25:37-42, 1983.

Weinstein BE: Evaluation and management of the hearing-impaired elderly. *Geriatrics* 45:75, 79-80, 83, 1990.

Weinstein BE: Age-related hearing loss: how to screen for it, and when to intervene. *Geriatrics* 49:40-45, 1994.

Other Measures:

Older Americans Resources and Services (OARS) Multidimensional Functional Assessment Questionnaire   i

Authors: OARS Program, 1975; revised 1988.

Source: OARS Program, Duke Center for the Study of Aging and Human Development, Duke University, Durham, North Carolina, http://www.geri.duke.edu/service/oars.htm. This online site provides information about the OARS Multidimensional Functional Assessment Questionnaire, training in the use of the questionnaire, and ordering information.

Targeted Population: Older adults.

Description: The Duke OARS Program, developed at the Duke Center for the Study of Aging and Human Development, was designed to determine the impact of services and alternative service programs on the functional status of older persons. One resulting instrument is the OARS Multidimensional Functional Assessment Questionnaire (OMFAQ). The first part of the OMFAQ measures five dimensions of functioning: social resources, economic resources, mental health, physical health, and ability to carry out activities of daily living. For each dimension the information obtained is summarized on a 6-point scale on which the values range from 1 (level of functioning excellent) to 6 (level of functioning totally impaired). The second part of the OMFAQ is a services assessment with inquiries about the extent of past and current use, type of provider, and perceived need for each of 24 generic services.

Scores: Several methods of scoring exist for the OMFAQ. Summary of the ratings for each of the five dimensions provides a total overall impairment score. Individual areas may also be scored to determine level of impairment within specific dimensions.

Accuracy: Extensive testing has been reported for the OMFAQ with demonstrated good reliability and validity (Fillenbaum & Smyer, 1981). This instrument is recommended by researchers as a superior measure for comprehensive assessment of personal functioning and service use (Bowling, 1997; McDowell & Newell, 1996).

Administration Time: 45 minutes by interview; training in administration is recommended to ensure uniformity of use.

References

Bowling A: *Measuring health: a review of quality of life measurement scales.* Philadelphia, 1997: Open University Press, pp 18-20.

Fillenbaum GG: *Multidimensional functional assessment: the OARS methodology—a manual,* ed 2. Durham, NC, 1978: Center for the Study of Aging and Human Development, Duke University.

Fillenbaum GG, Smyer MA: The development, validity and reliability of the OARS multidimensional functional assessment questionnaire: disability and pain scales. *J Gerontol* 36:428-433, 1981.

McDowell I, Newell C: *Measuring health: a guide to rating scales and questionnaires,* ed 2, 1996: Oxford University Press, pp. 464-472.

RISK ASSESSMENTS

Older adults are subject to many risks as a result of physical decline and inability to assert complete control over their environment. An increased risk for falling is common in the elderly; falls may lead to significant injuries and further decline. Elderly patients should be routinely screened for a history of falls and observed for any difficulties with balance or gait. Three measures to screen for impairment in gait and balance are included here, as well as two brief falls risk checklists.

Home and environmental surroundings present risks for falls and other accidents for the elderly when safety issues are not addressed. Two checklists for home and environmental assessment are reproduced here for completion during a home visit. A driving skills quiz is included for self-report evaluation of driving safety. Lastly, caring for the cognitively impaired elder produces stress for the caregiver, which may lead to various forms of elder abuse. The clinician needs to be aware of the older adult's living situation and assess for abuse potential routinely. Two brief questionnaires that assist the clinician in assessment for possible abuse are included.

Tinetti Balance and Gait Evaluation/Performance-Oriented Assessment of Mobility

Author: Tinetti ME, 1986.
Targeted Population: Older adults.
Description: The Tinetti Balance and Gait Evaluation, also known as *the Performance-Oriented Mobility Assessment*, is a widely used clinical measure of characteristics associated with falls. A 24-item (40-point) long version and a 16-item (28-point) short version exist; the short version is commonly used and is reprinted here. The short version assesses balance with nine items and gait with seven items. Each item contains performance indicators that are assigned point values of 0 to 2.
Scores: Item scores are summed for a balance scale score, a gait scale score, and a total score. A total score of <19 (of 28 points) indicates high risk for falling.
Accuracy: The Tinetti Balance and Gait Evaluation has shown good interrater reliability and concurrent validity (Tinetti, 1986) and predicts recurrent falls (Tinetti et al, 1986; Robbins et al, 1989). Raîch et al (2000) assessed the predictive validity of the long version to prospectively identify those at risk. A score of 36 or less (of 40 points) identified 7 of 10 of persons who experienced falls with 70% sensitivity and 52% specificity. The authors concluded that despite a rapid drop in sensitivity, the screening characteristics demonstrated by the Tinetti Balance and Gait Evaluation support its inclusion in periodic health examinations of older community dwellers.
Administration Time: 10-20 minutes by direct observation.

References

Raîch M, Hébert R, Prince F, et al: Screening older adults at risk of falling with the Tinetti balance scale. *Lancet* 356:1001-1002, 2000.

Robbins AS, Rubenstein LZ, Josephson KR, et al. Predictors of falls among elderly people. *Arch Intern Med* 149:1628-1633, 1989.

Tinetti ME: Performance-oriented assessment of mobility problems in elderly patients. *J Am Geriatr Soc* 34:119-126, 1986.

Tinetti ME, Williams TF, Mayewski R: Fall risk index for elderly patients based on number of chronic disabilities. *Am J Med* 80:429-434, 1986.

Get Up and Go Test

Authors: Mathias S et al, 1986.
Source: Mathias S, Nayak U, Isaacs B. Balance in elderly patients: the "Get Up and Go" test. *Arch Phys Med Rehabil* 67:387, 1986.
Targeted Population: Older adults.
Description: This test assesses balance in older adults. In this test, the patient is seated in a straight-backed, high-seat chair, placed 3 meters (10 feet) from a wall. The patient rises, stands still momentarily, walks toward the wall (using any customary walking aid), turns without touching the wall, returns to the chair, turns, and sits down. This activity is not timed. The clinician observes the patient and makes note of any balance or gait problems when the patient is seated, transferring, or ambulating. Abnormalities of gait and balance may include unsafe or incomplete transfers, poor sitting balance, difficulty rising or sitting down, staggering on turns, unnecessary slowness, hesitancy, excessive truncal sway, grabbing for support, and stumbling.
Scores: Performance on the Get Up and Go test is scored on the following scale: 1 = normal, 2 = very slightly abnormal, 3 = mildly abnormal, 4 = moderately abnormal, 5 = severely abnormal. "Normal" (1) means that the patient gave no evidence of being at risk of falling during the test or at any other time. "Severely abnormal" (5) means that the patient appeared at risk for a fall at any time during the test. Intermediate grades are selected subjectively by the clinician, based on the presence of undue slowness, hesitancy, abnormal movements of the trunk or upper limbs, staggering, or stumbling, which might place the patient at risk for falls in other situations. A score of 3 or greater indicates increased risk for falls.
Accuracy: The authors report agreement among observers from different medical backgrounds on the subjective scoring of the test. They also note good correlation with laboratory measures of gait.
Administration Time: <2 minutes by observation.

References

Fuller GF: Falls in the elderly. *Am Fam Physician* 61:2159-2168, 2173-2174, 2000.

Mathias S, Nayak USL, Isaacs B: Balance in elderly patients: the "Get Up and Go" test. *Arch Phys Med Rehabil* 67:387-389, 1986.

Timed Up and Go Test

Authors: Podsiadlo D, Richardson S, 1991.
Source: Podsiadlo D, Richardson S. The timed "Up and Go": a test of basic functional mobility for frail, elderly persons. *J Am Geriatric Soc* 39:142, 1991. Reprinted with permission Blackwell Publishing Ltd.
Targeted Population: Older adults.
Description: The timed Up and Go test is a modified, timed version of the *Get Up and Go* test (Mathias et al, 1986), which evaluates gait and balance. The patient is observed and timed while rising from an armchair, walking 3 meters, turning, walking back, and sitting down again. No physical assistance is given. The patient wears regular footwear and uses any customary walking aid. A stopwatch or wristwatch with a second hand is used to time this activity. The patient is allowed one practice trial and then three actual trials. The times from the three actual trials are averaged. This test is quick, requires no special equipment or training, and is easily included as part of the routine medical examination.
Scores: A score of <10 seconds = freely mobile, <20 seconds = mostly independent, 20 to 29 seconds = variable mobility, >30 seconds = impaired mobility. A score of 30 seconds or greater indicates that the patient has impaired mobility, requires assistance, and is at a high risk for falls.
Accuracy: The authors reported that the time score was reliable (interrater and intra-rater); correlated well with log-transformed scores on the Berg Balance Scale, gait speed, and Barthel Index of ADL; and appeared to predict the patient's ability to go outside alone safely.

The authors suggest that the timed Up and Go test is a reliable and valid test for quantifying functional mobility, which may also be useful in monitoring clinical change over time.

Administration Time: <2 minutes.

References

Fuller GF: Falls in the elderly. *Am Fam Physician* 61:2159-2168, 2173-2174, 2000.

Podsiadlo D, Richardson S: The timed "Up & Go": a test of basic functional mobility for frail elderly persons. *J Am Geriatr Soc* 39:142-148, 1991.

Risk Assessment Tool (RAT) for Falls Reassessment is Safe "Kare" (RISK) Tool

Authors: Brians LK, et al, 1991.

Targeted Population: Hospitalized adults, particularly the elderly.

Description: The Risk Assessment Tool (RAT) for Falls contains 26 items chosen for inclusion on the basis of analysis of causative factors of reported hospital falls and literature review of risks for falls. The evaluator checks the items that apply to the patient. The Reassessment is Safe "Kare" (RISK) Tool contains four items from the RAT that were found to be statistically associated with falls.

Scores: RAT: If four or more of the items are checked, the patient is considered to be at risk for falls. Additionally, if there is a history of falls before admission or history of confusion/disorientation, the patient is automatically considered at risk for falls.

RISK: A check for any of the four items identifies the patient at risk for falls. Additionally, if the patient at risk uses a wheelchair, he or she is considered to be at greater risk for falls.

Accuracy: The authors developed a study in which completed RATs were compared with incidence of falls. Only 4 of the 26 variables were statistically related to the falls. Based on this study, the RAT was shortened to four items and called *the RISK (Reassessment Is Safe "Kare") tool.*

Administration Time: RAT: <5 minutes; RISK: <1 minute.

Reference

Brians LK, Alexander K, Grota P, et al: The development of the RISK tool for fall prevention. *Rehabil Nurs* 16:67-69, 1991.

Guidelines for Home Safety Assessment

Authors: Stanhope M, Knollmueller RN, 2000.

Targeted Population: Older adults.

Description: Modified from guidelines for home safety assessment (Boling, 1998), this checklist assesses the home environment for physical and structural hazards, nutrition safety, fire prevention measures, crime protection, self-injury prevention measures, appropriate medication management, and wandering control (Stanhope & Knollmueller, 2000). Presence of any item is noted, and space is provided to record plan for improvement.

Administration Time: Varies; the assessment is completed during a patient home visit.

References

Boling PA: Safety in the home. In Yoshikawa TT, Cobbs EL, Brummel-Smith K, eds. *Practical ambulatory geriatrics* (p. 127). St. Louis, 1998: Mosby.

Stanhope M, Knollmueller RN. *Handbook of community-based and home health nursing practice.* St. Louis, 2000: Mosby, p. 14.

Environmental Assessment for the Elderly

Authors: Kane R et al, 1994.

Targeted Population: Older adults.

Description: This checklist from Kane et al (1994) assesses the home environment with a series of nine questions. Areas addressed include the following: rooms available to client, stairs, neighborhood safety, cleanliness, home insulation and ventilation, signs of neglect, and food supply. Also included are an extensive safety checklist and an extensive fall hazard checklist (Stanhope & Knollmueller, 2000).

Administration Time: Varies; the assessment is completed during a patient home visit.

References

Kane R, Ouslander J, Abrass I: *Essentials of clinical geriatrics*, ed 3. New York, 1994: McGraw-Hill.

Stanhope M, Knollmueller RN: *Handbook of community-based and home health nursing practice.* St. Louis, 2000: Mosby, p. 11-17.

Driving Skills Quiz

Source: Mayo Foundation for Medical Education and Research.

Targeted Population: Older adults.

Description: This questionnaire consists of 11 self-evaluation questions related to driving skills.

Scores: An answer of "yes" to one or more questions indicates that driving may need to be limited or a specific problem may need to be addressed. Answers of "yes" to most of the questions indicate the need to discontinue driving privileges.

Administration Time: 2-5 minutes by self-administration.

Reference

Mayo Foundation for Medical Education and Research: Driving: how safe are you behind the wheel? *Mayo Clinic Health Letter* 14:7, 1996.

Brief Abuse Screen for the Elderly (BASE)

Authors: Reis M et al, 1993.

Targeted Population: Primary care providers for older adults.

Description: This five-item questionnaire assists the clinician in assessing the likelihood of abuse. Questions are directed to the clinician, a family member, an intervener, or home care team member. Questions pertain to the possibility of abuse by a caregiver, a care receiver, or other person.

Scores: Questions regarding possible abuse are answered on a 5-point Likert-type scale ranging from 1 (no, not at all) to 5 (yes, definitely). If abuse is suspected, the estimated intervention time is also indicated on a scale ranging from 1 (immediately) to 5 (2 or more weeks). No other formal scoring is required.

Accuracy: Face validity was good with 86% to 90% agreement by three differently trained providers.

Administration Time: <1 minute.

References

Reis M, Nahmiash D: *When seniors are abused: a guide to intervention.* North York, Ontario, Canada, 1995, Captus Press.

Reis M, Nahmiash D, Schrier R: A brief abuse screen for the elderly (BASE): its validity and use. Paper presented at the 22nd Annual Scientific and Educational Meeting of the Canadian Association on Gerontology, Montreal, Quebec, Canada, October, 1993.

Caregiver Abuse Screen (CASE)

Authors: Reis M, Nahmiash D, 1995a.

Targeted Population: Caregivers of the elderly.

Description: The Caregiver Abuse Screen (CASE) contains eight items, specifically worded to be nonblaming, that identify caregivers who are more likely to be abusers. The CASE serves as an effective complement to the screening provided by the Brief Abuse Screen for the Elderly. The authors recommend using the CASE with all clients who are caregivers of seniors, regardless of whether abuse is suspected. The authors also report that the responses of caregivers on the CASE may be indicative of tendencies and stresses that could lead to subsequent abuse (Reis & Nahmiash, 1995a).

Scores: No formal scoring is performed; yes/no responses alert the clinician to stressors in the caregiver-receiver relationship.

Accuracy: The CASE demonstrated construct and predictive validity. When the CASE was administered to known abusers and control groups, overall scores for abusers were significantly higher than those for nonabusers (Reis & Nahmiash, 1995b).

Administration Time: <1 minute.

References

Reis M, Nahmiash D: *When seniors are abused: a guide to intervention.* North York, Ontario, Canada, 1995a: Captus Press.

Reis MF, Nahmiash D: Validation of the caregiver abuse screen (CASE). *Can J Aging* 14:45-60, 1995b.

COGNITIVE ASSESSMENT

Cognitive impairment affects many elderly persons, reducing their ability to function in employment and social settings and their ability to perform activities of daily living. Regular screening for cognitive impairment in older adults is an integral part of the multidimensional health assessment process. Early recognition of cognitive change allows the clinician to implement use of medications, behavioral modifications, and safety protocols, which promote maintenance of functional status for as long as possible.

The measurements included in this chapter can be used to assist the clinician in distinguishing normal cognitive status from moderate to severe dementia. However, the recognition of early subclinical behavioral changes presents a challenge to the primary care clinician. Early problems, such as decreases in concentration, short-term memory recall loss, and language deficits may be part of the normal aging process and may not necessarily represent the onset of dementia. Underlying depression, substance abuse, use of medications prescribed for other disorders, and nutritional deficits may complicate the diagnostic process and cause false-positive results on screening exams for dementia. Poor performance on a screening exam must also be tempered with clinician knowledge of limiting patient factors such as level of education, reading and writing abilities, hearing and vision difficulties, and personal belief systems. In contrast, changes in daily routine and social interactions, which may be elicited in the clinical exam, may reveal early signs of cognitive deterioration.

This chapter contains basic screening tools suitable for primary care practice. The reader is encouraged to become familiar with these tools and learn to recognize their inherent limitations. As with other assessment instruments, clinicians should not depend on a score from a screening tool to provide a definite diagnosis or to exclusively predict outcome. Because of the multitude of assessment tools for this subject, online resources for cognitive and agitation assessment tools not included in this text are cited at the end of the chapter.

Blessed Dementia Scale and Information-Memory-Concentration (IMC) Test

Authors: Blessed G et al, 1968.

Source: This test is reprinted here and is also available at http://www.strokecenter.org/trials/scales/blessed_dementia.html (Blessed Dementia Scale) and http://www.strokecenter.org/trials/scales/bd_imct.html (Information-Memory-Concentration Test).

Targeted Population: Older adults.

Description: The Blessed Dementia Scale and Information-Memory-Concentration (IMC) Test are frequently combined to identify dementia. The Dementia Scale contains 22 items measuring changes in performance of everyday activities; changes in self-care habits; and changes in personality, interests, and drive. Each item is scored 0 for normal competence, with higher scores for partial and total incapacities. The IMC Test includes standard questions on orientation, recent and remote memory, and concentration to identify dementia. Each item receives a positive score if the answer is correct.

Of note, the British terms contained in the IMC Test are replaced with corresponding terms in the United States. For use in the United States, *monarch* is replaced with *president*, *prime minister* with *vice-president*, and *Gateshead* with *Chicago*.

Scores: An overall score for the Dementia Scale ranges from 0 (normal) to 28 (extreme incapacity); a cognitive subscale omits items 12 to 22 (changes in personality, interests, and drive) and ranges from 0 (normal) to 17 (severely demented). An overall score on the IMC Test ranges from 0 (complete failure) to 37 (normal).

Accuracy: Reliability and validity evidence are weak for the Dementia Scale; McDowell and Newell (1996) note that the scale may have more clinical utility in estimating the level of care required. In contrast, the IMC Test shows good reliability and validity and a good overall estimate of intellectual functioning (McDowell & Newell, 1996). The test correlates well with other measures of mental status, including the Mini-Mental State Examination (MMSE) and Dementia Rating Scale.

Administration Time: Approximately 10 minutes for clinical evaluation (Dementia Scale) and 10 minutes for interview administration (IMC Test).

References

Blessed G, Tomlinson BE, Roth M: The association between quantitative measures of dementia and of senile change in the cerebral grey matter of elderly subjects. *Br J Psychiatry* 114:797-811, 1968.

McDowell I, Newell C: *Measuring health: a guide to rating scales and questionnaires*, ed 2. Oxford University Press, 1996, pp. 303-308.

FROMAJE Mental Status Guide

Author: Libow LS, 1980.

Targeted Population: Older adults.

Description: In this mental status test, the acronym *FROMAJE* is used to assist clinicians in recalling a brief, easily remembered tool. The acronym stands for Function, Reasoning, Orientation, Memory, Arithmetic, Judgment, and Emotional state. Each of the seven items contains questions related to that area of mental functioning. One to three points are assigned each item, with 1 point for adequate function and 3 points for severe dysfunction.

Scores: An overall score is obtained by summing the item scores. Interpretation of the overall score is as follows:

> 7-8 = No serious abnormality in behavior or mentation
> 9-10 = Mild dementia
> 11-12 = Moderate dementia
> >13 = Severe dementia

The author cautions that an E (emotional) rating of 3 points will produce a total of 9 points if the patient scores "normal" (1 point) on the other items. This score may be a false positive result for dementia, but it may indicate depression (Libow, 1980).

Accuracy: Dolamore et al (1994) reported good reliability and validity for the FROMAJE, and favorable comparison with the MMSE.

Administration Time: 10-20 minutes by interview.

References

Dolamore MJ, Libow LS, Mulvihill MN, et al: Mental status guide: FROMAJE for use with frail elders. *J Gerontol Nurs* 20:29-35, 48-49, 1994.

Libow LS. A rapidly administered, easily remembered mental status evaluation: FROMAJE. In Libow LS, Sherman FT, eds. *The core of geriatric medicine*, St. Louis, 1980: Mosby, pp. 85-91.

Set Test

Authors: Isaacs B, Akhtar AJ, 1972.

Source: This test is described here and is also available online at http://www.medal.org/ch18.html. From Isaccs B, Kennie AT: The Set Test: an aid to the detection of dementia in old people. *Br J Psychiatry* 123:467, 1973.

Targeted Population: Older adults.

Description: This brief test uses verbal recall to assess mental function. The subject is asked to name as many items as possible in four successive categories: colors, animals, fruits, and towns. The end point for each set is when the subject is able to name a total of 10 or more items, when the subject is unable to think of any new items, or the subject repeats items with no new additions. The authors recommend that the Set Test be administered periodically to monitor changes in mental functioning in the elderly.

Scores: One point is assigned for each item named in a set to a maximum of 10. Overall score is the sum of the set item scores with an overall maximum of 40. Scores <15 correspond to a clinical diagnosis of dementia. Scores ranging from 15 to 24 indicate a lesser degree of dementia. Scores >25 are reported as normal (Isaacs & Kennie, 1973).

Accuracy: The authors reported good correlation with other measures of mental functioning in the elderly.

Administration Time: <5 minutes by interview.

References

Isaacs B, Akhtar AJ: The Set Test: a rapid test of mental function in old people. *Age Aging* 1:222-226, 1972.

Isaacs B, Kennie AT: The Set Test: an aid to the detection of dementia in old people. *Br J Psychiatry* 123:467-470, 1973.

Clock Drawing Test (CDT)

Authors: Various authors, 1986 to present.

Source: Sunderland T, Hill JL, Mellow AM, et al: Clock drawing in Alzheimer's disease: a novel measure of dementia severity. *J Am Geriatric Soc* Aug:37(8):725-729, 1989. Reprinted with permission Blackwell Publications, Ltd.

Targeted Population: Older adults.

Description: For administration of the Clock Drawing Test (CDT), the subject is given a pen and piece of blank, white, 8½″ × 11″ paper with instructions to draw a clock and indicate the time as "ten past eleven" (Mendez et al, 1992). The instructions are repeated orally and in writing as often as necessary. After completion of the task, the drawing is analyzed by one of several scoring systems.

Various versions of these instructions exist; a predrawn circle may be presented to the subject or a different time may be indicated.

Scores: One drawback to the usefulness of this screening tool is the absence of a universally accepted scoring mechanism. Scoring of the clock drawing varies throughout the literature and ranges from a simple 4-point scoring system (Ishiai et al, 1993) to a complex 20-item analysis (Mendez et al, 1992). For reference, five of the scoring systems are described in Box 10-1. Of note, Shua-Haim et al (1996) devised a 6-point scoring system that was statistically shown to correlate with and predict the MMSE score.

Accuracy: Shulman (2000) performed a meta-analysis of CDT studies and reported an impressive mean sensitivity of 85% and a specificity of 85%. Correlations with the

---

Box 10-1 Clock Drawing Test Scoring Systems

MENDEZ 1992. CLOCK DRAWING INTERPRETATION SCALE (CDIS) WITH THE TIME "TEN MINUTES PAST ELEVEN."

Score "1" per Item

1. There is an attempt to indicate a time in any way.
2. All marks or items can be classified as either part of a closure figure, a hand, or a symbol for clock numbers.
3. There is a totally closed figure without gaps (closure figure).

Score Only if Symbols for Clock Numbers Are Present

4. A "2" is present and pointed out in some way for the time.
5. Most symbols are distributed as a circle without major gaps.
6. Three or more clock quadrants have one or more appropriate numbers per respective quadrant.
7. Most symbols are ordered in a clockwise or rightward fashion.
8. All symbols are totally within a closure figure.
9. An "11" is present and is pointed out in some way for time.
10. All numbers 1 to 12 are present.
11. There are no repeated or duplicated number symbols.
12. There are no substitutions for Arabic or Roman numerals.
13. The numbers do not go beyond the number 12.
14. All symbols lie about equally adjacent to a closure figure edge.
15. Seven or more of the same symbol type are ordered sequentially.

Score Only If One Or More Hands Are Present

16. All hands radiate from the direction of a closure figure center.
17. One hand is visibly longer than another hand.
18. There are two distinct and separable hands.
19. All hands are totally within a closure figure.
20. There is an attempt to indicate a time with one or more hands.

SUNDERLAND 1983. A PRIORI CRITERIA FOR EVALUATING CLOCK DRAWINGS

10-6 Drawing of clock face with number and circle generally intact:
   10 Hands in correct position (i.e., hours hand approaching 3 o'clock).

9 Slight errors in placement of hands.
8 More noticeable errors in placement of hour and minute hands.
7 Placement of hands is significantly off course.
6 Inappropriate use of clock hands (i.e., use of digital display or circling numbers despite repeated instructions).

5-1 Drawing of clock face with circle and numbers is NOT intact:
5 Crowding of numbers at one end of the clock or reversal of numbers. Hands may still be present in some fashion.
4 Further distortion of number sequence. Integrity of clock face is now gone (i.e., numbers are missing or placed outside of boundaries of the clock face).
3 Numbers and clock face are no longer obviously connected in the clock drawing. Hands are not present.
2 Drawing reveals some evidence of instructions being received but only vague representation of a clock.
1 Either no attempt or an uninterpretable effort is made.

LAM 1998. SCORING CRITERIA FOR CLOCK DRAWING TEST

Score	Description of clock
0	Correct time with normal spacing.
1	Slight impairment in spacing of lines or numbers.
2	Noticeable impairment in line spacing.
3	Incorrect spacing between numbers with subsequent inappropriate denotation of time.
4	Obvious errors in time denotation (arms misplaced, numbers in wrong place).
5	Abnormal clock face drawing with inaccurate time denotation (e.g., reversal of numbers, perseveration beyond 12, misplaced numbers, drawing only to one side, omission of most numbers).
6	Abnormal clock face drawing with inaccurate time denotation (e.g., reversal of numbers, perseveration beyond 12, misplaced numbers and drawing to one side and omission of most numbers).
7	A recognizable attempt to draw a clock face but no clear denotation of time.
8	Some evidence that a clock face is drawn.
9	Minimal evidence that a clock face is drawn.

Continued

| **Box 10-1** | Clock Drawing Test Scoring Systems—Cont'd |

10   No reasonable attempt to draw a clock face (presence of gross visual disturbance, hemiplegia, and severe psychotic state should be excluded from this score).

SHUA-HAIM 1996. SIMPLE SCORING SYSTEM

Award one point for each of the following:
  Approximate drawing of the clock face
  Presence of numbers in sequence
  Correct spatial arrangement of numbers
  Presence of clock hands
  Hands showing approximately the correct time
  Hands depicting the exact time
Using simple linear regression, the authors found the following formula to best approximate the

MMSE score in patients with the diagnosis of probable Alzheimer's disease:

$$MMSE = 2.4 \text{ (Clock Score)} + 12.7 \text{ (P} < .001)$$

The formula correlates to MMSE scores between 13 and 27. A clock score of zero predicts an MMSE score of 13 and below. A clock score of 6 correlates with an MMSE of 27 and higher.

ISHIAI 1993. CDT SIMPLE SCORING SYSTEM

A maximum of four points are awarded:
  One point each is awarded for the correct placement of the 3, the 6, and the 9 relative to the 12.
  One point is awarded for correct placement of the remaining numbers.

MMSE and other cognitive tests were high. High levels of interrater and test-retest reliability, positive predictive value, and sensitivity to cognitive change with good predictive validity are also recorded. The scoring systems have significant variability, but all report similar psychometric properties (Shulman, 2000; South et al 2001). The CDT has been used to screen executive cognitive dysfunction in the presence of normal findings on the MMSE (Juby et al, 2002), and it is recommended as a supplement to the standard MMSE for identification of older persons at high risk for cognitive decline over time (Ferrucci et al, 1996).

Although demonstrated to be able to distinguish cognitively normal older adults from those with at least mild dementia of the Alzheimer's type, the CDT has been criticized as a poor screen for very mild or questionable dementia, unable to distinguish between adults with normal cognitive ability and those with very mild or questionable dementia (Lee et al, 1996; Powlishta et al, 2002; Seigerschmidt et al, 2002).

Administration Time: 2-5 minutes.

References

Braunberger P: The Clock-Drawing Test, 2001. Available at http://www.neurosurvival.ca/ClinicalAssistant/scales/clock_drawing_test.htm

Ferrucci L, Cecchi F, Guralnik JM, et al: Does the Clock Drawing Test predict cognitive decline in older persons independent of the Mini-Mental State Examination? The FINE Study Group. Finland, Italy, The Netherlands Elderly. J Am Geriatr Soc 44:1326-1331, 1996.

Ishiai S, Sugishita M, Ichikawa T, et al: Clock-drawing test and unilateral spatial neglect. Neurology 43:106-110, 1993.

Juby A, Tench S, Baker V: The value of clock drawing in identifying executive cognitive dysfunction in people with a normal Mini-Mental State Examination score. Can Med Assoc J 167:859-864, 2002.

Lam LC, Chiu HF, Ng KO, et al: Clock-face drawing, reading and setting tests in the screening of dementia in Chinese elderly adults. J Gerontol B Psychol Sci Soc Sci 53:P353-P357, 1998.

Lee H, Swanwick GR, Coen RF, et al: Use of the clock drawing task in the diagnosis of mild and very mild Alzheimer's disease. Int Psychogeriatr 8:469-476, 1996.

Mendez MF, Ala T, Underwood KL: Development of scoring criteria for the clock drawing task in Alzheimer's disease. J Am Geriatr Soc 40:1095-1099, 1992.

Powlishta KK, Von Dras DD, Stanford A, et al: The clock drawing test is a poor screen for very mild dementia. Neurology 59:898-903, 2002.

Seigerschmidt E, Mösch E, Siemen M, et al: The clock drawing test and questionable dementia: reliability and validity. Int J Geriatr Psychiatry 17:1048-1054, 2002.

Shua-Haim J, Koppuzha G, Gross J: A simple scoring system for clock-drawing in patients with Alzheimer's disease. J Am Geriatr Soc 44:335, 1996.

Shulman KI: Clock-drawing: is it the ideal cognitive screening test? Int J Geriatr Psychiatry 15:548-561, 2000.

Shulman KI, Shedletsky R, Silver IL: The challenge of time: clock drawing and cognitive functioning in the elderly. Int J Geriatr Psychiatry 1:135-140, 1986.

South MB, Greve KW, Bianchini KJ, et al: Interrater reliability of three clock drawing test scoring systems. Appl Neuropsychol 8:174-179, 2001.

Sunderland T, Hill JL, Mellow AM, et al: Clock drawing in Alzheimer's disease. A novel measure of dementia severity. J Am Geriatr Soc 37:725-729, 1989.

6-Item Cognitive Impairment Test (6CIT)

Authors: Katzman R et al, 1983. Revised: Bullock R et al, 1999.

Source: This tool is reprinted in this text. Copyright for the revised 6-Item Cognitive Impairment Test (6CIT) is held by Kingshill (Version 2000). For information on this tool and access to this version, please visit http://www.kingshill-research.org/kresearch/6cit.ASP.

Targeted Population: Older adults.

Description: The 6CIT was developed by Katzman et al (1983) from the Blessed Information-Memory-Concentration Test. The six items were chosen on the basis of a positive correlation between scores and plaque counts obtained from the cerebral cortex samples from 38 subjects at autopsy. The items have been shown to discriminate among mild, moderate, and severe cognitive deficits.

Scores: Each of the six items is scored 0 if the answer is correct; a score of 2 to 4 is assigned for incorrect answers. The total score ranges from 0 to 28. A score of 8 or higher is an indicator of cognitive impairment.

Accuracy: The 6CIT was validated against the MMSE and was found to correlate well (Brooke & Bullock, 1999). The 6CIT was especially useful in identifying milder dementia with a higher sensitivity than that of the lengthier MMSE. A summary of the validation work for the 6CIT may be found online at http://www.kingshill-research.org/kresearch/validation.PDF.

Administration Time: 1-2 minutes.

References

Brooke P, Bullock R: Validation of the 6-item cognitive impairment test. *Int J Geriatr Psychiatry* 14:936-940, 1999.

Katzman R, Brown T, Fuld P, et al: Validation of a short Orientation-Memory-Concentration Test of cognitive impairment. *Am J Psychiatry* 140:734-739, 1983.

Hachinski Ischemic Score (HIS) for Multi-Infarct Dementia

Authors: Hachinski VC et al, 1975.

Source: The Hachinski Ischemic Score (HIS) for Multi-Infarct Dementia is reprinted here and is also available at http://www.strokecenter.org/trials/scales/hachinski.html.

Targeted Population: Older adults with possible vascular dementia.

Description: This tool is used to distinguish dementia of vascular causes from primary degenerative dementia. Thirteen clinical items are assessed for their presence in the patient's history.

Scores: Two points are scored for each of these clinical findings: abrupt onset, fluctuating course, history of strokes, focal neurologic symptoms, and focal neurologic signs. One point is assigned for each of the eight remaining features (Hachinski et al, 1975). The total score ranges from 0 to 18. A score of >7 indicates vascular (multi-infarct) dementia, a score of 4 to 7 indicates borderline/mixed dementia, and a score of <4 indicates primary degenerative dementia (Alzheimer's disease).

Rosen et al (1980) modified the scale by eliminating five features: fluctuating course (2 points), nocturnal confusion, relative preservation of personality, depression, and generalized atherosclerosis (1 point each), preserving the features that characterize those persons with vascular dementia. The total score for the modified screen ranges from 0 to 12; scores greater than zero represent increasing risk for vascular dementia. A cutoff point of 4 or greater was used in validation studies.

Accuracy: Moroney et al (1997) conducted a meta-analysis on patients with dementia. Analysis revealed that the best cutoff scores were ≤4 for Alzheimer's disease and ≥7 for multi-infarct dementia, as originally proposed, with a sensitivity of 89.0% and a specificity of 89.3%. The authors concluded that the HIS performed well in the differentiation between Alzheimer's disease and

multi-infarct dementia, the purpose for which it was originally designed, but that the clinical diagnosis of mixed dementia remains difficult. They suggest that further prospective studies of the HIS include additional clinical and neuroimaging variables to refine the scale and improve its ability to identify patients with mixed dementia.

Administration Time: 1-2 minutes if data are available.

References

Hachinski VC, Iliff LD, Silhka R: Cerebral blood flow in dementia. *Arch Neurol* 32:632-637, 1975.

Moroney JT, Bagiella E, Desmond DW, et al: Meta-analysis of the Hachinski Ischemic Score in pathologically verified dementias. *Neurology* 49:1096-1105, 1997.

Rosen WG, Terry RD, Fuld PA, et al: Pathological verification of ischemic score in differentiation of dementias. *Ann Neurol* 7:486-488, 1980.

Other Measures:
Mini-Mental State Examination (MMSE)

Author: Folstein M et al, 1975.

Source: The MMSE is no longer available for text publication. The MMSE is now published and sold by Psychological Assessment Resources, Inc., 16204 N. Florida Ave, Lutz, FL 33549; phone: 1-800-331-8378 or 1-813-968-3003; website: http://www.minimental.com/. The standard MMSE form published by Psychological Assessment Resources, Inc. is based on its original 1975 conceptualization, with minor subsequent modifications by the authors. MMSE kits are available and include an MMSE clinical guide, pocket norms card, user's guide, and test forms. The MMSE is also freely available at numerous online sites including http://www.medafile.com/mmses.htm, http://www.medal.org/adocs/docs_ch18/doc_ch18.03.html#A18.03.01, and http://www.family.georgetown.edu/welchjj/netscut/psych/minimental.html.

Targeted Population: Older adults.

Description: One of the most widely used tests of cognitive function, the MMSE is also well studied. The MMSE is a screening test only; diagnosis of dementia requires a full mental status examination with history and physical examination. The test contains 11 items in two parts. The first part requires verbal responses and assesses orientation, memory, and attention. The second part evaluates naming of objects, ability to follow oral and written commands, sentence writing, and ability to copy a complex polygon.

Scores: Points are assigned to correct responses. Total scores range from 0 to 30. The mean score for normal individuals is 27.6; for patients with dementia, the mean score is 9.7 (Folstein et al, 1975). The cutoff score ranges from 23 to 25 in multiple studies (McDowell & Newell, 1996). Cutoff scores may vary based on level of education. Scores at or less than the cutoff warrant further evaluation of cognitive function.

Accuracy: The MMSE has demonstrated good to excellent reliability (internal consistency, test-retest, and interrater) and validity (content and correlations with other cognitive function tests) in numerous studies (Tombaugh & McIntyre, 1992; McDowell & Newell, 1996). Predictive validity studies have shown that the MMSE has good ability to indicate when an individual becomes cognitively impaired. Some variation in scores was noted when educational levels were compared, with lower scores implying more cognitive impairment among those with higher education than among those with less education (Uhlmann & Larson, 1991). As education level increases, the specificity of the MMSE also rises, whereas the sensitivity decreases. Hence, cutoff scores may be lower in less educated persons. With the use of normative data, Crum et al (1993) provided cutoff scores of 19 for 0 to 4 years of education, 23 for 5 to 8 years of education, 27 for 9 to 12 years of education, and 29 for college level and beyond.

Administration Time: This test is not timed but takes approximately 10 minutes to administer.

References

Crum RM, Anthony JC, Bassett SS, et al: Population-based norms for the Mini-Mental State Examination by age and educational level. *JAMA* 269:2386-2391, 1993.

Folstein MF, Folstein SE, McHugh PR: "Mini-mental state": a practical method for grading the cognitive state of patients for the clinician. *J Psychiatr Res* 12:189-198, 1975.

McDowell I, Newell C: *Measuring health: a guide to rating scales and questionnaires*, ed 2. 1996, Oxford University Press, pp. 314-323.

Tombaugh TN, McIntyre NJ: The Mini-Mental State Examination: a comprehensive review. *J Am Geriatric Soc* 40:922-935, 1992.

Uhlmann RF, Larson EB: Effect of education on the Mini-Mental State Examination as a screening test for dementia. *J Am Geriatr Soc* 39:876-880, 1991.

Resources and References

Online Resources

Many other measures exist to screen for dementia; some are cited below. Scales that measure agitation in dementia may prove useful for primary care providers working with nursing home residents and are also cited here.

Dementia Scales

Brief Cognitive Rating Scale (BCRS). Available at http://www.geriatric-resources.com/html/bcrs.html.

Clifton Assessment Procedures for the Elderly (CAPE). Available at http://www.ehr.chime.ucl.ac.uk/demcare/cape.html.

Clinical Dementia Rating (CDR). Available at http://alzheimer.wustl.edu/adrc2/Education/CDR%20Inter-Page.html.

Dementia Rating Scale. Available at http://www.parinc.com/product.cfm?ProductID=539

Functional Assessment Staging. Available at http://www.geriatric-resources.com/html/fast.html

Global Deterioration Scale for Assessment of Primary Degenerative Dementia. Available at http://www.geriatric-resources.com/html/gds.html

Neecham Confusion Scale. Available at http://pccchealth.org/articles/neecham_scale.htm

Short Portable Mental Status Questionnaire. Available at http://nncf.unl.edu/alz/manual/sec1/portable.html

Agitation Scales

Agitated Behavior Scale. Available at http://www.ohiovalley.org/agitation/agbe.html

Brief Agitation Rating Scale (BARS) for Nursing Home Patients. Available at http://www.medal.org/ch18.html

Cohen-Mansfield Agitation Inventory. Available at http://www.medafile.com/zyweb/CMAI.htm, http://www.medal.org/ch18.html.

General Resources

Alzheimer's Association Resource List. Available at http://www.alz.org/Resources/ResourceLists.asp This site lists bibliographies and sources for assessment tools pertinent to Alzheimer's disease.

Alzheimer Research Forum. Available at http://www.alzforum.org/dis/dia/tes/default.asp.

A portion of this site is dedicated to the diagnosis of Alzheimer's disease, including laboratory tests, radiological testing, neuropsychologic tests, and other specific diagnostics. A group of cognitive assessment tools is included under neuropsychologic tests.

Duke University Center for the Study of Aging and Human Development. Available at http://www.geri.duke.edu/resource/resource.html.

This page provides links to other related medical information on the Internet. The Center for the Study for Aging and Human Development does not maintain the Web pages listed here, nor are they responsible for the content of the websites listed on this page.

Huffington Center on Aging: Geriatric Medicine Self-Instruction Modules Support. Available at http://www.geri-ed.com/modules/assess/idxlist.htm.

This module is one of a series of self-instructional modules in geriatric medicine offered by The Roy M. and Phyllis Gough Huffington Center on Aging, Baylor College of Medicine, Houston, Texas. The module includes advance directives and advance planning information, as well as numerous measures and tools for comprehensive geriatric assessment.

References

Burns A, Lawlor B, Craig S: *Assessment scales in old age psychiatry.* London, 1999: Martin Dunitz Ltd.

Ebersole P, Hess P: *Toward healthy aging: human needs and nursing response*, ed 5. St. Louis, 1998: Mosby

Gallo JJ, Fulmer T, Paveza GJ, et al: *Handbook of geriatric assessment*, ed 3. Rockville, MD, 2000: Aspen Publishers, Inc.

Yoshikawa TT, Cobbs EL, Brummel-Smith K. *Practical ambulatory geriatrics*. St. Louis, 1998: Mosby.

Instrumental Activities of Daily Living Scale (IADL)

Name: _____

Date: _____

D.O.B.: _____ Gender: Male   Female

Medical Record #: _____

Circle one statement in each category A-H that applies to subject.

A. Ability to use telephone

1. Operates telephone on own initiative; looks up and dials numbers, etc.   1

2. Dials a few well-known numbers   1

3. Answers telephone but does not dial   1

4. Does not use telephone at all.   0

B. Shopping

1. Takes care of all shopping needs independently   1

2. Shops independently for small purchases   0

3. Needs to be accompanied on any shopping trip.   0

4. Completely unable to shop.   0

C. Food Preparation

1. Plans, prepares and serves adequate meals independently   1

2. Prepares adequate meals if supplied with ingredients   0

3. Heats, serves and prepares meals or prepares meals but does not maintain adequate diet.   0

4. Needs to have meals prepared and served.   0

D. Housekeeping

1. Maintains house alone or with occasional assistance (e.g. "heavy work domestic help")   1

2. Performs light daily tasks such as dishwashing, bed making   1

3. Performs light daily tasks but cannot maintain acceptable level of cleanliness.   1

4. Needs help with all home maintenance tasks.   1

5. Does not participate in any housekeeping tasks.   0

E. Laundry

1. Does personal laundry completely   1

2. Launders small items; rinses stockings, etc.   1

3. All laundry must be done by others.   0

F. Mode of Transportation

1. Travels independently on public transportation or drives own car.   1

2. Arranges own travel via taxi, but does not otherwise use public transportation.   1

3. Travels on public transportation when accompanied by another.   1

4. Travel limited to taxi or automobile with assistance of another.   0

5. Does not travel at all.   0

G. Responsibility for own medications

1. Is responsible for taking medication in correct dosages at correct time.   1

2. Takes responsibility if medication is prepared in advance in separate dosage.   0

3. Is not capable of dispensing own medication.   0

H. Ability to Handle Finances

1. Manages financial matters independently (budgets, writes checks, pays rent and bills, goes to bank), collects and keeps track of income.   1

2. Manages day-to-day purchases, but needs help with banking, major purchases, etc.   1

3. Incapable of handling money.   0

OVERALL SCORE: 7-8 = high level independence
5-6 = moderate level independence
3-4 = moderate level dependence
1-2 = dependence

Adapted from Lawton MP, Brody EM: Assessment of older people: self-maintaining and instrumental activities of daily living, *Gerontologist* 9:179-186, 1969.

Structured Assessment of Independent Living Skills (SAILS)

Name: _____

Date: _____

Age: _____ Gender: Male   Female

Handedness: _____

Education: _____

Examiner: _____

SCORING FORM

Diagnosis:

Note: If patient is unable to complete task, assign maximum time of 60" unless otherwise indicated

MOTOR TASKS

Fine Motor Skills   Time   Score

1. Picks up coins   0 = drops two 1 = drops one 2 = slow 3 = normal (8")
2. Removes wrappers   0 = needs assistance 1 = tears one or more 2 = slow 3 = normal (35")
3. Cuts with scissors   0 = can't cut 1 = off line 2 = slow 3 = normal (32")
4. Folds letter and places in envelope   0 = can't fold 1 = doesn't fit 2 = slow 3 = normal (16")
5. Uses key in lock   0 = can't insert 1 = can't unlock 2 = slow 3 = normal (13")
   Subtotal:

Gross Motor Skills   Time   Score

1. Stands up from sitting   0 = unable   1 = uses arms of chair 2 = slow 3 = normal (2")
2. Opens and walks through door   0 = unable 1 = needs door held open 2 = slow 3 = normal (5")
3. Regular gait   0 = unable   1 = assistive device 2 = slow 3 = normal (6")
   Time   1) _____ 2) _____ Mean _____ Steps 1) _____ 2) _____ Mean _____
4. Tandem gait   0 = unable, steps off 4 or more times 1 = steps off 2-3 times
   2 = slow (1 step off allowed) 3 = normal (9")
   Time 1) _____ 2) _____ Mean _____ Steps off line 1) _____ 2) _____ Mean _____
5. Transfers object across room   0 = drops 1 = inaccurate placement 2 = slow 3 = normal (6")
   Time 1) _____ 2) _____ Mean _____
   Subtotal:

Dressing Skills   Time   Score

1. Puts on shirt (maximum = 120")   0 = can't put on or button 1 = misaligned
   2 = slow 3 = normal (86")
2. Buttons cuffs of shirt   0 = unable 1 = one cuff 2 = slow 3 = normal (45")
3. Puts on jacket   0 = can't put on 1 = needs help with zipper 2 = slow 3 = normal (27")
4. Ties shoelaces   0 = unable/wrong feet 1 = knot comes undone 2 = slow 3 = normal (9")
5. Puts on gloves   0 = unable 1 = one hand 2 = slow 3 = normal (21")
   Subtotal:

Eating Skills   Time   Score

1. Drinks from glass   0 = unable 1 = spits 2 = slow 3 = normal (3")
2. Transfers food with spoon   0 = unable 1 = drops 2 = slow 3 = normal (11")
3. Cuts with fork and knife   0 = unable 1 = drops 2 = slow 3 = normal (16")
4. Transfers food with fork   0 = unable 1 = drops 2 = slow 3 = normal (16")
5. Transfers liquid with spoon   0 = unable 1 = spills 2 = slow 3 = normal (13")
   Subtotal:

Total Motor Time _____   Total Motor Score _____

COGNITIVE TASKS

Expressive Language   Score

1. Quality of expression   0 = severe <25% 1 = moderate 25-90% 2 = mild 90-99% 3 = intact
2. Repetition   0 = no items 1 = 1 item 2 = 2 items 3 = all 3 items
3. Object naming   0 = 3 or less 1 = 4 items 2 = 5 items 3 = all 6 items
4. Writes legible note   0 = illegible 1 = 1 item 2 = 2 items 3 = all 3 items
5. Completes application form   0 = 3 or less 1 = 4 items 2 = 5 items 3 = all 6 items
   Subtotal: _____

Structured Assessment of Independent Living Skills (SAILS) - 2

Receptive language   Score

1. Reads and follows printed instructions   0 = none 1 = 1 item 2 = 2 items 3 = all 3 items
2. Understands written material   0 = none 1 = 1-4 items 2 = 5 items 3 = all 6 items
   Article 1: Correct 1) _____   2) _____   3) _____
   Article 2: Correct 1) _____   2) _____   3) _____
3. Understands common signs 0 = none 1 = 1 item 2 = 2 items 3 = all 3 items
4. Follows verbal directions 0 = none 1 = 1 item 2 = 2 items 3 = 3 items
   1) Touch shoulder 2) Hands on table, close eyes 3) Draw circle, hand pencil, fold paper
5. Identifies named objects 0 = none 1 = 1 item 2 = 2 items 3 = all 3 items
   Subtotal:

Time and Orientation   Score

1. States time on clock (6:14) 0 = off over 1 hour 1 = off within 1 hour 2 = off 10 minutes
   3 = correct within 1 minute
2. Calculates time interval (until 7:30) 0 = off 1 hour 1 = off within 1 hour 2 = off within 15 minutes
   3 = correct within 1 minute
3. States time of alarm setting (8:15) 0 = off 1 hour 1 = off within 1 hour 2 = off within 15 minutes
   3 = correct within 1 minute
4. Locates current date on calendar 0 = incorrect month 1 = correct month 2 = correct week
   3 = correct date
5. Correctly reads calendar 0 = none 1 = 1 item 2 = 2 items 3 = all 3 items
   1) Fridays   2) Day of 15th   3) 2nd Monday
   Subtotal:

Money-Related Skills   Score

1. Counts money   0 – none 1 – 1 item 2 – 2 items 3 = all 3 items
   1) 35 cents _____   2) 95 cents _____   3) $1.41 _____
2. Makes change   0 = none 1 = 1 item 2 = 2 items 3 = all 3 items
   1) ($.75 from $1.00) = $.25 _____   2) ($.41 from $.50) = $.09 _____
   3) ($2.79 from $5.00) = $2.21 _____
3. Understands monthly utility bill 0 = none 1 = 1 item 2 = 2 items 3 = all 3 items
   1) (Light Co.) _____   2) ($38.46) _____   3) (3/6/87) _____
4. Writes check 0 – 2 or less 1 – 3 items 2 – 4 items 3 = all 5 items
   1) Date 2) Payee 3) Numerical amount 4) Written amount 5) Signature
5. Understands chequebook 0 = none 1 = 1 item 2 = 2 items 3 = all 3 items
   1) Checks on August 11 2) Check #355 3) Balance ($440.40)
   Subtotal:

Total Cognitive Score _____

Instrumental Activities   Score

1. Uses telephone book 0 = none 1 = 1 item 2 = 2 items 3 = all 3 items
2. Dials telephone number 0 = cannot handle phone 1 = misdials number
   2 = needs help to read 3 – correctly reads and dials
3. Understands medication label 0 = none 1 = 1 item 2 = 2 items 3 = all 3 items
4. Opens medication container 0 = can't open two 1 = can't open one 2 = needs cue 3 = normal
5. Follows simple recipe 0 = unable 1 = 1 step 2 = 2 steps 3 = all 3 steps
   Subtotal:

Social Interaction   Score

1. Responds to greeting and farewell 0 = none 1 = 1 item 2 = 2 items 3 = all 3 items
2. Responds to request for information 0 = none 1 = 1 item 2 = 2 items 3 = all 3 items
3. Responds to social directives 0 = none 1 = 1 item 2 = 2 items 3 = all 3 items
4. Requests needed information 0 = none 1 = 1 item 2 = 2 items 3 = all 3 items
5. Understanding non-verbal expression 0 = none 1 = 1 item 2 = 2 items 3 = all 3 items
   Subtotal:

GRAND TOTAL SCORE _____

From Mahurin RK, DeBettignies BH, Pirozzolo FJ: Structured assessment of independent living skills: preliminary report of a performance measure of functional abilities in dementia, *J Gerontol* 46(2):58-66, 1991.

Five-Item Instrumental Activities of Daily Living Questionnaire

Name: _____

Date: _____

Address: _____

Phone: _____

D.O.B.: _____Gender: Male   Female

Medical Record #: _____

1. Can you get to places out of walking distance. . .
   1 Without help (can travel alone on buses, taxis, or drive your own car)?
   0 With some help (need someone to help you or go with you when traveling), or are you unable to travel unless emergency arrangements are made for a specialized vehicle like an ambulance?
   — Not answered

2. Can you go shopping for groceries or clothes [assuming she or he has transportation]. . .
   1 Without help (taking care of all shopping needs yourself, assuming you had transportation)?
   0 With some help (need someone to go with you on all shopping trips), or are you completely unable to do any shopping?
   — Not answered

3. Can you prepare your own meals. . .
   1 Without help (plan and cook full meals yourself)?
   0 With some help (can prepare some things but unable to cook full meals yourself), or are you completely unable to prepare any meals?
   — Not answered

4. Can you do your housework. . .
   1 Without help (can scrub floors, etc.)?
   0 With some help (can do light housework but need help with heavy work), or are you completely unable to do any housework?
   — Not answered

5. Can you handle your own money. . .
   1 Without help (write checks, pay bills, etc.)?
   0 With some help (manage day-to-day buying but need help with managing your checkbook and paying your bills), or are you completely unable to handle money?
   — Not answered

Total Score _____

Adapted from the Older American Resources and Services (OARS) multidimensional functional assessment questionnaire. From Fillenbaum GG: Screening the elderly: a brief instrumental activities of daily living measure, *J Am Geriatric Soc* 33:706, 1995. Reprinted with permission Blackwell Publishing, Ltd.

Hearing Handicap Inventory for the Elderly-Screening Version (HHIE-S)*

Name: _____

Date: _____

Address: _____

Phone: _____

D.O.B.: _____ Gender: Male   Female

Medical Record #: _____

	Yes (4)	Sometimes (2)	No (0)
E-1. Does a hearing problem cause you to feel embarrassed when meeting new people?	_____	_____	_____
E-2. Does a hearing problem cause you to feel frustrated when talking to members of your family?	_____	_____	_____
S-3. Do you have difficulty hearing when someone speaks in a whisper?	_____	_____	_____
E-4. Do you feel handicapped by a hearing problem?	_____	_____	_____
S-5. Does a hearing problem cause difficulty when visiting friends, relatives, or neighbors?	_____	_____	_____
S-6. Does a hearing problem cause you to attend religious services less often than you would like?	_____	_____	_____
E-7. Does a hearing problem cause you to have arguments with family members?	_____	_____	_____
S-8. Does a hearing problem cause you difficulty when listening to TV or radio?	_____	_____	_____
E-9. Do you feel that any difficulty with your hearing limits or hampers your personal or social life?	_____	_____	_____
S-10. Does a hearing problem cause you difficulty when in a restaurant with relatives or friends?	_____	_____	_____

E = emotional response S = social/situational response

*Range of total points, 0-40; 0-8, no self-perceived handicap; 10-22, mild to moderate handicap; 24-40, significant handicap

From Ventry IM, Weinstein BE: Identification of elderly people with hearing problems, *ASHA* July 25:37, 1983. Copyright by the American-Speech-Language-Hearing Association. Reprinted with permission.

Tinetti Balance and Gait Evaluation/Performance-Oriented Assessment of Mobility

Name: _____

Date: _____

Address: _____

Phone: _____

D.O.B.: _____ Gender: Male   Female

Medical Record #: _____

Balance

Instructions: Subject is seated in a hard, armless chair. The following maneuvers are tested:

1. Sitting balance
   0 = Leans or slides in chair
   1 = Steady, safe

2. Arise
   0 = Unable without help
   1 = Able but uses arm to help
   2 = Able without use of arms

3. Attempts to arise
   0 = Unable without help
   1 = Able, but requires more than one attempt
   2 = Able to arise with one attempt

4. Immediate standing balance (first 5 seconds)
   0 = Unsteady (staggers, moves feet, marked trunk sway)
   1 = Steady but uses walker/cane or grabs other object for support
   2 = Steady without walker or cane or other support

5. Standing balance
   0 = Unsteady
   1 = Steady, but wide stance (medial heels > than 4" apart) or uses cane/walker or other support
   2 = Narrow stance without support

6. Nudge (subject at maximum position with feet as close together as possible. Examiner pushes lightly on subject's sternum with palm of hand 3 times.)
   0 = Begins to fall
   1 = Staggers, grabs, but catches self
   2 = Steady

7. Eyes closed (at maximum position #6)
   0 = Unsteady
   1 = Steady

8. Turn 360°
   0 = Discontinuous steps
   1 = Continuous steps
   0 = Unsteady (grabs, staggers)
   1 = Steady

9. Sit down
   0 = Unsafe (misjudged distance; falls into chair)
   1 = Uses arms or not a smooth motion
   2 = Safe, smooth motion

_____/16_____ BALANCE SCORE

Tinetti Balance and Gait Evaluation/Performance-Oriented Assessment of Mobility - 2

Gait
Instructions: Subject stands with examiner. Walks down hallway or across room, first at his/her usual pace, then back at a "rapid but safe" pace (using usual walking aid such as cane/walker).

10. Initiation of gait (immediately after told 'go')
    0 = Any hesitancy or multiple attempts to start
    1 = No hesitancy

11. Step length and height (right foot swing)
    0 = Does not pass L. stance foot with step
    1 = Passes L. stance foot
    0 = R. foot does not clear floor completely with step
    1 = R. foot completely clears floor

12. Step length and height (left foot swing)
    0 = Does not pass R. stance foot with step
    1 = Passes R. stance foot
    0 = L. foot does not clear floor completely with step
    1 = L. foot completely clears floor

13. Step symmetry
    0 = R. and L. step length not equal (estimate)
    1 = R. and L. step length appear equal

14. Step continuity
    0 = Stopping or discontinuity between steps
    1 = Steps appear continuous

15. Path (estimated in relation to floor tiles, 12" wide. Observe excursion of one foot over about 10 feet of course.)
    0 = Marked deviation
    1 = Mild/moderate deviation or uses a walking aid
    2 = Straight without walking aid

16. Trunk
    0 = Marked sway or uses walking aid
    1 = No sway but flexion of knees or back or spreads arms out while walking
    2 = No sway, no flexion, no use of arms and no walking aid

17. Walk stance
    0 = Heels apart
    1 = Heels almost touching while walking

_____/12_____ GAIT SCORE

_____/28_____ TOTAL MOBILITY SCORE (BALANCE AND GAIT)

From Tinetti ME: Performance-oriented assessment of mobility problems in elderly patients, *J Am Geriatric Soc* 34:119-126, 1986. Reprinted with permission Blackwell Publishing, Ltd.

Risk Assessment Tool (RAT) for Falls

Name: _____

Date: _____

Address: _____

Phone: _____

D.O.B.: _____ Gender: Male   Female

Medical Record #: _____

Directions: Place a check mark in front of elements that apply to your patient. The decision of whether or not a patient is at risk for falls is based on your nursing judgment. GUIDELINE: A patient who has a check mark in front of an element with an asterisk (*) or four or more of the other elements would be identified as at risk for falls.

General Data

_____ Age over 60
_____ History of falls prior to admission*
_____ Postoperative/admit for operation
_____ Smoker

Physical Condition

_____ Dizziness/imbalance
_____ Unsteady gait
_____ Diseases/problems affecting weight-bearing joints
_____ Weakness
_____ Paresis
_____ Seizure disorder
_____ Impairment of vision
_____ Impairment of hearing
_____ Diarrhea
_____ Urinary frequency

Mental Status

_____ Confusion/disorientation*
_____ Impaired memory or judgment
_____ Inability to understand or follow directions

Medications

_____ Diuretics or diuretic effects
_____ Hypotensive or CNS suppressants (narcotic, sedative, psychotropic, hypnotic, tranquilizer, antihypertensive, antidepressant)
_____ Medication that increases GI motility (laxative, enema)

Ambulatory Devices Used

_____ Cane
_____ Crutches
_____ Walker
_____ Wheelchair
_____ Geri chair
_____ Braces

From Brians LK, Alexander K, Grota P, et al: The development of the RISK tool for fall prevention. Reprinted from *Rehabilitation Nursing* 16: 67, 1991 with permission of the Association of Rehabilitation Nurses, 4700 West Lake Avenue, Glenview, IL, 60025-1485. Copyright 1997.

Reassessment Is Safe "Kare" (RISK) Tool

Name: _____

Date: _____

Address: _____

Phone: _____

D.O.B.: _____   Gender: Male   Female

Medical Record #: _____

Directions: Place a check in front of any element that applies to your patient. A patient who has a check mark in front of any of the first four elements would be identified as at risk for falls. In addition, when a high-risk patient has a check mark in front of the element "Uses a wheelchair," he or she is considered to be at greater risk for falls.

_____ Unsteady gait/dizziness/imbalance   _____ Uses a wheelchair

_____ Impaired memory or judgment

_____ Weakness

_____ History of falls

From Brians LK, Alexander K, Grota P, et al: The development of the RISK tool for fall prevention. Reprinted from *Rehabilitation Nursing* 16: 67, 1997 with permission of the Association of Rehabilitation Nurses, 4700 West Lake Avenue, Glenview, IL, 60025-1485. Copyright 1997.

Guidelines for Home Safety Assessment

Name: _____

Date: _____

Address: _____

Phone: _____

D.O.B.: _____ Gender: Male   Female

Medical Record #: _____

	Okay (y/n)	Plan to improve
Basic structure		
Intact roof		
Solid floors and stairs		
Functioning toilet (or outhouse)		
Source of fresh water		
Wheelchair ramp		
Temperature control		
Fan/air conditioner		
Proper use of heating pads		
Proper water heater temperature		
Adequate heat/insulation		
Nutrition		
Kitchen condition/food storage		
Evidence of alcohol use		
Pests		
Fire prevention and response		
Use of kerosene heaters		
Use of open gas burners on stove for heat		
Smoking in bed		
Use of oxygen		
Dangerous electrical wiring		
Smoke alarms		
Exit plans in case of fire		
Self-injury/violence prevention		
Locks		
Method of calling for help		
Proximity of neighbors		
Surrounding criminal activity		
Emergency phone numbers by telephone		
Loaded guns/knives		
Household toxins		
Water/bathtub		
Power tools		
Medication management		
Duplicate medicines, outdated drugs, pill box		
Correct labeling		
Storage safety, accessibility, refrigeration		
Caregiver familiarity		
Wandering control (for confused clients)		
Doortop latches, special locks		
Fenced yards with hidden latches		
Identification bracelets		
Electronic wandering alarms		

From Stanhope M, Knollmueler RN: *Handbook of community-based and home health nursing practice: tools for assessment, intervention, and education,* ed 3. Modified from Yoshikawa TT, Cobbs EL, Brummel-Smith K: *Practical Ambulatory Geriatrics,* St Louis, 1998, Mosby.

Environmental Assessment for the Elderly

Name: _____

Date: _____

Address: _____

Phone: _____

D.O.B.: _____ *Gender: Male   Female*

Medical Record #: _____

1. How many rooms are available to client?
   Own bedroom   _____   If shared, with whom?   _____
   Bathroom   _____
   Kitchen   _____
   Living/sitting room _____

2. Must client climb stairs to enter or leave house?
   Yes _____   No _____
   If yes, are they well lit and in good repair?
   Yes _____   No _____

3. Is neighborhood dangerous?
   Yes _____   No _____

4. Is house clean?
   Yes _____   No _____

5. Does house seem adequately insulated and ventilated?
   Yes _____   No _____

6. Are there signs of neglect?
   Old food in refrigerator   _____
   Unwashed dishes   _____
   Accumulated dirty clothing   _____
   Other (describe):   _____

7. Is there a sufficient supply of food for at least several days?
   Yes _____   No _____

8. Safety checklist

a. Can the client:	Yes	No
Lock and unlock the door	_____	_____
Reach light switches	_____	_____
Call for help (telephone and numbers accessible)	_____	_____
Safely transfer from bed, chair, toilet, tub	_____	_____

b. Are there obvious dangers:		
Overloaded electrical outlets	_____	_____
Frayed electrical wires	_____	_____
Poor lighting	_____	_____
Cluttered furniture	_____	_____
Unsafe furniture	_____	_____
Frayed carpets or broken floors	_____	_____
Missing or broken smoke alarm	_____	_____

From Kane R, Ouslander J, Abrass I: *Essentials of clinical geriatrics*, ed 3, New York, 1994, McGraw-Hill. Reprinted with permission McGraw-Hill Companies.

Driving Skills Quiz

Name: _____

Date: _____

Address: _____

Phone: _____

D.O.B.: _____ Gender: Male   Female

Medical Record #: _____

If you answer yes to one or more of the following questions, you may want to limit your driving or take steps to improve a problem.

If you answer yes to most of the questions, it may be time to consider letting someone else do your driving for you.

The quiz is based in part on an American Association of Retired Persons publication.

- Does driving make you feel nervous or physically exhausted?

- Do you have difficulty seeing pedestrians, signs and vehicles?

- Do cars frequently seem to appear from nowhere?

- At night, does the glare from oncoming headlights temporarily "blind" you?

- Do you find intersections confusing?

- Are you finding it harder to judge the distance between cars?

- Do you have difficulty coordinating your hand and foot movements?

- Are you slower than you used to be in reacting to dangerous situations?

- Do you sometimes get lost in familiar neighborhoods?

- Do other drivers often honk at you?

- Have you had an increased number of traffic violations, accidents or near-accidents in the past year?

From Mayo Foundation for Medical Education and Research: Driving: how safe are you behind the wheel? *May Clinic Health Letter* 14(4):7, 1996. Based in part on materials developed by AARP. Visit www.aarp.org/drive for more information.

Brief Abuse Screen for the Elderly (BASE)

Name: _____

Address: _____

Phone: _____

D.O.B.: _____ Gender: *Male* *Female*

Medical Record #: _____

Please respond to every question (as well as you can estimate) concerning all clients 60 years or over who are caregivers (regular helper of any kind) or care-receivers:

1. Is the client an elderly person who has a caregiver? ☐ Yes ☐ No

2. Is the client a caregiver of an elderly person? ☐ Yes ☐ No

3. Do you suspect abuse? (see also #4)

   a) By a caregiver? Comments: _____

1	2	3	4	5
No, not at all	**only slightly, doubtful**	**possibly, somewhat**	**probably, quite likely**	**yes, definitely**

   b) By a care-receiver? Comments: _____

1	2	3	4	5
No, not at all	**only slightly, doubtful**	**possibly, somewhat**	**probably, quite likely**	**yes, definitely**

   c) By someone else? Specify: _____

1	2	3	4	5
No, not at all	**only slightly, doubtful**	**possibly, somewhat**	**probably, quite likely**	**yes, definitely**

4. If any answer except "no, not at all", indicate what kind(s) of abuse(s) is (are) suspected.

   a) ☐ physical

   b) ☐ psychosocial

   c) ☐ financial

   d) ☐ neglect (includes passive and active)

5. If abuse is suspected, how soon do you estimate that intervention is needed?

1	2	3	4	5
Immediately	**within 24 hrs.**	**24-72 hrs.**	**1 week**	**2 or more weeks**

_____   _____

Signature and Designation   Date

From Reis M, Nahmiash D: *When seniors are abused: a guide to intervention*, Concord, Ontario, 1995, Captus Press. Reprinted with permission of Captus Press, Inc, Units 14 and 15, 1600 Steeles Avenue, West Concord, Ontario, Canada L4K 4M4. Email: info@captus.com; Internet: http://www.captus.com.

Caregiver Abuse Screen (CASE)

Name: _____

Date: _____

Address: _____

Phone: _____

D.O.B.: _____ Gender: Male   Female

Medical Record #: _____

Please answer the following questions as a helper or caregiver:

1. Do you sometimes have trouble making (_____) control his/her temper or aggression?   ☐ Yes   ☐ No

2. Do you often feel that you are being forced to act out of character or do things you feel bad about?   ☐ Yes   ☐ No

3. Do you find it difficult to manage (_____'s) behaviour?   ☐ Yes   ☐ No

4. Do you sometimes feel that you are forced to be rough with (_____)?   ☐ Yes   ☐ No

5. Do you sometimes feel that you can't do what is really necessary or what should be done for (_____)?   ☐ Yes   ☐ No

6. Do you often feel that you have to reject or ignore (_____)?   ☐ Yes   ☐ No

7. Do you often feel so tired and exhausted that you cannot meet (_____'s) needs?   ☐ Yes   ☐ No

8. Do you often feel that you have to yell at (_____)?   ☐ Yes   ☐ No

From Reis M, Nahmiash D: *When seniors are abused: a guide to intervention*, Concord, Ontario, 1995, Captus Press. Reprinted with permission of Captus Press, Inc, Units 14 and 15, 1600 Steeles Avenue, West Concord, Ontario, Canada L4K 4M4. Email: info@captus.com; Internet: http://www.captus.com.

Blessed Dementia Scale and Information-Memory Concentration (IMC) Test

Name: _____

Date: _____

Address: _____

Phone: _____

D.O.B.: _____ Gender: Male   Female

Medical Record #: _____

Changes in performance of everyday activities

1. Inability to perform household tasks	1	½	0
2. Inability to cope with small sums of money	1	½	0
3. Inability to remember short list of items, e.g. in shopping	1	½	0
4. Inability to find way about indoors	1	½	0
5. Inability to find way about familiar streets	1	½	0
6. Inability to interpret surroundings (e.g. to recognize whether in hospital, or at home, to discriminate between patients, doctors and nurses, relatives and hospital staff etc)	1	½	0
7. Inability to recall recent events (e.g. recent outings, visits of relatives or friends to hospital, etc.)	1	½	0
8. Tendency to dwell in the past	1	½	0

Changes in habits

9. Eating:

Cleanly with proper utensils	0
Messily with spoon only	2
Simple solids, e.g. biscuits	2
Has to be fed	3

10. Dressing:

Unaided	0
Occasionally misplaced buttons, etc.	1
Wrong sequence, commonly forgetting items	2
Unable to dress	3

11. Complete sphincter control | 0
Occasional wet beds	1
Frequent wet beds	2
Doubly incontinent	3

Changes in personality, interests, drive

No change	0
12. Increased rigidity	1
13. Increased egocentricity	1
14. Impairment of regard for feelings of others	1
15. Coarsening of affect	1
16. Impairment of emotional control, e.g. increased petulance and irritability	1
17. Hilarity in inappropriate situations	1
18. Diminished emotional responsiveness	1
19. Sexual misdemeanour (appearing de novo in old age)	1
Interests retained	0
20. Hobbies relinquished	1
21. Diminished initiative or growing apathy	1
22. Purposeless hyperactivity	1

Total _____

Ascertain from relative/friend. Applies to last 6 months. Score lies between 0 (fully preserved capacity) and +28 (extreme incapacity)

Information–Memory–Concentration Test

Information test-Score for correct response shown; incorrect responses score 0.

Name	1
Age	1
Time (hour)	1
Time of day	1
Day of week	1
Date	1
Month	1
Season	1
Year	1
Place—	
Name	1
Street	1
Town	1
Type of place (e.g. home, hospital, etc.)	1
Recognition of persons (cleaner, doctor, nurse, patient, relative; any two available)	2

Total _____

Memory:

(1) personal

Date of birth	1
Place of birth	1
School attended	1
Occupation	1
Name of sibs or Name of wife	1
Name of any town where patient had worked	1
Name of employers	1

(2) non-personal

Date of World War I[1]	1
Date of World War II[1]	1
Monarch[2]	1
Prime Minister[3]	1

(3) Name and address (5-minute recall)

Mr. John Brown	
42 West Street	
Gateshead[4]	5

Concentration

Months of year backwards	2	1	0
Counting 1-20	2	1	0
Counting 20-1	2	1	0

Total _____

Scores lie between 0 (complete failure) and +37 (full marks)
1. ½ for approximation within 3 years.
2. President in U.S. version.
3. Vice-President in U.S. version.
4. Chicago in U.S. version.

From Blessed G, Tomlinson BF, Roth M: The association between quantitative measures of dementia and of senile change in the cerebral grey matter of elderly subjects, *Br J Psychiatry* 114:797-811, 1968.

FROMAJE Mental Status Guide

Name: _____

Date: _____

Address: _____

Phone: _____

D.O.B.: _____ *Gender: Male   Female*

Medical Record #: _____

Spend some time with the patient in general discussion. State who you are and that you would like to spend 15 to 20 minutes with the patient, asking questions that will give you further understanding of how he or she is functioning. After establishing some comfort and rapport, proceed with the interview. By this time you will know whether a communication problem exists, such as dysarthria, aphasia, a hearing problem, or a language barrier.

A score of 1 to 3 is given for each of the seven sections; a score of 1 indicates an appropriate answer. A total score of 8 or less indicates normality (Libow, 1977, 1980). A total score of 9 or more reflects dementia; higher scores suggest worse cognitive capacity.

Function. It is necessary to seek the opinion of two primary caregivers who know the individual well (eg, nurses, relatives, friends). Questions should elicit how that person would—without any physical illness and purely on the basis of that person's social and mental function—cope with social responsibilities (eg, hygiene, managing finances).

Without home help of any form	Score 1
With part-time home help	Score 2
With 24-hour home help	Score 3

To gain further insight, one may ask the primary caregivers questions related to social function, which may help resolve conflicting opinions.

Reasoning. These questions comprise proverb interpretation and similarity discernment.
Proverbs:
The early bird catches the worm.
People who live in glass houses should not throw stones.

Similarities:
An apple and an orange; how are they similar?
A table and a chair; how are they similar?
Begin with either proverb interpretation or similarity discernment. If the interviewee responds to your satisfaction, it is not necessary to complete the other subsection. Two questions must be asked, at least. An equivocal answer in one subsection should lead the interviewer to ask questions from the other subsection.

A good, abstract answer in either section	Score 1
Concreteness (eg, an apple and an orange both taste nice or the proverb means that you should not live in a glass house)	Score 2
No answer, unintelligible, or obviously nonsensical	Score 3

Orientation. Brief questions employed here relate to time, place, and person.

Time: What is the day, month and year?
Place: Where are you now?
Person: What is your full name?
In an institutional environment, minor inaccuracies do not necessarily indicate a dementing illness. For example, if the day is Friday, and the answer is Thursday, this is allowed. Equally, if it is March and the answer is February, or if the month has recently changed, this too may be accepted as normal. However, if the answer to where are you now is, "in a hotel," this is not acceptable—whereas the response, "a hospital," may be.

A good answer with one or two minor errors (as above)	Score 1
Answers between 1 and 3; partial answers	Score 2
No answer, nonsensical, or inaccurate	Score 3

FROMAJE Mental Status Guide - 2

Memory. These questions relate to immediate, recent, and distant memory.

Immediate: Repeat these numbers: 4, 12, 18. Remember these as you will be asked for them again in a minute or so.
Recent: Where were you yesterday? What did you have for your breakfast today? (This answer requires corroboration).
Distant: Where and in what year were you born?
(Now ask the interviewee to recall the numbers)
Errors in remembering where the individual was yesterday are usually considered abnormal, but lapses in memory regarding content of the morning's breakfast are not. Many immigrant elders do not know their date of birth and allowances must be made if this is suspected. One small error here, with all else correct, would be acceptable. Failure to recall one number is allowed, and if hearing is poor, two.

A good answer, with one or two minor errors, as outlined above	Score 1
Answers between 1 and 3; partial answers	Score 2
A poor answer, as for the other sections	Score 3

Arithmetic. The questions test basic mathematic ability.

Count from 1 to 10.
Count back from 100 to 90.
If you have $100 and spend $7, what will you have left? If you spend $7 more, how much will you have?
If the interviewee can answer the serial sevens or count backwards, it is permissible to leave out the 1 to 10. Allow extra time to interviewees because arithmetic function generally is slower for them than for younger persons. Missing one number on the forwards or backwards counting may be acceptable. Allowing for time, incomplete serial sevens is not accepted as normal.

If the answers are correct	Score 1
Answers between 1 and 3, even if counting is correct	Score 2
A poor answer, no answer, or inaccurate	Score 3

Judgment. This section searches for socially appropriate, self-preservation ability, and complements the Function and Reasoning sections. Like the Reasoning section, this is a test of right and left hemispheric function. At least two questions should be asked.

If you needed help at night, how would you obtain it?
If there was a fire in your wastepaper basket, what would you do about it?
If you had trouble with your neighbor, how would you improve the situation?
A socially unacceptable answer, even if it has some logic, is not allowed, and would score 2. Answers may vary, depending upon the circumstances, but senseless answers would score 3.

A good, socially acceptable and sensible answer	Score 1
Socially unacceptable or concrete-type answer	Score 2
A poor, illogical, or unintelligible answer	Score 3

Emotion. In this final section, few questions must be asked of the interviewee, but a score of 1 or 2 (not 3) is given depending upon the appropriateness of the mood, psyche, or emotional state at the time of the interview. Evidence of depression (eg, mood, sleeplessness, anorexia) or paranoia should be sought.

If the interviewee is acting appropriately (judged by his or her circumstances) and is not significantly anxious or depressed	Score 1
Inappropriate emotion, significant anxiety, or depression	Score 2

NOTE: Maximum possible score in this screening tool is 20 points, which would indicate severe dementia.
Scoring: 7-8 = no serious abnormality 9-10 = mild dementia 11-12 = moderate dementia >13 = severe dementia

From Libow LS: A rapidly administered, easily remembered mental status evaluation: FROMAJE. In Libow LS, Sherman FT, editors: *The core of geratric medicine*, St Louis, 1980, Mosby, pp. 85-91.

6-item Cognitive Impairment Test (6CIT)

Name: _____

Date: _____

Address: _____

Phone: _____

D.O.B.: _____   *Gender: Male   Female*

Medical Record #: _____

(Note: Circle with correct answer)

1. What year is it?	Correct (0)	Incorrect (4)
2. What month is it?	Correct (0)	Incorrect (3)

Ask your patient to remember the following address (Memory Phase):
John / Brown / 42 / West Street / Chicago

3. What time is it? (within an hour)	Correct (0)	Incorrect (3)	
4. Count backwards from 20 to 1	Correct (0)	1 error (2)	More than 1 error (4)
5. Months of the year backwards	Correct (0)	1 error (2)	More than 1 error (4)
6. Repeat the Memory Phase	Correct (0)	1 error (2)	2 errors (4)
	3 errors (6)	4 errors (8)	All incorrect (10)

Score:

(A score of 8 or more is an indicator of cognitive impairment. Explore causative factors)

Hachinski Ischemic Score (HIS) for Multi-Infarct Dementia

Name: _____

Date: _____

Address: _____

Phone: _____

D.O.B.: _____ *Gender: Male   Female*

Medical Record #: _____

	Score
Abrupt onset	2
Stepwise deterioration	1
Fluctuating course	2
Nocturnal confusion	1
Relative preservation of personality	1
Depression	1
Somatic complaints	1
Emotional incontinence	1
History of hypertension	1
History of strokes	2
Generalized atherosclerosis	1
Focal neurological symptoms	2
Focal neurological signs	2

(A score of greater than 7 suggests a vascular component to the dementia.)

From Hachinski VC, Iliff LD, Silhka E, et al: Cerebral blood flow in dementia, *Arch Neurol* 32:632-637, 1975.

CHAPTER 11

Health Status Measures

Lorraine Loretz and Eric Cardin

Chapter Contents

Introduction to Measures of Health Status

Health status measures, or health-related quality of life measures, were gradually conceived as a result of a shift in thinking on the definition of health in the 20th century. Health, originally defined as absence of disease, was examined by measurement indices such as morbidity and mortality statistics, survival rates, employment disability rates, and physical functioning. Although these measures are still used today, the concept of health as total social, psychologic, and physical well-being, as defined by the World Health Organization in 1946, has led to increased use and development of more subjective indicators of health. Quality-of-life measurement from the patient's perspective has added a new dimension to the statistical indices. Outcome assessments attempt to grade the quality of life by examining functional abilities, psychologic well-being, social health, pain status, and general satisfaction with life. By incorporating these indicators of positive health into the overall picture of patient outcomes, the clinician obtains a clearer picture of the value of therapies, procedures, and rehabilitation efforts.

Health status instruments, which began development as research tools in the later part of the 20th century, are now often used to monitor progress during rehabilitation, to document the effects of disability, and to track recovery from surgery or disease. Thousands of such tools have been developed in recent years as clinicians, health and disability insurance plans, pharmaceutical companies, and employers sought methods to monitor and improve health care. Health status measures may be grouped into general areas of commonality described in Box 11-1. There may be significant overlap for many tools into two or more general categories. Most measures deal specifically with one or several of these general areas; few tools that can effectively evaluate all areas of

health without being cumbersome and time-consuming exist. The refinement of existing tools and development of new ones continue to progress globally as more and more clinicians and researchers appreciate the value of assessing health in the context of personal quality of life.

Commonly used health status measures have generally been tested in a variety of settings and populations for reliability, validity, sensitivity, and specificity. Ongoing research continues to test instruments, with efforts made to modify or further develop an instrument when reliability and validity measurements reveal gaps or weaknesses in tool items. The numerous studies for each tool vary widely in the populations evaluated, analyses of item responses, comparison of groups, and comparison with other tools. The focus of this text is to provide the reader with access to tools; as such, a brief summary of accuracy information is presented, and the reader is directed to further resources for in-depth examination of reliability and validity findings. For further information on health status measures, the reader may consult one of the fine review texts by Bowling (1997, 2001), McDowell and Newell (1996), or Turk and Melzack (2001).

Chapter Contents

This chapter contains well-known measures of health status in two general categories of instruments: quality-of-life measures and functional ability/disability measures. The overwhelming number of such instruments prevents the inclusion of most available measures; the most commonly used measures and those most pertinent for use in primary care practice have been selected for this text. Each measure is reprinted here, or the reader is directed to the source for purchase or downloading.

Health status measures specific to evaluation of the elderly may be found in Chapter 10. Measures of psychological well-being are included with other psychologic tools in Chapter 9. Pain scales are included in Chapter 12. Disease-specific measures may be found in Chapter 15. Measures involving social health are included in Chapter 16.

QUALITY-OF-LIFE AND WELL-BEING MEASURES

Spitzer's Quality of Life (QL) Index

Authors: Spitzer WL et al, 1981.

Source: Reprinted in this text, Spitzer's Quality of Life (QL) Index is also available at http://www.medal.org/ch1.html.

Targeted Population: Adults with cancer and chronic disease.

Description: Developed to assess health outcomes among persons with cancer and other chronic disease, this widely used measure can also be applied to other clinical situations involving illness. There are five items on this

---

Box 11-1 Health Measurement Areas

FUNCTIONAL ABILITY AND DISABILITY

Instruments measure physical disability and handicap:
　Activities of daily living (ADL) scales
　Instrumental activities of daily living (IADL) scales

PSYCHOLOGICAL WELL-BEING

Instruments measure cognitive functioning and
　mental status:
　Measures of cognitive impairment and dementia
　Depression and anxiety measurements

SOCIAL HEALTH

Tools measure degree of social support and
　social isolation:
　Social adjustment scales
　Measures of subjective social well-being and
　　role function
　Social support scales

PAIN MEASUREMENTS

Tools measure presence of pain and effect on quality
　of life:
　Unidimensional and multidimensional pain scales
　　measure intensity and sensation
　Pain tools based on observed behavior

GENERAL HEALTH STATUS AND QUALITY OF LIFE

General health measures seek subjective information
　about the perceived quality of life:
　Health profiles (includes a set of scores) and indices
　　(a single score summary)
　Many include sections on physical functioning and
　　disability.
　These tools often have extensive validity and
　　reliability testing.

LIFE SATISFACTION

Measures of well-being in relation to happiness,
　satisfaction, and morale

POPULATION-SPECIFIC MEASURES

Measurement tools from any of the above categories
　that focus on a single population, disease, injury, or
　condition

---

brief tool, related to five domains of function: activity level (including occupation), activities of daily living (ADL), health, support, and outlook. The patient responds according to his or her perception of wellness during the past week for each domain. Additionally, there is the Spitzer Quality of Life Uniscale, an optional visual analogue scale for overall quality of life assessment, with parameters ranging from "lowest quality" to "highest quality."

Scores: Scores of 0, 1, or 2 are selected for each domain based on which parameter most closely matches the patient's current condition. The QL Index is the sum of the scores for the five domains. Scores range from 0 to 10, with high scores better than low scores. Scores of 0 to 3 are considered very low scores. A patient is often reassessed at intervals of weeks to months to monitor the trend of quality-of-life experience.

Accuracy: The QL Index was initially judged to have content validity and has shown statistically significant correlation with other global functioning indices (Spitzer et al, 1981; Gough et al, 1983; Mor, 1987). However, later analyses have called into question the validity of the index, suggesting that the scale did not appropriately address quality-of-life issues for patients with cancer and demonstrated variations in reproducibility (Slevin et al, 1988). The QL Index does not discriminate differences in global quality of life in healthy people (Spitzer et al, 1981), and there is the added confusion of several dimensions contained within each of the five items. Despite these shortcomings, the QL Index remains widely used and accepted by clinicians. The brevity of the tool, its ease in administration, and general limitation to physical functioning make this tool best used for monitoring global long-term progress of seriously ill patients (Wood-Dauphinee & Williams, 1991).

Administration Time: 1 to 2 minutes by proxy administration.

References

Gough IR, Furnival CM, Schilder L, et al: Assessment of the quality of life of patients with advanced cancer. *Eur J Cancer Clin Oncol* 19:1161-1165, 1983.

Mor V: Cancer patients' quality of life over the disease course: lessons from the real world. *J Chronic Dis* 40:535-544, 1987.

Slevin ML, Plant H, Lynch D, et al: Who should monitor quality of life, the doctor or the patient? *Br J Cancer* 57:109-112, 1988.

Spitzer WO, Dobson AJ, Hall J, et al: Measuring the quality of life of cancer patients: a concise QL-Index for use by physicians. *J Chronic Dis* 34:585-597, 1981.

Wood-Dauphinee S, Williams JI: The Spitzer Quality-of-Life Index: its performance as a measure. In Osoba D, ed. *Effect of cancer on quality of life*, Boca Raton, FL, 1991: CRC Press, pp. 169-184.

COOP Functional Assessment Charts

Authors: Nelson EC, Wasson J, 1987.

Source: The nine COOP Charts are copyrighted by the Dartmouth College/COOP Project 1995, Dartmouth Medical School, Butler Building, HB 7265, Hanover, NH 03755; phone: 603-650-1220; fax: 603-650-1331. The charts are available and permitted for personal use at http://www.dartmouth.edu/~coopproj/figure1.html.

Targeted Population: Adults.

Description: This tool consists of nine charts that measure a patient's overall functional health. Each COOP chart consists of a title, a question referring to the status of the patient over the past 2 to 4 weeks, and five response choices. Each response is illustrated by a drawing that depicts a level of functioning or well-being along a 5-point ordinal scale (Nelson et al, 1998, 1987). The charts represent four domains of health: function (physical fitness, daily activities, and social activities), health perceptions (quality of life, overall health, and change in health), symptoms and feelings (pain, emotional status), and social support (McDowell & Newell, 1996). The charts were designed for use in clinical primary care settings.

Scores: Scores for each chart range from 1 to 5, with 1 representing the most favorable level of health, and 5 representing the least favorable level of health with severe limitations.

Accuracy: The COOP charts have been tested extensively in many clinical settings with large samples. Studies have revealed the charts to be useful, to be accepted by staff and patients, and to have provided information that led to changes in management (Landgraf et al, 1990; Nelson et al, 1990). McDowell and Newell (1996) cite numerous studies that support the reliability and the convergent, divergent, and discriminatory validity of the charts.

Administration Time: ~2 to 5 minutes by self-administration.

References

Landgraf JM, Nelson EC, Hays RD, et al: Assessing function: does it really make a difference? A preliminary evaluation of the acceptability and utility of the COOP Function Charts. In Lipkin M, ed: *Functional status measurement in primary care* (pp. 150-165). New York, 1990: Springer-Verlag.

McDowell I, Newell C: *Measuring health: a guide to rating scales and questionnaires*, ed 2. New York, 1996: Oxford University Press, pp. 410-417.

Nelson EC, Wasson JH, Johnson DJ, et al: Dartmouth COOP functional health assessment charts: brief measures for clinical practice, 1998. Available at http://www.dartmouth.edu/~coopproj/more_charts.html.

Nelson EC, Wasson J, Kirk J, et al: Assessment of function in routine clinical practice: description of the COOP Chart method and preliminary findings. *J Chronic Dis* 40(suppl 1):55S-63S, 1987.

Nelson EC, Landgraf JM, Hays RD, et al. The COOP Function Charts: a system to measure patient function in physicians' offices: In Lipkin M, ed. *Functional status measurement in primary care* (pp. 97-131). New York, 1990: Springer-Verlag.

The Duke Health Profile

Author: Parkerson GR, et al, 1990.

Source: The developers of the Duke Health Profile (DUKE) encourage its use by others. The measure is copyrighted; however, permission to use it for clinical and research purposes is granted on request, usually without charge. For further information, contact the Department of

Community and Family Medicine, Duke University Medical Center, Durham, NC 27710; phone: 919-681-3043; e-mail: parke001@mc.duke.edu. The Duke Instrument Packet contains a master copy of the instrument including royalty-free permission to use and reproduce, the *DUKE User's Guide for Duke Health Measures*, and research reference materials. This packet may be ordered from http://www.outcomes-trust.org/instruments.htm.

Targeted Population: Adults.

Description: The DUKE is a brief and practical measure for self-reported health-related quality of life and functional health status. This tool consists of 17 items covering six health scales (physical, mental, social, general, perceived health, and self-esteem) and four dysfunction scales (anxiety, depression, pain, and disability). The physical, mental, social, and perceived health scales and the disability scale are independent of each other in that none of their items are shared, whereas the other scales have shared items. The DUKE has been used mostly for primary care patients but can also be used for patients with chronic conditions or subjects in research studies.

Scores: Each item has only three response options. Each response is assigned a raw score; all items for each scale are summed. If one or more responses is missing, then scores cannot be calculated for any scale that involves that item (Parkerson et al, 1990). The total raw score for each scale is divided by the maximum raw score and multiplied by 100 to provide a score ranging from 0 to 100. High scores for health measures indicate good health. High scores for dysfunction measures indicate poor health. Scoring for the 10 scales of the DUKE can be done manually or by computer.

Accuracy: Reliability and validity reports are mixed because of the lack of specificity in the component scales, absence of completely independent measures, and a physical health scale that is not comparable with other measures (McDowell & Newell, 1996). Despite these findings, the DUKE is an excellent tool when it is used as a general outcome measure in primary care.

Administration Time: 2-5 minutes by self-administration.

References

McDowell I, Newell C: *Measuring health: a guide to rating scales and questionnaires*, ed 2. New York, 1996: Oxford University Press, pp. 420-424.

Parkerson GR Jr: *User's guide for the Duke Health Profile (DUKE)*. Durham, NC, 1994: Duke University Medical Center.

Parkerson GR, Broadhead WE, Tse C-KJ: The Duke Health Profile: a 17-item measure of health and dysfunction. *Med Care* 28:1056-1072, 1990.

Parkerson GR, Broadhead WE, Tse C-KJ. 1995. Health status and severity of illness as predictors of outcomes in primary care. *Med Care* 33:53-66, 1995.

Arthritis Impact Measurement Scales 2 (AIMS2) and Arthritis Impact Measurement Scales 2–Short Form (AIMS2-SF)

Authors: Arthritis Impact Measurement Scales 2 (AIMS2): Meenan RF et al, 1992; Arthritis Impact Measurement Scales 2–Short Form (AIMS2-SF): Guillemin F et al, 1997.

Source: The AIMS2 is reprinted in this text. Information about the AIMS2, the AIMS2-SF and permission for use are available at http://www.qolid.org/public/aims/cadre/. The full AIMS2 may be viewed online at http://www.qolid.org/public/aims/cadre/aims2.pdf. The AIMS2-SF may be viewed online at http://www.medal.org/ch37.html.

Targeted Population: Adults.

Description: The AIMS2 was developed from the Arthritis Impact Measurement Scales (AIMS), originally published by Meenan et al (1980). The AIMS was designed to measure changes in global health, pain, mobility, and social function in patients with arthritis. Over time, the AIMS has been refined, tested, translated, and modified to become one of the most widely used outcome measures in arthritis research. Application to clinical settings has been ongoing, and with the AIMS2-SF, a concise, yet valid, instrument is available for routine clinical use (Ren et al, 1999).

The original AIMS had 45 items and nine subscales assessing mobility, physical activity, dexterity, household activity, social activities, ADL, pain, depression, and anxiety. The revised version, AIMS2, contains 57 questions derived from the original AIMS plus 44 more questions dealing with satisfaction with health, the impact of arthritis on function, and patient priorities for improvement (Meenan et al, 1992). The nine subscales were renamed, and three more subscales were added (arm function, social support, and work). The AIMS2-SF was developed to evaluate patients more quickly, yet preserve content validity. It contains 26 items with five subscales (physical, symptoms, affect, social interaction, and role) (Guillemin et al, 1997).

Scores: Each item is scored on a 5-point scale ranging from always functions (0) to never functions (4) or similar descriptors. The patient chooses the response most closely approximating the past month's experiences. Higher scores indicate greater limitations. Complete administration, scoring and interpretation information is available online at: http://www.qolid.org/public/aims/cadre/guide.pdf.

Accuracy: Both the AIMS2 and AIMS2-SF have shown good to excellent reliability and validity, including internal consistency and test-retest reliability, in multiple studies (Bowling, 2001; Ren et al, 1999). The AIMS2-SF has psychometric properties similar to those of the AIMS2 (Guillemin et al, 1997), and the AIMS2 and AIMS2-SF have shown substantial to near-perfect agreement (Haavardsholm et al, 2000).

Administration Time: By self-administration: 20 minutes for AIMS2; 5-10 minutes for AIMS2-SF.

References

Bowling A: *Measuring disease*, ed 2. Philadelphia, 2001: Open University Press, pp. 233-235.

Guillemin F, Coste J, Pouchot J, et al: The AIMS2-SF: a short form of the Arthritis Impact Measurement Scales 2. French Quality of Life in Rheumatology Group. *Arthritis Rheum* 40:1267-1274, 1997.

Haavardsholm EA, Kvien TK, Uhlig T, et al: A comparison of agreement and sensitivity to change between AIMS2 and a short form of AIMS2 (AIMS2-SF) in more than 1,000 rheumatoid arthritis patients. *J Rheumatol* 27:2810-2816, 2000.

McDowell I, Newell C: *Measuring health: a guide to rating scales and questionnaires*, ed 2. New York, 1996: Oxford University Press, pp. 383-393.

Meenan RF, Gertman PM, Mason JH: Measuring health status in arthritis. The arthritis impact measurement scales. *Arthritis Rheum* 23: 146-152, 1980.

Meenan RF, Mason JH, Anderson JJ, et al: AIMS2: the content and properties of a revised and expanded Arthritis Impact Measurement Scales health status questionnaire. *Arthritis Rheum* 35:1-10, 1992.

Ren XS, Kazis L, Meenan R: Short-form Arthritis Impact Measurement Scales 2: tests of reliability and validity among patients with osteoarthritis. *Arthritis Care Res* 12:163-171, 1999.

Other Measures:

Sickness Impact Profile   i

Author: Bergner M, et al, 1976; Revised 1981.

Source: Copyright is held by Johns Hopkins University, 1977. The Medical Outcomes Trust provides Sickness Impact Profile (SIP) purchasing information at http://www.outcomes-trust.org. The SIP is sold as an instrument packet that contains a master copy of the instrument (including royalty-free permission to use and reproduce), a SIP user manual, technical notes, and reviews.

Targeted Population: Adults.

Description: This 136-item health status questionnaire provides a descriptive profile of changes in a person's behavior as a result of sickness. The SIP contains 12 categories (sleep and rest, eating, work, home management, recreation and pastimes, ambulation, mobility, body care and movement, social interaction, alertness behavior, emotional behavior, communication) and two overall domains (physical and psychosocial) (Bergner et al, 1975, 1976, 1981).

The SIP is available in eight languages; references are listed at http://www.vtpu.org.au/resources/translatedinstruments/mi/mi-sip.php.

Scores: Respondents check the items that apply to them and are related to their health. For each category, the scores are summed and expressed as a percentage of the maximum score possible. Higher scores represent greater dysfunction. An overall score, 2 domain scores, and 12 category scores may be calculated; items are weighted according to a standardized weighting scheme.

Accuracy: The SIP has been comprehensively tested and validated; it was developed with multiple field trials over 6 years. McDowell and Newell (1996) have summarized psychometric data; test-retest reliability, internal consistency, and interrater reliabilities have been reported as excellent. The SIP has compared favorably with most leading health status measures, although some studies suggest that it is not sensitive to small changes in a

patient's status. The SIP is often used as the "gold standard" against which other health status instruments are evaluated.

Administration Time: 20 to 30 minutes, by self-administration or interview.

References

Bergner M, Bobbitt RA, Carter WB, et al: The Sickness Impact Profile: development and final revision of a health status measure. *Med Care* 19:787-805, 1981.

Bergner M, Bobbitt RA, Kressel S, et al: The Sickness Impact Profile: conceptual formulation and methodology for the development of a health status measure. *Int J Health Serv* 6:393-415, 1976.

Gilson BS, Gilson JS, Bergner M, et al: The Sickness Impact Profile: development of an outcome measure of health care. *Am J Public Health* 65:1304-1310, 1975.

McDowell I, Newell C: *Measuring health: a guide to rating scales and questionnaires*, ed 2. New York, 1996: Oxford University Press, pp. 431-438.

Medical Outcomes Study Short Form 36 (MOS SF-36) and Medical Outcomes Study Short Form 12 (MOS SF-12)   i

Author: Ware JE, 1992.

Source: Co-copyright and trademark holders for the Medical Outcomes Study Short Form 36 (MOS SF-36) and Medical Outcomes Study Short Form 12 (MOS SF-12) are the Medical Outcomes Trust (MOT), the Health Assessment Lab, and QualityMetric Incorporated. Information regarding licensing, use, and ordering may be found online at http://www.qualitymetric.com/products/descriptions/sflicenses.shtml. The forms may be viewed at http://www.qualitymetric.com/products/SurveyInfo.shtml. The MOS SF-36, MOS SF-12, and other quality-of-life forms may also be viewed at http://www.rand.org/health/surveys.html.

Targeted Population: Adolescents (age 14 and older) and adults.

Description: Developed from the work at the Rand Corporation in Santa Monica, California, the MOS SF-36 measures health status and outcomes from the patient's point of view. The MOS SF-36 contains 36 items that measure eight dimensions: physical activities (10 items), role limitations caused by physical health problems (4 items), role limitations caused by emotional problems (3 items), social limitations (2 items), pain (2 items), general health perceptions (5 items), vitality and fatigue (4 items), and mental health (5 items). There is one question in which subjects are asked to compare current health to that of 1 year previously to provide an estimate of change in health status. The MOS SF-36 is one of the most well-known health status instruments and is used around the world.

The MOS SF-12 was developed to be a much shorter, yet valid, alternative to the MOS SF-36 for use in large surveys of general and specific populations, as well as for use in large longitudinal studies of health outcomes. The 12 items in the MOS SF-12 are a subset of those in the

MOS SF-36; the MOS SF-12 includes one or two items from each of the eight dimensions. Both standard (4-week) and acute (1-week) recall versions are available. **Scores:** Each item has a different scoring format, ranging from a simple "yes/no" response to Likert-type scales. An equation with weighted scores is used to obtain item scores; mean scores may be calculated for subscales. The scoring method is complex, is described fully in the user's manual, and can be done with automated software. An overall score is not reported.

Accuracy: The MOS SF-36 and MOS SF-12 are well-developed, concise instruments with excellent core descriptions of reliability and validity (McHorney et al, 1993, 1994). Many studies detailing the good to excellent reliability and validity of these tools are reviewed by McDowell and Newell (1996) and Bowling (1997). The MOS SF-36 has become a standard against which other instruments are measured.

Administration Time: 5 to 15 minutes by self-administration or by trained interviewer.

References

Bowling A: *Measuring health: a review of quality of life measurement scales.* Philadelphia, 1997: Open University Press, pp. 57-61.

McDowell I, Newell C: *Measuring health: a guide to rating scales and questionnaires,* ed 2. New York, 1996: Oxford University Press, pp. 446-456.

McHorney CA, Ware JE Jr, Lu JFR, et al: The MOS 36-item Short-Form Health Survey (SF-36): II. Psychometric and clinical tests of validity in measuring physical and mental health constructs. *Med Care* 31:247-263, 1993.

McHorney CA, Ware JE Jr, Raczek AE, et al: The MOS 36-item Short-Form Health Survey (SF-36): III. Tests of date quality, scaling assumptions, and reliability across diverse patient groups. *Med Care* 32:40-66, 1994.

Ware JE, Sherbourne CD: The MOS 36-item Short-Form Health Survey (SF-36). I. Conceptual framework and item selection. *Med Care* 30:473-483, 1992.

Nottingham Health Profile (NHP)   **i**

Authors: Hunt SM et al, 1981.

Source: Contact S. McKenna for permission for use: Dr. Stephen McKenna, Galen Research, Enterprise House, Manchester Science Park, Lloyd Street North, Manchester M15 6SE, UK. This tool may be viewed online at http://www.medal.org/ch1.html.

Targeted Population: Adults.

Description: The Nottingham Health Profile (NHP) provides a brief indication of a patient's perceived emotional, social, and physical health problems (Hunt et al, 1981, 1985). It serves to identify how people feel when they experience ill health. There are 45 items, 38 in part I and 7 in part II. Six domains consist of items for physical mobility (8 items), pain (8 items), social isolation (5 items), emotional reactions (9 items), energy (3 items), and sleep (5 items). This tool, which is more frequently used in Europe, is suitable for use in primary care clinical settings.

Scores: Each item is weighted on the basis of findings from previous studies. The maximum sum of the items in each domain is 100. The higher the score, the greater is the health problem. Scores are presented as profiles rather than overall scores. A mean score may be calculated across all items within each domain. The overall score is the mean across all items.

Accuracy: Extensive testing has indicated good reliability, test-retest/reproducibility, internal consistency, and validity for the NHP (MacDowell & Newell, 1996; Jenkinson et al, 1988). Disadvantages revolve around its limitations in measurement of function (some disabilities are not measured), inadequate index of mental distress, and inability to detect small improvements in health (Bowling, 1997).

Administration Time: 5 to 10 minutes by self-administration.

References

Bowling A: *Measuring health: a review of quality of life measurement scales.* Philadelphia, 1997: Open University Press, pp. 43-47.

Hunt SM, McEwen J, McKenna SP: Measuring health status: a new tool for clinicians and epidemiologists. *J Royal Coll Gen Pract* 35:185-188, 1985.

Hunt SM, McKenna SP, McEwen J, et al: The Nottingham Health Profile: subjective health status and medical consultations. *Soc Sci Med (A)* 15:221-229, 1981.

Jenkinson C, Fitzpatrick R, Argyle M: The Nottingham Health Profile: an analysis of its sensitivity in differentiating illness groups. *Soc Sci Med* 27:1411-1414, 1988.

McDowell I, Newell C: *Measuring health: a guide to rating scales and questionnaires,* ed 2. New York, 1996: Oxford University Press, pp. 438-446.

FUNCTIONAL ABILITY AND DISABILITY MEASURES

In addition to the instruments reviewed in the following sections, there are many disability indices developed for use with site-specific orthopedic injuries, pain, and disabilities. The volume of measures available is beyond the scope of this text; for further listing of disability indices, the reader is directed to references at the American Academy of Orthopaedic Surgeons website http://www.aaos.org/wordhtml/research/bjdecad/list01.htm, or other online resources listed at the end of the chapter.

Barthel Index

Authors: Mahoney FI, Barthel DW, 1965.

Source: The Barthel Index is reprinted here and is also available online at http://www.strokecenter.org/trials/scales/barthel.pdf. Copyright for the Barthel Index is held by the Maryland State Medical Society. It may be used freely for noncommercial purposes with citation by Mahoney and Barthel (1965). Permission is required to modify the Barthel Index or use it for commercial purposes.

Targeted Population: Adults in long-term care or rehabilitation settings.

Description: Designed for use with patients who have been hospitalized for long terms, the Barthel Index is intended to measure the functional ability of a patient, to monitor progress in mobility and self-care over time, and to assess nursing care needs. This 10-item tool measures the following domains: feeding, transfer mobility to and from bed, personal hygiene tasks, use of toilet, bathing, walking on level surface, ascending/descending stairs, dressing, bowel continence, and bladder continence. Tasks for daily community living, such as cooking or shopping, are omitted. A variety of versions of this measure exist; other versions are modified in number of items, item grouping, or scoring.

Scores: Each item is weighted; the sum of the items equals the Barthel Index score. The score ranges from 0 to 100, with 100 indicating complete independent performance in all domains. An "independent" assessment implies that the patient must not require assistance before, during, or after completion of a task.

Accuracy: This tool is often used as part of neurologic, psychiatric, or rehabilitation evaluations. Reliability and validity testing have shown good to excellent results (Collin et al, 1988; Wade, 1992; McDowell & Newell, 1996). Some investigators have suggested that the Barthel Index is less appropriate for disabled people who live at home, may require supplementation with a broader measure for more accurate assessments, and may be improved by expanding the numbers of categories used for each ADL function (Bowling, 2001). Despite the brevity of the scale, it is sensitive enough to accurately assess basic needs for care, for which it was designed.

Administration Time: 1-5 minutes by observer assessment or self-report.

References

Bowling A: *Measuring disease*, ed 2. Philadelphia, 2001: Open University Press, pp. 196-198.

Collin C, Wade DT, Davies S, et al: The Barthel ADL Index: a reliability study. *Int Disabil Stud* 10:61-63, 1988.

Mahoney FI, Barthel DW: Functional evaluation: the Barthel Index. *Maryland State Med J* 14:61-65, 1965.

McDowell I, Newell C: *Measuring health: a guide to rating scales and questionnaires*, ed 2. New York, 1996: Oxford University Press, pp. 56-63.

Wade DT : *Measurement in neurological rehabilitation*. Oxford, 1992: Oxford University Press.

Katz Index of Activities of Daily Living

Author: Katz S et al, 1963; Revised 1976.

Source: The Katz Index is reprinted in this text and may also be viewed online at http://www.upstate.edu/geriatric_education/assessment.html, as well as at other Internet sites.

Targeted Population: Adults, especially the elderly.

Description: The Katz Index of Activities of Daily Living (ADL) was developed to evaluate elderly and chronically ill patients for functional ability in performing essential life activities. Six activities are assessed: bathing, dressing, toileting, transferring from bed to chair, continence, and feeding. The patient is assessed in each of these functions, and on the basis of the pattern for independence or dependence, one of eight grades is assigned. The grade is then used in assessing prognosis and guiding rehabilitation. The index does not measure instrumental activities such as housework, managing finances, or shopping.

Scores: Each activity is rated on a 3-point scale of independence. The 3-point scales are then translated into a dependent/independent classification by using guidelines developed by Katz et al (1970). The patient's overall performance is then summarized on an 8-point scale describing the level of independent activities. A simplified scoring system is used to count the number of activities in which the patient is dependent; total scores range from 0 (independent in all functions) to 6 (dependent in all functions).

Accuracy: The Katz Index was the first ADL scale published, and as such, continues to be widely used. Little formal reliability or validity testing has been reported, but its utility in evaluating the functional status of the elderly has been universally recognized. The index is not sensitive to low levels of disability, nor does it take environment into account; hence, it may be inappropriate for use in general practice or among patients with minor illness. Although the Katz Index has historical importance, more sensitive and comprehensive measures for functional ability evaluation now exist.

Administration Time: The activities are best assessed over a 2-week period by observation and interview.

References

Katz S, Akpom CA: Index of ADL. *Med Care* 14:116-118, 1976.

Katz S, Downs TD, Cash HR, et al: Progress in development of the Index of ADL. *Gerontologist* 10:20-30, 1970.

Katz S, Ford AB, Moskowitz RW, et al: Studies of illness in the aged. The Index of ADL: a standardized measure of biological and psychological function. *JAMA* 185:914-919, 1963.

McDowell I, Newell C: *Measuring health: a guide to rating scales and questionnaires*, ed 2. New York, 1996: Oxford University Press, pp. 63-67.

Functional Status Index (FSI)

Author: Jette AM, 1978, 1980.

Source: The Functional Status Index (FSI) 18-item form is included in this chapter and is also available at http://www.medicalexercisespecialist.com/functional_scales/Functionals.pdf. A review of this tool is also available at http://measurementexperts.org/instrument/instrument_reviews.asp.

Targeted Population: Adults living in the community.

Description: The FSI was developed to assess the functional status of adults with arthritis. The FSI measures the degree of dependence, pain, and difficulty in performing five categories of activities: mobility, personal care, home chores, hand activities, and social activities (Jette, 1980a). A 45-item form and an 18-item form of the FSI are available; the 18-item form is included here. Each of the 18 items is assessed in three domains: level of assistance required to complete task, degree of pain associated with the task, and level of difficulty in completing the task. Task performance is considered over the past 7 days.

Scores: The rating scale for level of independence (assistance) ranges from unable or unsafe to do the activity (5 points) to independent (1 point). Pain and difficulty domains are scored on a 4-point scale with 1 point each assigned to "no pain" and "no difficulty" and 4 points each given for "severe pain" and "severe difficulty." Scores for each domain range from 18 to 90 (assistance) and 18 to 72 (pain and difficulty). Lower scores for each domain and overall indicate a higher level of functioning; higher scores indicate a greater degree of disability.

Accuracy: Reliability studies have demonstrated good to excellent results, including studies on internal consistency, test-retest reliability, and inter-rater agreement (Jette, 1980b; Jette, 1987; Jette & Deniston, 1978; McDowell & Newell, 1996). Validity studies indicate that the FSI has good sensitivity in detecting improvements in functioning, including social functioning (Bowling, 2001). McDowell and Newel (1996) suggest that more validity data be collected before extensive use of this index is implemented. From a clinician's perspective, however, this tool delivers a clear picture of changes in basic functional ability and pain.

Administration Time: 20 to 30 minutes by administrator interview for the 18-item FSI.

References

Bowling A: *Measuring disease*, ed 2. Philadelphia, 2001: Open University Press, pp. 235-237.

Jette AM: Functional capacity evaluation: an empirical approach. *Arch Phys Med Rehabil* 61:85-89, 1980a.

Jette AM: Functional Status Index: reliability of a chronic disease evaluation instrument. *Arch Phys Med Rehabil* 61:395-401, 1980b.

Jette AM: The Functional Status Index: reliability and validity of a self-report functional disability measure. *J Rheumatol* 14(suppl 15):15-21, 1987.

Jette AM, Deniston OL: Inter-observer reliability of a functional status assessment instrument. *J Chronic Dis* 31:573-580, 1978.

McDowell I, Newell C: *Measuring health: a guide to rating scales and questionnaires*, ed 2. New York, 1996: Oxford University Press, pp. 84-88.

Functional Independence Measure (FIM™)

Authors: Hamilton BB, Granger CV, 1987.

Source: Copyright for the Functional Independence Measure (FIM™) is held by Uniform Data System for Medical Rehabilitations (UDS$_{MR}$^{SM}). For further information on the FIM™, please contact Uniform Data System for Medical Rehabilitations, 232 Parker Hall, University at Buffalo, 3435 Main St, Buffalo, NY 14214-3007; phone: 716-829-2076; fax: 716-829-2080; E-mail: fimnct@ubvms.cc.buffalo.edu or info@udsmr.org; website: http://www.udsmr.org.

A complete description of the FIM and an Internet forum for discussion of the FIM are available at http://www.tbims.org/combi/FIM/index.html.

A review of the FIM with administration and scoring instructions may be found at http://www.sci-queri. research.med.va.gov/fim.htm.

Targeted Population: Adults; a pediatric version (WeeFIM) is also available.

Description: Used to monitor patient progress and to assess outcomes of rehabilitation, the FIM is the central measure of the Uniform Data System for Medical Rehabilitation (UDS) (Hamilton et al, 1987; Keith et al, 1987). Formed by a national task force in 1983, the UDS seeks to maintain the world's leading outcomes database for all phases of medical rehabilitation and to lead medical rehabilitation research related to severity, disability, and measure of outcomes. With the FIM, the UDS system has successfully achieved this goal, and it is widely subscribed to by rehabilitation facilities in the United States and Europe (Deutsch et al, 2002). The FIM instrument is viewed as a brief disability measure rather than a general health instrument; it is appropriate for use as a patient assessment tool, as well as an evaluative instrument. This tool has become the standard of care for outcomes measurement in the rehabilitation community.

The FIM is composed of 18 items that are rated on a 7-point scale representing gradations of functioning from independence (7) to complete dependence (1). The 18 items assess independence in domains of self-care, sphincter control, mobility, locomotion, communication, and social cognition. The amount of assistance required by a person with a disability to perform these basic life activities safely and effectively within his or her living environment is assessed. Administration and scoring techniques are provided in training workshops conducted by UDS.

Scores: A total score is the sum of the individual item scores and ranges from 18 (total assistance) to 126 (independent).

Accuracy: The FIM has been tested for reliability and validity with excellent results (McDowell & Newell, 1996). The physical components of the FIM compare favorably with the best among the other ADL instruments, whereas the cognitive and social communication domains may have low sensitivity. Documentation for the FIM is outstanding, and the instrument benefits from continued refinement by UDS.

Administration Time: 30 minutes to administer and score by trained clinicians or nonclinicians.

References

Deutsch A, Fiedler RC, Granger CV, et al: The Uniform Data System for Medical Rehabilitation report of patients discharged from comprehensive medical rehabilitation programs in 1999. *Am J Phys Med Rehabil* 81:133-142, 2002.

Hamilton BB, Granger CV, Sherwin FS, et al: A uniform national data system for medical rehabilitation (pp. 137-147). In Fuhrer MJ, ed: *Rehabilitation outcomes: analysis and measurement*. Baltimore, 1987: Paul H. Brookes.

Keith RA, Granger C, Hamilton BB, et al: The Functional Independence Measure: a new tool for rehabilitation. In Eisenberg MG, Grzesiak RC, eds: *Advances in clinical rehabilitation*, vol 1 (pp. 6-18), 1987.

McDowell I, Newell C: *Measuring health: a guide to rating scales and questionnaires*, ed 2. New York, 1996: Oxford University Press, pp. 115-121.

Pain Disability Index (PDI)

Author: Pollard CA, 1984.

Source: The Pain Disability Index (PDI) is reprinted here and is also available online at http://www.medal.org/ch37.html.

Targeted Population: Adults.

Description: The PDI is a brief, self-report instrument for measuring the impact that pain has on the ability of a person to participate in essential life activities. The index may be used for initial patient evaluation and to monitor patients over time to judge the effectiveness of interventions. The PDI measures seven domains of life activity that may be disrupted by chronic pain: family/home responsibilities, recreation, social activity, occupation, sexual behavior, self-care, and life support activity. Each of the domain activities is defined for the patient on the instrument. For each domain, a visual analogue scale with numbers 0 (no disability) to 10 (total disability) is presented for patient rating. The patient circles the number on the scale that best represents the level of disability caused by the overall pain present in his or her life.

Scores: Scores for each domain are summed and range from 0 (no disability) to 70 (total disability), which is the *pain disability index*. The higher the index, the greater is the disability caused by pain.

Accuracy: Reliability and validity studies indicate that the PDI has modest test-retest reliability and discriminates between patients with low and high levels of disability (Tait et al, 1990; Chibnall & Tait, 1994). Jerome and Gross (1991) found that the discretionary activities were more likely than the obligatory factors to distinguish working and nonworking persons with pain, as well as depressed and nondepressed patients. Turk and Melzack (2001) caution that the face-apparent nature of the tool and possible patient biases (e.g., toward increased disability) in reporting may affect the validity of the instrument.

Administration Time: 1 to 2 minutes by self-administration.

References

Chibnall JT, Tait RC: The Pain Disability Index: factor structure and normative data. *Arch Phys Med Rehabil* 75:1082-1086, 1994.

Pollard CA: Preliminary validity study of the pain disability index. *Percept Mot Skills* 59:974, 1984.

Tait RC, Pollard CA, Margolis RB, et al: The Pain Disability Index: psychometric and validity data. *Arch Phys Med Rehabil* 68:438-441, 1987.

Tait RC, Chibnall JT, Krause S: The pain disability index: psychometric properties. *Pain* 40:171-182, 1990.

Jerome A, Gross RT: Pain Disability Index: construct and discriminant validity. *Arch Phys Med Rehabil* 72:920-922, 1991.

Turk DC, Melzack R, editors: *Handbook of pain assessment*, ed 2 (p. 372). New York, 2001: Guilford Press.

Other Measures:

Stanford Health Assessment Questionnaire (HAQ)

Author: Fries JF, 1980.

Source: The Health Assessment Questionnaire (HAQ) instrument and instructions are available for viewing and downloading at http://www.aramis.stanford.edu/HAQ.html. The HAQ is copyrighted only so it will remain unmodified; however, the authors consider the tool to be in the public domain. There is no charge for permission to use this instrument. This site also includes an extensive list of references regarding this measure.

Targeted Population: Adults.

Description: The HAQ was originally developed in 1978 by James F. Fries, MD, and colleagues at Stanford University (Fries et al, 1980, 1982). Developed as a comprehensive measure of outcome in patients with a wide variety of rheumatic diseases, the HAQ has also been used as a generic instrument for self-reported patient outcomes. It has become the dominant instrument for evaluation of health status for many diseases, including arthritis. It is widely used throughout the world to measure difficulty in performing ADL.

The "full five dimension" HAQ is a comprehensive instrument that catalogues patient outcomes in four domains: disability, discomfort and pain, drug side effects, and dollar costs. The "2-page" or "short" HAQ includes the first two domains: The HAQ Disability Index (HAQDI) and the Pain Scale. The "short" HAQ is frequently used independently; data for these domains are based on the past week's experiences. The HAQDI assesses patients' usual abilities in eight categories: dressing and grooming, arising, eating, walking, hygiene, reach, grip, and common daily activities. Patients score the degree of difficulty they have in completing items within subcategories.

Scores: Items in the HAQDI are scored on a 4-point scale with 0 points assigned to "without any difficulty" and 3 points given for "unable to do." The total HAQDI score is a summation of the total category scores (6 minimum required) divided by the number of categories scored. The score yields a "Functional Disability Index" of 0 to 3, indicating the level of functional limitations.

Siegert et al (1984) suggested the following interpretations of overall scores: 0.0 to 0.5, the patient is completely self-sufficient; 0.5 to 1.25, the patient is reasonably self-sufficient and experiences some minor and even major difficulties in performing ADL; 1.25 to 2.0, the patient is still self-sufficient but has many major problems with ADL; 2.0 to 3.0, the patient may be called severely handicapped.

The Pain Scale is scored on a 15-cm visual analogue scale labeled from 0 (no pain) to 100 (very severe pain). The patient's mark on the scale is measured in centimeters from the left and multiplied by 0.2 to give a value of 0 to 3.

Criticism of the HAQ's scoring centers on loss of precision as a result of counting only the highest score in each category. Thus the HAQ summarizes the patient's major difficulty but does not use all the information collected, resulting in comparative insensitivity to measuring change.

Accuracy: Numerous studies reveal the HAQ to have strong reliability and validity, including internal consistency, test-retest reliability, and correlation with other prominent disability instruments (Bruce & Fries, 2003; MacDowell & Newell, 1996). Because of its rigorous testing and descriptive nature, this instrument has been widely used for outcomes measurement in rheumatology. **Administration Time:** 5 minutes for the "short" HAQ; 20 to 30 minutes for the full HAQ by self-report or administration. The questionnaire is typically mailed to patients for completion every 6 months to track progress.

References

Bruce B, Fries JF: The Stanford Health Assessment Questionnaire: a review of its history, issues, progress, and documentation. *J Rheumatol* 30:167-178, 2003. Available at http://www.aramis.stanford.edu/downloads/JRheumatol_new%20HAQ.pdf

Fries JF, Spitz P, Kraines RG, et al: Measurement of patient outcome in arthritis. *Arthritis Rheum* 23:137-145, 1980.

Fries JF, Spitz PW, Young DY: The dimensions of health outcomes: the Health Assessment Questionnaire, disability and pain scales. *J Rheumatol* 9:789-793, 1982.

McDowell I, Newell C: *Measuring health: a guide to rating scales and questionnaires,* ed 2. New York, 1996: Oxford University Press, pp. 106-115.

Siegert CE, Vleming LJ, Vandenbroucke JP, et al: Measurement of disability in Dutch rheumatoid arthritis patients. *Clin Rheumatol* 3:305-309, 1984.

Online Resources

Quality of Life Instruments Database (QOLID): http://www.qolid.org/ This extensive database identifies and describes quality-of-life (QOL) and patient-reported outcomes (PRO) instruments and facilitates access to the measures. Basic information on more than 1000 instruments is available to the public; access to copies of the instruments, translations, and user manuals is available for a subscription fee. Instruments are grouped by generic terms, alphabetical listing, pathology/disease category, targeted population, and author's name. A 10-criteria search engine is also available.

The Jason Program: http://www.jasonprogram.org/tools.htm. This site provides links to tools suitable for palliative care. Resources include pain rating scales and forms, quality-of-life measures, handheld software, prescribing information, protocols, and order sheets.

The Medical Algorithms Project: http://www.medal.org/ch1.html. The Medical Algorithms Project; developed by Quanta Healthcare Solutions, Inc, 2002, provides access to tools and algorithms published for professional use. Chapter 1 includes full access to many quality-of-life instruments and performance measures. Chapter 37 includes numerous occupational medicine and disability assessment tools pertinent for a variety of primary care topics (http://www.medal.org/ch37.html).

Center on Outcome Measurement in Brain Injury (COMBI): http://www.tbims.org/combi/index.html. This online resource provides detailed information and support regarding outcome measures for brain injuries. More than 20 instruments are reviewed, ranging from disability assessment tools to family needs assessment.

Spitzer's Quality of Life (QL) Index

Score each heading 2, 1, or 0 according to your most recent assessment of the patient.

Activity — *During the last week, the patient*

- has been working or studying full-time or nearly so, in usual occupation; or managing own household; or participating in unpaid or voluntary activities, whether retired or not — 2
- has been working or studying in usual occupation or managing own household or participating in unpaid or voluntary activities; but requiring major assistance or a significant reduction in hours worked or a sheltered situation or was on sick leave — 1
- has not been working or studying in any capacity and not managing own household — 0

Daily living — *During the last week, the patient*

- has been self-reliant in eating, washing, toileting, and dressing; using public transport or driving own car — 2
- has been requiring assistance (another person or special equipment) for daily activities and transport but performing light tasks — 1
- has not been managing personal care or light tasks and/or has not been leaving own home or institution at all — 0

Health — *During the last week, the patient*

- has been appearing to feel well or reporting feeling "great" most of the time — 2
- has been lacking energy or not feeling entirely "up to par" more than just occasionally — 1
- has been feeling very ill or "lousy," seeming weak and washed out most of the time or was unconscious — 0

Support — *During the last week*

- the patient has been having good relationships with others and receiving strong support from at least one family member and/or friend — 2
- support received or perceived has been limited from family and friends and/or by the patient's condition — 1
- support from family and friends occurred infrequently or only when absolutely necessary or patient was unconscious — 0

Outlook — *During the past week the patient*

- has usually been appearing calm and positive in outlook, accepting and in control of personal circumstances, including surroundings — 2
- has sometimes been troubled because not fully in control of personal circumstances or has been having periods of obvious anxiety or depression — 1
- has been seriously confused or very frightened or consistently anxious and depressed or unconscious — 0

QL-Index total

How confident are you that your scoring of the preceding dimensions is accurate? Please ring [circle] the appropriate category.

Absolutely confident 1	Very confident 2	Quite confident 3	Not very confident 4	Very doubtful 5	Not at all confident 6

From Spitzer WO, Dobson AJ, Hall J, et al: Measuring the quality of life of cancer patients: A concise QL-index for use by physicians, *J Chronic Dis* 34:591, 1981.

COOP Functional Assessment Charts

Patient Name: _____

Date: _____

PHYSICAL FITNESS

During the past 4 weeks . . .
What was the hardest physical activity you could do for at least 2 minutes?

Very heavy, (for example) • Run, fast pace • Carry a heavy load upstairs or uphill (25 lbs/10 kgs)		1
Heavy, (for example) • Jog, slow pace • Climb stairs or a hill moderate pace		2
Moderate, (for example) • Walk, medium pace • Carry a heavy load level ground (25 lbs/10 kgs)		3
Light, (for example) • Walk, medium pace • Carry light load on level ground (10 lbs/5 kgs)		4
Very light, (for example) • Walk, slow pace • Wash dishes		5

FEELINGS

During the past 4 weeks . . .
How much have you been bothered by emotional problems such as feeling anxious, depressed, irritable or downhearted and blue?

Not at all		1
Slightly		2
Moderately		3
Quite a bit		4
Extremely		5

DAILY ACTIVITIES

During the past 4 weeks . . .
How much difficulty have you had doing your usual activities or task, both inside and outside the house because of your physical and emotional health?

No difficulty at all		1
A little bit of difficulty		2
Some difficulty		3
Much difficulty		4
Could not do		5

COOP Functional Assessment Charts - 2

SOCIAL ACTIVITIES

During the past 4 weeks. . .
Has your physical and emotional health limited your social activities with family, friends, neighbors or groups?

1	Not at all
2	Slightly
3	Moderately
4	Quite a bit
5	Extremely

PAIN

During the past 4 weeks. . .
How much bodily pain have you generally had?

1	No pain
2	Very mild pain
3	Mild pain
4	Moderate pain
5	Severe pain

CHANGE IN HEALTH

How would you rate your overall health now compared to 4 weeks ago?

1	Much better
2	A little better
3	About the same
4	A little worse
5	Much worse

COOP Functional Assessment Charts - 3

QUALITY OF LIFE

How have things been going for you during the past 4 weeks?

Very well: could hardly be better	1
Pretty Good	2
Good and bad parts about equal	3
Pretty bad	4
Very bad: could hardly be worse	5

SOCIAL SUPPORT

During the past 4 weeks. . .
Was someone available to help you if you needed and wanted help? For example if you
– felt very nervous, lonely, or blue
– got sick and had to stay in bed
– needed someone to talk to
– needed help with daily chores
– needed help just taking care of yourself

Yes, as much as I wanted	1
Yes, quite a bit	2
Yes, some	3
Yes, a little	4
No, not at all	5

OVERALL HEALTH

During the past 4 weeks. . .
How would you rate your health in general?

Excellent	1
Very good	2
Good	3
Fair	4
Poor	5

The Duke Health Profile

Note: The scores shown are used in calculating the seven health measures. In calculating the four negative measures, the scoring for items 2, 4, 5, 7, 10-14 and 17 is reversed (see scoring). The scores are omitted from the version completed by the respondent.

Instructions:
Here are a number of questions about your health and feelings. Please read each question carefully and check (✔) your best answer. You should answer the questions in your own way. There are no right or wrong answers.

	Yes, describes me exactly	Somewhat describes me	No, doesn't describe me at all
1. I like who I am	2	1	0
2. I am not an easy person to get along with	0	1	2
3. I am basically a healthy person	2	1	0
4. I give up too easily	0	1	2
5. I have difficulty concentrating	0	1	2
6. I am happy with my family relationships	2	1	0
7. I am comfortable being around people	2	1	0

Today would you have any physical trouble or difficulty:	None	Some	A Lot
8. Walking up a flight of stairs	2	1	0
9. Running the length of a football field	2	1	0

During the *past week:*

How much trouble have you had with:	None	Some	A Lot
10. Sleeping	2	1	0
11. Hurting or aching in any part of your body	2	1	0
12. Getting tired easily	2	1	0
13. Feeling depressed or sad	2	1	0
14. Nervousness	2	1	0

During the *past week:*

How often did you:	None	Some	A Lot
15. Socialize with other people (talk or visit with friends or relatives)	0	1	2
16. Take part in social, religious, or recreation activities (meetings, ... church, movies, sports, parties)	0	1	2

During the *past week:*

How often did you:	None	1-4 Days	5-7 Days
17. Stay in your home, a nursing home, or hospital because .... of sickness, injury, or other health problem	2	1	0

The Duke Health Profile - 2

NOTE: This page is to be used only by personnel responsible for calculating scores.

MANUAL METHOD OF SCORING THE DUKE*

Copyright © 1989 by the Department of Community and Family Medicine,
Duke University Medical Center, Durham N.C., U.S.A.

PHYSICAL HEALTH SCORE

Item	Raw Score
8 =	_____
9 =	_____
10 =	_____
11 =	_____
12 =	_____
Sum =	_____

$\div 10 = $ _____ $\times 100 = $ ☐

GENERAL HEALTH SCORE

Physical Health score = _____
Mental Health score = _____
Social Health score = _____
Sum = _____ $\div 3 = $ ☐

MENTAL HEALTH SCORE

Item	Raw Score
1 =	_____
4 =	_____
5 =	_____
13 =	_____
14 =	_____
Sum =	_____

$\div 10 = $ _____ $\times 100 = $ ☐

PERCEIVED HEALTH SCORE

Item	Raw Score
3 =	_____

$\div 2 = $ _____ $\times 100 = $ ☐

SOCIAL HEALTH SCORE

Item	Raw Score
2 =	_____
6 =	_____
7 =	_____
15 =	_____
16 =	_____
Sum =	_____

$\div 10 = $ _____ $\times 100 = $ ☐

SELF-ESTEEM SCORE

Item	Raw Score
1 =	_____
2 =	_____
4 =	_____
6 =	_____
7 =	_____
Sum =	_____

$\div 10 = $ _____ $\times 100 = $ ☐

(Change these 6 item raw scores as follows: if 0, change to 2; if 2, change to 0; if 1, no change)

ANXIETY SCORE

Item	Raw Score	Revised
2 =	_____ ,	_____
5 =	_____ ,	_____
7 =	_____ ,	_____
10 =	_____ ,	_____
12 =	_____ ,	_____
14 =	_____ ,	_____
Sum =	_____	

$\div 12 = $ _____ $\times 100 = $ ☐

(Change this item raw score as follows: if 0, change to 2; if 2, change to 0; if 1, no change)

PAIN SCORE

Item	Raw Score	Revised
11 =	_____ ,	_____

$\div 2 = $ _____ $\times 100 = $ ☐

(Change these 5 item raw scores as follows: if 0, change to 2; if 2, change to 0; if 1, no change)

DEPRESSION SCORE

Item	Raw Score	Revised
4 =	_____ ,	_____
5 =	_____ ,	_____
10 =	_____ ,	_____
12 =	_____ ,	_____
13 =	_____ ,	_____
Sum =	_____	

$\div 10 = $ _____ $\times 100 = $ ☐

(Change this item raw score as follows: if 0, change to 2; if 2, change to 0; if 1, no change)

DISABILITY SCORE

Item	Raw Score	Revised
17 =	_____ ,	_____

$\div 2 = $ _____ $\times 100 = $ ☐

*Raw score = last digit of the numeral adjacent to the blank checked by the respondent for each item. For example, the raw score for item 10 is "1" if the second blank is checked (Blanked numeral = 101).

Missing values: If one or more responses are missing within one of the ten measures, a score cannot be calculated for that particular measure.

From Parkerson GR, Broadhead WE, Tse C-KJ: The Duke Health Profile: A 17-item measure of health and dysfunction, *Med Care* 28:1070, 1990. With permission.

Arthritis Impact Measurement Scale-2 (AIMS2)

Name: _____

Address: _____

| Number | Street | Apt# |

City   State   Zip

Phone: _____ Today's Date: _____

Area Code   Number   Month   Day   Year

ID _____ 1-4/

Adm# _____ 5-6/

Card   #1   7/*

Instructions: Please answer the following questions about your health. Most questions ask about your health during the past month. There are no right or wrong answers to the questions and most can be answered with a simple check (X). Please answer every question.

Please check (**X**) the most appropriate answer for each question.
These questions refer to **MOBILITY LEVEL.**

DURING THE PAST MONTH . . .	All Days (1)	Most Days (2)	Some Days (3)	Few Days (4)	No Days (5)	AIMS
1. How often were you physically able to drive a car or use public transportation?	___	___	___	___	___	8/
2. How often were you out of the house for at least part of the day?	___	___	___	___	___	9/
3. How often were you able to do errands in the neighborhood?	___	___	___	___	___	10/
4. How often did someone have to assist you to get around outside your home?	___	___	___	___	___	11/
5. How often were you in a bed or chair for most or all of the day?	___	___	___	___	___	12/

AIMS

These questions refer to **WALKING AND BENDING.**

DURING THE PAST MONTH . . .	All Days (1)	Most Days (2)	Some Days (3)	Few Days (4)	No Days (5)	
6. Did you have trouble doing vigorous activities such as running, lifting heavy objects, or participating in strenuous sports?	___	___	___	___	___	13/
7. Did you have trouble either walking several blocks or climbing a few flights of stairs?	___	___	___	___	___	14/
8. Did you have trouble bending, lifting or stooping?	___	___	___	___	___	15/
9. Did you have trouble either walking one block or climbing one flight of stairs?	___	___	___	___	___	16/
10. Were you unable to walk unless assisted by another person or by a cane, crutches, or walker?	___	___	___	___	___	17/

AIMS

These questions refer to **HAND AND FINGER FUNCTION.**

DURING THE PAST MONTH . . .	All Days (1)	Most Days (2)	Some Days (3)	Few Days (4)	No Days (5)	
11. Could you easily write with a pen or pencil?	___	___	___	___	___	18/
12. Could you easily button a shirt or blouse?	___	___	___	___	___	19/
13. Could you easily turn a key in a lock?	___	___	___	___	___	20/
14. Could you easily tie a knot or a bow?	___	___	___	___	___	21/
15. Could you easily open a new jar of food?	___	___	___	___	___	22/

AIMS

These questions refer to **ARM FUNCTION.**

DURING THE PAST MONTH . . .	All Days (1)	Most Days (2)	Some Days (3)	Few Days (4)	No Days (5)	
16. Could you easily wipe your mouth with a napkin?	___	___	___	___	___	23/
17. Could you easily put on a pullover sweater?	___	___	___	___	___	24/
18. Could you easily comb or brush your hair?	___	___	___	___	___	25/
19. Could you easily scratch your lower back with your hand?	___	___	___	___	___	26/
20. Could you easily reach shelves that were above your head?	___	___	___	___	___	27/

AIMS

Please check (**X**) the most appropriate answer for each question.
These questions refer to **SELF-CARE TASKS.**

DURING THE PAST MONTH . . .	Always (1)	Very Often (2)	Sometimes (3)	Almost Never (4)	Never (5)	
21. Did you need help to take a bath or shower?	___	___	___	___	___	28/
22. Did you need help to get dressed?	___	___	___	___	___	29/
23. Did you need help to use the toilet?	___	___	___	___	___	30/
24. Did you need help to get in or out of bed?	___	___	___	___	___	31/

AIMS

These questions refer to **HOUSEHOLD TASKS.**

DURING THE PAST MONTH . . .	Always (1)	Very Often (2)	Sometimes (3)	Almost Never (4)	Never (5)	
25. If you had the necessary transportation, could you go shopping for groceries without help?	___	___	___	___	___	32/
26. If you had kitchen facilities, could you prepare your own meals without help?	___	___	___	___	___	33/
27. If you had household tools and appliances, could you do your own housework without help?	___	___	___	___	___	34/
28. If you had laundry facilities, could you do your own laundry without help?	___	___	___	___	___	35/

AIMS

These questions refer to **SOCIAL ACTIVITY.**

DURING THE PAST MONTH . . .	All Days (1)	Most Days (2)	Some Days (3)	Few Days (4)	No Days (5)	
29. How often did you get together with friends or relatives?	___	___	___	___	___	36/
30. How often did you have friends or relatives over to your home?	___	___	___	___	___	37/
31. How often did you visit friends or relatives at their homes?	___	___	___	___	___	38/
32. How often were you on the telephone with close friends or relatives?	___	___	___	___	___	39/
33. How often did you go to a meeting of a church, club, team, or other group?	___	___	___	___	___	40/

AIMS

These questions refer to **SUPPORT FROM FAMILY AND FRIENDS.**

DURING THE PAST MONTH . . .	Always (1)	Very Often (2)	Sometimes (3)	Almost Never (4)	Never (5)	
34. Did you feel that your family or friends would be around if you needed assistance?	___	___	___	___	___	41/
35. Did you feel that your family or friends were sensitive to your personal needs?	___	___	___	___	___	42/
36. Did you feel that your family or friends were interested in helping you solve problems?	___	___	___	___	___	43/
37. Did you feel that your family or friends understood the effects of your arthritis?	___	___	___	___	___	44/

AIMS

These questions refer to **ARTHRITIS PAIN.**

DURING THE PAST MONTH . . .	Severe (1)	Moderate (2)	Mild (3)	Very Mild (4)	None (5)	
38. How would you describe the arthritis pain you usually had?	___	___	___	___	___	45/

Please check (**X**) the most appropriate answer for each question.

	All Days (1)	Most Days (2)	Some Days (3)	Few Days (4)	No Days (5)	
39. How often did you have severe pain from your arthritis?	_____	_____	_____	_____	_____	46/
40. How often did you have pain in two or more joints at the same time?	_____	_____	_____	_____	_____	47/
41. How often did your morning stiffness last more than one hour from the time you woke up?	_____	_____	_____	_____	_____	48/
42. How often did your pain make it difficult for you to sleep?	_____	_____	_____	_____	_____	49/

AIMS

These questions refer to **WORK.**

	Paid work (1)	House work (2)	School work (3)	Unemployed (4)	Disabled (5)	Retired (6)	
DURING THE PAST MONTH . . .							
43. What has been your main form of work?	_____	_____	_____	_____	_____	_____	50/

If you answered unemployed, disabled, or retired, please skip the next four questions and go to the next page.

	All Days (1)	Most Days (2)	Some Days (3)	Few Days (4)	No Days (5)	
DURING THE PAST MONTH . . .						
44. How often were you unable to do any paid work, housework, or school work?	_____	_____	_____	_____	_____	51/
45. On the days that you did work, how often did you have to work a shorter day?	_____	_____	_____	_____	_____	52/
46. On the days that you did work, how often were you unable to do your work as carefully and accurately as you would like?	_____	_____	_____	_____	_____	53/
47. On the days that you did work, how often did you have to change the way your paid work, housework, or school work is usually done?	_____	_____	_____	_____	_____	54/

AIMS

These questions refer to **LEVEL OF TENSION.**

	Always (1)	Very Often (2)	Sometimes (3)	Almost Never (4)	Never (5)	
DURING THE PAST MONTH . . .						
48. How often have you felt tense or high-strung?	_____	_____	_____	_____	_____	55/
49. How often have you been bothered by nervousness or your nerves?	_____	_____	_____	_____	_____	56/
50. How often were you able to relax without difficulty?	_____	_____	_____	_____	_____	57/
51. How often have you felt relaxed and free of tension?	_____	_____	_____	_____	_____	58/
52. How often have you felt calm and peaceful?	_____	_____	_____	_____	_____	59/

AIMS

These questions refer to **MOOD.**

	Always (1)	Very Often (2)	Sometimes (3)	Almost Never (4)	Never (5)	
DURING THE PAST MONTH . . .						
53. How often have you enjoyed the things you do?	_____	_____	_____	_____	_____	60/
54. How often have you been in low or very low spirits?	_____	_____	_____	_____	_____	61/
55. How often did you feel that nothing turned out the way you wanted it to?	_____	_____	_____	_____	_____	62/
56. How often did you feel that others would be better off if you were dead?	_____	_____	_____	_____	_____	63/
57. How often did you feel so down in the dumps that nothing would cheer you up?	_____	_____	_____	_____	_____	64/

Please check (**X**) the most appropriate answer for each question.
These questions refer to **SATISFACTION WITH EACH HEALTH AREA.**

DURING THE PAST MONTH . . .	Very Satisfied (1)	Somewhat Satisfied (2)	Neither Satisfied Nor Dis- satisfied (3)	Somewhat Dissatisfied (4)	Very Dissatisfied (5)	
58. How satisfied have you been with each of these areas of your health?						
MOBILITY LEVEL (example: do errands)	____	____	____	____	____	65/
WALKING AND BENDING (example: climb stairs)	____	____	____	____	____	66/
HAND AND FINGER FUNCTION (example: tie a bow)	____	____	____	____	____	67/
ARM FUNCTION (example: comb hair)	____	____	____	____	____	68/
SELF-CARE (example: take bath)	____	____	____	____	____	69/
HOUSEHOLD TASKS (example: housework)	____	____	____	____	____	70/
SOCIAL ACTIVITY (example: visit friends)	____	____	____	____	____	71/
SUPPORT FROM FAMILY (example: help with problems)	____	____	____	____	____	72/
ARTHRITIS PAIN (example: joint pain)	____	____	____	____	____	73/
WORK (example: reduce hours)	____	____	____	____	____	74/
LEVEL OF TENSION (example: felt tense)	____	____	____	____	____	75/
MOOD (example: down in dumps)	____	____	____	____	____	76/

These questions refer to **ARTHRITIS IMPACT ON EACH AREA OF HEALTH.**

DURING THE PAST MONTH . . .	Not A Problem For Me (0)	Due Entirely To Other Causes (1)	Due Largely To Other Causes (2)	Due Partly To Arthritis And Partly To Other Causes (3)	Due Largely To My Arthritis (4)	Due Entirely To My Arthritis (5)	
59. How much of your problem in each area of health was due to your arthritis?							
MOBILITY LEVEL (example: do errands)	____	____	____	____	____	____	8/
WALKING AND BENDING (example: climb stairs)	____	____	____	____	____	____	9/
HAND AND FINGER FUNCTION (example: tie a bow)	____	____	____	____	____	____	10/
ARM FUNCTION (example: comb hair)	____	____	____	____	____	____	11/
SELF-CARE (example: take bath)	____	____	____	____	____	____	12/
HOUSEHOLD TASKS (example: housework)	____	____	____	____	____	____	13/
SOCIAL ACTIVITY (example: visit friends)	____	____	____	____	____	____	14/
SUPPORT FROM FAMILY (example: help with problems)	____	____	____	____	____	____	15/
ARTHRITIS PAIN (example: joint pain)	____	____	____	____	____	____	16/
WORK (example: reduce hours)	____	____	____	____	____	____	17/
LEVEL OF TENSION (example: felt tense)	____	____	____	____	____	____	18/
MOOD (example: down in dumps)	____	____	____	____	____	____	19/

ID 1-4/
Adm# 5-6/
Card #2   7/

AIMS

You have now answered questions about different AREAS OF YOUR HEALTH. These areas are listed below. Please check (**X**) up to THREE AREAS in which you would **MOST LIKE TO SEE IMPROVEMENT.** Please read all 12 areas of health choices before making your decision:

check = 1
blank = 0

60. AREAS OF HEALTH — THREE AREAS FOR IMPROVEMENT

Area		
MOBILITY LEVEL (example: do errands)	_____	20/
WALKING AND BENDING (example: climb stairs)	_____	21/
HAND AND FINGER FUNCTION (example: tie a bow)	_____	22/
ARM FUNCTION (example: comb hair)	_____	23/
SELF-CARE (example: take bath)	_____	24/
HOUSEHOLD TASKS (example: housework)	_____	25/
SOCIAL ACTIVITY (example: visit friends)	_____	26/
SUPPORT FROM FAMILY (example: help with problems)	_____	27/
ARTHRITIS PAIN (example: joint pain)	_____	28/
WORK (example: reduce hours)	_____	29/
LEVEL OF TENSION (example: felt tense)	_____	30/
MOOD (example: down in dumps)	_____	31/

Please make sure that you have checked no more than THREE AREAS for improvement.

AIMS

These questions refer to your **CURRENT** and **FUTURE HEALTH.**

	Excellent (1)	Good (2)	Fair (3)	Poor (4)	
61. In general would you say that your HEALTH NOW is excellent, good, fair, or poor?	_____	_____	_____	_____	64/

	Very Satisfied (1)	Somewhat Satisfied (2)	Neither Satisfied Nor Dis-satisfied (3)	Somewhat Dissatisfied (4)	Very Dissatisfied (5)	
62. How satisfied are you with your HEALTH NOW?	_____	_____	_____	_____	_____	32/

	Not A Problem For Me (0)	Due Entirely To Other Causes (1)	Due Largely To Other Causes (2)	Due Partly To Arthritis And Partly To Other Causes (3)	Due Largely To My Arthritis (4)	Due Entirely To My Arthritis (5)	
63. How much of your problem with your HEALTH NOW is due to your arthritis?	_____	_____	_____	_____	_____	_____	34/

Please check (**X**) the most appropriate answer for each question.

	Excellent (1)	Good (2)	Fair (3)	Poor (4)	
64. In general do you expect that your HEALTH 10 YEARS FROM NOW will be excellent, good, fair, or poor?	____	____	____	____	35/

	No Problem At All (1)	Minor Problem (2)	Moderate Problem (3)	Major Problem (4)	
65. How big a problem do you expect your arthritis to be 10 YEARS FROM NOW?	____	____	____	____	36/

AIMS

This question refers to **OVERALL ARTHRITIS IMPACT.**

	Very Well (1)	Well (2)	Fair (3)	Poor (4)	Very Poorly (5)	
66. CONSIDERING ALL THE WAYS THAT YOUR ARTHRITIS AFFECTS YOU, how well are you doing compared with other people your age?	____	____	____	____	____	37/

67. What is the main kind of arthritis that you have?

check = 1
blank = 0

Rheumatoid Arthritis	_____	38/
Osteoarthritis/Degenerative Arthritis	_____	39/
Systemic Lupus Erythematosis	_____	40/
Fibromyalgia	_____	41/
Scleroderma	_____	42/
Psoriatic Arthritis	_____	43/
Reiter's Syndrome	_____	44/
Gout	_____	45/
Low Back Pain	_____	46/
Tendonitis/Bursitis	_____	47/
Osteoporosis	_____	48/
Other	_____	49/

68. How many years have you had arthritis?   _____   50-51/

	All Days (1)	Most Days (2)	Some Days (3)	Few Days (4)	No Days (5)	
DURING THE PAST MONTH . . .						
69. How often have you had to take MEDICATION for your arthritis?	____	____	____	____	____	52/

AIMS

70. Is your health currently affected by any of the following medical problems?

		Yes (1)	No (2)	
High blood pressure _____		____	____	53/
Heart disease _____		____	____	54/
Mental illness _____		____	____	55/
Diabetes _____		____	____	56/
Cancer_____		____	____	57/
Alcohol or drug use _____		____	____	58/
Lung disease_____		____	____	59/

Please check (**X**) yes or no for each question.

	Yes (1)	No (2)	
Kidney disease _____	_____	_____	60/
Liver disease _____	_____	_____	61/
Ulcer or other stomach disease _____	_____	_____	62/
Anemia or other blood disease _____	_____	_____	63/

	Yes (1)	No (2)	
71. Do you take medicine every day for any problem other than your arthritis? _____	_____	_____	64/
72. Did you see a doctor more than three times last year for any problem other than arthritis? _____	_____	_____	65/

AIMS

Please provide the following information about yourself:

73. What is your age at this time? _____ 66-67/

74. What is your sex?

Male (1) _____ 68/
Female (2) _____

75. What is your racial background?

White (1) _____ 69/
Black (2) _____
Hispanic (3) _____
Asian or Pacific Islander (4) _____
American Indian or Alaskan Native (5) _____
Other (6) _____

76. What is your current marital status?

Married (1) _____ 70/
Separated (2) _____
Divorced (3) _____
Widowed (4) _____
Never married (5) _____

77. What is the highest level of education you received?
Less than seven years of school (1) _____ 71/
Grades seven through nine (2) _____
Grades ten through eleven (3) _____
High school graduate (4) _____
One to four years of college (5) _____
College graduate (6) _____
Professional or graduate school (7) _____

78. What is your approximate family income including wages, disability payment, retirement income and welfare? 72/

Less than $10,000 (1) _____
$10,000-$19,999 (2) _____
$20,000-$29,999 (3) _____
$30,000-$39,999 (4) _____
$40,000-$49,999 (5) _____
$50,000-$59,999 (6) _____
$60,000-$69,999 (7) _____
More than $70,000 (8) _____

Thank you for completing this questionnaire.

Arthritis Impact Measurement Scales 2–Short Form (AIMS2-SF)

Questions:	All Days	Most	Some	Few	No
(1) How often were you physically able to drive a car or use public transportation?					
(2) How often were you in a bed or chair for most or all of the day?					
(3) Did you have trouble doing vigorous activities such as running, lifting heavy objects, or participating in strenuous sports?					
(4) Did you have trouble either walking several blocks or climbing a few flights of stairs?					
(5) Were you unable to walk unless assisted by another person or by a cane, crutches, or walker?					
(6) Could you easily write with a pen or pencil?					
(7) Could you easily button a shirt or blouse?					
(8) Could you easily turn a key in a lock?					
(9) Could you easily comb or brush your hair?					
(10) Could you easily reach shelves that were above your head?					
(11) Did you need help to get dressed?					
(12) Did you need help to get in or out of bed?					
(13) How often did you have severe pain from your arthritis?					
(14) How often did your morning stiffness last more than 1 hour from the time you woke up?					
(15) How often did your pain make it difficult for you to sleep?					
(16) How often have you felt tense or high-strung?					
(17) How often have you been bothered by nervousness or your nerves?					
(18) How often have you been in low or very low spirits?					
(19) How often have you enjoyed the things you do?					
(20) How often did you feel a burden to others?					
(21) How often did you get together with friends or relatives?					
(22) How often were you on the telephone with close friends or relatives?					
(23) How often did you go to a meeting of a church, club, team, or other group?					
(24) Did you feel that your family or friends were sensitive to your personal needs?					
If you are unemployed, disabled, or retired, END of questionnaire. ELSE:					
(25) How often were you unable to do any paid work, housework, or schoolwork?					
(26) On the days that you did work, how often did you have to work a shorter day?					

Responses: based on findings during the past 4 weeks

Response	Points if unable to function	Points if able to function
all days or always	4	0
most days or very often	3	1
some days or sometimes	2	2
few days or almost never	1	3
no days or never	0	4

total score =
= SUM (points for all 24 or 26 items)

Subscales:
(1) physical: 1 2 3 4 5 6 7 8 9 10 11 12 24
(2) symptoms: 13 14 15
(3) affect: 16 17 18 20
(4) social interaction: 19 21 22 23
(5) role: 25 and 26

The scores can be rescaled to cover 0 (no impact perfect health) to 10 (maximum worst health).

Barthel Index

Date of Visit: _____

Patient Name: _____

Medical Record #: _____

Date of Birth: _____ *Age:* _____ *Gender:* Male   Female

Activity	Score

Feeding
0 = unable
5 = needs help cutting, spreading butter, etc., or requires modified diet
10 = independent   _____

Bathing
0 = dependent
5 = independent (or in shower)   _____

Grooming
0 = needs help with personal care
5 = independent face/hair/teeth/shaving (implements provided)   _____

Dressing
0 = dependent
5 = needs help but can do about half unaided
10 = independent (including buttons, zips, laces, etc.)   _____

Bowels
0 = incontinent (or needs to be given enemas)
5 = occasional accident
10 = continent   _____

Bladder
0 = incontinent, or catheterized and unable to manage alone
5 = occasional accident
10 = continent   _____

Toilet Use
0 = dependent
5 = needs some help, but can do something alone
10 = independent (on and off, dressing, wiping)   _____

Transfers (bed to chair and back)
0 = unable, no sitting balance
5 = major help (one or two people, physical), can sit
10 = minor help (verbal or physical)
15 = independent   _____

Mobility (on level surfaces)
0 = immobile or <50 yards
5 = wheelchair independent, including corners, >50 yards
10 = walks with help of one person (verbal or physical) >50 yards
15 = independent (but may use any aid; for example, stick) >50 yards _____

Stairs
0 = unable
5 = needs help (verbal, physical, carrying aid)
10 = independent   _____

Total (0-100): _____

The Barthel ADL Index: Guidelines

1. The index should be used as a record of what a patient does, not as a record of what a patient could do.
2. The main aim is to establish degree of independence from any help, physical or verbal, however minor and for whatever reason.
3. The need for supervision renders the patient not independent.
4. A patient's performance should be established by using the best available evidence. The patient, friends/relatives, and nurses are the usual sources of information, but direct observation and common sense are also important. However, direct testing is not needed.
5. Usually the patient's performance over the preceding 24-48 hours is important, but occasionally longer periods will be relevant.
6. Middle categories imply that the patient supplies over 50 percent of the effort.
7. Use of aids to be independent is allowed.

From Mahoney R, Barthel D: Functional evaluation: The Barthel Index, *Maryland State Medical Journal* 14: 61-65, 1965. Used with permission.

Katz Index of Activities of Daily Living

Date of Visit: _____

Patient Name: _____

Medical Record #: _____

Date of Birth: _____ *Age:* _____ *Gender:* Male   Female

For each area of functioning listed below, check description that applies. (The word "assistance" means supervision, direction, or personal assistance.)

BATHING - either sponge bath, tub bath, or shower.

☐

Receives no assistance (gets in and out of tub by self if tub is usual means of bathing)

☐

Receives assistance in bathing only one part of the body (such as back or a leg)

☐

Receives assistance in bathing more than one part of the body (or not bathed)

DRESSING - gets clothes from clothes closets and drawers -including underclothes and outer garments and uses fasteners (including braces if worn)

☐

Gets clothes and gets completely dressed without assistance

☐

Gets clothes and gets dressed without assistance except for assistance in tying shoe

☐

Receives assistance in getting clothes or in getting dressed or stays partly or completely undressed

TOILETING - going to the "toilet room" for bowel and urine elimination; cleaning self after elimination, and arranging clothes

☐

Goes to "toilet room," cleans self, and arranges clothes without assistance (may use object for support such as cane, walker, or wheelchair and may manage night bedpan or commode, emptying same in morning)

☐

Receives assistance in going to "toilet room" or in cleansing self or in arranging clothes after elimination or in use of night bedpan or commode

☐

Doesn't go to room termed "toilet" for the elimination process

TRANSFER

☐

Moves in and out of bed as well as in and out of chair without assistance (may be using object for support such as cane or walker)

☐

Moves in and out of bed or chair with assistance

☐

Doesn't get out of bed

CONTINENCE

☐

Controls urination and bowel movement completely by self

☐

Has occasional "accidents"

☐

Supervision helps keep control, catheter is used, or is incontinent

FEEDING

☐

Feeds self without assistance

☐

Feeds self except for getting help in cutting meat or buttering bread

☐

Receives assistance in feeding or is fed partly or completely by using tubes or intravenous fluids

From Katz S, Downs TD, Cash HR, et al: Progress in the development of the Index of ADL, *Gerontologist* 10:23, 1970.

The Index of Independence in Activities of Daily Living: Scoring and Definitions (Katz)

The Index of Independence in Activities of Daily Living is based on an evaluation of the functional independence or dependence of patients in bathing, dressing, going to toilet, transferring, continence, and feeding. Specific definitions of functional independence and dependence appear below the index.

A —Independent in feeding, continence, transferring, going to toilet, dressing, and bathing.

B —Independent in all but one of these functions.

C —Independent in all but bathing and one additional function.

D —Independent in all but bathing, dressing, and one additional function.

E —Independent in all but bathing, dressing, going to toilet, and one additional function.

F —Independent in all but bathing, dressing, going to toilet, transferring, and one additional function.

G —Dependent in all six functions.

Other —Dependent in at least two functions, but not classifiable as C, D, E, or F.

Independence means without supervision, direction, or active personal assistance, except as specifically noted below. This is based on actual status and not on ability. A patient who refuses to perform a function is considered as not performing the function, even though he is deemed able.

Bathing (sponge, shower or tub)

Independent: assistance only in bathing a single part (as back or disabled extremity) or bathes self completely

Dependent: assistance in bathing more than one part of body; assistance in getting in or out of tub or does not bathe self

Dressing

Independent: gets clothes from closets and drawers; puts on clothes, outer garments, braces; manages fasteners; act of tying shoes is excluded

Dependent: does not dress self or remains partly undressed

Going to toilet

Independent: gets to toilet; gets on and off toilet; arranges clothes; cleans organs of excretion (may manage own bedpan used at night only and may or may not be using mechanical supports)

Dependent: uses bedpan or commode or receives assistance in getting to and using toilet

Transfer

Independent: moves in and out of bed independently and moves in and out of chair independently (may or may not be using mechanical supports)

Dependent: assistance in moving in or out of bed and/or chair; does not perform one or more transfers

Continence

Independent: urination and defecation entirely self-controlled

Dependent: partial or total incontinence in urination or defecation; partial or total control by enemas, catheters, or regulated use of urinals and/or bedpans

Feeding

Independent: gets food from plate or its equivalent into mouth (precutting of meat and preparation of food, as buttering bread, are excluded from evaluation)

Dependent: assistance in act of feeding (see above): does not eat at all or receives parenteral feeding

From Katz S, Downs TD, Cash HR, et al: Progress in the development of the Index of ADL, *Gerontologist* 10:23, 1970.

Functional Status Index (FSI)

Date of Visit: _____

Patient Name: _____

Medical Record #: _____

Date of Birth: _____ *Age:* _____ *Gender:* Male   Female

Assistance
- 1 – Independent
- 2 – Uses Devices
- 3 – Uses Human Assistance
- 4 – Uses Devices and Human Assistance
- 5 – Unable or Unsafe to do the Activity

Pain
- 1 – No Pain
- 2 – Mild Pain
- 3 – Moderate Pain
- 4 – Severe Pain

Difficulty
- 1 – No Difficulty
- 2 – Mild Difficulty
- 3 – Moderate Difficulty
- 4 – Severe Difficulty

Activity	Assistance	Pain	Difficulty
Mobility			
Walking Outside	_____	_____	_____
Climbing up Stairs	_____	_____	_____
Rising from Chair	_____	_____	_____
Personal Care			
Put on Pants	_____	_____	_____
Button Shirt/Blouse	_____	_____	_____
Wash Whole Body	_____	_____	_____
Put on Shirt/Blouse	_____	_____	_____
Home Chores			
Vacuum Rug	_____	_____	_____
Reach Low Cupboard	_____	_____	_____
Do Laundry	_____	_____	_____
Do Yardwork	_____	_____	_____
Hand Activities			
Writing	_____	_____	_____
Open Container	_____	_____	_____
Dial Phone	_____	_____	_____
Social Activities			
Perform your job	_____	_____	_____
Drive a Car	_____	_____	_____
Attend meetings	_____	_____	_____
Visit Friends/Family	_____	_____	_____

Jette AM, Deniston OL: Inter-observer reliability of a functional status assessment instrument, *J Chronic Dis* 31:573-580, 1978.

FIM™ Instrument

LEVELS	7 Complete Independence (timely, safely) 6 Modified Independence (device)	**NO HELPER**
	Modified Dependence 5 Supervision (subject = 100%) 4 Minimal Assistance (subject = 75%+) 3 Moderate Assistance (subject = 50%+) **Complete Dependence** 2 Maximal Assistance (subject =25%+) 1 Total Assistance (subject = less than 25%)	**HELPER**

Self-Care
A. Eating
B. Grooming
C. Bathing
D. Dressing - Upper Body
E. Dressing - Lower Body
F. Toileting

Sphincter Control
G. Bladder Management
H. Bowel Management

Transfers
I. Bed, Chair, Wheelchair
J. Toilet
K. Tub, Shower

Locomotion
L. Walk/Wheelchair
M. Stairs

ADMISSION   DISCHARGE   FOLLOW-UP

W Walk   C Wheelchair   B Both

Motor Subtotal Score

Communication
N. Comprehension
O. Expression

A Auditory   V Visual   B Both

Social Cognition
P. Social Interaction
Q. Problem Solving
R. Memory

Cognitive Subtotal Score

TOTAL FIM™ SCORE

NOTE: Leave no blanks. Enter 1 if patient is not testable due to risk.

The Functional Independence Measure (FIM™): Items and Levels of Function

SELF-CARE

Eating. Includes use of suitable utensils to bring food to mouth, chewing and swallowing, once meal is appropriately prepared.

Grooming. Includes oral care, hair grooming, washing hands and face, and either shaving or applying makeup.

Bathing. Includes bathing the body from the neck down (excluding the back), tub, shower or sponge/bed bath. Performs safely.

Dressing—Upper Body. Includes dressing above the waist as well as donning and removing prosthesis or orthosis when applicable.

Dressing—Lower Body. Includes dressing from the waist down as well as donning or removing prosthesis or orthosis when applicable.

Toileting. Includes maintaining perineal hygiene and adjusting clothing before and after toilet or bed pan use. Performs safely.

SPHINCTER CONTROL

Bladder Management. Includes complete intentional control of urinary bladder and use of equipment or agents necessary for bladder control.

Bowel Management. Includes complete intentional control of bowel movement and use of equipment or agents necessary for bowel control.

MOBILITY

Transfers: Bed, Chair, Wheelchair. Includes all aspects of transferring to and from bed, chair, and wheelchair, and coming to a standing position, if walking is the typical mode of locomotion.

Transfer: Toilet. Includes getting on and off a toilet.

Transfers: Tub or Shower. Includes getting into and out of a tub or shower stall.

LOCOMOTION

Walking or Using Wheelchair. Includes walking, once in a standing position, or using a wheelchair, once in a seated position, on a level surface.

Check most frequent mode of locomotion. If both are about equal, check W *and* C. If initiating a rehabilitation program, check the mode for which training is intended.
( ) W = Walking ( ) C = Wheelchair

Stairs. Goes up and down 12 to 14 stairs (one flight) indoors.

COMMUNICATION

Comprehension. Includes understanding of either auditory or visual communication (e.g., writing, sign language, gestures).

Check and evaluate the most usual mode of comprehension. If both are about equally used, check A *and* V.
( ) A = Auditory ( ) V = Visual

Expression. Includes clear vocal or nonvocal expression of language. This item includes both intelligible speech or clear expression of language using writing or a communication device.

Check and evaluate the most usual mode of expression. If both are about equally used, check V *and* N.
( ) V = *Vocal* ( ) N = *Nonvocal*

SOCIAL COGNITION

Social Interaction. Includes skills related to getting along and participating with others in therapeutic and social situations. It represents how one deals with one's own needs together with the needs of others.

Problem Solving. Includes skills related to solving problems of daily living. This means making reasonable, safe, and timely decisions regarding financial, social and personal affairs and initiating, sequencing and self-correcting tasks and activities to solve the problems.

Memory. Includes skills related to recognizing and remembering while performing daily activities in an institutional or community setting. It includes ability to store and retrieve information, particularly verbal and visual. A deficit in memory impairs learning as well as performance of tasks.

DESCRIPTION OF THE LEVELS OF FUNCTION AND THEIR SCORES

INDEPENDENT—Another person is not required for the activity (NO HELPER).

7 COMPLETE INDEPENDENCE—All of the tasks described as making up the activity are typically performed safely, without modification, assistive devices, or aids, and within a reasonable time.

6 MODIFIED INDEPENDENCE—Activity requires any one or more than one of the following: an assistive device, more than reasonable time, or there are safety (risk) considerations.

DEPENDENT—Another person is required for either supervision or physical assistance in order for the activity to be performed, or it is not performed (REQUIRES HELPER).

MODIFIED DEPENDENCE—The subject expends half (50%) or more of the effort. The levels of assistance required are:

5 Supervision or setup—Subject requires no more help than standby, cuing or coaxing, without physical contact. Or, helper sets up needed items or applies orthoses.

4 Minimal contact assistance—With physical contact the subject requires no more help than touching, and subject expends 75% or more of the effort.

3 Moderate assistance—Subject requires more help than touching, or expends half (50%) or more (up to 75%) of the effort.

COMPLETE DEPENDENCE—The subject expends *less* than half (*less* than 50%) of the effort. Maximal or total assistance is required, or the activity is not performed. The levels of assistance required are:

2 Maximal assistance—Subject expends less than 50% of the effort, but at least 25%.

1 Total assistance—Subject expends less than 25% of the effort.

Pain Disability Index (PDI)

Date of Visit: _____

Patient Name: _____

Medical Record #: _____

Date of Birth: _____ *Age:* _____ *Gender:* Male Female

The rating scales below are designed to measure the degree to which several aspects of your life are presently disrupted by chronic pain. In other words, we would like to know how much your pain is preventing you from doing what you would normally do, or from doing it as well as you normally would. Respond to each category by indicating the *overall* impact of pain in your life, not just when the pain is at its worst.

For each of the seven categories of life activity listed, please circle the number on the scale which describes the level of disability you typically experience. A score of 0 means no disability at all, and a score of 10 signifies that all of the activities in which you would normally be involved have been totally disrupted or prevented by your pain.

1. *Family/Home Responsibilities.* This category refers to activities related to the home or family. It includes chores and duties performed around the house (e.g., yard work) and errands or favors for other family members (e.g., driving the children to school).

   0   1   2   3   4   5   6   7   8   9   10
   no disability   total disability

2. *Recreation.* This category includes hobbies, sports, and other similar leisure time activities.

   0   1   2   3   4   5   6   7   8   9   10
   no disability   total disability

3. *Social Activity.* This category refers to activities which involve participation with friends and acquaintances other than family members. It includes parties, theater, concerts, dining out, and other social functions.

   0   1   2   3   4   5   6   7   8   9   10
   no disability   total disability

4. *Occupation.* This category refers to activities that are a part of or directly related to one's job. This includes nonpaying jobs as well, such as that of a housewife or volunteer worker.

   0   1   2   3   4   5   6   7   8   9   10
   no disability   total disability

5. *Sexual Behavior.* This category refers to the frequency and quality of one's sex life.

   0   1   2   3   4   5   6   7   8   9   10
   no disability   total disability

6. *Self Care.* This category includes activities which involve personal maintenance and independent daily living (eg, taking a shower, driving, getting dressed, etc).

   0   1   2   3   4   5   6   7   8   9   10
   no disability   total disability

7. *Life-Support Activity.* This category refers to basic life-supporting behaviors such as eating, sleeping, and breathing.

   0   1   2   3   4   5   6   7   8   9   10
   no disability   total disability

From Pollard CA: Preliminary validity of the pain disability index, *Perceptual and Motor Skills* 59:974, 1984. Copyright Perceptual and Motor Skills.

Pain Scales

Chapter Contents

ICON KEY: ▤ Tool Printed ⊘ Tool on CD-ROM ∞ Customizable Tool **i** Information and Resources Provided for Further Acquisition

Introduction to Pain Scales

The literature is rich with pain assessment tools and scales. From pediatric oncology to surgical specialties to gerontology, clinicians have developed numerous measures with which to assess pain intensity and quality. The American Pain Society has issued guidelines for pain assessment and treatment, which emphasize the need for timely and effective assessment and treatment of pain by primary care providers (Fox et al, 2000). The American Pain Society clinical practice guidelines for the management of acute pain, and cancer pain and other types of pain, and clinical guidelines published by the U.S. Agency for Health Care Policy and Research (now the Agency for Healthcare Research and Quality [AHRQ]) (Car et al, 1992; Bigos et al, 1994; Jacox et al, 1994) have guided clinicians in the continued development of reliable assessment tools and pain management.

Documentation of pain scores in a consistent manner promotes identification of unrelieved pain and allows for monitoring improvement in pain management. The most effective pain scales are those that are easy to administer, are liked by patients and providers, and are reliable and valid in measuring pain (Keck et al, 1996). Pain scales are just one segment of the assessment process for patients with pain. In effective pain management, pain scores are used in conjunction with assessment of treatment side effects, mental well-being, and functional quality-of-life measures.

Unidimensional scales are used for reporting on a single aspect of pain, most commonly its intensity. These scales are widely used for the clinical evaluation of pain in many settings. Advantages include ease of administration, minimal training time, and valid, reliable results in most populations (Ferrell, 2000). The use of unidimensional pain scales may be more appropriate for evaluation of acute pain than for chronic pain (Ho et al, 1996). Since chronic pain is more complex in terms of social effects, degree of support, mental status, and disability issues, the assessment of chronic pain often requires more complex evaluation tools.

Multidimensional tools, such as the McGill Pain Questionnaire or health status instruments, seek information about pain quality in several domains and assess the impact of pain on activities of daily living. Although multidimensional scales provide more in-depth pain assessment, disadvantages include length of the tools, increased time to administer, and difficulty in scoring in a clinical setting (Ferrell, 2000).

Pain measures can be categorized as patient self-report scales, behavioral observations, or physiologic measures:

Self-Report Pain Scales. Self-report pain scales are considered to be the best measure because of the subjective experience of pain. Categories of self-report pain tools in which descriptions of various aspects of the dimensions of pain are used have been reported by Beyer et al (1990) and are listed in Table 12-1.

Behavioral Measures. Behavioral measures of pain rely on observation by health care professionals or surrogates to rate the severity of pain. Pain behavior tools describe pain indicators, such as body movements, cry, facial expression, consolability, and changes in usual behavior. They have been shown to be psychometrically sound when used with the general population; changes with treatment effects have also been demonstrated (Herr & Garand, 2001). Behavioral scales may be used for patients with difficulty in verbally reporting their pain because of immaturity (infants and children younger than 3 years), cognitive impairment, or language barriers. In pediatric patients, discrepancies have been found between behavioral measures and the child's self-report of pain (LaMontagne et al, 1991); parental observations have been shown to be more accurate that those of health care professionals (Beyer et al, 1990). Improvement in the accuracy of behavioral measures of pain has been shown

Table 12-1   Types of Self-Report Pain Tools Grouped by Pain Aspects

Aspects of Pain	Examples of Pain Scales
Location	Body outline tool
Intensity	Visual analogue scale, color analogue scale, poker chip scale, pain ladder, pain thermometer, numeric rating scales, verbal descriptor scale, pictorial scales, word graphic scale
Quality	McGill Pain Questionnaires, Brief Pain Inventory–Revised, health status instruments
Timing	History of pain, pain diary, daily sensation log diary, pain periodicity charts

to occur when standardized, multidimensional assessment tools are used; when staff education is provided; and when the tools are used in conjunction with a self-report measure (Colwell et al, 1996).

Physiologic Measures. Physiologic measures include autonomic changes (e.g., heart rate, blood pressure, heart rate variability) and hormonal-metabolic measures, such as plasma or salivary sampling of hormones (e.g., cortisol, epinephrine). The major disadvantage to these measures is that they are nonspecific: changes unrelated to pain may occur, or changes may be related to fear and anxiety during painful procedures. Physiologic measures are often used in combination with behavioral observations to assess pain in patients with cognitive or verbal impairment, or for pediatric patients.

Recommendations for Use in Specific Patient Populations

Adults

In adults, self-report measures such as visual or numeric scales are the most widely used tools to assess pain intensity or pain relief. Adults generally report pain honestly; infrequently, concerns may arise if the patient perceives a benefit to overreporting or underreporting pain. A multidimensional tool may be used, time permitting, if more detailed information about pain quality or impact on general health status is desired.

Pediatric

With children, as with adults, self-report measures are the preferred tool and should be used whenever children are able to communicate (McGrath et al, 1996). Choice of a pain instrument will be based on a combination of reliability and validity, availability of the scale, ease of use and scoring, age of the child, and child preferences.

Pain specialists and published clinical guidelines are in agreement that, in addition to self-report scales, changes in children's behavior, appearance, activity level, and vital signs should be noted, because these may indicate a change in the pain intensity (Royal College of Nursing, 1999). If a self-report pain measure cannot be used because of youth or disability, multiple measures such as behavioral and physiologic scales, may be used to assess intensity, quality, location, and pattern of pain. Parents tend to underestimate their children's pain, but parents' ratings are closer to children's own ratings than are nurses' ratings (Franck et al, 2000). Neonates and very young children may be assessed for pain with one of the many behavioral scales that grade body movements, facial expression, cry, vocalizations, and response to others.

Geriatric

Herr and Garand (2001) have published a thorough review of pain assessment issues in the elderly and note that it is critical to determine the patient's ability to use a self-report pain scale and to find a tool that can be consistently used with each assessment. Alterations in cognitive, sensory-perceptual, and motor abilities may interfere with the ability to communicate or to quantify the pain experience. Communication problems may also affect persons without these impairments, such as non–English-speaking patients. Persons with cognitive impairment may be able to report pain reliably at the moment or when prompted; pain recall and periodicity over time may be less reliable. Failure to recognize and treat pain can be a pitfall in treating older patients with cognitive impairment.

Numeric rating scales, the verbal descriptor scale, pictorial pain scales, and the visual analogue scale have shown acceptable validity for the older adult patient who is able to hear, read, and understand directions for using a self-report measure for pain assessment. The verbal descriptor scale and numeric rating scales are preferred by older adults, making them good first-choice measures (Herr & Garand, 2001; Carey et al, 1997). Adults with mild to moderate cognitive impairment may report pain intensity adequately by using the pain thermometer, verbal descriptor scale, or the faces pictorial scale (Ferrell et al, 1995; Weiner et al, 1998). If the patient has severe cognitive deficits, other methods of assessment are necessary, including observation of alterations in usual alert and social behavior such as confusion, social withdrawal, or apathetic behavior.

Reliability and Validity

Pain cannot be measured objectively by physiologic or clinical signs. Because there are no independent biologic markers of pain, the validity of pain scales is based largely on face value, the concurrence with other known scales, and the experience in many populations over several years (Ferrell, 2000). The pain scales included in this chapter have established psychometric properties and enjoy wide use in clinical practice for a variety of patient populations. Studies that demonstrate the reliability and validity of selected pain scales are cited in Table 12-2.

Contents of this Chapter

The pain scales included in this chapter are described in the following sections. Table 12-2 contains a summary of some widely known pain scales. Online access, if available, is noted for each tool. Pain scales may be laminated for use as convenient pocket tools in the clinical setting. Assessment of the "5th vital sign" during routine examinations or a more focused pain assessment for a particular condition is facilitated by quick access to an easy-to-use tool. An example of a pain scale ruler ready for lamination may be found online at http://www.ndhcri.org/pain/Tools/Wong-Baker_Faces_Pain_Rating_Scale.pdf. This ruler includes the Wong-Baker Faces Rating Scale, a color visual analogue scale, and a numeric rating scale.

In addition to the pain measures included in this chapter, pain scales for target diagnoses such as back pain, headache, and neuropathic pain have also been developed. Many validated tools that assess the effect that pain has on the quality of life are also available. Headache assessment is included in Chapter 15; disability measures and other health status tools are grouped separately in Chapter 11. Other measures are too numerous for inclusion in this text, please refer to Online References and Resources for further information.

Resources and References
Online Resources

18 Multi-language Pain Assessment Scales: http://www.partnersagainstpain.com/index-pc.aspx?sid=12&aid=7692.

American Pain Society: The American Pain Society is a multidisciplinary organization of basic and clinical scientists, practicing clinicians, policy analysts, and others. The mission of the American Pain Society is to advance pain-related research, education, treatment and professional practice. Website: http://www.ampainsoc.org.

The Medical Algorithms Project: The Medical Algorithms Project; developed by Quanta Healthcare Solutions, Inc, 2002, provides access to tools and algorithms published for professional use. Chapter 44 (Pediatrics) includes a section of tools for "Assessing Pain in Pediatric Patients", available at http://www.medal.org/ch44.html. Chapter 37 (Occupational Medicine & Disability Assessment) includes a section of tools for "Pain Evaluation" available at http://www.medal.org/ch37.html.

Pain as the 5th Vital Sign: This Veteran's Administration program includes tips on performing pain screenings, and offers guidelines for the completion of comprehensive pain assessments; available at http://www.va.gov/oaa/pocketcard/pain.asp.

Royal College of Nursing, 1999: Clinical Practice Guidelines: The recognition and assessment of acute pain in children with an excellent review of pediatric pain assessment tools is included at this site. National electronic Royal College of Nursing available online at: http://www.nelh.nhs.uk/guidelinesdb/html/front/Acute PainInChildren.html.

References

Abstracts of the 20th Annual Scientific Meeting, American Pain Society, April 19-22, 2001: Diagnosis, assessment, and reviews, *J Pain* 2:1-9.

American Geriatric Society Panel on Chronic Pain in Older Persons: The management of chronic pain in older persons, *J Am Geriatr Soc* 46:635-651, 1998.

Beyer JE, McGrath PJ, Berde C: Discordance between self-report and behavioral pain measures in children aged 3-7 years after surgery, *J Pain Symptom Manage* 5:350-356, 1990.

Bigos S, Bower O, Braen G, et al: *Acute Low Back Problems in Adults.* Clinical Practice Guideline No. 14 (AHCPR Publication No. 94-0642). Rockville, MD, Agency for Health Care Policy and Research, US Department of Health and Human Services, Public Health Service, December 1994. Available at http://www.ahcpr.gov/clinic/cpgonline.htm.

Car DB, Jacox AK, Chapman CR, et al: *Acute Pain Management: Operative or Medical Procedures and Trauma.* Clinical Practice Guideline No 1 (AHCPR Publication No. 92-0032). Rockville, MD, Agency for Health Care Policy and Research, US Department of Health and Human Services, Public Health Service, February 1992. Available at http://www.ahcpr.gov/clinic/cpgonline.htm.

Carey SJ, Turpin C, Smith J, et al: Improving pain management in an acute care setting: The Crawford Long Hospital of Emory University experience, *Orthop Nurs* 16:29, 1997.

Colwell C, Clark L, Perkins R: Postoperative use of pediatric pain scales: Children's self-report versus nurse assessment of pain intensity and affect, *J Pediatr Nurs* 11:375-381, 1996.

Fox CD, Berger D, Fine PG, et al: *Pain assessment and treatment in the managed care environment: A Position Statement from the American Pain Society.* Approved by the APS Board of Directors on January 11, 2000. Available at http://www.ampainsoc.org/managedcare/position.htm.

Ferrell BA: Pain management, *Clin Geriatr Med* 16:853-874, 2000.

Ferrell BA, Ferrell BR, Rivera L: Pain in cognitively impaired nursing home patients, *J Pain Symptom Manage* 10:591-598, 1995.

Franck LS, Greenberg CS, Stevens B: Pain assessment in infants and children, *Pediatr Clin North Am* 47:487-512, 2000.

Herr KA, Garand L: Assessment and measurement of pain in older adults, *Clin Geriatr Med* 17:457-478, vi, 2001.

Ho K, Spence J, Murphy MF: Review of pain-measurement tools, *Ann Emerg Med* 27:427-432, 1996.

Jacox A, Car DB, Payne R, et al: *Management of Cancer Pain.* Clinical Practice Guideline No. 9 (AHCPR Publication No. 94-0592). Rockville, MD, Agency for Health Care Policy and Research, US Department of Health and Human Services, Public Health Service, March 1994. Available at http://www.ahcpr.gov/clinic/cpgonline.htm.

Keck J, Gerkensmeyer J, Joyce B, et al: Reliability and validity of the FACES and Word Descriptor scales to measure pain in verbal children, *J Pediatr Nurs* 11:368-374, 1996.

LaMontagne LL, Johnson BD, Hepworth JT: Children's ratings of postoperative pain compared to ratings by nurses and physicians, *Issues Comprehensive Pediatr Nurs* 14:241-247, 1991.

Margoles MS, Weiner R, editors: *Chronic pain: assessment, diagnosis, and management,* Boca Raton, FL, 1999, CRC Press.

McGrath PA: *Pain in children: nature, assessment, and treatment,* New York, 1990, Guilford Press.

McGrath PA, Seifert C, Speechley K, et al: A new analogue scale for assessing children's pain: an initial validation study, *Pain* 64:435-443, 1996.

Royal College of Nursing: Clinical Practice Guidelines, 1999. Available at http://www.nelh.nhs.uk/guidelinesdb/html/front/AcutePainIn Children.html.

Turk DC, Melzack R, editors: *Handbook of pain assessment,* ed 2, New York, 2001, Guilford Press.

Weiner D, Peterson B, Keefe F: Evaluating persistent pain in long term care residents: what role for pain maps? *Pain* 76:249-257, 1998.

DESCRIPTIVE, NUMERIC, AND VISUAL ANALOGUE PAIN INTENSITY SCALES

The three scales described in the following sections are used most frequently to assess acute pain and are described in general reference texts and review articles on pain. They are quick and easy to administer, involve minimal work in scoring, and are preferred by most adults and clinicians.

Verbal Descriptor Scale (VDS)

Targeted Population: Older children and adults.

Description: The Verbal Descriptor Scale (VDS) consists of a list of phrases that represent different levels of pain intensity (e.g., "no pain," "slight pain," "mild pain," "moderate pain," "severe pain," "very severe pain," and "the most intense pain imaginable") on which the patient checks the most accurate descriptor. It has shown good reliability and validity for adults, including those with mild to moderate cognitive impairment. The VDS is the preferred pain scale for many older adults. Patients must interpret and express their pain in verbal terms, so the VDS is best suited for more articulate patients (Herr & Garand, 2001).

Administration Time: <1 minute by self-administration or interview.

Reference

Herr KA, Garand L: Assessment and measurement of pain in older adults. *Clin Geriatr Med* 17:457-78, vi, 2001.

Numeric Rating Scale (NRS)

Source: The scale is reprinted here for clinical use. The "18 Multi-language Pain Assessment Scales," translations of the Numeric Rating Scale (NRS), are available online at http://www.partnersagainstpain.com/index-pc.aspx?sid=12&aid= 7692.

Targeted Population: Adolescents and adults.

Description: Numeric rating scales ask the patient to rate his or her pain from 0 to 10, with 0 representing no pain and 10 representing the worst possible pain. Some scales use variations such as 0 to 5 or 0 to 20. The NRS may be positioned either vertically or horizontally; a vertical presentation is easier for persons with impaired abstract thinking to use. The scale is reliable and valid for assessment of pain for a range of medical conditions and clinical settings. Healthy older adults prefer the NRS over the Visual Analogue Scale (VAS) (Carey et al, 1997; Herr & Garand, 2001). The NRS can also be used orally with a simple, verbal descriptor question: "On a scale of 0 to 10, if 0 means no pain and 10 means the worst pain you can imagine, how much is your pain now?"

Scores: It is generally agreed that scores between 1 and 4 indicate a mild level of pain intensity, scores of 5 and 6 are consistent with moderate levels of pain, and scores of 7 or higher signify severe pain.

Administration Time: <1 minute by self-administration or interview.

Table 12-2 Selected Pain Scales

Name/Online Source	Scale Description	Age Range/Qualifiers	Validity/References
Self-Report Scales			
Verbal Descriptor Scale (VDS)	A list of phrases that represent different levels of pain intensity (e.g., "no pain," "slight pain," "mild pain," "moderate pain," "severe pain," "very severe pain," and "the most intense pain imaginable"); score may be descriptive or assigned a numeric value.	Literate children and adults; is the preferred pain scale for many older adults	Reliable and valid; Herr & Garand, 2001; Keck et al, 1996
Numeric Rating Scale (NRS)	Patient rates his/her pain from 0 to 10 (or 5 or 20), with 0 representing no pain and 10 (or 5 or 20) representing the worst possible pain.	5 years and older; is the preferred pain scale for many older healthy adults	Reliable and valid; Herr & Garand, 2001; Ho et al, 1996; Price et al, 1994
Visual Analogue Scale (VAS)	A single horizontal or vertical 10-cm line anchored by descriptors of pain at each end; patient marks the line at any point between "no pain" and "worst pain imaginable."	5 years and older; other scales are preferred by older adults	Reliable and valid, less so in younger children or adults with cognitive impairment. Ferrell, 2000; Herr & Garand, 2001; Ho et al, 1996; McCormack et al, 1988
Pain Thermometer (PT)	A variation of the VDS; picture of a thermometer along a continuum of adjectives describing pain or numeric rating marked from 0 to 10.	5 years and older; preferred tool for patients with moderate to severe cognitive deficits or abstract thinking or verbal communication difficulties; older adults prefer PT to the VAS or the NRS	Reliable and valid, even in persons with substantial levels of cognitive impairment; learning effect may emerge; Herr & Garand, 2001; Szyfelbein et al, 1985
Colored Analog Scale (CAS)	Horizontal or vertical ruler on which increasing intensity of red signifies more pain; numerical ratings are on the back	4 years and older; can be used at younger ages than VAS; converges to VAS at older ages	Reliable and valid, comparable to VAS and Faces Pain Scale; Bulloch & Tenenbein, 2002; McGrath et al, 1996
Poker Chip Tool	Four red poker chips; child chooses chips from 0 (no hurt) to 4 (most hurt one could have); ask how many "pieces of hurt" he has. Alternatively, child may place poker chips in a receptacle to indicate how much pain he/she is experiencing.	4.5-13.0 years	Reliable and valid; Beyer & Wells, 1989; Hester et al, 1990
Wong/Baker Faces Rating Scale http://www3.us.elsevierhealth.com/WOW/faces.html	Cartoon drawings of facial expressions ranging from no pain to intense pain (crying). Subject selects the drawing that fits his/her level of pain.	3 years +	Reliable and valid; Bieri et al, 1990; Carey et al, 1997; Keck et al, 1996; Wong & Baker, 1988
Oucher Scale	Six photographs depicting facial expression of no hurt to biggest hurt; includes numerical 0-100 scale. Subject selects the photo image that fits his/her level of pain.	3-12 years	Reliable and valid; Beyer, 1984; Beyer et al, 1990; Beyer et al, 1992

(Continued)

Table **12-2** Selected Pain Scales—Cont'd

Name/Online Source	Scale Description	Age Range/Qualifiers	Validity/References
Faces Pain Scale–Revised (FPS-R) http://www.painsourcebook.ca/pdfs/pps92.pdf	A set of simple line drawings of faces without smiles or tears, expressing "no pain" to "worst pain." Subject selects the drawing that fits his/her level of pain.	3 years +	Reliable and valid; Bieri et al, 1990; Bulloch & Tenenbein, 2002; Goodenough et al, 1997; Herr et al, 1998; Hicks et al, 2001; Hunter et al, 2000
Body Outline Tool	Line drawing of body, unclothed; subject marks an "X" or colors painful area; different colors can be used to signify levels of pain intensity	4 years +	Reliable and valid; Ho et al, 1996; Savedra et al, 1989c; Van Cleve & Savedra, 1993
McGill Pain Questionnaire (MPQ) and Short Form MPQ http://www.health-sciences.ubc.ca/whiplash.bc/bc/mcgill.htm	Four groups with 20 categories of 78 descriptor words are used to indicate the quality of pain. Each word has a rank value within its category; the values are summed for a "pain rating index." Also included are a VAS or VDS and body outline diagram. SF-MPQ has 15 pain descriptor words, rated 0 (none) to 3 (severe), and a VAS or VDS.	Adults with pain in all settings	Reliable and valid; Holroyd et al, 1992; Katz & Melzack, 1999; Lowe et al, 1991; Melzack, 1975, 1987
Brief Pain Inventory–Short Form http://www.mdanderson.org/pdf/bpisf.pdf	Severity of pain, location of pain, amount of pain relief, and impact of pain on daily functions are assessed on numeric rating scales; parameters are assessed for current, past and average pain. A body outline for location of pain and a line for pain medications/treatments are included.	Adult patients with cancer pain and pain caused by other chronic diseases	Reliable and valid; Cleeland, 1989, 1991; Cleeland et al, 1996; Serlin et al, 1995; Tittle et al, 2003
Adolescent Pediatric Pain Tool (APPT)	Body outline, word-graphic rating scale, and pain descriptor list measure location, quality, intensity, onset, duration, and pattern of a child's pain.	8-17 years	Reliable and valid; Savedra et al, 1993; Savedra & Tesler, 1989; Savedra et al, 1989a, 1989b Tesler et al, 1991
Behavioral Measures			
Objective Pain Score (OPS) (aka Objective Pain Scale) http://www.medal.org/ch44.html	Systolic blood pressure, crying, movement, agitation, and complaints of pain are assessed and scored on a 0-2 scale. Total score ranges from 0 to 10; higher scores indicate pain.	4 months-18 years	Reliable and valid; Hannallah et al, 1987 (no testing); Broadman et al, 1988; Morton, 1997; Norden et al, 1991a, 1991b
Children's Hospital of Eastern Ontario Pain Scale (CHEOPS) http://www.medal.org/ch44.html	Six parameters are assessed: crying, facial expression, verbalizations, torso activity, whether and how child touches wound, leg position; points range from 0 to 3 for each behavior within each parameter. A score >4 indicates pain.	1-7 years	Reliable and valid; excellent interrater reliability; Barrier et al, 1989; Beyer et al, 1990: did not correlate well with self-report scales; McGrath et al, 1985
Neonatal Infant Pain Scale (NIPS) http://www.medal.org/ch44.html	Facial expression, cry, breathing patterns, arms, legs, and state of arousal are assessed and scored. Each parameter has a score of 0 to 1 or 2; total scores range from 0 to 7.	Preterm and term neonates	Reliable and valid per authors; Lawrence et al, 1993

CRIES (Crying, Requires oxygen, Increased vital signs, Expression, Sleep) Scale for Neonatal Postoperative Pain Assessment: http://www.medal.org/ch44.html	Five parameters are assessed: Crying, Requires oxygen, Increased vital signs, Expression, and Sleep. Each has a score of 0-2; sum of subscores ranges from 0 to 10. Higher scores indicate more pain.	Neonates: 32-60 weeks' gestation	Reliable and valid; Krechel & Bildner, 1995
Behavioral Pain Score (BPS) http://www.medal.org/ch44.html	An abbreviated form of CHEOPS; three behavioral parameters are assessed: facial expression, cry, and movements, scored 0 to 2 or 3. Total score range is 0 to 8; higher numbers indicate more pain.	3-36 months	Data on reliability and validity not available; Robieux & Kumar, 1991
Riley Infant Pain Scale (RIPS) http://www.medal.org/ch44.html	Six parameters (facial, body movement, sleep, verbal/touch, consolability, and response to movements/touch) are scored on a 0-3 scale; total score ranges from 0 to 18; higher scores indicate more pain.	Preverbal infants and children with cerebral palsy	Reliable (specific, not sensitive) and valid; Joyce et al, 1994; Schade et al, 1996
FLACC (Face Legs Activity Cry Consolability) Behavioral Scale for Postoperative Pain in Young Children http://www.medal.org/ch44.html	Five categories of pain behaviors—facial expression, leg movement, activity, cry, and consolability—are scored on a 0- to 2-point scale. Total score range is 0 to 10; higher score reflects discomfort and pain.	2 months-7 years; reliable for children with cognitive impairment	Reliable and valid; high interrater reliability; Merkel et al, 1997; Voepel-Lewis et al, 2002; Willis et al, 2003
Toddler-Preschooler Postoperative Pain Scale (TPPPS) http://www.medal.org/ch44.html	Seven behavioral descriptors for three categories of behavior (verbal, facial, bodily movements) are used to assess acute pain following procedures. Each behavior descriptor scores 0 or 1, depending on presence in a 5-minute period; total scores range from 0 to 7.	1-5 years	Reliable and valid per authors; Tarbell et al, 1992
Physiologic Measures			
Autonomic measures (e.g., heart rate, blood pressure, heart rate spectral analyses)	Scores changes in heart rate, blood pressure, or measures of heart rate variability (e.g., "vagal tone").	All ages	Can be used at all ages; useful for patients receiving mechanical ventilation; nonspecific: changes can occur unrelated to pain; unreliable in infants; Buttner & Finke, 2000
Hormonal-metabolic measures	Plasma or salivary sampling of hormones (e.g., cortisol, epinephrine)	All ages	Can be used at all ages; nonspecific; changes can occur unrelated to pain; inconvenient, cannot provide "real-time" information; Ho et al, 1996

(Continued)

Table **12-2** Selected Pain Scales—Cont'd

REFERENCES

Barrier G, Attia J, Mayer MN, et al: Measurement of post-operative pain and narcotic administration in infants using a new clinical scoring system. *Intensive Care Med* 15(suppl 1): S37-39, 1989.

Beyer JE: *The Oucher: a user's manual and technical report.* Charlottesville, 1984: University of Virginia Alumni Patent Foundation.

Beyer JE, Denyes MJ, Villarruel AM: The creation, validation, and continuing development of the Oucher: a measure of pain intensity in children. *J Pediatr Nurs* 7:335-346, 1992.

Beyer JE, McGrath PJ, Berde C: Discordance between self-report and behavioral pain measures in children aged 3-7 years after surgery. *J Pain Symptom Manage* 5:350-356, 1990.

Beyer J, Wells N: The assessment of pain in children. *Pediatr Clin North Am* 36:837-854, 1989.

Bieri D, Reeve R, Champion GD, et al: The Faces Pain Scale for the self-assessment of the severity of pain experienced by children: development, initial validation and preliminary investigation for ratio scale properties. *Pain* 41:139-150, 1990.

Broadman LM, Rice LH, Hannallah RS: Comparison of a physiological and a visual analogue pain scale in children. *Can J Anaesth* 35:S137-S138, 1988.

Bulloch B, Tenenbein M: Validation of 2 pain scales for use in the pediatric emergency department. *Pediatrics* 110:e33, 2002.

Buttner W, Finke W: Analysis of behavioural and physiological parameters for the assessment of postoperative analgesic demand in newborns, infants and young children: a comprehensive report on seven consecutive studies. *Paediatr Anaesth* 10:303-318, 2000.

Carey SJ, Turpin C, Smith J, et al: Improving pain management in an acute care setting: The Crawford Long Hospital of Emory University experience. *Orthop Nurs* 16:29-36, 1997.

Cleeland CS: Measurement of pain by subjective report. In: Chapman CR, Loeser JD, editors. Advances in Pain Research and Therapy, vol 12: *Issues in pain measurement.* New York: Raven Press, pp. 391-403, 1989.

Cleeland CS: Brief Pain Inventory © (BPI). University of Wisconsin—Madison, 1991, Pain Research Group.

Cleeland CS, Nakamura Y, Mendoza TR, et al: Dimensions of the impact of cancer pain in a four country sample: New information from multidimensional scaling. *Pain* 67:267-273, 1996.

Ferrell BA: Pain management. *Clin Geriatr Med* 16:853-874, 2000.

Goodenough B, Addicoat L, Champion GD, et al: Pain in 4- to 6-year-old children receiving intramuscular injections: a comparison of the Faces Pain Scale with other self-report and behavioral measures. *Clin J Pain* 13:60-73, 1997.

Hannallah RS, Broadman LM, Belman AS, et al: Comparison of caudal and ilioinguinal/iliohypogastric nerve blocks for control of post-orchiopexy pain in pediatric ambulatory surgery. *Anesthesiology* 66: 832-834, 1987.

Herr KA, Garand L: Assessment and measurement of pain in older adults. *Clin Geriatr Med* 17: 457-478, vi, 2001.

Herr KA, Mobily PR, Kohout FJ, et al: Evaluation of the Faces Pain Scale for use with the elderly. *Clin J Pain* 14:29-38, 1998.

Hester NO, Foster R, Kristensen K: Measurement of pain in children: generalizability and validity of the Pain Ladder and the Poker Chip Tool. In: Tyler DC, Krane EJ, editors. *Advances in pain research therapy.* New York, 1990: Raven Press Ltd.

Hicks CL, von Baeyer CL, Spafford P, et al: The Faces Pain Scale–Revised: toward a common metric in pediatric pain measurement. *Pain* 93:173-183, 2001.

Ho K, Spence J, Murphy MF: Review of pain-measurement tools. *Ann Emerg Med* 27:427-432, 1996.

Holroyd KA, Holm JE, Keefe FJ, et al: A multi-center evaluation of the McGill Pain Questionnaire: results from more than 1700 chronic pain patients. *Pain* 48:301-311, 1992.

Hunter M, McDowell L, Hennessy R, et al: An evaluation of the Faces Pain Scale with young children. *J Pain Symptom Manage* 20:122-129, 2000.

Joyce BA, Schade JG, Keck JF, et al: Reliability and validity of preverbal pain assessment tools. *Issues Comprehensive Pediatr Nurs* 17:121-135, 1994.

Katz J, Melzack R: Measurement of pain. *Surg Clin North Am* 79:231-252, 1999.

Keck J, Gerkensmeyer J, Joyce B, et al: Reliability and validity of the FACES and Word Descriptor scales to measure pain in verbal children. *J Pediatr Nurs* 11:368-374, 1996.

Krechel SW, Bildner J: CRIES: a new neonatal postoperative pain measurement score. Initial testing and reliability. *Paediatr Anaesth* 5:53-61, 1995.

Lawrence J, Alcock D, McGrath P, et al: The development of a tool to assess neonatal pain. *Neonatal Network* 12:59-65, 1993.

Lowe NK, Walker SN, MacCallum RC: Confirming the theoretical structure of the McGill Pain Questionnaire in acute clinical pain. *Pain* 46:53-60, 1991.

McCormack HM, Horne DJ, Sheather S: Clinical applications of visual analogue scales: a critical review. *Psychol Med* 18:1007-1019, 1988.

McGrath PJ, Johnson G, Goodman JT, et al: The CHEOPS: a behavioral scale to measure postoperative pain in children. In: Chapman J, Fields HL, Dubner R, et al, editors. *Advances in pain research and therapy vol 9* (pp. 395-402). New York, 1985: Raven Press.

McGrath PA, Seifert C, Speechley K, et al: A new analogue scale for assessing children's pain: an initial validation study. *Pain* 64:435-443, 1996.

Melzack R: The McGill Pain Questionnaire: major properties and scoring methods. *Pain* 1:277-299, 1975.

Melzack R: The short-form McGill Pain Questionnaire. *Pain* 30:191-197, 1987.

Merkel SI, Voepel-Lewus T, Shayevitz JR, et al: The FLACC: a behavioral scale for scoring postoperative pain in young children. *Pediatr Nurs* 23:293-297, 1997.

Morton NS: Pain assessment in children. *Paediatr Anaesth* 7:267-272, 1997.

Norden J, Hannallah RS, Getson P, et al: Concurrent validation of an objective pain scale for infants and children [abstract]. *Anesthesiology* 75(3a):A934, 1991a.

Norden J, Hannallah RS, Getson P, et al: Reliability of an objective pain scale in children. *Anesth Analg* 72:S199, 1991b.

Price DD, Bush FM, Long S, et al: A comparison of pain measurement characteristics of mechanical visual analogue and simple numerical rating scales. *Pain* 56:217-226, 1994.

Robieux I, Kumar R: Assessing pain and analgesia with a lidocaine-prilocaine emulsion in infants and toddlers during venipuncture. *J Pediatr* 118:971-973, 1991.

Savedra MC, Holzemer WL, Tesler MD, et al: Assessment of postoperation pain in children and adolescents using the adolescent pediatric pain tool. *Nurs Res* 42:5-9, 1993.

Savedra MC, Tesler MD: Assessing children's and adolescents' pain. *Pediatrician* 16:24-29, 1989.

Savedra MC, Tesler MD, Holzemer WL, et al: *Adolescent pediatric pain tool (APPT) preliminary user's manual*. San Francisco, 1989a: University of California. For information contact savedra@linex.com.

Savedra MC, Tesler MD, Holzemer WL, et al: Pain location: validity and reliability of body outline markings by hospitalized children and adolescents. *Res Nurs Health* 12:307-314, 1989b.

Schade JG, Joyce BA, Gerkensmeyer J, et al: Comparison of three preverbal scales for post operative pain assessment in a diverse pediatric sample. *J Pain Symptom Manage* 12:348-359, 1996.

Serlin RC, Mendoza TR, Nakamura Y, et al: When is cancer pain mild, moderate or severe? Grading pain severity by its interference with function. *Pain* 61:277-284, 1995.

Szyfelbein SK, Osgood PF, Carr DB: Pain thermometer. In McGrath PA, editor: *Pain in children: nature, assessment, and treatment*. New York, 1990: Guilford Press.

Tarbell SE, Cohen IT, Marsh JL: The Toddler-Preschooler Postoperative Pain Scale: an observational scale for measuring postoperative pain in children aged 1-5. Preliminary report. *Pain* 50:273-280, 1992.

Tesler MD, Savedra MC, Holzemer WL, et al: The word-graphic rating scale as a measure of children's and adolescents' pain intensity. *Res Nurs Health* 14:361-371, 1991.

Tittle MB, McMillan SC, Hagan S: Validating the Brief Pain Inventory for use with surgical patients with cancer. *Oncol Nurs Forum* 30(2 part 1):325-330, 2003.

Van Cleve LJ, Savedra MC: Pain location: validity and reliability of body outline markings by 4 to 7-year-old children who are hospitalized. *Pediatr Nurs* 19:217-220, 1993.

Voepel-Lewis T, Merkel S, Tait AR, et al: The reliability and validity of the Face, Legs, Activity, Cry, Consolability observational tool as a measure of pain in children with cognitive impairment. *Anesth Analg* 95:1224-1229, 2002.

Willis MHW, Merkel SI, Voepel-Lewis T, et al: FLACC behavioral pain assessment scale: a comparison with the child's self-report. *Pediatr Nurs* 29:195-198, 2003.

Wong D, Baker C: Pain in children: comparison of assessment scales. *Pediatr Nurs* 14:9-17, 1988.

References

Carey SJ, Turpin C, Smith J, et al: Improving pain management in an acute care setting: The Crawford Long Hospital of Emory University experience. *Orthop Nurs* 16:29, 1997.

Herr KA, Garand L: Assessment and measurement of pain in older adults. *Clin Geriatr Med* 17:457-78, vi, 2001.

Visual Analogue Scales (VAS)

Targeted Population: Adolescents and adults.

Description: The Visual Analogue Scales (VAS) consist of a horizontal or vertical 10-cm line, with the left-hand or lower side labeled "no pain" and the right-hand or upper side labeled "most intense pain imaginable" (or similar descriptor). The patient indicates his or her level of pain or discomfort by placing a mark on the horizontal or vertical line. Visual analogue scales were not preferred by many older adults in some studies (Carey et al, 1997). If the scales are used to measure pain in persons with mild abstract cognitive impairment, a vertical presentation of the 10-cm line, as included in this text, is preferable to a horizontal presentation (Herr & Garand, 2001).

Scores: The score is determined by measuring the position of the mark on the scale with a centimeter ruler.

Administration Time: <1 minute.

References

Carey SJ, Turpin C, Smith J, et al: Improving pain management in an acute care setting: The Crawford Long Hospital of Emory University experience. *Orthop Nurs* 16:29, 1997.

Herr KA, Garand L: Assessment and measurement of pain in older adults. *Clin Geriatr Med* 17:457-78, vi, 2001.

PICTORIAL PAIN SCALES

Pictorial or "faces" pain scales consist of a series of progressively distressed facial expressions; they were originally developed for use with children. The patient chooses the face that symbolizes the severity of his or her current pain. Although they are particularly helpful for assessing pain in young children, the pictorial pain scales have also shown good reliability with and are preferred by older adults.

Wong/Baker Faces Rating Scale

Authors: Wong D, Baker C, 1988.

Source: The Wong/Baker Faces Rating Scale is available online at: http://www3.us.elsevierhealth.com/WOW/faces.html (scale), http://www3.us.elsevierhealth.com/WOW/facesPermission.html (permission for use), http://www.us.elsevierhealth.com/WOW/facesTranslations.html (translations).

Targeted Population: Persons age 3 years and older, especially children.

Description: This pictorial pain scale developed by Wong and Baker (1988) contains cartoon faces arranged from a very happy, smiling face depicting "no pain" to a tearful, sad face depicting "worst pain." The Wong/Baker

Faces Scale is the preferred scale for younger children and is easily understood by all age groups.

Scores: The patient indicates the pictorial face that corresponds to the level of his or her pain. Scores range from 0 (no pain) to 5 (most severe pain).

Accuracy: The Wong/Baker Faces Scale has demonstrated reliability and validity when tested against the visual analogue scales and others (Keck et al, 1996; Carey et al, 1997; Bieri et al, 1990).

Administration Time: <1 minute.

References

Bieri D, Reeve R, Champion GD, et al: The Faces Pain Scale for the self-assessment of the severity of pain experienced by children: development, initial validation and preliminary investigation for ratio scale properties. *Pain* 41:139-150, 1990.

Carey SJ, Turpin C, Smith J, et al: Improving pain management in an acute care setting: The Crawford Long Hospital of Emory University experience. *Orthop Nurs* 16:29, 1997.

Keck J, Gerkensmeyer J, Joyce B, et al: Reliability and validity of the FACES and Word Descriptor scales to measure pain in verbal children. *J Pediatr Nurs* 11:368-374, 1996.

Wong D, Baker C: Pain in children: comparison of assessment scales. *Pediatr Nurs* 14:9-17, 1988.

Oucher Scale

Authors: Beyer JE et al, 1992.

Targeted Population: Children, 3 to 12 years old.

Description: The Oucher Scale was developed by Beyer et al (1992) to assist 3- to 12-year-olds in describing the intensity of pain. Six photographs depicting facial expressions of "no hurt" to "biggest hurt" are presented, along with a numerical 0-100 scale. Three scales are available, depicting white, Hispanic, and African-American children, respectively.

Scores: The patient indicates the photograph that corresponds to the level of his or her pain. The chosen photograph corresponds to a number on the vertical numerical scale (10-100). The vertical numerical scale may be used by children who can count to 100.

Accuracy: Construct validity of the Oucher Scale has been reported for children ages 3 to 12 years (Beyer & Knott, 1998; Beyer et al, 1992).

Administration Time: <1 minute.

References

Beyer JE, Denyes MJ, Villarruel AM: The creation, validation, and continuing development of the Oucher: a measure of pain intensity in children. *J Pediatr Nurs* 7:335-346, 1992.

Beyer JE, Knott CB: Construct validity estimation for the African-American and Hispanic versions of the Oucher Scale. *J Pediatr Nurs* 13:20-31, 1998.

The Faces Pain Scale–Revised (FPS-R)

Authors: Hicks CL et al, 2001. Adapted from Bieri D et al, 1990.

Source: The Faces Pain Scale–Revised is reprinted here and may also be found (in English and French) online at http://www.painsourcebook.ca/pdfs/pps92.pdf.

Targeted Population: Children and adults.

Description: The Faces Pain Scale–Revised (FPS-R) was adapted from the Faces Pain Scale (Bieri et al, 1990) for easier linear scoring. The six images are simple line drawings of faces without smiles or tears, expressing "no pain" to "worst pain." It is easy to administer; the patient indicates which face most closely represents his or her pain intensity.

Scores: The chosen face is scored as 0, 2, 4, 6, 8, or 10 by counting left to right. A score of 0 = "no pain"; 10 = "very much pain."

Accuracy: The FPS-R is reliable and valid for use with younger children in parallel with numerical self-rating scales (0 to 10); for use with older children; with behavioral observation scales for those unable to provide self-report; and for use with the elderly (Hicks et al, 2001; Herr et al, 1998; Bieri et al, 1990).

Administration Time: <1 minute.

References

Bieri D, Reeve R, Champion GD, et al: The Faces Pain Scale for the self-assessment of the severity of pain experienced by children: development, initial validation and preliminary investigation for ratio scale properties. *Pain* 41:139-150, 1990.

Herr KA, Mobily PR, Kohout FJ, et al: Evaluation of the Faces Pain Scale for use with the elderly. *Clin J Pain* 14:29-38, 1998.

Hicks CL, von Baeyer CL, Spafford P, et al: The Faces Pain Scale–Revised: toward a common metric in pediatric pain measurement. *Pain* 93:173-183, 2001.

MULTIDIMENSIONAL SCALES

McGill Pain Questionnaires (MPQ)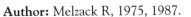

Author: Melzack R, 1975, 1987.

Source: The long and short versions of the McGill Pain Questionnaire (MPQ) are reprinted in this text. The short-form MPQ (SF-MPQ) may also be found online at http://health-sciences.ubc.ca/whiplash.bc/mcgill.htm/ and http://www.med.umich.edu/obgyn/repro-endo/Lebovicresearch/PainSurvey.pdf.

Targeted Population: Adults.

Description: The MPQ is a well-known tool for the thorough evaluation of pain. Developed by Melzack (1975, 1987), this qualitative tool has long (MPQ) and short (SF-MPQ) versions. The MPQ identifies 78 key words that describe the different qualities of pain and places them into 20 categories. The categories are sorted into four major groups: sensory (42 words in 10 categories), affective (14 words in 5 categories), evaluative (5 words in one category), and miscellaneous (17 words in 4 categories). Each word is assigned a rank value within its category based on its position in the word set. A 0- to 5-point verbal descriptive scale (VDS) or a VAS is also completed to indicate the overall pain intensity at the time of administration of the questionnaire. A body outline is included for the patient to mark locations of pain, with the words *internal* and *external* added. The course of pain over time is also assessed with nine words.

The SF-MPQ consists of a 15-word descriptor list (11 sensory and 4 affective words); each word is rated on an intensity scale as 0 = none, 1 = mild, 2 = moderate, and 3 = severe (Melzack, 1987). The VDS and VAS are also included on the short form for determining pain intensity. A body outline tool is sometimes included with the SF-MPQ.

Scores: The sum of the rank values of the words chosen becomes the *pain rating index (PRI)*. The score on the VDS or VAS, which indicates the overall pain intensity, is termed the *present pain intensity (PPI)*.

Accuracy: Katz and Melzack (1999) have provided a summary of the studies demonstrating the reliability, validity, and consistency of the MPQ. The MPQ is easily understood by older adults, and it shows good concurrent validity with other pain intensity scales (Ho et al, 1996). Neither version of the MPQ, however, has been systematically evaluated for use among persons with cognitive impairment; therefore, is not recommended for that population (Herr & Garand 2001). The MPQ has shown consistency and reliability in the evaluation of both acute and chronic pain (Holroyd et al, 1992; Lowe et al, 1991), although a meta-analysis by Wilkie et al (1990) revealed that higher affective scores appeared to differentiate chronic painful conditions from acute painful conditions.

Administration Time: MPQ: 10 to 25 minutes by self-report or interview. SF-MPQ: ~5 minutes by self-report or interview.

References

Herr KA, Garand L: Assessment and measurement of pain in older adults. *Clin Geriatr Med* 17: 457-478, vi, 2001.

Ho K, Spence J, Murphy MF: Review of pain-measurement tools. *Ann Emerg Med* 27:427-432, 1996.

Holroyd KA, Holm JE, Keefe FJ, et al: A multi-center evaluation of the McGill Pain Questionnaire: results from more than 1700 chronic pain patients. *Pain* 48:301-311, 1992.

Katz J, Melzack R: Measurement of pain. *Surg Clin North Am* 79:231-252, 1999.

Lowe NK, Walker SN, MacCallum RC: Confirming the theoretical structure of the McGill Pain Questionnaire in acute clinical pain. *Pain* 46:53-60, 1991.

Melzack R: The McGill Pain Questionnaire: major properties and scoring methods. *Pain* 1:277-299, 1975.

Melzack R: The short-form McGill Pain Questionnaire. *Pain* 30:191-197, 1987.

Wilkie DJ, Savedra MC, Holzemier WL, et al: Use of the McGill Pain Questionnaire to measure pain: a meta-analysis, *Nurs Res* 39:36-41, 1990.

Brief Pain Inventories (BPI)

Author: Cleeland CS, 1991.

Source: The BPI — Short Form is reprinted here. More information about the BPI may be found online at: http://www.mapi-research-inst.com/pdf/art/qol9_4.pdf. The long and short versions of the BPI are available online through the University of Texas, M.D. Anderson Cancer Center, Department of Symptom Research at http://www.mdanderson.org/departments/prg/ and clicking on "symptom assessment tools," following links to "The Brief Pain Inventory (BPI)", then the short or long forms as preferred. Permission to use these tools must be obtained from the author with agreement to not alter its format; permission is granted free of charge at http://www.mdanderson.org/departments/prg/ and clicking on "symptom assessment tools," following links to "The Brief Pain Inventory (BPI)," then "permission form."

Targeted Population: Adults with chronic disease.

Description: The Brief Pain Inventories were developed by Cleeland (1991) from the Wisconsin Brief Pain Questionnaire (Daut et al, 1983) for assessment of the severity of pain and the impact of pain on daily functions in patients with cancer pain and pain due to other chronic diseases. Both the short and long versions of this tool assess severity of pain, location of pain, amount of pain relief, and impact of pain on daily functions using numeric rating scales (Cleeland & Ryan, 1994). A body outline for location of pain and a line for pain medications/treatments are included. The long form also provides space for documentation of demographic information, history of the illness, alleviating and exacerbating factors, detailed history on pain medication usage and satisfaction, and a verbal descriptor pain scale. The BPI has been translated into several languages.

Scores: There is no scoring algorithm, but the arithmetic mean of the 4 severity items can be used as measures of pain severity and the arithmetic mean of the 7 interference items can be used as a measure of pain interference.

Accuracy: The BPI has been extensively validated in the cancer population and has demonstrated good reliability and validity (Serlin et al, 1995; Cleeland et al, 1996; Tittle et al, 2003).

Administration Time: 5 minutes for the short form and 10 minutes for the long form, administered by self-report or interview.

References

Cleeland CS: Brief Pain Inventory © (BPI). University of Wisconsin-Madison, 1991, Pain Research Group.

Cleeland CS, Ryan KM: Pain assessment: global use of the Brief Pain Inventory, *Ann Acad Med Singapore* 23:129-138, 1994.

Cleeland CS, Nakamura Y, Mendoza TR, et al: Dimensions of the impact of cancer pain in a four country sample: New information from multidimensional scaling, *Pain* 67:267-273, 1996.

Daut RL, Cleeland CS, Flanery RC: Development of the Wisconsin Brief Pain Questionnaire to assess pain in cancer and other diseases, *Pain* 17:197-210, 1983.

Serlin RC, Mendoza TR, Nakamura Y, et al: When is cancer pain mild moderate or severe? Grading pain severity by its interference with function, *Pain* 61:277-284, 1995.

Tittle MB, McMillan SC, Hagan S: Validating the Brief Pain Inventory for use with surgical patients with cancer, *Oncology Nursing Forum* 30(2 part 1):325-330, 2003.

BEHAVIORAL OR COMBINED BEHAVIORAL-PHYSIOLOGIC SCALES

Tools that measure pain-related behavior are often used for children who are unable to self-report. These tools are also used to supplement self-report or physiologic measures. For best accuracy, administrators of the measure should have training in use of the scale and use it concurrently with a self-report measure if possible.

Children's Hospital of Eastern Ontario Pain Scale (CHEOPS)

Authors: McGrath PJ et al, 1985.

Source: The Children's Hospital of Eastern Ontario Pain Scale (CHEOPS) is reprinted in this text and is also available online at http://www.anes.ucla.edu/pain/assessment_tool-cheops.htm.

Targeted Population: Children, ages 1 to 7 years.

Description: Recommended for children ages 1 to 7 years old, this tool measures six parameters of behavior: cry, facial expression, verbalizations, torso activity, whether and how child touches wound, and leg position. Three to six behaviors are listed for each parameter; points range from 0 to 3 for each behavior.

Scores: Points for each of the behaviors are summed; a total score >4 indicates pain.

Accuracy: CHEOPS has demonstrated validity and interrater reliability (McGrath et al, 1985; Barrier et al, 1989), although Beyer et al (1990) found that it did not correlate well with self-report scales.

Administration Time: 1 to 2 minutes by trained observer.

References

Barrier G, Attia J, Mayer MN, et al: Measurement of post-operative pain and narcotic administration in infants using a new clinical scoring system. *Intensive Care Med* 15(suppl 1):S37-S39, 1989.

Beyer JE, McGrath PJ, Berde C: Discordance between self-report and behavioral pain measures in children aged 3-7 years after surgery. *J Pain Symptom Manage* 5:350-356, 1990.

McGrath PJ, Johnson G, Goodman JT, et al: The CHEOPS: a behavioral scale to measure postoperative pain in children. In: Chapman J, Fields HL, Dubner R, et al, editors. *Advances in pain research and therapy,* vol 9, New York, 1985, Raven Press, pp. 395-402.

Neonatal Infant Pain Scale (NIPS)

Authors: Lawrence J et al, 1993.

Source: The Neonatal Infant Pain Scale (NIPS) is reprinted in this text and is also available online at http://www.anes.ucla.edu/pain/assessment_tool-nips.htm.

Targeted Population: Infants.

Description: NIPS scores behavioral measures of infants based on facial expression, cry, breathing patterns, movement of arms and legs, and state of arousal.

Scores: Each parameter is scored 0 or 1, except cry, which is scored 0, 1, or 2; the maximum score is 7. A score greater than 3 indicates pain.

Accuracy: The NIPS is an objective and replicable tool for use in assessing pain or pain-elicited distress in infants (Blauer & Gerstmann, 1998; Lawrence et al, 1993). NIPS has been used in many studies to evaluate infant pain and in studies that validate other infant pain scales (Hudson-Barr et al, 2002).

Administration Time: 1 to 2 minutes by trained observer.

References

Blauer T, Gerstmann D: A simultaneous comparison of three neonatal pain scales during common NICU procedures. *Clin J Pain* 14:39-47, 1998.

Hudson-Barr D, Capper-Michel B, Lambert S, et al: Validation of the Pain Assessment in Neonates (PAIN) scale with the Neonatal Infant Pain Scale (NIPS). *Neonatal Network* 21:15-21, 2002.

Lawrence J, Alcock D, McGrath P, et al: The development of a tool to assess neonatal pain. *Neonatal Network* 12:59-65, 1993.

OTHER PAIN MEASURES

Body Outline Tool

Targeted Population: Children.

Description: This line drawing may be used for pain assessment in children. A child may choose a crayon and color on the diagram to show where he or she hurts. The marks may be made as big or small as necessary to indicate the location and/or intensity of pain.

Scores: The drawing provides information as to the location of the pain and indication of severity. It may serve to facilitate communication and discussion about pain.

Administration Time: 1 to 5 minutes by self-administration.

Geriatric Pain Assessment Form

Authors: Stein WM, Ferrell BA, 1996.

Targeted Population: Older adults.

Description: This one-page form (Stein & Ferrell, 1996) contains space for documentation of primary diagnoses, medications, and nonpharmacologic pain treatments. Pain-focused information may be entered on a scale for pain intensity, a body outline for pain location, and a visual analogue scale. Space in which to record pain descriptors; maneuvers that exacerbate or alleviate pain; and the effects of pain on mood, sleep, and activities of daily living is included. Lastly, lines for documentation of the Mini-Mental Status Exam (MMSE) score, a depression scale score, and a gait and balance assessment appear on the form.

Scores: Scores for various screens are grouped on this form, providing a helpful summary of the pain history for the older patient.

Reference

Stein WM, Ferrell BA: Pain in the nursing home. *Clin Geriatr Med* 12:601-613, 1996.

Visual Analogue Scale (VAS)

The Worst Imaginable Pain

No Pain

Numeric Rating Scale (NRS)

| 20 |
| 19 |
| 18 |
| 17 |
| 16 |
| 15 |
| 14 |
| 13 |
| 12 |
| 11 |
| 10 |
| 9 |
| 8 |
| 7 |
| 6 |
| 5 |
| 4 |
| 3 |
| 2 |
| 1 |
| 0 |

Verbal Descriptor Scale (VDS)

The most intense pain imaginable

Very severe pain

Severe pain

Moderate pain

Mild pain

Slight pain

No pain

Wong/Baker Faces Rating Scale

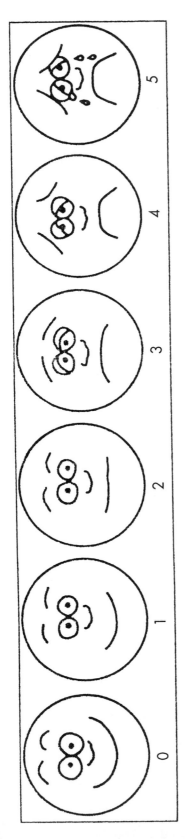

Wong/Baker Faces Rating Scale. Explain to the patient that each face is for a person who feels happy because he has no pain (hurt) or sad because he has some or a lot of pain. **Face 0** is very happy because the person doesn't hurt at all. **Face 1** hurts just a little bit. **Face 2** hurts a little more. **Face 3** hurts a little more. **Face 4** hurts a whole lot. **Face 5** hurts as much as you can imagine, although you don't have to be crying to feel this bad. Ask the patient to choose the face that best describes how he or she is feeling. *Recommended for persons 3 years and older.*

384

Oucher Faces Rating Scale

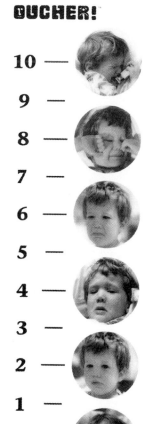

OUCHER!

10 —
9 —
8 —
7 —
6 —
5 —
4 —
3 —
2 —
1 —
0 —

http://www.oucher.org

**Oucher Scale
(Caucasian)**

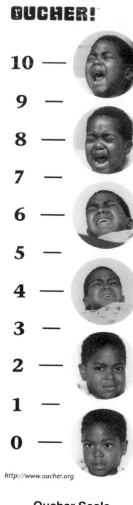

OUCHER!

10 —
9 —
8 —
7 —
6 —
5 —
4 —
3 —
2 —
1 —
0 —

http://www.oucher.org

**Oucher Scale
(African-American)**

OUCHER!

10 —
9 —
8 —
7 —
6 —
5 —
4 —
3 —
2 —
1 —
0 —

http://www.oucher.org

**Oucher Scale
(Hispanic)**

The Caucasian version of the Oucher was developed and copyrighted in 1983 by Judith E. Beyer, PhD, RN, currently at the University of Missouri-Kansas City School of Nursing. The African-American and Hispanic versions were developed and copyrighted in 1990 by Mary J. Denyes, PhD, RN, Wayne State University, and Antonio M. Villarruel, PhD, RN, University of Michigan. Cornelia Porter, PhD, RN, and Charlotta Marshall, MSN, RN, contributed to the development of the African-American scale.

Faces Pain Scale – Revised (FPS-R)

In the following instructions, say "hurt" or "pain," whichever seems right for a particular child.

"These faces show how much something can hurt. This face *[point to left-most face]* **shows <u>no pain</u>. The faces show more and more pain** *[point to each from left to right]* **up to this one** *[point to right-most face]*—**it shows <u>very much pain</u>. Point to the face that shows how much you hurt** *[right now]*."

Score the chosen face 0, 2, 4, 6, 8, or 10, counting left to right, so '0' = 'no pain' and '10' = 'very much pain.'
Do not use words like happy and sad. This scale is intended to measure how children feel inside, not how their face looks.

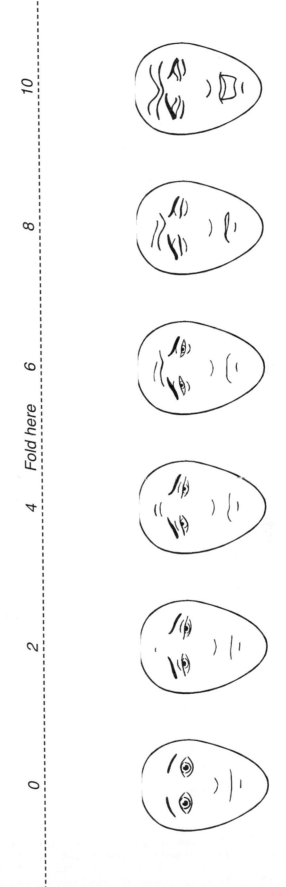

| 0 | 2 | 4 | Fold here 6 | 8 | 10 |

From Hicks CL, von Baeyer CL, Spafford P, et al: The Faces Pain Scale—revised: toward a common metric in pediatric pain measurement, *Pain* 93:173-183, 2001. Scale adapted from Bieri D, Reeve R, Champion GD, et al: The Faces pain Scale for the self-assessment of the severity of pain experienced by children: development, initial validation and preliminary investigation for ratio scale properties, *Pain* 41:139-150, 1990. Permission granted by the International Association for the Study of Pain.

McGill Pain Questionnaire (MPQ)

Patient's Name: _____ Date: _____ Time: _____ AM/PM

PRI: S _____ A _____ E _____ M _____ PRI(T) _____ PPI _____
　(1-10)　　　　　(11-15)　　　　　(16)　　　　　(17-20)　　　　　(1-20)

1	FLICKERING ___ QUIVERING ___ PULSING ___ THROBBING ___ BEATING ___ POUNDING ___

2 JUMPING ___
 FLASHING ___
 SHOOTING ___

3 PRICKING ___
 BORING ___
 DRILLING ___
 STABBING ___
 LANCINATING ___

4 SHARP ___
 CUTTING ___
 LACERATING ___

5 PINCHING ___
 PRESSING ___
 GNAWING ___
 CRAMPING ___
 CRUSHING ___

6 TUGGING ___
 PULLING ___
 WRENCHING ___

7 HOT ___
 BURNING ___
 SCALDING ___
 SEARING ___

8 TINGLING ___
 ITCHY ___
 SMARTING ___
 STINGING ___

9 DULL ___
 SORE ___
 HURTING ___
 ACHING ___
 HEAVY ___

10 TENDER ___
 TAUT ___
 RASPING ___
 SPLITTING ___

11 TIRING ___
 EXHAUSTING ___

12 SICKENING ___
 SUFFOCATING ___

13 FEARFUL ___
 FRIGHTFUL ___
 TERRIFYING ___

14 PUNISHING ___
 GRUELLING ___
 CRUEL ___
 VICIOUS ___
 KILLING ___

15 WRETCHED ___
 BLINDING ___

16 ANNOYING ___
 TROUBLESOME ___
 MISERABLE ___
 INTENSE ___
 UNBEARABLE ___

17 SPREADING ___
 RADIATING ___
 PENETRATING ___
 PIERCING ___

18 TIGHT ___
 NUMB ___
 DRAWING ___
 SQUEEZING ___
 TEARING ___

19 COOL ___
 COLD ___
 FREEZING ___

20 NAGGING ___
 NAUSEATING ___
 AGONIZING ___
 DREADFUL ___
 TORTURING ___

PPI
0 NO PAIN ___
1 MILD ___
2 DISCOMFORTING ___
3 DISTRESSING ___
4 HORRIBLE ___
5 EXCRUCIATING ___

BRIEF ___　RHYTHMIC ___　CONTINUOUS ___
MOMENTARY ___　PERIODIC ___　STEADY ___
TRANSIENT ___　INTERMITTENT ___　CONSTANT ___

E = EXTERNAL
I = INTERNAL

Mark or comment on the above figure
where you have your pain or problems.

COMMENTS:

Indicate on this line how bad your pain is—at the left end of line means no pain at all, at right end means worst pain possible.

No
pain _____ Worst possible
　　　　　　　　　　　　　　　　　　　　　　　　　　　　　　pain

The descriptors fall into four major groups: Sensory, 1 to 10; Affective, 11-15; Evaluative, 16; and Miscellaneous, 17-20. The rank value for each descriptor is based on its position in the word set. The sum of the rank values is the pain rating index (PRI). The present pain intensity (PPI) is based on a scale of 0 to 5.

Adapted from Melzack R: The McGill Pain Questionnaire: major properties and scoring methods, *Pain* 1(3):277-299, 1975.

McGill Pain Questionnaire and Pain Diagram—Short Form

(Reproduced with permission of author © Dr. Ron Melzack, for publication and distribution)

Date: _____

Name: _____

Check the column to indicate the level of your pain for each word, or leave blank if it does not apply to you.___

		Mild	Moderate	Severe
1	Throbbing	_____	_____	_____
2	Shooting	_____	_____	_____
3	Stabbing	_____	_____	_____
4	Sharp	_____	_____	_____
5	Cramping	_____	_____	_____
6	Gnawing	_____	_____	_____
7	Hot-burning	_____	_____	_____
8	Aching	_____	_____	_____
9	Heavy	_____	_____	_____
10	Tender	_____	_____	_____
11	Splitting	_____	_____	_____
12	Tiring-Exhausting	_____	_____	_____
13	Sickening	_____	_____	_____
14	Fearful	_____	_____	_____
15	Cruel-Punishing	_____	_____	_____

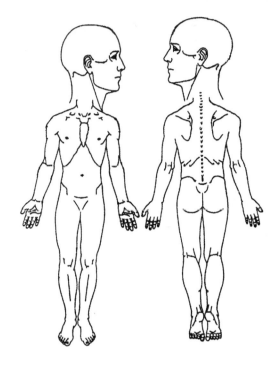

Mark or comment on the above figure where you have your pain or problems.

Indicate on this line how bad your pain is—at the left end of line means no pain at all, at right end means worst pain possible.

No Pain	_____	Worst Possible Pain

S	/33	A	/12	VAS	/10

From Melzack R: The short form McGill Pain Questionnaire, *Pain* 30:191-197, 1987.

STUDY ID# _____   HOSPITAL # _____

DO NOT WRITE ABOVE THIS LINE

Brief Pain Inventory

Date: _____/_____/_____   Time:_____

Name: _____ _____ _____

            Last   First   Middlle Initial

1.   Throughout our lives, most of us have had pain from time to time (such as minor headaches, sprains, and toothaches). Have you had pain other than these every-day kinds of pain today?

                 1.   Yes   2.   No

2.   On the diagram, shade in the areas where you feel pain. Put an X on the area that hurts the most.

3.   Please rate your pain by circling the one number that best describes your pain at its worst in the last 24 hours.

0	1	2	3	4	5	6	7	8	9	10
No Pain										Pain as bad as you can imagine

4.   Please rate your pain by circling the one nuimber that best describes your pain at its least in the last 24 hours.

0	1	2	3	4	5	6	7	8	9	10
No Pain										Pain as bad as you can imagine

5.   Please rate your pain by circling the one number that best describes your pain on the average.

0	1	2	3	4	5	6	7	8	9	10
No Pain										Pain as bad as you can imagine

6.   Please rate your pain by circling the one number that tells how much pain you have right now.

0	1	2	3	4	5	6	7	8	9	10
No Pain										Pain as bad as you can imagine

7. What treatments or medications are you receiving for your pain?

_____

_____

8. In the last 24 hours, how much relief have pain treatments or medications provided? Please circle the one percentage that most shows how much relief you have received.

0%	10%	20%	30%	40%	50%	60%	70%	80%	90%	100%
No Relief										Complete Relief

9. Circle the one number that describes how, during the past 24 hours, pain has interfered with your:

A. General Activity

0	1	2	3	4	5	6	7	8	9	10
Does not Interfere										Completely Interferes

B. Mood

0	1	2	3	4	5	6	7	8	9	10
Does not Interfere										Completely Interferes

C. Walking Ability

0	1	2	3	4	5	6	7	8	9	10
Does not Interfere										Completely Interferes

D. Normal Work (includes both work outside the home and housework)

0	1	2	3	4	5	6	7	8	9	10
Does not Interfere										Completely Interferes

E. Relations with other people

0	1	2	3	4	5	6	7	8	9	10
Does not Interfere										Completely Interferes

F. Sleep

0	1	2	3	4	5	6	7	8	9	10
Does not Interfere										Completely Interferes

G. Enjoyment of life

0	1	2	3	4	5	6	7	8	9	10
Does not Interfere										Completely Interferes

Children's Hospital of Eastern Ontario Pain Scale (CHEOPS)

(Recommended for children 1-7 years old) — A score greater than 4 indicates pain.

Item	Behavioral		Definition
Cry	No Cry	1	Child is not crying.
	Moaning	2	Child is moaning or quietly vocalizing silent cry.
	Crying	2	Child is crying, but the cry is gentle or whimpering.
	Scream	3	Child is in full-lunged cry; sobbing; may be scored with complaint or without complaint.
Facial	Composed	1	Neutral facial expression.
	Grimace	2	Score only if definite negative facial expression.
	Smiling	0	Score only if definite positive facial expression.
Child Verbal	None	1	Child not talking.
	Other complaints	1	Child complains, but not about pain, e.g., "I want to see Mommy" or "I am thirsty."
	Pain complaints	2	Child complains about pain.
	Both complaints	2	Child complains about pain and about other things, e.g., "It hurts; I want my Mommy."
	Positive	0	Child makes any positive statement or talks about other things without complaint.
Torso	Neutral	1	Body (not limbs) is at rest; torso is inactive.
	Shifting	2	Body is in motion in a shifting or serpentine fashion.
	Tense	2	Body is arched or rigid.
	Shivering	2	Body is shuddering or shaking involuntarily.
	Upright	2	Child is in a vertical or upright position.
	Restrained	2	Body is restrained.
Touch	Not touching	1	Child is not touching or grabbing at wound.
	Reach	2	Child is reaching for but not touching wound.
	Touch	2	Child is gently touching wound or wound area.
	Grab	2	Child is grabbing vigorously at wound.
	Restrained	2	Child's arms are restrained.
Legs	Neutral	1	Legs may be in any position but are relaxed; includes gentle swimming or separate-like movement.
	Squirm/kicking	2	Definitive uneasy or restless movements in the legs and/or striking out with foot or feet.
	Drawn up/tensed	2	Legs tensed and/or pulled up tightly to body and kept there.
	Standing	2	Standing, crouching or kneeling.
	Restrained	2	Child's legs are being held down.

From McGrath PJ, Johnson G, Goodman JT, et al: The CHEOPS: a behavioral scale to measure postoperative pain in children. In: Chapman J, Fields HL, Dubner R, et al, editors. *Advances in pain research and therapy*, vol 9, New York, 1985, Raven Press.

Neonatal/Infant Pain Scale (NIPS)

(Recommended for children less than 1 year old) – A score greater than 3 indicates pain.

Pain Assessment		
Facial Expression		
0	Relaxed muscles	Restful face, neutral expression
1	Grimace	Tight facial muscles; furrowed brow, chin, jaw, (negative facial expression-nose, mouth and brow)
Cry		
0	No Cry	Quiet, not crying
1	Whimper	Mild moaning, intermittent
2	Vigorous Cry	Loud scream; rising, shrill, continuous (Note: Silent cry may be scored if baby is intubated as evidenced by obvious mouth and facial movement.
Breathing Patterns		
0	Relaxed	Usual pattern for this infant
1	Change in Breathing	Indrawing, irregular, faster than usual; gagging; breath holding
Arms		
0	Relaxed/Restrained	No muscular rigidity; occasional random movements of arms
1	Flexed/Extended	Tense, straight arms; rigid and/or rapid extension, flexion
Legs		
0	Relaxed/Restrained	No muscular rigidity; occasional random leg movement
1	Flexed/Extended	Tense, straight legs; rigid and/or rapid extension, flexion
State of Arousal		
0	Sleeping/Awake	Quiet, peaceful sleeping or alert random leg movement
1	Fussy	Alert, restless, and thrashing

From Lawrence J, Alcock D, McGrath P, et al: The development of a tool to assess neonatal pain, *Neonatal Network* 12:59-65, 1993.

Body Outline Tool

Date of Visit: _____

Patient Name: _____

Medical Record #: _____

Date of Birth: _____ *Age:* _____ *Gender:* Male   Female

Please choose a crayon and color on the picture where you hurt.

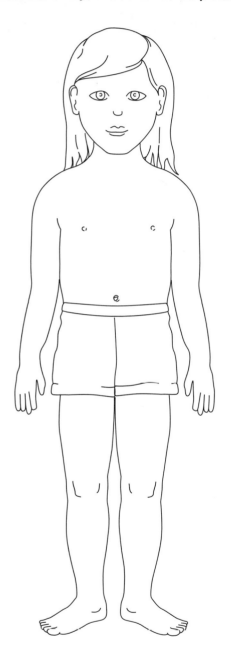 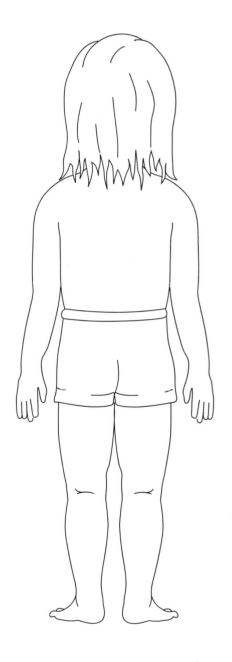

Geriatric Pain Assessment Sheet

Date of Visit: _____

Patient Name: _____

Medical Record #: _____

Date of Birth: _____ *Age:* _____ *Gender:* Male   Female

Primary Diagnoses: _____   _____   _____

_____   _____   _____

Medications & Schedule: _____   _____   _____

_____   _____   _____

_____   _____   _____

Non-Pharmacologic Pain Treatments: _____

_____

Success of Above: _____

_____

Pain Intensity: Now: 0   1   2   3   4   5
            None   Mod   Severe

Worst in 24 Hours:

0   1   2   3   4   5
None   Mod   Severe

Pain Descriptors:

_____

_____

Pain Location:

Right   Left   Left   Right

Maneuvers That Exacerbate:

_____

_____

_____

Maneuvers That Alleviate:

_____

_____

Visual Analog Scale (Place an X on Scale to Indicate Pain Severity)

Effects of Pain on: Mood: _____   Sleep: _____

ADLS/IADLS: _____

MMSE Score: _____   Depression Scale Score: _____

Gait & Balance Assessment: _____

From Stein WM, Ferrell BA: Pain in the nursing home, *Clin Geratr Med* 12:601, 1996.

CHAPTER 13

Wound Classification Systems and Risk Assessment Tools

Chapter Contents

WOUND CLASSIFICATION SYSTEMS

Classification systems have been designed as a way to communicate the description of an ulceration of the skin. Skin ulceration is a localized area of tissue necrosis most often caused by unrelieved pressure, vascular disease, neuropathy, infection, or a combination of these. Use of a classification system for skin ulcers by a large, diverse population of clinicians improves communication among providers, allowing for treatment planning and consistent monitoring of treatment progress. Wound classification systems have also been shown to have value as predictors of outcome.

Many standard wound classification systems have been proposed since the 1970s and have specifically been designed to categorize either pressure ulcers or diabetic foot ulcers (Box 13-1). The classification systems differ in the variables used in describing the status of wounds.

These variables include depth of wound, presence of infection, and presence of peripheral vascular disease. Most wound classification systems (Shea, 1975; Wagner, 1981; National Pressure Ulcer Advisory Panel [NPUAP], 1989; Yarkony-Kirk, 1990) are based primarily on wound depth, with partial or no mention of presence of infection or peripheral vascular disease. Some recent classification systems incorporate all variables into the staging of ulceration, providing a more consistent and complete assessment algorithm.

Wound care specialists advise caution in evaluation of wounds with eschars and wounds in dark-skinned individuals. An eschar may overlay a deeper lesion; thus, debridement may be necessary to determine the extent of the ulceration. Erythema may be masked in dark-skinned individuals; careful examination is recommended. Once the status of a wound is accurately graded by using one of the classification systems, it is recommended to document the name of the system along with the grade

Box 13-1 Wound Classification Systems

Shea Grading System for Pressure Ulcerations
(Shea, 1975)*
Wagner Wound Classification (Wagner, 1981)
National Pressure Ulcer Advisory Panel (NPUAP)
Staging System for Pressure Ulcerations
(National Pressure Ulcer Advisory Panel, 1989)*
Yarkony-Kirk Scale for Pressure Ulcers
(Yarkony et al, 1990)*
Sessing Scale for Pressure Ulcer Healing
(Ferrell et al, 1995)*
University of Texas Diabetic Wound Classification
System (Lavery et al, 1996)*
Depth-Ischemia Classification of Diabetic Foot Lesions
(Brodsky, 1999)
OASIS Status for a Pressure Ulcer (Wound Ostomy and
Continence Nurse Society, 2001)*
Pressure Ulcer Scale for Healing (PUSH)
(Stotts, et al, 2001)†

*Tools may be found online at http://www.medal.org/ch21.html.
†Tool may be found online at http://www.npuap.org.

(e.g., "Wagner, Grade 3"; "UT [University of Texas], Grade II-C"). This documentation will facilitate improved interprofessional communication among members of the health care team.

Included in this chapter are the widely used NPUAP Pressure Ulcer Classification System, the Pressure Ulcer Scale for Healing (PUSH Tool), the popular Wagner Wound Classification, and the comprehensive University of Texas Diabetic Wound Classification System. Other classification systems may be found online, as indicated, or in the list of references and resources at the end of the chapter.

National Pressure Ulcer Advisory Panel (NPUAP) Staging System for Pressure Ulcerations

Authors: Agency for Health Care Policy and Research (AHCPR), 1992. Updated by NPUAP, 1998.
Source: The NPUAP Staging System is reprinted here; more information is available online at http://www.npuap.org.
Description: This commonly used pressure ulcer classification system describes skin changes as stages based on the sole criteria of wound depth. The first stage of this system describes *erythema* as a precursor to actual skin loss. The NPUAP Staging System reprinted here is from the AHCPR Guidelines, which are consistent with the recommendations of the NPUAP Consensus Development Conference, with stage I guidelines updated by NPUAP in 1998.
Scores: Four stages are described on the basis of wound depth.

References

Agency for Health Care Policy and Research: Panel for the Prediction and Prevention of Pressure Ulcers in Adults. *Pressure ulcers in adults:*

Prediction and prevention. Clinical Practice Guideline No. 3 (AHCPR Publication No. 92-0047). Rockville, MD, 1992, AHCP Research, Public Health Service, US Department of Health and Human Services.

National Pressure Ulcer Advisory Panel: Stage I assessment in darkly pigmented skin, 1998. Available at http://www.npuap.org.

Pressure Ulcer Scale for Healing (PUSH Tool) i

Authors: National Pressure Ulcer Advisory Panel (NPUAP): Stotts NA et al, 2001.
Source: The Pressure Ulcer Scale for Healing (PUSH) Tool is copyrighted to the NPUAP; the tool may be accessed and used for education, research, and practice purposes. The NPUAP recommends use of the PUSH Tool at "regular intervals." For more information about the PUSH Tool and to download the PUSH tool, please access http://www.npuap.org.
Description: The goal of the PUSH Tool is to quickly and reliably capture the key assessments necessary to determine whether a pressure ulcer is getting better or worse over time. This excellent tool is used to monitor the three critical parameters that are the most indicative of healing: surface area, exudate, and type of wound tissue.
Scores: A subscore is categorized for each of these ulcer characteristics. The subscores are then added to obtain the total score. A comparison of total scores measured over time provides an indication of the improvement or deterioration in pressure ulcer healing.
Accuracy: The PUSH Tool has been validated by two multisite retrospective studies and a pilot test conducted by the Health Care Financing Administration (HCFA) (Stotts et al, 2001).

References

Stotts NA, Rodeheaver GT, Thomas DR, et al: An instrument to measure healing in pressure ulcers: development and validation of the pressure ulcer scale for healing (PUSH). *J Gerontol* 56: M795-M799, 2001.

Wagner Wound Classification

Authors: Meggitt B, 1976; Wagner FW, 1981.
Description: This diabetic foot ulcer grading system, first described by Meggitt (1976) and popularized by Wagner (1981), describes six wound *grades* that are primarily based on wound depth. Infection is included as a component of Grade 3. End-stage vascular disease (gangrene) is the predominant component in Grades 4 and 5. There is no indication of infection or vascular status of wounds in Grades 0 to 2.

The Wagner diabetic foot grading system was designed to describe the "natural history" of the diabetic foot ulceration as it progressed from intact skin under or over a bony prominence to ulceration, abscess, osteomyelitis, and gangrene. More recently, critical revisions of the Wagner Wound Classification have incorporated vascular and infection status into the grading of diabetic foot lesions (Lavery et al, 1996; Brodsky, 1999; Smith, 2003). However, the Wagner Wound Classification continues to be the system most widely used by clinicians for grading of diabetic foot wounds.

References

Brodsky JW: The diabetic foot. In Mann RA, editor. *Surgery of the foot and ankle,* ed 7, (vol, pp. 895-969). St Louis, 1999, Mosby.

Lavery LA, Armstrong DG, Harkless LB: Classification of diabetic foot wounds. *J Foot Ankle Surg* 35:528-531, 1996.

Meggitt B: Surgical management of the diabetic foot. *Br J Hosp Med* 16:227-332, 1976.

Smith RG: Validation of Wagner's classification: a literature review. *Ostomy Wound Manage* 49:54-62, 2003.

Wagner FW: The dysvascular foot: a system for diagnosis and treatment. *Foot Ankle* 2:64-122, 1981.

University of Texas Diabetic Wound Classification System

Authors: Lavery LA et al, 1996.

Source: This system is reprinted in this text and is also available online at http://www.medal.org/ch21.html.

Description: The diabetic wound classification system of the University of Texas Health Science Center, San Antonio, assesses ulcer depth, the presence of wound infection, and the presence of clinical signs of lower-extremity ischemia. This system uses four *grades* of ulcer depth (0 to 3); within each grade are four *stages* (A to D), based on ischemia or infection, or both.

Accuracy: Armstrong et al (1998) demonstrated that outcomes deteriorated with increasing grade and stage of wounds when the University of Texas Wound Classification System was used. The University of Texas system has been statistically shown to be a better predictor of outcome, compared with the Wagner Wound Classification, in that the addition of staging to the grade classification enhances the prognostic power of the tool in assessing risk for amputation and prediction of ulcer healing (Armstrong et al, 1998; Oyibo et al, 2001; Smith, 2003).

References

Armstrong DG, Lavery LA, Harkless LB: Validation of a diabetic wound classification system. The contribution of depth, infection, and ischemia to risk of amputation. *Diabetes Care* 21:855-859, 1998.

Lavery, LA, Armstrong DG, Harkless LB: Classification of diabetic foot wounds. *J Foot Ankle Surg* 35:528-531, 1996.

Oyibo SO, Jude EB, Tarawneh I, et al: A comparison of two diabetic foot ulcer classification systems: the Wagner and the University of Texas wound classification systems. *Diabetes Care* 24:84-88, 2001.

Smith RG: Validation of Wagner's classification: a literature review. *Ostomy Wound Manage* 49:54-62, 2003.

RISK ASSESSMENT TOOLS FOR PRESSURE ULCERS

Development of pressure ulcers is a serious and common problem of the immobile, chronically ill patient. Elderly persons who are confined to bed or a chair are predominantly at risk. Such patients may be hospitalized, reside in long-term care facilities, or be cared for at home.

Box 13-2	Risk Assessment Tools for Pressure Ulcers

Norton Scale for Predicting Risk of Pressure Ulcer (Norton, 1962)
Waterlow Pressure Sore Risk Scale (Waterlow, 1985)
Braden Scale for Predicting Risk of Pressure Ulcer (Bergstrom et al, 1987)
Gosnell Scale for Predicting Risk of Pressure Ulcer (Gosnell, 1989)
Cornell Ulcer Risk Score (CURS) (Eachempati et al, 2001)

These tools may be found online at http://www.medal.org/ch21.html.

Once pressure ulcers occur, morbidity is likely and may lead to death. Prevention of the development of pressure ulcers is facilitated by early detection of risk factors. Risk factors include immobility, loss of sensory perception, incontinence, impaired nutritional status, and friction/shearing forces.

Various tools have been developed to predict risk of pressure ulcers (Box 13-2). Included in this chapter are the Braden Scale for Predicting Pressure Sore Risk and the Norton Pressure Ulcer Prediction Scale. Both are widely used and have been recommended by the Agency for Health Care Policy and Research (1992) for predicting risk of pressure sores. Other tools may be found online, as indicated in Box 13-2.

Norton Pressure Ulcer Prediction Scale

Authors: Norton D et al, 1962.

Description: The Norton Pressure Ulcer Prediction Scale is a 5-item instrument that assesses general physical condition, mental condition, activity, mobility, and incontinence.

Scores: Each item is assigned a score from 1 (least favorable) to 4 (most favorable). The total score is the sum of the subscale scores. A normal score is 20; a total score of 14 or below indicates risk.

Accuracy: The Norton scale has been used as the risk assessment tool in many studies; however, its predictive accuracy is only 0% to 37% (Patterson & Bennett, 1995). Modifications to the Norton scale have been suggested, including addition of a category for nutrition and clarification of the terms good, fair, poor, and very bad (Kanj et al, 1998). Results of another study suggest that use of the activity and mobility subscales alone is sufficient to assess the risk of pressure ulcers in hospitalized patients (Perneger et al, 1998). Despite these criticisms, the Norton scale is widely used and is recommended by the Agency for Health Care Policy and Research (1992).

References

Agency for Health Care Policy and Research: Panel for the Prediction and Prevention of Pressure Ulcers in Adults. *Pressure ulcers in adults: Prediction and prevention. Clinical Practice Guideline No. 3*

(AHCPR Publication No. 92-0047). Rockville, MD, 1992, AHCP Research, Public Health Service, US Department of Health and Human Services.

Kanj LF, Wilking SV, Phillips TJ: Pressure ulcers. *J Am Acad Dermatol* 38:517-536, 1998.

Norton D: Calculating the risk: reflections on the Norton Scale. *Decubitus* 2:24-31, 1989.

Norton D, McLaren R, Exton-Smith AN: *An investigation of geriatric nursing problems in hospitals.* London: 1962, Corporation for the Care of Old People.

Patterson JA, Bennett RG: Prevention and treatment of pressure sores. *J Am Geriatr Soc* 43:919-927, 1995.

Perneger TV, Gaspoz JM, Raë AC, et al: Contribution of individual items to the performance of the Norton pressure ulcer prediction scale. *J Am Geriatr Soc* 46:1282-1286, 1998.

Braden Scale for Predicting Pressure Sore Risk

Authors: Bergstromn N et al, 1987a, 1987b.

Source: The Braden Scale is reprinted here and is also available online at http://www.bradenscale.com/braden.pdf, http://www.webmedtechnology.com/public/BradenScale-skin.pdf, and http://www.rohoinc.com/pdf/braden.pdf. The tool is copyright protected; permission for use may be granted at no charge to professionals who agree not to resell it or to profit from its use. Permission is readily given to those using the tool in research, scholarly publications, or programs of prevention in clinical agencies. For more information and permission for use, see http://www.bradenscale.com/.

Description: Created in 1988, the Braden Scale assesses six areas of risk for development of pressure ulcers: levels of sensory perception, activity, mobility, skin moisture, friction/shear, and nutrition.

Scores: Each risk area is assigned a score from 1 (least favorable) to 4 (most favorable), with the exception of the friction and shear subscale, which is rated from 1 to 3. The total score is the sum of the six subscale scores. A normal score is 23; a score less than 16 indicates high risk for pressure sore development. Bergstrom et al (1998) established 18 as the critical cutoff score for predicting risk in a variety of settings. Braden and Bergstrom (1996) recommend that all patients be assessed on admission and 24 to 48 hours later, followed by ongoing assessment.

Accuracy: Depending on the population studied, the sensitivity of this scoring system ranges from 79% to 100%; the specificity, from 64% to 90%; and the positive predictive value, from 37% to 54%; interrater reliability is high (Braden & Bergstrom, 1994; Bergstrom et al, 1996; Bergstrom et al, 1987a, 1987b; Patterson & Bennett, 1995). Registered nurses were shown to be able to use the Braden Scale more reliably than nurse aides and licensed practical nurses (Bergstrom et al, 1987).

References

Braden BJ, Bergstrom N: Predictive validity of the Braden Scale for pressure sore risk in a nursing home population. *Res Nurs Health* 17:459-470, 1994.

Braden BJ, Bergstrom N: Risk assessment and risk-based programs of prevention in various settings. *Ostomy Wound Manage* 42(10A suppl):6S-12S, 1996.

Bergstrom N, Braden B, Kemp M, et al: Multi-site study of incidence of pressure ulcers and the relationship between risk level, demographic characteristics, diagnoses, and prescription of preventive interventions. *J Am Geriatr Soc* 44:22-30, 1996.

Bergstrom N, Braden B, Kemp M, et al: Predicting pressure ulcer risk: a multisite study of the predictive validity of the Braden Scale. *Nurs Res* 47:61-69, 1998.

Bergstrom N, Braden BJ, Laguzza A, et al: The Braden Scale for predicting pressure sore risk. *Nurs Res* 36:205-210, 1987a.

Bergstrom N, Demuth PJ, Braden BJ: A clinical trial of the Braden Scale for predicting pressure sore risk. *Nurs Clin North Am* 22:417-428, 1987b.

Patterson JA, Bennett RG: Prevention and treatment of pressure sores. *J Am Geriatr Soc* 43:919-927, 1995.

References

Agency for Health Care Policy and Research: Panel for the Prediction and Prevention of Pressure Ulcers in Adults. *Pressure ulcers in adults: Prediction and prevention. Clinical Practice Guideline No. 3* (AHCPR Publication No. 92-0047). Rockville, MD, 1992, AHCP Research, Public Health Service, US Department of Health and Human Services.

Bergstrom N, Braden BJ, Laguzza A, et al: The Braden Scale for predicting pressure sore risk. *Nurs Res* 36:205-210, 1987a.

Brodsky JW: The diabetic foot. In Mann, RA, editor. *Surgery of the foot and ankle,* ed 7, (vol, pp. 895-969). St Louis, 1999, Mosby.

Eachempati SR, Hydo LJ, Barie PS: Factors influencing the development of decubitus ulcers in critically ill surgical patients. *Crit Care Med* 29:1678-1682, 2001.

Ferrell BA, Artinian BM, Sessing D: The Sessing Scale for assessment of pressure ulcer healing. *J Am Geriatric Soc* 43:37-40, 1995.

Gosnell DJ: Pressure sore risk assessment: a critique. Part I: The Gosnell scale. *Decubitus* 2:32-38, 1989.

Lavery LA, Armstrong DG, Harkless LB: Classification of diabetic foot wounds. *J Foot Ankle Surg* 35:528-531, 1996.

National Pressure Ulcer Advisory Panel: Pressure ulcers prevalence cost and risk assessment: consensus development conference statement. *Decubitus* 2:24-28, 1989.

Norton D, McLaren R, Exton-Smith AN: *An investigation of geriatric nursing problems in hospitals.* London: 1962, Corporation for the Care of Old People.

Shea JD: Pressure sores: classification and management. *Clin Orthop Related Res* 112:89-100, 1975.

Stotts NA, Rodeheaver GT, Thomas DR, et al: An instrument to measure healing in pressure ulcers: development and validation of the pressure ulcer scale for healing (PUSH). *J Gerontol* 56:M795-M799, 2001.

Wagner FW: The dysvascular foot: a system for diagnosis and treatment. *Foot Ankle* 2:64-122, 1981.

Waterlow J: Pressure sores: a risk assessment card. *Nurs Times* 81:49-55, 1985.

Wound Ostomy and Continence Nurse Society. Spring 2001. OASIS *Guidance Document: status for a pressure ulcer.* Available at http://www.wocn.org/

Yarkony GM, Mathews P, Carlson C: Classification of pressure ulcers. *Arch Dermatol* 126:1218-1219, 1990.

National Pressure Ulcer Advisory Panel (NPUAP)
Staging System for Pressure Ulcerations

Stage I: Nonblanchable erythema of intact skin, the heralding lesion of skin ulceration. In individuals with darker skin, discoloration of the skin, warmth, edema, induration, or hardness may also be indicators.

Stage II: Partial-thickness skin loss involving epidermis, dermis, or both. The ulcer is superficial and presents clinically as an abrasion, blister, or shallow crater.

Stage III: Full-thickness skin loss involving damage to or necrosis of subcutaneous tissue that may extend down to, but not through, underlying fascia. The ulcer presents clinically as a deep crater with or without undermining of adjacent tissue.

Stage IV: Full-thickness skin loss with extensive destruction, tissue necrosis, or damage to muscle, bone, or supporting structures (e.g., tendon, joint capsule). Undermining and sinus tracts may also be associated with stage 4 pressure ulcers.

National Pressure Ulcer Advisory Panel, 1998. Web site: http://www.npuap.org.

Wagner Wound Classification

Grade 0:   No open lesion. Pre- or post-ulcerative lesion with intact skin

Grade 1:   Partial- or full-thickness superficial ulcer

Grade 2:   Full-thickness ulcer open to tendon, ligament, bone, or joint capsule

Grade 3:   Full-thickness ulcer open to bone with abscess or osteomyelitis

Grade 4:   Full-thickness ulcer with partial foot gangrene, wet or dry, with or without cellulitis

Grade 5:   Whole foot gangrene, nonsalvageable

From Wagner FW, Jr: A dysvascular foot: a system for diagnosis and treatment, *Foot Ankle* 2:64-122, 1981. Reprinted with permission.

University of Texas Diabetic Wound Classification System

	Grade			
	0	**I**	**II**	**III**
A Nonischemic clean wounds	Preulcerative or postulcerative lesion completely epithelialized	Superficial wound, not involving tendon, capsule, or bone	Wound penetrating to tendon or capsule	Wound penetrating to bone or joint
B Infected nonischemic wounds	Preulcerative or postulcerative lesion, completely epithelialized with infection	Superficial wound, not involving tendon, capsule, or bone with infection	Wound penetrating to tendon or capsule with infection	Wound penetrating to bone or joint with infection
C Ischemic wounds	Preulcerative or postulcerative lesion, completely epithelialized with ischemia	Superficial wound, not involving tendon, capsule, or bone with ischemia	Wound penetrating to tendon or capsule with ischemia	Wound penetrating to bone or joint with ischemia
D Infected ischemic wounds	Preulcerative or postulcerative lesion, completely epithelialized with infection and ischemia	Superficial wound, not involving tendon, capsule, or bone with infection and ischemia	Wound penetrating to tendon or capsule with infection and ischemia	Wound penetrating to bone or joint with infection and ischemia

From Lavery LA, Armstrong DG, Harkless LB: Classification of diabetic foot wounds, *J Foot Ankle Surg* 35:528-531, 1996. Reproduced with permission.

Norton Pressure Ulcer Prediction Scale

Name	Date	Physical condition		Mental condition		Activity		Mobility		Incontinent		Total score
		Good	4	Alert	4	Ambulant	4	Full	4	Not	4	
		Fair	3	Apathetic	3	Walk/help	3	Slightly limited	3	Occasional	3	
		Poor	2	Confused	2	Chairbound	2	Very limited	2	Usually/Urine	2	
		Very bad	1	Stupor	1	Stupor	1	Immobile	1	Doubly	1	

Interpretation: maximum score 20; minimum score 5; at risk for pressure ulcer if score ≤ 14

From Norton D, McLaren R, Exton-Smith AN: *An investigation of geriatric nursing problems in hospitals*, 1962. Copyright: National Corporation for the Care of Old People (now Centre for Policy on Ageing), London, England. Reprinted with permission.

Braden Scale for Predicting Pressure Sore Risk

Patient's Name _____   Evaluator's Name _____   Date of Assessment _____

	1	2	3	4				
SENSORY PERCEPTION ability to respond meaningfully to pressure-related discomfort	**1. Completely Limited** Unresponsive (does not moan, flinch, or grasp) to painful stimuli, due to diminished level of consciousness or sedation. OR limited ability to feel pain over most of body.	**2. Very Limited** Responds only to painful stimuli. Cannot communicate discomfort except by moaning or restlessness OR has a sensory impairment which limits the ability to feel pain or discomfort over ½ of body.	**3. Slightly Limited** Responds to verbal commands, but cannot always communicate discomfort or the need to be turned. OR has some sensory impairment which limits ability to feel pain or discomfort in 1 or 2 extremities.	**4. No Impairment** Responds to verbal commands. Has no sensory deficit which would limit ability to feel or voice pain or discomfort.				
MOISTURE exposed to moisture	**1. Constantly Moist** Skin is kept moist almost constantly by perspiration, urine, etc. Dampness is detected every time patient is moved or turned.	**2. Very Moist** Skin is often, but not always moist. Linen must be changed at least once a shift.	**3. Occasionally Moist** Skin is occasionally moist, requiring an extra linen change approximately once a day.	**4. Rarely Moist** Skin is usually dry, linen only requires changing at routine intervals.				
ACTIVITY degree of physical activity	**1. Bedfast** Confined to bed.	**2. Chairfast** Ability to walk severely limited or non-existent. Cannot bear own weight and/or must be assisted into chair or wheelchair.	**3. Walks Occasionally** Walks occasionally during day, but for very short distances, with or without assistance. Spends majority of each shift in bed or chair.	**4. Walks Frequently** Walks outside room at least twice a day and inside room at least once every two hours during waking hours				
MOBILITY ability to change and control body position	**1. Completely Immobile** Does not make even slight changes in body or extremity position without assistance	**2. Very Limited** Makes occasional slight changes in body or extremity position but unable to make frequent or significant changes independently.	**3. Slightly Limited** Makes frequent though slight changes in body or extremity position independently.	**4. No Limitation** Makes major and frequent changes in position without assistance.				
NUTRITION usual food intake pattern	**1. Very Poor** Never eats a complete meal. Rarely eats more than ⅓ of any food offered. Eats 2 servings or less of protein (meat or dairy products) per day. Takes fluids poorly. Does not take a liquid dietary supplement OR is NPO and/or maintained on clear liquids or IV's for more than 5 days.	**2. Probably Inadequate** Rarely eats a complete meal and generally eats only about ½ of any food offered. Protein intake includes only 3 servings of meat or dairy products per day. Occasionally will take a dietary supplement. OR receives less than optimum amount of liquid diet or tube feeding	**3. Adequate** Eats over half of most meals. Eats a total of 4 servings of protein (meat, dairy products) per day. Occasionally will refuse a meal, but will usually take a supplement when offered OR is on a tube feeding or TPN regimen which probably meets most of nutritional needs	**4. Excellent** Eats most of every meal. Never refuses a meal. Usually eats a total of 4 or more servings of meat and dairy products. Occasionally eats between meals. Does not require supplementation.				
FRICTION & SHEAR	**1. Problem** Requires moderate to maximum assistance in moving. Complete lifting without sliding against sheets is impossible. Frequently slides down in bed or chair, requiring frequent repositioning with maximum assistance. Spasticity, contractures or agitation leads to almost constant friction	**2. Potential Problem** Moves feebly or requires minimum assistance. During a move skin probably slides to some extent against sheets, chair, restraints or other devices. Maintains relatively good position in chair or bed most of the time but occasionally slides down.	**3. No Apparent Problem** Moves in bed and in chair independently and has sufficient muscle strength to lift up completely during move. Maintains good position in bed or chair.					
								Total Score

Nutrition Tools

Chapter Contents

Chapter Contents

This chapter consists of tools used in assessment and counseling of nutrition-related issues. Tools include weight screening tables and a validated nutritional assessment tool. Various food guide pyramids, which can help the clinician to tailor the diet to preferred eating styles, are included.

Body Mass Index 📄⊘

The body mass index (BMI) table measures BMI for heights 58 to 76 inches and weights from 91 to 443 pounds. BMI defines the degree of adiposity as measured by the following formula: Weight (lb)/Height (in^2). BMI provides general guidelines for the measure of body fatness for adults with underweight (BMI of <18.5), normal weight (BMI of 18.5-24.9), overweight (BMI of 25-29.9), and obesity (BMI of 30 or greater).

Tables are available at http://www.nhlbi.nih.gov/guidelines/obesity/bmi_tbl.htm and are reprinted here.

Height and Weight Assessment 📄⊘

Common reference standards are often used to compare body weight with height to determine the appropriate range of ideal body weights. These include the Metropolitan Life Insurance Tables. The 1999 table is reprinted here and is also available at http://www.bcbst.com/MPManual/HW.htm.

Ideal body weight may also be calculated by the Hamwi Method. For medium-sized adults, the ideal body weight for males is 106 lb for the first 5 feet of height and an additional 6 lb for every inch over 5 feet; the ideal body weight for females is 100 lb for the first 5 feet of height and an additional 5 lb for every inch over 5 feet.

If the body frame is light (small), then the calculated weight should be reduced by 10%. If the frame is heavy (large), then the calculated weight should be increased by 10%.

Mini Nutritional Assessment (MNA) 📄⊘

Author: Guigoz Y et al, 1996.
Source: The Mini Nutritional Assessment (MNA) is reprinted in this text. This tool—as well as an online user guide, scoring instructions, and discussion—may be found at http://www.mna-elderly.com/index.htm.
Targeted Population: Older adults.

Description: The MNA is a tool allowing rapid evaluation of the nutritional status of the frail elderly. The MNA is composed of 18 simple and rapidly measured items.

Scores: Each item is scored from 0 to 3 points as defined by responses to item questions. Item scores are summed for a total score, which ranges from 0 to 30. Thresholds were selected by cross-tabulations of serum albumin levels and MNA scoring levels from cross-validation results. Scores indicate malnutrition as follows: ≥24 points = well-nourished; 17 to 23.5 points = at risk for malnutrition; <17 points = malnourished.

Accuracy: The initial developmental study included two criteria used to validate the findings with excellent correlation for both parameters: clinical status (physician-conducted independent nutritional assessment) and comprehensive nutritional assessment. The MNA has been tested for concurrent validity in differing populations with excellent results at matching the clinical status (well-nourished or undernourished) with MNA score (Garry et al, 1982; Stuck et al, 1993).

Administration Time: Less than 15 minutes by proxy administration.

References

Garry PJ, Goodwin JS, Hunt WC, et al: Nutritional status in a healthy elderly population: dietary and supplemental intake. *Am J Clin Nutr* 36:319-331, 1982.

Guigoz Y, Vellas B, Garry PJ: Assessing the nutritional status of the elderly: The Mini Nutritional Assessment as part of the geriatric evaluation. *Nutr Rev* 54:S59-S65, 1996.

Stuck AE, Siu AL, Wieland GD, et al: Comprehensive geriatric assessment: a meta-analysis of controlled trials. *Lancet* 342:1032–1036, 1993.

FOOD GUIDE PYRAMIDS

Dietary guidelines are created by various health organizations with the goal of providing recommendations for caloric intake and exercise levels, which promote the achievement and maintenance of ideal weight. Guidelines also seek to ensure nutrient adequacy and promote food choices that have favorable findings in prevention of chronic diseases. Food guide pyramids translate the essential ingredients detailed in dietary guidelines into the kinds and amounts of food to be eaten each day. Pyramids have been tailored to meet the eating preferences of a variety of populations, while incorporating the essential nutrients and calories into an achievable, understandable diet.

USDA Food Guide Pyramid

The traditional Food Guide Pyramid, based on the USDA Food Guide Pyramid Dietary Guidelines, guides the user to food choices from six general food groups, recommending the number of servings the user should eat from each part of the pyramid every day. It is a general guide that lets the user choose a customized, healthful diet. The Pyramid calls for eating a variety of foods to get needed nutrients and the amount of calories to maintain healthy weight. The U.S. Department of Agriculture (USDA) Food Guide Pyramid is available at http://www. schoolmeals.nal.usda.gov/py/pmap.htm.

Food Guide Pyramid for Young Children

This pyramid is an adaptation of the original USDA Food Guide Pyramid, released in 1992. The adaptations, based on actual food patterns of young children, simplify the educational messages and focus on food preferences and nutritional requirements of young children (2 to 6 years old). The Food Guide Pyramid for Young Children is available at http://www.usda.gov/cnpp/KidsPyra/.

Willett's Healthy Eating Pyramid

Author: Willetts W, 2001.

Recent evidence suggests that adherence to the USDA Dietary Guidelines for Americans is associated with only a small reduction in major chronic disease risk (McCullough et al, 2002). Walter Willett's Healthy Eating Pyramid is an alternative to the traditional US Food Guide Pyramid. Willett suggests that when the recommendations are followed closely, it will result in significantly reduced risk for major chronic diseases (Willett, 2001). Based on research at the Harvard School of Public Health and the Harvard Medical School, this new Food Guide Pyramid was developed along with healthy eating guidelines. The Pyramid focuses on reduction of total caloric intake, reduction or elimination of trans-fats, promotion of carbohydrates with low glycemic indices, proper ratios of monounsaturated and polyunsaturated fats, and daily exercise. Walter Willett's Healthy Eating Pyramid is available at http://www.hsph.harvard.edu/now/aug24/.

References

McCullough ML, Feskanich D, Stampfer MJ, et al: Diet quality and major chronic disease risk in men and women: moving toward improved dietary guidance. *Am J Clin Nutr* 76:1261-1271, 2002.

Willett W: *Eat, drink and be healthy*. New York, 2001, Simon and Schuster.

Food Guide Pyramid for Vegetarian Meal Planning

In response to the prevalence of vegetarian diets, the American Dietetic Association (ADA) released a position statement in 1997, with a "Food Guide Pyramid for Vegetarian Meal Planning." The ADA stated that appropriately planned vegetarian diets are healthful and nutritionally adequate and provide health benefits in the prevention and treatment of certain diseases. The Food Guide Pyramid for Vegetarian Meal Planning is available at http://www.vrg.org/nutrition/adapyramid.htm.

Box **14-1** Ethnic Cultural Food Pyramids*
Asian Diet Pyramid
Bilingual Food Guide Pyramids in over 30 different languages
Arabic Food Pyramid
Chinese Food Pyramid
Cuban Food Pyramid
Indian Food Pyramid
Italian Food Pyramid
Mexican Food Pyramid
Portuguese Food Pyramid
Russian Food Pyramid
Thai Food Pyramid
Japanese Food Pyramid
Mediterranean Diet Pyramid
Native American Food Guide
Spanish Daily Food Guide Flyer

*From the U.S. Department of Agriculture. Available at http://www.nal.usda.gov/fnic/etext/000023.html#xtocid2381818

Box **14-2** Food Pyramids for Special Audiences
Interactive Food Guide Pyramid for Kids*
Food Guide Pyramid Quiz for Preschool Nutrition*
Pyramid Tracker for Kids age 7-10*
Food Guide Pyramid Concentration Game*
Modified Food Guide Pyramid for People Over 70 Years*
Vegetarian Diet Pyramid*
Prader-Willi Food Pyramid: http://www.pwsausa.org/syndrome/foodpyramid.htm
Beverage Guide Pyramid From the Processed Apple Institute: http://www.applejuice.org/SmartSip.html#d
Food Guide Pyramid for Children with Diabetes: http://www.castleweb.com/Diabetes/d_08_800.htm
Vegetarian Food Guide Pyramid from VegSource: http://www.vegsource.com/nutrition/pyramid.htm
Food Guide Pyramid for Older Adults: http://nutrition.tufts.edu/consumer/pyramid.html
Activity Pyramid: http://www.nmclites.edu/wellness/activity-pyr.htm

*From the U.S. Department of Agriculture. Available at http://www.nal.usda.gov/fnic/etext/000023.html#xtocid2381818

Reference

Messina VK, Burke KI: Position of The American Dietetic Association: vegetarian diets. *J Am Diet Assoc* 97:1317-1321, 1997.

Other Food Guide Pyramid Resources:

Ethnic/Cultural and Specialized Food Pyramids

The Food and Nutrition Information Center (FNIC) is located at the National Agricultural Library (NAL), part of the USDA and the Agricultural Research Service (ARS).

Their award-winning website, http://www.nal.usda.gov/fnic/index.html, contains tools and resources for nutrition counseling, including child care nutrition, food safety, resources for the Women, Infants and Children (WIC) Program, a resource system for healthy school meals, and food stamps nutrition education information.

Specialized food pyramids found on this site include ethnic/cultural food pyramids (Box 14-1), food pyramids for special audiences (Box 14-2), and the Mayo Clinic Healthy Weight Pyramid.

Body Mass Index

BMI (Height in inches)	Normal						Overweight					Obese										Extreme Obesity															
	19	20	21	22	23	24	25	26	27	28	29	30	31	32	33	34	35	36	37	38	39	40	41	42	43	44	45	46	47	48	49	50	51	52	53	54
	Body Weight (pounds)																																			
58	91	96	100	105	110	115	119	124	129	134	138	143	148	153	158	162	167	172	177	181	186	191	196	201	205	210	215	220	224	229	234	239	244	248	253	258
59	94	99	104	109	114	119	124	128	133	138	143	148	153	158	163	168	173	178	183	188	193	198	203	208	212	217	222	227	232	237	242	247	252	257	262	267
60	97	102	107	112	118	123	128	133	138	143	148	153	158	163	168	174	179	184	189	194	199	204	209	215	220	225	230	235	240	245	250	255	261	266	271	276
61	100	106	111	116	122	127	132	137	143	148	153	158	164	169	174	180	185	190	195	201	206	211	217	222	227	232	238	243	248	254	259	264	269	275	280	285
62	104	109	115	120	126	131	136	142	147	153	158	164	169	175	180	186	191	196	202	207	213	218	224	229	235	240	246	251	256	262	267	273	278	284	289	295
63	107	113	118	124	130	135	141	146	152	158	163	169	175	180	186	191	197	203	208	214	220	225	231	237	242	248	254	259	265	270	278	282	287	293	299	304
64	110	116	122	128	134	140	145	151	157	163	169	174	180	186	192	197	204	209	215	221	227	232	238	244	250	256	262	267	273	279	285	291	296	302	308	314
65	114	120	126	132	138	144	150	156	162	168	174	180	186	192	198	204	210	216	222	228	234	240	246	252	258	264	270	276	282	288	294	300	306	312	318	324
66	118	124	130	136	142	148	155	161	167	173	179	186	192	198	204	210	216	223	229	235	241	247	253	260	266	272	278	284	291	297	303	309	315	322	328	334
67	121	127	134	140	146	153	159	166	172	178	185	191	198	204	211	217	223	230	236	242	249	255	261	268	274	280	287	293	299	306	312	319	325	331	338	344
68	125	131	138	144	151	158	164	171	177	184	190	197	203	210	216	223	230	236	243	249	256	262	269	276	282	289	295	302	308	315	322	328	335	341	348	354
69	128	135	142	149	155	162	169	176	182	189	196	203	209	216	223	230	236	243	250	257	263	270	277	284	291	297	304	311	318	324	331	338	345	351	358	365
70	132	139	146	153	160	167	174	181	188	195	202	209	216	222	229	236	243	250	257	264	271	278	285	292	299	306	313	320	327	334	341	348	355	362	369	376
71	136	143	150	157	165	172	179	186	193	200	208	215	222	229	236	243	250	257	265	272	279	286	293	301	308	315	322	329	338	343	351	358	365	372	379	386
72	140	147	154	162	169	177	184	191	199	206	213	221	228	235	242	250	258	265	272	279	287	294	302	309	316	324	331	338	346	353	361	368	375	383	390	397
73	144	151	159	166	174	182	189	197	204	212	219	227	235	242	250	257	265	272	280	288	295	302	310	318	325	333	340	348	355	363	371	378	386	393	401	408
74	148	155	163	171	179	186	194	202	210	218	225	233	241	249	256	264	272	280	287	295	303	311	319	326	334	342	350	358	365	373	381	389	396	404	412	420
75	152	160	168	176	184	192	200	208	216	224	232	240	248	256	264	272	279	287	295	303	311	319	327	335	343	351	359	367	375	383	391	399	407	415	423	431
76	156	164	172	180	189	197	205	213	221	230	238	246	254	263	271	279	287	295	304	312	320	328	336	344	353	361	369	377	385	394	402	410	418	426	435	443

Source: Adapted from Clinical Guidelines on the Identification, Evaluation, and Treatment of Overweight and Obesity in Adults: The Evidence Report.

HEIGHT AND WEIGHT ASSESSMENT

Women

Height (feet/inches)	Small Frame	Medium Frame	Large Frame
4'10"	102-111	109-121	118-131
4'11"	103-113	111-123	120-134
5'0"	104-115	113-126	122-137
5'1"	106-118	115-129	125-140
5'2"	108-121	118-132	128-143
5'3"	111-124	121-135	131-147
5'4"	114-127	124-138	134-151
5'5"	117-130	127-141	137-155
5'6"	120-133	130-144	140-159
5'7"	123-136	133-147	143-163
5'8"	126-139	136-150	146-167
5'9"	129-142	139-153	149-170
5'10"	132-145	142-156	152-173
5'11"	135-148	145-159	155-176
6'0"	138-151	148-162	158-179

Weights at ages 25-59 based on lowest mortality weight in pounds according to frame (in indoor clothing weighing 3 lbs., shoes with 1" heel)

Men

Height (feet/inches)	Small Frame	Medium Frame	Large Frame
5'2"	128-134	131-141	138-150
5'3"	130-136	133-143	140-153
5'4"	132-138	135-145	142-156
5'5"	134-140	137-148	144-160
5'6"	136-142	139-151	146-164
5'7"	138-145	142-154	149-168
5'8"	140-148	145-157	152-172
5'9"	142-151	148-160	155-176
5'10"	144-154	151-163	158-180
5'11"	146-157	154-166	161-184
6'0"	149-160	157-170	164-188
6'1"	152-164	160-174	168-192
6'2"	155-168	164-178	172-197
6'3"	158-172	167-182	176-202
6'4"	162-176	171-187	181-207

Weights at ages 25-59 based on lowest mortality weight in pounds according to frame (in indoor clothing weighing 3 lbs., shoes with 1" heel)

NESTLÉ NUTRITION SERVICES

Mini Nutritional Assessment (MNA)

Last name: _____   First name: _____   Sex: _____   Date: _____

Age: _____   Weight, kg: _____   Height, cm: _____   I.D. Number: _____

Complete the screen by filling in the boxes with the appropriate numbers.
Add the numbers for the screen. If score is 11 or less, continue with the assessment to gain a Malnutrition Indicator Score.

Screening

A Has food intake declined over the past 3 months due to loss of appetite, digestive problems, chewing or swallowing difficulties?
0 = severe loss of appetite
1 = moderate loss of appetite
2 = no loss of appetite ☐

B Weight loss during last 3 months
0 = weight loss greater than 3 kg (6.6 lbs)
1 = does not know
2 = weight loss between 1 and 3 kg (2.2 and 6.6 lbs)
3 = no weight loss ☐

C Mobility
0 = bed or chair bound
1 = able to get out of bed/chair but does not go out
2 = goes out ☐

D Has suffered psychological stress or acute disease in the past 3 months
0 = yes   2 = no ☐

E Neuropsychological problems
0 = severe dementia or depression
1 = mild dementia
2 = no psychological problems ☐

F Body Mass Index (BMI) (weight in kg) / (height in m)²
0 = BMI less than 19
1 = BMI 19 to less than 21
2 = BMI 21 to less than 23
3 = BMI 23 or greater ☐

Screening score (subtotal max. 14 points) ☐ ☐

12 points or greater   Normal – not at risk – no need to complete assessment
11 points or below   Possible malnutrition – continue assessment

Assessment

G Lives independently (not in a nursing home or hospital)
0 = no   1 = yes ☐

H Takes more than 3 prescription drugs per day
0 = yes   1 = no ☐

I Pressure sores or skin ulcers
0 = yes   1 = no ☐

J How many full meals does the patient eat daily?
0 = 1 meal
1 = 2 meals
2 = 3 meals ☐

K Selected consumption markers for protein intake
• At least one serving of dairy products (milk, cheese, yogurt) per day?   yes ☐ no ☐
• Two or more servings of legumes or eggs per week?   yes ☐ no ☐
• Meat, fish or poultry every day   yes ☐ no ☐
0.0 = if 0 or 1 yes
0.5 = if 2 yes
1.0 = if 3 yes ☐ . ☐

L Consumes two or more servings of fruits or vegetables per day?
0 = no   1 = yes ☐

M How much fluid (water, juice, coffee, tea, milk…) is consumed per day?
0.0 = less than 3 cups
0.5 = 3 to 5 cups
1.0 = more than 5 cups ☐ . ☐

N Mode of feeding
0 = unable to eat without assistance
1 = self-fed with some difficulty
2 = self-fed without any problem ☐

O Self view of nutritional status
0 = views self as being malnourished
1 = is uncertain of nutritional state
2 = views self as having no nutritional problem ☐

P In comparison with other people of the same age, how does the patient consider his/her health status?
0.0 = not as good
0.5 = does not know
1.0 = as good
2.0 = better ☐ . ☐

Q Mid-arm circumference (MAC) in cm
0.0 = MAC less than 21
0.5 = MAC 21 to 22
1.0 = MAC 22 or greater ☐ . ☐

R Calf circumference (CC) in cm
0 = CC less than 31   1 = CC 31 or greater ☐

Assessment (max. 16 points) ☐ ☐ . ☐

Screening score ☐ ☐

Total Assessment (max. 30 points) ☐ ☐ . ☐

Malnutrition Indicator Score

17 to 23.5 points   at risk of malnutrition ☐

Less than 17 points   malnourished ☐

Ref.: Guigoz Y, Vellas B and Garry P.J. 1994. Mini Nutritional Assessment: A practical assessment tool for grading the nutritional state of elderly patients. *Facts and Research in Gerontology.* Supplement #2:15-59.
Rubenstein LZ, Harker J, Guigoz Y and Vellas B. Comprehensive Geriatric Assessment (CGA) and the MNA: An Overview of CGA, Nutritional Assessment, and Development of a Shortened Version of the MNA. In: "Mini Nutritional Assessment (MNA): Research and Practice in the Elderly". Vellas B, Garry PJ and Guigoz Y , editors. Nestlé Nutrition Workshop Series. Clinical & Performance Programme, vol. 1. Karger, Bâle, in press.

Food Guide Pyramid

A Guide to Daily Food Choices

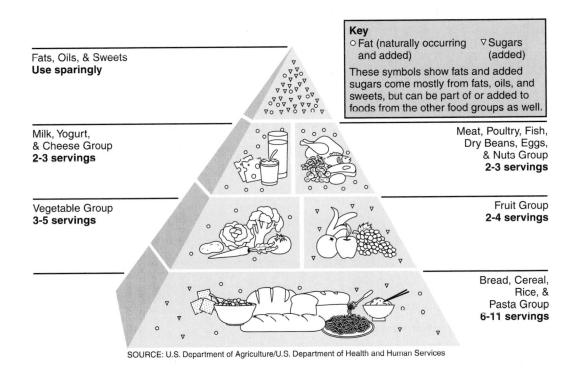

Fats, Oils, & Sweets
Use sparingly

Key
○ Fat (naturally occurring   ▽ Sugars
and added)   (added)

These symbols show fats and added
sugars come mostly from fats, oils, and
sweets, but can be part of or added to
foods from the other food groups as well.

Milk, Yogurt,
& Cheese Group
2-3 servings

Meat, Poultry, Fish,
Dry Beans, Eggs,
& Nuts Group
2-3 servings

Vegetable Group
3-5 servings

Fruit Group
2-4 servings

Bread, Cereal,
Rice, &
Pasta Group
6-11 servings

SOURCE: U.S. Department of Agriculture/U.S. Department of Health and Human Services

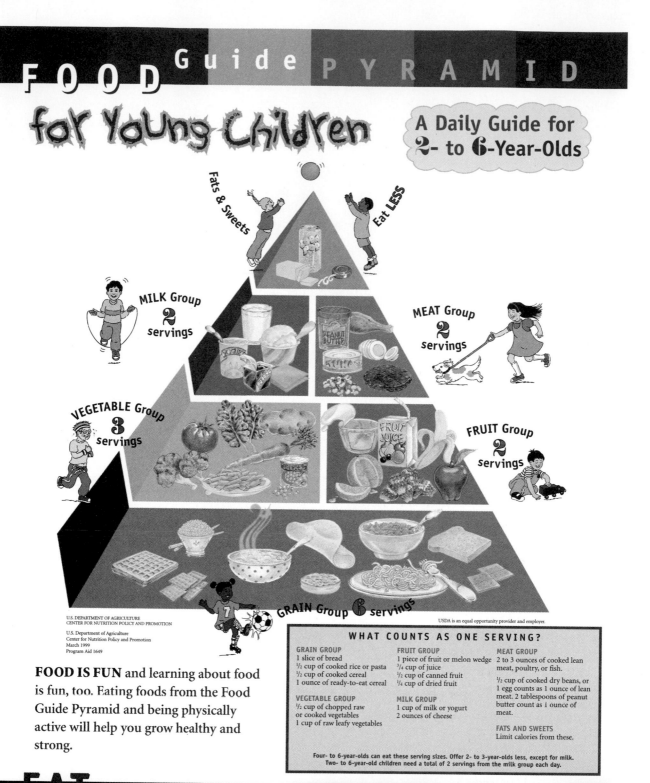

FOOD Guide PYRAMID

for Young Children

A Daily Guide for 2- to 6-Year-Olds

Fats & Sweets — Eat LESS

MILK Group 2 servings

MEAT Group 2 servings

VEGETABLE Group 3 servings

FRUIT Group 2 servings

GRAIN Group 6 servings

U.S. DEPARTMENT OF AGRICULTURE
CENTER FOR NUTRITION POLICY AND PROMOTION

U.S. Department of Agriculture
Center for Nutrition Policy and Promotion
March 1999
Program Aid 1649

USDA is an equal opportunity provider and employer.

FOOD IS FUN and learning about food is fun, too. Eating foods from the Food Guide Pyramid and being physically active will help you grow healthy and strong.

WHAT COUNTS AS ONE SERVING?

GRAIN GROUP
1 slice of bread
½ cup of cooked rice or pasta
½ cup of cooked cereal
1 ounce of ready-to-eat cereal

VEGETABLE GROUP
½ cup of chopped raw or cooked vegetables
1 cup of raw leafy vegetables

FRUIT GROUP
1 piece of fruit or melon wedge
¾ cup of juice
½ cup of canned fruit
¼ cup of dried fruit

MILK GROUP
1 cup of milk or yogurt
2 ounces of cheese

MEAT GROUP
2 to 3 ounces of cooked lean meat, poultry, or fish.

½ cup of cooked dry beans, or 1 egg counts as 1 ounce of lean meat. 2 tablespoons of peanut butter count as 1 ounce of meat.

FATS AND SWEETS
Limit calories from these.

Four- to 6-year-olds can eat these serving sizes. Offer 2- to 3-year-olds less, except for milk. Two- to 6-year-old children need a total of 2 servings from the milk group each day.

EAT a variety of FOODS AND ENJOY!

Willett's Healthy Eating Pyramid

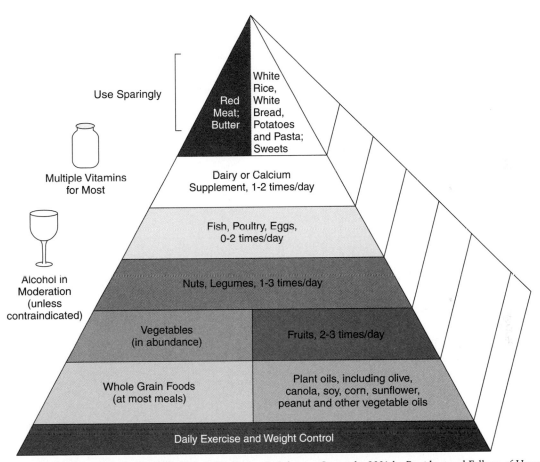

From Willett WC: *Eat, Drink, and Be Healthy*, New York, 2001, Simon & Schuster. Copyright 2001 by President and Fellows of Harvard College. Reprinted with permission.

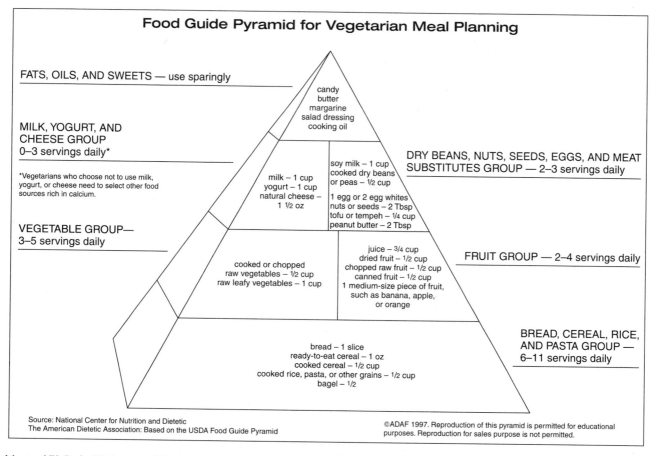

Food Guide Pyramid for Vegetarian Meal Planning

FATS, OILS, AND SWEETS — use sparingly

candy
butter
margarine
salad dressing
cooking oil

MILK, YOGURT, AND
CHEESE GROUP
0–3 servings daily*

*Vegetarians who choose not to use milk,
yogurt, or cheese need to select other food
sources rich in calcium.

milk – 1 cup
yogurt – 1 cup
natural cheese –
1 ½ oz

soy milk – 1 cup
cooked dry beans
or peas – ½ cup

1 egg or 2 egg whites
nuts or seeds – 2 Tbsp
tofu or tempeh – ¼ cup
peanut butter – 2 Tbsp

DRY BEANS, NUTS, SEEDS, EGGS, AND MEAT
SUBSTITUTES GROUP — 2–3 servings daily

VEGETABLE GROUP—
3–5 servings daily

cooked or chopped
raw vegetables – ½ cup
raw leafy vegetables – 1 cup

juice – ¾ cup
dried fruit – ½ cup
chopped raw fruit – ½ cup
canned fruit – ½ cup
1 medium-size piece of fruit,
such as banana, apple,
or orange

FRUIT GROUP — 2–4 servings daily

bread – 1 slice
ready-to-eat cereal – 1 oz
cooked cereal – ½ cup
cooked rice, pasta, or other grains – ½ cup
bagel – ½

BREAD, CEREAL, RICE,
AND PASTA GROUP —
6–11 servings daily

Source: National Center for Nutrition and Dietetic
The American Dietetic Association: Based on the USDA Food Guide Pyramid

©ADAF 1997. Reproduction of this pyramid is permitted for educational
purposes. Reproduction for sales purpose is not permitted.

Messina VK, Burke KI: Position of the American Dietetic Association: vegetarian diets, *J Am Diet Assoc* 97:1317-1321, 1997.

Copyright 1997 American Dietetic Association. Used with permission.

CHAPTER 15

System-Specific Assessment Tools

Chapter Contents

ICON KEY: 📄 Tool Printed ⊘ Tool on CD-ROM ∞ Customizable Tool **i** Information and Resources Provided for Further Acquisition

Chapter Contents—cont'd

ICON KEY: 📄 Tool Printed   ⬭ Tool on CD-ROM   ∞ Customizable Tool   **i** Information and Resources Provided for Further Acquisition

Introduction

Thousands of instruments, tools. and measures have been developed within specialty areas of health care. So many resources and instruments exist that they would fill several textbooks. Included in this chapter is a small sampling of the many specialty measures available. Tools were selected for inclusion on the basis of usefulness in a primary care practice, brevity, validity, and availability; the selection is by no means comprehensive.

Tools included here are categorized into cardiology, optometry, otolaryngology, neurology, gastroenterology, and urology and sexual function specialties. A small selection of tools that may be of use in a primary care practice are reviewed and made available within these categories. Space constraints and copyright protections have prevented the reproduction of the many measures available, and decisions about whether to include or eliminate a tool from this chapter were difficult to make. Many other tools exist, both within these categories and within other specialties such as pulmonology, orthopedics, rehabilitation medicine, gynecology, oncology, dermatology, and endocrinology. Fortunately, today's information technology permits access to many of these resources, which were once available only within original publications or textbooks.

Online Multispecialty Resources

Online medical and nursing resources have proliferated over the past several years. Websites now include links to specific instruments, specialty collections, professional organizations, online journals, government agencies, and medical libraries. Many of these resources have been cited in previous chapters; following are several online resources containing a broad spectrum of multispecialty information.

Free Medical Journals.com: The Free Medical Journals Site is dedicated to the promotion of free access to medical journals over the Internet. More than 1320 journals sorted by specialty, title, and language and "new journals" are available through links on this site. A "Journal Alert" feature allows the reader to be notified about new free journals. Available at http://www.freemedicaljournals.com/

Measurement Excellence Initiative–MEI Compendium: This Resource Center under the Veterans Administration Health Services and Research Development (HSR&D) Service is also known as the *Measurement Excellence and Training Resource Information Center*, or METRIC. The website provides reviews and listings of assessment instruments pertinent to research and clinical practice. Reviews provide practical information, research contacts, bibliography, factors and norms, and reliability and validity evidence for each measure. Available at http://www.measurementexperts.org/.

The Medical Algorithms Project: Cited previously throughout this text, this project contains hundreds of useful health care algorithms, rating scales, and references. A medical algorithm is any computation, formula, survey, measure, or look-up table that is useful in health care. More than 5100 algorithms, organized into 45 chapters, are available as spreadsheets. The algorithms have been collected from the biomedical literature, including research journals and textbooks. Available at http://www.medal.org/

UMass HealthNet: A project of the UMass Medical School, UMass Memorial Health Care, and cooperating agencies, this site provides direct access to measures, tools, organizations, and online resources in multispecialty areas. Available at http://www.healthnet. umassmed.edu/

WEB DIRxTIONS: This companion website offers convenient hyperlinks to the content available in printed directories published by the editors of WEB DIRxTIONS, which has been publishing MDWEB.COMpendium®, PATIENTWEB.COMpendium®, and WEB.COMpendium™ for 5 years. This independent company publishes content on more than 18 different medical/health topics. These peer-reviewed directories include essential websites for health care professionals and patients. The health care professional edition websites are rated overall for content and usability and specifically for characteristics such as continuing education credits, interactivity, forum for feedback, multilingual capability, fees, registration, and corporate sponsorship. Available at http://www.webdirxtions.com/

CARDIOLOGY

Heart Failure

New York Heart Association (NYHA) Classification for Congestive Heart Failure (CHF)   📄⬭

This well-known system, known as the *New York Heart Association Congestive Heart Failure (NYHA CHF) Classification* or *NYHA Functional Classification*, was developed in the 1970s and last revised in 1994 (American Heart Association [AHA], 1994). Although general wording of the classification has been modified in numerous publications, the basic system has classified functional capacity to estimate prognosis for patients with heart failure in clinical practice. While more recent classification and staging of heart failure has been published by the American College of Cardiology and AHA (Hunt et al, 2001), the NYHA CHF Classification continues to be widely used to describe functional limitations. It is now used in conjunction with the recent

| Box 15-1 | **New York Heart Association Functional Classification for Congestive Heart Failure (NYHA CHF)** |

Class I: No limitation of physical activity. Ordinary physical activity does not cause undue fatigue, palpitation, dyspnea, or angina.
Class II: Slight limitation of physical activity. Ordinary physical activity results in fatigue, palpitation, dyspnea, or angina.
Class III: Marked limitation of physical activity. Comfortable at rest, but less than ordinary physical activity results in fatigue, palpitation, dyspnea, or angina.
Class IV: Unable to carry on any physical activity without discomfort. Symptoms are present at rest. With any physical activity, symptoms increase.

Adapted from American Heart Association, Criteria Committee: AHA medical/scientific statement. 1994 revisions to classification of functional capacity and objective assessment of patients with diseases of the heart, *Circulation* 90:644-645, 1994.

American College of Cardiology (ACC)/AHA Classification Stages, which emphasize both the evolution and progression of the disease.

The NYHA Functional Classification (Box 15-1) subjectively measures the severity of disease by the presence of symptoms. Since the development of this classification, conceptual and clinical understanding of heart failure has progressed and changed such that treatment protocols go beyond the goal of limiting symptoms associated with physical activity. The NYHA classification continues to be used in conjunction with newer heart failure staging, to provide a clearer picture of the severity of symptoms.

American College of Cardiology (ACC)/American Heart Association (AHA) 2001 Guidelines: Stages of Heart Failure

Advances in cardiology made during the 1990s included better diagnostic capabilities, recognition of the significance of left ventricular dysfunction in the absence of symptoms, and improved treatment options for early stages of heart failure and for those at risk for heart failure. The concept of heart failure as a functional disease, in which patients go "in and out of failure" has changed and evolved to an understanding of its nature as a chronic disease characterized by progressive deterioration. Recognition of cellular processes that occur in the absence of symptoms has led to development of treatment protocols that may prevent further deterioration rather than focus solely on the elimination of symptoms.

A new approach to the classification of heart failure has been developed by expert committee members and jointly released by the ACC and AHA (Hunt et al, 2001) (Table 15-1). This approach objectively identifies the patient's stage of disease and links appropriate treatment

| Table 15-1 | **American College of Cardiology (ACC)/American Heart Association (AHA) 2001 Guidelines: Stages of Heart Failure** |

Stage	Description	Examples
A	Patients at high risk of developing HF because of the presence of conditions that are strongly associated with the development of HF. Such patients have no identified structural or functional abnormalities of the pericardium, myocardium, or cardiac valves and have never shown signs or symptoms of HF.	Systemic hypertension; coronary artery disease; diabetes mellitus; history of cardiotoxic drug therapy or alcohol abuse; personal history of rheumatic fever; family history of cardiomyopathy.
B	Patients who have developed structural heart disease that is strongly associated with the development of HF but who have never shown signs or symptoms of HF.	Left ventricular hypertrophy or fibrosis; left ventricular dilatation or hypocontractility; asymptomatic valvular heart disease; previous myocardial infarction.
C	Patients who have current or prior symptoms of HF associated with underlying structural heart disease.	Dyspnea or fatigue due to left ventricular systolic dysfunction; asymptomatic patients who are undergoing treatment for prior symptoms of HF.
D	Patients with advanced structural heart disease and marked symptoms of HF at rest despite maximal medical therapy and who require specialized interventions.	Patients who are frequently hospitalized for HF and cannot be safely discharged from the hospital; patients in the hospital awaiting heart transplantation; patients at home receiving continuous intravenous support for symptom relief or being supported with a mechanical circulatory assist device; patients in a hospice setting for the management of HF.

American College of Cardiology (ACC/AHA) 2001 Guidelines: Stages of Heart Failure. Copyright 2002 by the American College of Cardiology and American Heart Association, Inc. Reprinted with permission.
HF, Heart failure.

for each stage. Unlike the NYHA Functional Classification, in which a patient may present with acute symptoms only to experience regression to a less symptomatic class after treatment, the ACC/AHA stages are progressive only. Patients do not experience regression to a lesser stage; stages are based on progression of structural cardiac changes that may be slowed or stopped, but not reversed, by treatment.

Four stages of heart failure have been designated. Stage A identifies the patient who is at high risk for heart failure but has no structural disorder of the heart; stage B refers to a patient with a structural disorder of the heart who has never had symptoms of heart failure; stage C denotes the patient with past or current symptoms of heart failure associated with underlying structural heart disease; and stage D designates the patient with end-stage disease who requires specialized treatment strategies (Hunt et al, 2001). Large clinical trials have demonstrated that pharmacologic interventions can reduce the morbidity and mortality rates associated with heart failure. Treatment of patients at risk for heart failure (stages A and B) before symptoms have developed and even before the appearance of left ventricular dysfunction, may inhibit or halt pathogenesis of cardiac remodeling, resulting in reduced morbidity and progression of disease. Guidelines and suggested therapies for treatment at each stage are found in the ACC/AHA Guidelines document, which is available online (Hunt et al, 2001).

FACES Screening Tool for Heart Failure

Adapted from the Heart Failure Society of America, FACES (Box 15-2) is a mnemonic that cues the provider to questions regarding symptoms of heart failure.

Cardiac Risk Indices

Known coronary artery disease (CAD) and risk factors for cardiovascular disease increase the risk of major perioperative cardiovascular complications. The preoperative cardiac evaluation assesses the patient's medical status, including presence of CAD or risk factors such as hypertension, congestive heart failure, valvular heart disease, and arrhythmias. Once these factors have been identified, the clinician makes recommendations regarding

Box **15-2**	FACES Screening Tool for Heart Failure

> **F** – Do you ever feel **F**atigue?
> **A** – Have you experienced an altered **A**ctivity or exercise pattern?
> **C** – Do you feel any **C**ongestion in your chest?
> **E** – Do you ever get **E**dema (swelling)?
> **S** – Are you ever **S**hort of breath?

Adapted from the Heart Failure Society of America, 2002. Available at http://www.abouthf.org/hf_awareness_materials.htm.

preoperative cardiac testing and perioperative management that promotes risk reduction.

Over the past 3 decades, risk stratification indices and clinical guidelines that reflected the current cardiovascular standard of care have been developed (Cohn & Goldman, 2003). Goldman's Cardiac Risk Index (Goldman et al, 1977) was the first index developed from a large, prospective, multivariate analysis of patients undergoing noncardiac surgery. This original index identified major cardiovascular complications (cardiac death, ventricular tachycardia, confirmed myocardial infarction, pulmonary edema) as end points. Nine independent risk predictors of these cardiac complications were identified, weighted, and summed to produce four categories of surgical risk. The Cardiac Risk Index has been validated in a number of studies.

Subsequent indices were, in part, based on Goldman's Index. Each succeeding risk index applied newer clinical studies available at the time; as more clinical information and outcomes studies became available, the guidelines correspondingly evolved. Significant indices that are still in use today include those by Detsky (1986), Larsen (1987), and Pederson (1990). The past decade has seen only three advances in formal risk stratification measures: the ACC/AHA guidelines (Eagle et al, 2002), the American College of Physicians (ACP) guidelines (Palda et al, 1997), and the Revised Cardiac Risk Index (Lee et al, 1999).

The ACC/AHA guidelines are reviewed and the corresponding stepwise algorithm for ordering appropriate preoperative cardiac screening tests is reprinted in Chapter 7. The Revised Cardiac Risk Index (Lee et al, 1999) is reprinted in this chapter. This index is a simplified tool that accurately identifies patients at greater risk for cardiac complications; its ease of use makes it particularly applicable for primary care practice.

Revised Cardiac Risk Index

Authors: Lee TH et al, 1999.

Targeted Population: Patients undergoing major noncardiac surgery.

Description: The Revised Cardiac Risk Index (Box 15-3), a revision of the Goldman criteria (Goldman et al, 1977), identifies six independent predictors of major cardiac complications in patients undergoing elective major noncardiac surgical procedures.

Scores: One point is assigned for the presence of each of six independent predictors (high-risk type of surgery, history of ischemic heart disease, history of congestive heart failure, history of cerebrovascular disease, preoperative treatment with insulin, and preoperative serum creatinine level >2.0 mg/dL). Patients are assigned to one of four classes (classes I to IV) based on the sum of points assigned. Rates of major cardiac complications have been determined for each class from a prospective study.

| Box **15-3** | Revised Cardiac Risk Index |

Each risk factor is assigned one point
1. **High-risk surgical procedures**
   - Intraperitoneal
   - Intrathoracic
   - Suprainguinal vascular
2. **History of ischemic heart disease**
   - History of myocardial infarction
   - History of positive exercise test
   - Current complaint of chest pain considered secondary to myocardial ischemia
   - Use of nitrate therapy
   - ECG with pathological Q waves
3. **History of congestive heart failure**
   - History of congestive heart failure
   - Pulmonary edema
   - Paroxysmal nocturnal dyspnea
   - Bilateral rales or S3 gallop
   - Chest radiograph showing pulmonary vascular redistribution
4. **History of cerebrovascular disease**
   - History of transient ischemic attack or stroke
5. **Preoperative treatment with insulin**
6. **Preoperative serum creatinine > 2.0 mg/dL**

Risk of Major Cardiac Event*

Points	Class	Risk
0	I	0.4%
1	II	0.9%
2	III	6.6%
3 or more	IV	11%

Adapted from Lee TH, Marcantonio ER, Mangione CM, et al: Derivation and prospective validation of a simple index for prediction of cardiac risk of major noncardiac surgery, *Circulation* 100(10): 1043-1049, 1999.
ECG, Electrocardiogram.
*"Major cardiac event" includes myocardial infarction, pulmonary edema, ventricular fibrillation, primary cardiac arrest, and complete heart block.

Accuracy: Rates of major cardiac complications were determined for two cohorts, a derivation cohort (n = 2893), which was used to develop this index, and a validation cohort (n = 1422) (Lee et al, 1999). Factors that best correlated with cardiac complications were identified. Thorough statistical analysis selected for the final six predictors of cardiac risk; an equal-weight model was found to perform no differently than a variable-weight model; thus predictors were assigned equal weight for the final index. The index performed more accurately than two well-known, previously published indices, those of Goldman et al (1977) and Detsky et al (1986). The index was also found to be superior to a vascular surgery index (Lee et al, 1999) for risk assessment in the general population and for vascular surgery, but neither index performed well for patients undergoing abdominal aortic aneurysm surgery. The Revised Cardiac Index is recommended as the index of choice for stratifying risk of

cardiac complications and is best used with clinical guidelines such as those published by the ACC/AHA (Goldman, 2001; Cohn & Goldman, 2003).
Administration Time: <2 minutes from medical history.

References

Cohn SL, Goldman L: Preoperative risk evaluation and perioperative management of patients undergoing noncardiac surgery, *Med Clin North Am* 87:111-136, 2003.

Detsky AS, Abrams HB, Forbath N, et al: Cardiac assessment for patients undergoing noncardiac surgery. A multifactorial clinical risk index, *Arch Intern Med* 146:2131-2134, 1986.

Goldman L: Assessing and reducing cardiac risks of noncardiac surgery, *Am J Med* 110:320-323, 2001.

Goldman L, Caldera DL, Nussbaum SR, et al: Multifactorial index of cardiac risk in noncardiac surgical procedures, *N Engl J Med* 297: 845-850, 1977.

Lee TH, Marcantonio ER, Mangione CM, et al: Derivation and prospective validation of a simple index for prediction of cardiac risk of major noncardiac surgery, *Circulation* 100:1043-1049, 1999.

Online Cardiology Resources

American College of Cardiology (ACC): The official site of the ACC provides a framework of evidence-based clinical statements and guidelines developed by leaders in the field of cardiovascular medicine to help address contemporary practice issues. Guidelines include practice guidelines (including pocket guidelines and guidelines in PDA format), performance measures, consensus documents, policy statements, and consensus conference reports. Practice guidelines include *ACC/AHA Guideline Update for Perioperative Cardiovascular Evaluation for Noncardiac Surgery; ACC/AHA Practice Guidelines for Evaluation and Management of Chronic Heart Failure in the Adult; ACC/AHA/ESC Guidelines for the Management of Patients with Atrial Fibrillation; Coronary Artery Bypass Graft Surgery; Management of Patients with Unstable Angina and Non-ST-Segment Elevation Myocardial Infarction; ACC/AHA Guidelines for the Management of Patients with Acute Myocardial Infarction; ACC/AHA Practice Guidelines for Implantation of Cardiac Pacemakers and Antiarrhythmia Devices; ACC/AHA/ACP-ASIM Practice Guidelines for Management of Patients with Chronic Stable Angina; and ACC/AHA Practice Guidelines for Management of Patients with Valvular Heart Disease.* Available at http://www.acc.org/

American College of Physicians: American College of Physicians Position Paper: Guidelines for assessing and managing the perioperative risk from coronary artery disease associated with major noncardiac surgery. *Ann Intern Med* 127:309-312,1997. Available at http://www.annals.org/cgi/content/full/127/4/309.

Goldman and Detsky Risk Calculators: Available at http://www.vasgbi.com/riskdetsky.htm.

National Heart, Lung and Blood Institute (NHLBI): Under the Department of Health and Human Services, National Institutes of Health, the NHLBI maintains a website that includes current clinical practice guidelines for a variety of cardiopulmonary conditions. Guidelines include *The Seventh Report of the Joint National Committee on Prevention, Detection, Evaluation, and Treatment of High Blood Pressure* (JNC 7); *Clinical Guidelines on Cholesterol Management in Adults* (ATP III); *Guidelines for the Diagnosis and Management of Asthma; Clinical Guidelines on Overweight and Obesity.* Extensive resources include guidelines, fact sheets, and other publications on a wide range of clinical conditions under these topics: Heart and Vascular Information, Lung Information, Blood Information, and Sleep Information. *Interactive Tools and Resources* includes free, downloadable applications for Palm OS devices, health assessment tools, slide shows, and downloadable slide sets. Available at http://www.nhlbi.nih.gov/guidelines/index.htm.

Pharmacologic Management of Chronic Heart Failure (CHF)–Pocket Guide: This useful CHF Pocket Card is published by the Veterans Administration National Clinical Practice Guidelines (CPG) Council. The card includes the ACC/AHA Staging, New York Heart Association Functional Classification, and 2003 guidelines for treatment of congestive heart failure with specific oral medication recommendations. Available at http://www.oqp.med.va.gov/cpg/CHF/G/CHFPoc508.pdf.

Preoperative Cardiac Risk Assessment: This clinical teaching module, from the Divisions of General Internal Medicine and Lane Medical Library at Stanford University, includes the Goldman Index and the Revised Cardiac Risk Index; preoperative risk assessments by functional status, electrocardiography, echocardiography, radionuclide ventriculography determined ejection fraction, thallium scanning, and history of myocardial infarction; and optimal prophylaxis protocols for postoperative thromboembolism. Available at http://www.ctm.stanford.edu/preop_consult/ preop_consultp5.html.

The Medical Algorithms Project: Chapter 6: Cardiovascular System: This project includes tools for hemodynamic measurements; cardiac risk assessment; and evaluation of coronary heart disease, myocardial infarction, congestive heart failure, hypertension, valvular disease, peripheral vascular disease, and other cardiovascular conditions. This project contains hundreds of useful health care algorithms, rating scales, and references. The algorithms have been collected from the biomedical literature, including research journals and textbooks. Available at http://www.medal.org/ch6.html.

Cardiology References

American Heart Association, Criteria Committee: AHA medical/scientific statement. Revisions to classification of functional capacity and objective assessment of patients with diseases of the heart. *Circulation* 90:644-645, 1994.

Cohn SL, Goldman L: Preoperative risk evaluation and perioperative management of patients with coronary artery disease, *Med Clin North Am* 87:111-136, 2003.

Detsky AS, Abrams HB, Forbath N, et al: Cardiac assessment for patients undergoing noncardiac surgery. A multifactorial clinical risk index, *Arch Intern Med* 146:2131-2134, 1986.

Eagle KA, Berger PB, Calkins H, et al: ACC/AHA guideline update for perioperative cardiovascular evaluation for noncardiac surgery–executive summary: a report of the American College of Cardiology/American Heart Association Task Force on Practice Guidelines (Committee to Update the 1996 Guidelines on Perioperative Cardiovascular Evaluation for Noncardiac Surgery), *J Am Coll Cardiol* 39:542-553, 2002. Available at http://www.acc.org/clinical/guidelines/perio/update/pdf/perio_update.pdf and http://www.americanheart.org/downloadable/heart/1013454973885perio_update.pdf.

Hunt SA, Baker DW, Chin MH, et al: *ACC/AHA guidelines for the evaluation and management of chronic heart failure in the adult: a report of the American College of Cardiology/American Heart Association Task Force on Practice Guidelines (Committee to Revise the 1995 Guidelines for the Evaluation and Management of Heart Failure).* 2001. American College of Cardiology Web site. Available at http://www.acc.org/clinical/ guidelines/failure/hf_index.htm.

Larsen SF, Olesen KH, Jacobsen E, et al: Prediction of cardiac risk in non-cardiac surgery, *Eur Heart J* 8:179-185, 1987.

Palda VA, Detsky AS: Perioperative assessment and management of risk from coronary artery disease, *Ann Intern Med* 127:313-328, 1997.

Pedersen T, Eliasen K, Henriksen E: A prospective study of risk factors and cardiopulmonary complications associated with anaesthesia and surgery: risk indicators of cardiopulmonary morbidity, *Acta Anaesthesiol Scand* 34:144-155, 1990.

OPTOMETRY AND OTOLARYNGOLOGY

Snellen Visual Acuity Chart   i

The Snellen alphabet chart is the most commonly used tool for screening far (distant) vision. The chart contains letters arranged in lines of gradually diminished size. At the beginning of each line is a fraction that indicates the visual acuity for that line. The numerator represents the distance in feet between the patient and the chart (standard is 20 feet). The denominator is the distance in feet from which a person with normal vision can read the letters. Normal vision is designated as 20/20. The larger the denominator, the poorer is the vision. At the end of each line is another fraction, with the numerator as the distance in feet from which a person with normal vision can read the letters. The denominator is the distance in meters from which a person with normal vision can read the letters. Large, standard-size numbers (1 to 11) mark the very end of each line, indicating the number of that line for reference. Green and red bars are present following lines 6 and 8, respectively. A Snellen "E" chart, with the letter E placed at random rotations in graduated lines, is available for patients who cannot read. A picture chart is available for preschool children.

For the purpose of testing visual acuity, the patient is positioned 20 feet in front of the Snellen eye chart, in good lighting. The patient covers one eye at a time with a card and reads progressively smaller letters until he or she can go no further. Each eye is tested, and findings are recorded for each eye and then for the two eyes together. The smallest complete line that the patient can read accurately without missing any letters is recorded. If the patient is able to read some but not all letters of the next smaller line, this may be indicated as "+ number of letters" read correctly on the next line (for example, 20/40 +2). The patient may be allowed to use his or her glasses or contact lenses, if available, to determine the best corrected vision. The Snellan eye chart (standard size 22″ high × 11″ wide), may be purchased for office use from any medical or optometric supply vendor.

Rosenbaum Chart

The Rosenbaum chart is used to screen near vision. Similar to the Snellen chart in design, the Rosenbaum chart contains rows of numbers, rotated E's, and X's, and O's. To the right of the rows are two columns. The first column indicates the standard point size of the type, and the second column corresponds to Jaeger scale typeset for each row. At the far right is a column of fractions indicating the visual acuity for each row. Instructions for use are written below the rows. At the bottom of the card is a pupil gauge with diameter measurements of 2 to 9 mm.

For the purpose of testing near vision, the patient holds the card in good light 14 inches from the eye.

The patient reads progressively smaller rows until he or she can no longer read accurately. Each eye is tested separately while the patient is wearing myopic or hyperopic corrective lenses, if these are used. Patients with presbyopia may read through bifocal segments to obtain the best corrected near vision. The smallest complete line that the patient can read accurately without missing any letters is recorded. A Rosenbaum Pocket Vision Screener is reprinted here for lamination and personal use. The chart (standard size $6\,^3/_8''$ high × 3″ wide) may also be purchased from any medical or optometric supply vendor.

Jaeger Charts are a series of passages written in typescripts of different graduated sizes, from very small (J1) to very large (J14), which are designed to test near vision acuity. Patients with normal vision should be able to read the smallest print in good lighting at a comfortable reading distance. Failure to read below a J6 chart with optimally corrected vision represents a 50% loss of visual acuity. Variations have been shown to exist for character size, character and word spacing, and print quality from computer-generated sources of Jaeger reading cards (Batey, 1996). It is recommended that the clinician purchase Jaeger reading cards from a medical or optometric vendor.

Reference

Batey JE: *Jaeger vs Computer,* American Society for Nondestructive Testing, Inc, 1996. Available at http://www.asnt.org/publications/materialseval/basics/septemberbasics/septembe.htm.

Amsler Grid

Age-related macular degeneration (AMD) blurs sharp, central vision necessary for "straight-ahead" activities such as reading, sewing, and driving. AMD is a leading cause of vision loss in Americans 60 years of age and older. There is no pain associated with AMD; it may progress quickly or advance so slowly that patients notice little change in their vision. The Amsler Grid is a tool used to screen the central visual field. It can detect early and sometimes subtle visual changes in a variety of macular diseases such as AMD and diabetic macular edema. It can also be used to monitor changes in vision once they have been detected.

The grid contains straight lines that resemble graph paper and is available with a white or black background; white is more commonly used. At the center of the grid is a black dot used as a fixation point. To use the grid, the patient holds the tool at normal reading distance while wearing usual reading glasses. Each eye is tested separately in good light. The patient stares at the central dot and notes the presence of any line distortion, scotoma, or loss of vision. An Amsler Grid is reprinted here for lamination and personal use. The grid (standard size $5\,^1/_2'' \times 8''$) may also be purchased from any medical or optometric supply vendor. Free Amsler Grid Cards are available from The Macular Degeneration Network (http://www.maculardegeneration.org/WetDry/WetamslerMain.html).

Self-Assessment Hearing Test

This one-page self-assessment questionnaire is designed to screen patients for hearing loss. Ten simple questions with a yes/no answer format identify common symptoms associated with hearing loss. Patients may complete the questionnaire in the office or at home and may be referred for audiologic evaluation if indicated.

Burke Dysphagia Screening Test (BDST)

Source: The Burke Dysphagia Screening Test (BDST) is reprinted here (Box 15-4) and is also described online at http://www.medal.org/ch8.html.

Targeted Population: Patients in the rehabilitative phase after stroke.

Description: The BDST identifies patients at risk of aspiration pneumonia, recurrent upper airway obstruction, and death. Seven items are noted to be present or absent.

Scores: A positive test result exists if at least one of the seven items is present. The test result is considered negative if all of the items are absent.

Accuracy: The BDST was validated in patients in the rehabilitation phase after a stroke at an inpatient stroke rehabilitation unit (DePippo et al, 1994). Main outcome measures were pneumonia, recurrent upper airway obstruction, and death. The BDST identified 11 of 12 patients who subsequently developed one of the endpoint measures. The relative risk for the occurrence of any of the complications was 7.65 times greater for those who did not pass the BDST.

Administration Time: <2 minutes from patient history and bedside swallow test.

Box 15-4 Burke Dysphagia Screening Test

1. Has the patient had a bilateral stroke?	Yes	No
2. Has the patient had a stroke involving the brainstem?	Yes	No
3. Does the patient have a history of pneumonia during the acute stroke phase?	Yes	No
4. Does the patient have coughing associated with feeding or during a 3 ounce water swallow test?	Yes	No
5. Does the patient persistently fail to consume at least one half of meals?	Yes	No
6. Is prolonged time required for feeding the patient?	Yes	No
7. Is a non-oral feeding program in progress for the patient?	Yes	No

Score: A 'yes' response to one or more items is a positive screen.
From DePippo KL, Holas MA, Reding MJ: The Burke dysphagia screening test: validation of its use in patients with stroke, *Arch Phys Med Rehabil* 75(2):1284-1286, 1994. Reprinted with permission from American Congress of Rehabilitation Medicine and the American Academy of Physical Medicine and Rehabilitation.

Reference

DePippo KL, Holas MA, Reding MJ: The Burke dysphagia screening test: validation of its use in patients with stroke. *Arch Phys Med Rehabil* 75:1284-1286, 1994.

Epworth Sleepiness Scale (ESS)

Author: Johns MW, 1991.

Source: The Epworth Sleepiness Scale (ESS) is reprinted here and is also available at many locations online including http://www.stanford.edu/~dement/epworth.html and http://www.smmc.com/sleep/sleepweek/epworth.html.

Targeted Population: Adults.

Description: This self-administered questionnaire is a quantitative subjective measurement of sleepiness. Eight hypothetical situations are rated on a 4-point scale for dozing probability.

This simple survey provides a measurement of the subject's general level of daytime sleepiness and is widely used by sleep professionals in the evaluation of sleep disorders.

Scores: For each activity, the patient rates his or her chances of falling asleep while engaged in the activity. Scores range from 0 (never dozing in a situation) to 3 (always dozing). Scores for the eight items are summed. Total ESS scores above 10 suggest chronic sleepiness and scores above 12 confirm its presence.

Accuracy: Total ESS scores significantly distinguished healthy subjects from patients in various diagnostic groups including those with obstructive sleep apnea syndrome, narcolepsy, and idiopathic hypersomnia (Johns, 1991). Reliability and internal consistency of the ESS were reported to be high when patients with obstructive sleep apnea syndrome were compared with healthy control subjects (Johns, 1992). The ESS has also been validated in Chinese (Chen et al, 2002). Chervin and Aldrich (1999) reported a significant association with self-rated problem sleepiness but not with Multiple Sleep Latency Test (MSLT) scores or objective measures of sleep apnea severity. However, Johns (2000) compared three commonly used tests for sleepiness (the MSLT, the maintenance of wakefulness test [MWT], and the ESS) and showed that the ESS was the most discriminating test.

Administration Time: <2 minutes by self-administration.

References

Chen NH, Johns MW, Li HY, et al: Validation of a Chinese version of the Epworth sleepiness scale, *Qual Life Res* 11:817-821, 2002.

Chervin RD, Aldrich MS: The Epworth Sleepiness Scale may not reflect objective measures of sleepiness or sleep apnea, *Neurology* 52:125-131, 1999.

Johns MW: A new method for measuring daytime sleepiness: The Epworth Sleepiness Scale, *Sleep* 14:540-545, 1991.

Johns MW: Reliability and factor analysis of the Epworth Sleepiness Scale, *Sleep* 15:376-381, 1992.

Johns MW: Sensitivity and specificity of the multiple sleep latency test (MSLT), the maintenance of wakefulness test and the Epworth sleepiness scale: failure of the MSLT as a gold standard, *J Sleep Res* 9:5-11, 2000.

Online Optometry/Otolaryngology Resources

American Academy of Otolaryngology–Head and Neck Surgery: Available at http://www.entnet.org/

Suppleyes Optometry: This vendor specializes in optometric supplies and carries a variety of laminated eye charts for professional use. Available at http://www.suppleyes.net/

The Medical Algorithms Project: Chapter 8: Pulmonary and Acid-Base: This chapter includes tools for evaluation of sleep apnea, dysphagia, and pulmonary conditions. This project contains hundreds of useful health care algorithms, rating scales, and references. The algorithms have been collected from the biomedical literature, including research journals and textbooks. Available at http://www.medal.org/ ch8.html.

NEUROLOGY

Glasgow Coma Scale

Authors: Teasdale G, Jennett B, 1974.

Source: The Glasgow Coma Scale is reprinted here (Table 15-2) and is also available online at http://www.cdc.gov/masstrauma/resources/gcscale.htm.

Targeted Population: Adults and children; a Modified Glasgow Coma Scale (Table 15-3) is used for children younger than 5 years.

Description: The Glasgow Coma Scale was designed to quantify the depth and duration of coma and impaired consciousness. Assessment of the cerebral cortex and brainstem functions is based on three responses to stimuli: eye opening response, verbal response, and motor response. This scale is the scoring system most widely used in assessing the level of consciousness after traumatic brain injury and other causes of unresponsiveness. Of note, in the assessment of trauma, factors including shock, hypoxemia, drug use, alcohol intoxication, and metabolic disturbances alter level of consciousness and interfere with the scale's ability to accurately reflect the severity of a traumatic brain injury. Spinal cord injuries will make the motor scale invalid; severe orbital trauma may make eye opening impossible to assess.

Scores: For each category, the patient's best response is matched to the criteria for scoring. The three category scores are summed to produce the Glasgow Coma Score. Scores range from 3 (minimum-deepest coma) to 15 (maximum-normal). Impaired consciousness is rated as mild (scores 13-15), moderate (scores 9-12), and severe (scores 3-8); scores <8 are associated with significant risk of death.

If a response category is limited by injury or intervention (such as endotracheal tube [Verbal Response], orbital trauma [Eye-Opening Response], spinal cord trauma [Motor Response]), the score may be documented by its individual components. Thus a patient with a spinal cord injury might be scored as "E4 V5 M-spinal cord injury."

Accuracy: The Glasgow Coma Scale has a relatively high degree of interobserver reliability and correlates well with outcome after severe brain injury. Education on proper administration of the stimuli and assessment of

Table **15-2** Glasgow Coma Scale		
Assessed Behaviors	**Criteria for Scoring**	**Scores**
Eye-Opening Response	Spontaneous opening with blinking at baseline	4
	To verbal stimuli, command, speech	3
	To pain only (not applied to face)	2
	No response	1
Verbal Response	Oriented	5
	Confused conversation, but able to answer questions	4
	Inappropriate words	3
	Incoherent	2
	No response	1
Motor Response	Obeys commands for movement	6
	Purposeful movement to painful stimulus	5
	Withdraws in response to pain	4
	Flexion in response to pain (decorticate posturing)	3
	Extension response in response to pain (decerebrate posturing)	2
	No response	1

Add the numbers from each category. Maximum score = 15, minimum score = 3.

From Teasdale G, Jennett B: Assessment of coma and impaired consciousness: a practical scale, *Lancet* 2:81-84, 1974.

response is important for accurate and consistent scoring (Teasdale et al, 1978; Rowley & Fielding, 1991).
Administration Time: <2 minutes.

References:

Reilly PL, Simpson DA, Sprod R, et al: Assessing the conscious level in infants and young children: a paediatric version of the Glasgow Coma Scale, *Childs Nerv Syst* 4:30-33, 1988.

Rowley G, Fielding K: Reliability and accuracy of the Glasgow Coma Scale with experienced and inexperienced users, *Lancet* 337:535-538, 1991.

Teasdale G, Jennett B: Assessment of coma and impaired consciousness: a practical scale, *Lancet* 2:81-84, 1974.

Teasdale G, Kril-Jones R, van der Sande J: Observer variability in assessing impaired consciousness and coma, *J Neurol Neurosurg Psychiatry* 41:603-610, 1978.

Migraine Disability Assessment (MIDAS) Questionnaire   i

Authors: Stewart WF et al, 1999b.
Source: The Migraine Disability Assessment (MIDAS) Questionnaire is available online for downloading at http://www.migraine-disability.net/. This source, the Migraine Disability Website, is designed to offer information to both patients and health care professionals. A range of educational materials provides information on how MIDAS and disability assessment are helping to improve migraine management. The MIDAS is also available at http://www.achenet.org/women/midas.php and http://www.uhs.berkeley.edu/home/healthtopics/pdf/assessment.pdf.
Targeted Population: Adults and children with headache.

Description: MIDAS consists of five scored questions that measure headache-related disability and two additional unscored questions on pain intensity and headache frequency. The authors recommend use of the MIDAS Questionnaire to improve physician-patient communication about headache-related disability and influence health care delivery for patients with migraine. The tool is particularly suited to primary care because of its brevity and simplicity of use and scoring (Stewart et al, 2001, 1999b).
Scores: The number of days in the previous 3 months for which activities were missed because of headache are counted for each of five questions. The overall MIDAS score (expressed as number of days) is obtained by summing the answers to the five questions. The MIDAS score is classified into four grades of severity that predict treatment needs: grade I (score 0-5) = minimal or infrequent

Table **15-3** Modified Glasgow Coma Scale–(verbal response modified for young children)		
Verbal Response	Appropriate words, smiles, fixes and follows	5
	Consolable crying	4
	Persistently irritable	3
	Restless, agitated	2
	None	1

Eye-Opening and Motor Responses are scored as for adults. Adapted from Reilly PL, Simpson DA, Sprod R, et al: Assessing the conscious level in infants and young children: a paediatric version of the Glasgow Coma Scale, *Childs Nerv Systm* 4:30-33, 1988.

disability with little or no treatment needs, specific migraine therapy is indicated; grade II (score 6-10) = mild or infrequent disability with moderate treatment needs; grade III (score 11-20) = moderate disability with urgent treatment needs; grade IV (score ≥21) = severe disability with very urgent treatment needs.

Accuracy: The MIDAS Questionnaire has shown good internal consistency, test-retest reliability, and validity; and scores correlate with physicians' clinical judgment regarding patients' pain, disability, and need for medical care (Stewart et al, 2001; Lipton et al, 2001; Stewart et al, 1999a, 1999b). Evaluation of the relationship between headache features (attack frequency, pain intensity, pain quality, and associated symptoms) and MIDAS score suggest that the MIDAS Questionnaire captures information about disability that is not inherent to other headache features and is independent of gender and work status (Stewart et al, 2003). Bigal et al (2003) also demonstrated that patients with chronic migraine had remarkable impairment of their daily activities, as reflected by high MIDAS scores.

Administration Time: <2 minutes by self-administration.

References

Bigal ME, Rapoport AM, Lipton RB, et al: Assessment of migraine disability using the Migraine Disability Assessment (MIDAS) Questionnaire: a comparison of chronic migraine with episodic migraine, *Headache* 43:336, 2003.

Lipton RB, Stewart WF, Sawyer J, et al: Clinical utility of an instrument assessing migraine disability: the Migraine Disability Assessment (MIDAS) Questionnaire, *Headache* 41:854-861, 2001.

Stewart WF, Lipton RB, Dowson AJ, et al: Development and testing of the Migraine Disability Assessment (MIDAS) Questionnaire to assess headache-related disability, *Neurology* 56(suppl 1):S20-S28, 2001.

Stewart WF, Lipton RB, Kolodner K: Migraine Disability Assessment (MIDAS) score: relation to headache frequency, pain intensity, and headache symptoms, *Headache* 43:258-265, 2003.

Stewart WF, Lipton RB, Kolodner K, et al: Reliability of the Migraine Disability Assessment (MIDAS) score in a population-based sample of headache sufferers, *Cephalalgia* 19:107-114, 1999a.

Stewart WF, Lipton RB, Whyte J, et al: An international study to assess reliability of the Migraine Disability Assessment (MIDAS) score, *Neurology* 53:988-994, 1999b.

Headache Diary

Headache is a complex condition that may result in a variety of disability issues. Successful treatment of the headache reduces disability and allows the patient to resume normal life. Treatment failure may occur for a number of reasons (Box 15-5), but its likelihood is diminished by obtaining a thorough history. A headache diary can track triggers, headache patterns, and monitor treatment effectiveness, which may be critical to making the appropriate diagnosis and prescribing the best treatment for headache conditions.

The components of a headache diary need to elicit information critical to diagnosing and monitoring treatment progress for headache conditions. Key elements in the headache diary include the temporal profile of

---

Box 15-5 Possible Reasons for Treatment Failure for Headache

1. The diagnosis is incomplete or incorrect:
   - A secondary headache disorder goes undiagnosed
   - A primary headache disorder present is misdiagnosed (hemicrania continua, paroxysmal hemicrania, hypnic headache)
   - The number of headache disorders is not clear (two or more headache disorders are present and at least one goes unrecognized)
2. Important exacerbating factors have been missed:
   - Acute headache medication or caffeine overuse
   - Hormonal triggers
   - Dietary or lifestyle triggers
   - Psychosocial factors
   - Use of other medications that trigger headache
3. Pharmacotherapy has been inadequate:
   - Ineffective drug
   - Excessive initial doses
   - Inadequate final doses
   - Inadequate duration of treatment
   - Combination therapy required
   - Poor absorption
   - Noncompliance
4. Nonpharmacologic treatment has been inadequate, patient may need:
   - Physical medicine (nerve block or trigger point injections, physical therapy)
   - Cognitive behavioral therapy
5. Other factors:
   - Unrealistic expectations by the patient
   - Comorbid and concomitant conditions
   - Inpatient treatment may be required

From Lipton RB, Silberstein SD, Saper JR, et al: Why headache treatment fails, *Neurology* 60:1064-1070, 2003.

---

headache onset and progression; quality descriptors of the headache (including visual, prodromal, and autonomic symptoms and sensory changes); localization of the pain; sleep-wake times; concurrent events or provoking activity (potential triggers include amount of sleep, certain foods and additives, use of hormones or other medications, exertion of any type including sexual activity, and other stressors); relieving factors (including rest, positioning, avoidance of triggering factors, use of ice or heat, and massage); and consideration of other disorders such as dental procedures, ocular disturbances, sinus disease, and nasopharyngeal carcinoma (Lipton et al, 2003; Purdy, 2001).

Headache diaries can be found in abundance online by using any search engine. A headache diary that incorporates the features mentioned previously is included in this chapter.

References

Lipton RB, Silberstein SD, Saper JR, et al: Why headache treatment fails, *Neurology* 60:1064-1070, 2003.

Purdy RA: Clinical evaluation of a patient presenting with headache, *Med Clin North Am* 85:847-863, v., 2001.

Berg Balance Scale

Authors: Berg K et al, 1989.

Source: The Berg Balance Scale form is reprinted in this text. The scale is also available for downloading at the Center for Gerontology and Health Care Research website at http://www.chcr.brown.edu/Balance.htm.

Targeted Population: Adults.

Description: The Berg Balance Scale contains 14 items that describe a position or movement. Equipment required for testing consists of a stopwatch or watch with a second hand; a ruler or other indicator of 2, 5, and 10 inches (5, 12 and 25 cm); chairs of reasonable height; and a step or a stool of average step height. The administrator instructs the patient on the requested position or movement and scores ability to complete the task with a 5-level scale.

Scores: Each of the 14 items is scored from 0 to 4, with lower numbers describing decreased ability. The lowest response category that applies for each item is scored. For most items, the subject is asked to maintain a given position for a specific time. Progressively more points are deducted if the time or distance requirements are not met, if the subject's performance warrants supervision, or if the subject touches an external support or receives assistance from the examiner. The item scores are summed for a total score. Total scores range from a minimum of 0 to a maximum of 56. Interpretation of scores relates to mobility level: 0 to 20 = wheelchair bound, 21 to 40 = walking with assistance, 41 to 56 = independent. The scores are often used to monitor changes during rehabilitation after injury or stroke.

Accuracy: The Berg Balance Scale is used extensively and reliably in rehabilitation, nursing home, and research settings to assess functional limitations in balance and/or mobility (Thomas, 2001; Wee et al, 2003; Berg et al, 1992b). The scale has demonstrated validity when compared with laboratory and other clinical measures of balance and mobility within a geriatric population (Berg et al, 1992a) for estimating approximate length of stay and eventual discharge destination from stroke rehabilitation (Wee et al, 2003) and for predicting outcome after acquired brain injury (Feld, 2001). The total Berg score contributes significantly to the prediction of falls with high sensitivity and specificity (Lajoie & Gallagher, 2004).

Administration Time: 15 to 30 minutes by health care personnel.

References

Berg KO, Maki BE, Williams JI, et al: A comparison of clinical and laboratory measures of postural balance in an elderly population, *Arch Phys Med Rehabil* 73:1073-1083, 1992a.

Berg K, Wood-Dauphinee S, Williams JI, et al: Measuring balance in the elderly: preliminary development of an instrument, *Physiotherapy Canada* 41:304-311, 1989.

Berg K, Wood-Dauphinee S, Williams JI, et al: Measuring balance in the elderly: validation of an instrument, *Can J Pub Health* 2:S7-S11, 1992b.

Feld JA: Berg balance scale and outcome measures in acquired brain injury, *Neurorehabil Neural Repair* 15: 239-244, 2001.

Lajoie Y, Gallagher SP: Predicting falls within the elderly community: comparison of postural sway, reaction time, the Berg balance scale and the Activities-specific Balance Confidence (ABC) scale for comparing fallers and non-fallers, *Arch Gerontol Geriatr* 38:11-26, 2004.

Thomas RL: Physical therapy intervention with the geriatric client in the nursing home, *Clin Fam Pract* 3:535-559, 2001.

Wee JY, Wong H, Palepu A: Validation of the Berg Balance Scale as a predictor of length of stay and discharge destination in stroke rehabilitation, *Arch Phys Med Rehabil* 84:731-735, 2003.

Abnormal Involuntary Movement Scale (AIMS)

Authors: Guy W, 1976; modified by Munetz MR, Benjamin S, 1988.

Source: The Abnormal Involuntary Movement Scale (AIMS) is reproduced here and can be obtained online by using any search engine.

Targeted Population: Patients who may be experiencing dyskinetic movement, patients taking neuroleptic medications.

Description: AIMS is the benchmark scale for assessment and recording of tardive dyskinesia and the most widely used assessment tool to establish the presence and severity of involuntary movements. It is a 12-item instrument that is used to assess abnormal involuntary movements associated with antipsychotic drugs, such as tardive dystonia and chronic akathisia, as well as "spontaneous" motor disturbance related to the illness itself. The scale is preceded by an "Examination Procedure," which the clinician follows for item administration. Using the guide, the clinician rates three objective categories of movements: Facial and Oral Movements (four areas), Extremity Movements (two areas), and Trunk Movements (one area). The clinician then rates a fourth category, Global Judgments, that contains three areas of subjective assessment. Dental problems and use of dentures are noted following the rating categories. The AIMS examination has been widely recommended for periodic screening for tardive dyskinesia and follow-up of patients with the disorder. Munetz and Benjamin (1988) state that the AIMS examination is best conducted within the context of an ongoing treatment program and should be part of the informed consent process required for patients treated with neuroleptic drugs.

Scores: Scores for the three Movement and single Global Judgment categories are based on a 5-point scale (0 = none, 4 = severe). Scores may be reported for each of these categories. Two methods of scoring AIMS have been reported. When AIMS was first introduced, the authors directed that movements (items 8, 11, and 12) be scored one point less in severity if they did not occur spontaneously. Later, Munetz and Benjamin (1988) recommended omission of this guideline; studies have shown the instrument to have good statistical properties when this rule is omitted. Schooler and Kane (1982) proposed three criteria for a diagnosis of probable tardive dyskinesia: exposure to neuroleptics for a total of at least 3 months, a score of 2 for at least two body areas OR a score of 3 for at least one body area, and the exclusion of other causes for abnormal movement.

Accuracy: Interrater reliability is good; however, Lane et al (1985) demonstrated that experienced raters had generally higher levels of agreement than inexperienced raters. Research suggests that routine clinical use of the AIMS examination may improve the early detection of tardive dyskinesia, which could result in a decrease in the morbidity associated with this disorder (Munetz & Schulz, 1986).

Administration Time: 5 to 10 minutes by clinician administration; may be integrated into a routine clinical evaluation.

References

Guy W. *ECDEU assessment manual for psychopharmacology*, revised ed. Washington, DC, 1976, US Department of Health, Education, and Welfare.

Lane RD, Glazer WM, Hansen TE, et al: Assessment of tardive dyskinesia using the Abnormal Involuntary Movement Scale, *J Nerv Ment Dis* 173:353-357, 1985.

Munetz MR, Benjamin S: How to examine patients using the Abnormal Involuntary Movement Scale, *Hosp Community Psychiatry* 39: 1172-1177, 1988.

Munetz MR, Schulz SC: Screening for tardive dyskinesia, *J Clin Psychiatry* 47:75-77, 1986.

Schooler NR, Kane JM: Research diagnoses for tardive dyskinesia, *Arch Gen Psychiatry* 39:486-487, 1982.

Online Neurology Resources

The Internet Stroke Center: This website is a nonprofit, educational service of the Stroke Center at Barnes–Jewish Hospital, Washington University Medical Center, and the Cerebrovascular Diseases Section of the Department of Neurology at Washington University School of Medicine in St. Louis. Included on this site is information obtained from published accounts, meeting presentations, Internet searches, and direct correspondence regarding stroke research and clinical care. A complete selection of scales and measures pertaining to stroke are available at this site. These include measures in categories of Prehospital Assessment, Acute Assessment, Functional Assessment, and Outcome Assessment, as well as other diagnostic and screening tests related to stroke. Available at http://www.strokecenter.org/trials/scales/index.htm.

The Medical Algorithms Project: Chapter 17: Neurology: This chapter includes measures for assessment of coma, multiple sclerosis, stroke, sleep, headache, neuralgia, dementia, spinal cord injuries, epilepsy, and other conditions. This project contains hundreds of useful health care algorithms, rating scales, and references. The algorithms have been collected from the biomedical literature, including research journals and textbooks. http://www.medal.org/ch17.html.

GASTROENTEROLOGY

Rhodes Index of Nausea, Vomiting, and Retching

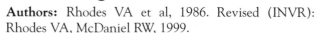

Authors: Rhodes VA et al, 1986. Revised (INVR): Rhodes VA, McDaniel RW, 1999.

Targeted Population: Adults.

Description: The Rhodes Index of Nausea, Vomiting, and Retching (INVR) is an eight-item instrument used to assess nausea and vomiting over the previous 12 hours. Originally designed as a six-item scale (Rhodes et al, 1983), the Rhodes Inventory of Nausea and Vomiting–Form 2 (INV-2) was expanded to eight items based on the study of patterns of nausea and vomiting in patients receiving chemotherapy (Rhodes et al, 1986). Eight 5-point self-report items measure the patient's perception of duration of nausea, frequency of nausea, distress from nausea, frequency of vomiting, amount of vomiting, distress from vomiting, frequency of retching, and distress from retching. The INV-2 arranges the eight items as a choice of five sentences for each item, which describe the level of symptoms. The revised index, INVR, contains eight introductory statements of the same symptom components as the INV-2; and patients complete the statement with the selection of one of five possible responses. The possible responses on the INVR are presented in the same order as the complete sentences of the original INV-2. The patient evaluates symptoms every 12 hours on the 5-point scale.

Scores: The Likert-type scale for each item is scored from 0 (indicating minimal or no symptom) to 4 (representing the worst symptom). Item scores are summed for a total score with a range of 0 to 32. In addition to the total score, subscale scores for symptom experience, symptom occurrence and symptom distress as a whole and for nausea, vomiting, and retching independently may be tallied. Most clinicians consider the patient's Distress Score of 1 or higher sufficient to warrant additional symptom management. Although the Occurrence Scores are important, the Distress Score provides a better index of the patient's perception (Rhodes, personal communication, February 16, 2004).

Accuracy: The INV-2 has demonstrated strong reliability and validity and has been used extensively in oncology, obstetrics, postanesthesia, and medical and surgical units to monitor and manage patients' symptoms (Lacroix et al, 2000; Rhodes et al, 1984; Rhodes et al, 1987, Rhodes & McDaniel, 1997; Rhodes & McDaniel, 1999; Zhou et al, 2001). The INVR was shown to be as reliable as the INV-2 and is more user friendly for both patients and health care providers (Rhodes & McDaniel, 1999).

Administration Time: <2 minutes by self-report.

References

Lacroix R, Eason E, Melzack R: Nausea and vomiting during pregnancy: a prospective study of its frequency, intensity, and patterns of change, *Am J Obstet Gynecol* 182:931-937, 2000.

Rhodes VA, Watson PM, Johnson MH: A self-report tool for assessing nausea and vomiting, *Oncol Nurs Forum* 10:11-13, 1983.

Rhodes VA, Watson PM, Johnson MH: Association of chemotherapy related nausea and vomiting with pretreatment and posttreatment anxiety, *Oncol Nurs Forum* 13:41-47, 1986.

Rhodes VA, McDaniel RW: Measuring nausea, vomiting, and retching. In Frank-Stromborg M, Olsen SJ, editors. *Instruments for assessing clinical problems* (pp. 509-517). Sudbury, MA, 1997, Jones & Bartlett.

Rhodes VA, McDaniel RW: The Index of Nausea, Vomiting, and Retching: a new format of the Index of Nausea and Vomiting, *Oncol Nurs Forum* 26:889-894, 1999.

Rhodes VA, Watson PM, Johnson M: Development of reliable and valid measures of nausea and vomiting, *Cancer Nurs* 7:33-41, 1984.

Rhodes VA, Watson PM, Johnson MH, et al: Patterns of nausea, vomiting, and distress in patients receiving antineoplastic drug protocols, *Oncol Nurs Forum* 14:35-43, 1987.

Zhou Q, O'Brien B, Soeken K: Rhodes Index of Nausea and Vomiting–Form 2 in pregnant women. A confirmatory factor analysis, *Nurs Res* 50:251-257, 2001.

Constipation Assessment Scale (CAS)

Author: McMillan SC, 1989.

Source: The Constipation Assessment Scale (CAS) is reprinted in this text, is in the public domain, and is available online at http://www.medal.org/ch10.html.

Targeted Population: Adults.

Description: This tool contains eight items that assess the incidence and severity of constipation, help identify patients with this problem, and monitor their responses to therapy. Items include abdominal distention or bloating, change in amount of gas passed rectally, less frequent bowel movements, oozing liquid stool, rectal fullness or pressure, rectal pain with bowel movement, small volume of stool, and inability to pass stool. Items are rated based on recall of symptoms over the past 3 days.

Scores: Patients rate each of the previously mentioned items in severity by choosing one of three answers. Points are assigned to the responses: no problem = 0; some problem = 1; severe problem = 2. Total score is the sum of points for all eight findings. Total scores range from 0 (minimum, no constipation) to 16 (maximum, worst possible constipation). The higher the score, the worse the constipation. Broussard (1998) modified the score for pregnant women by using a 5-point scale, scored 0 to 4, providing a total score range of 0 to 32 (0 to 8 = no or minimal; 9 to 17 = minimal to moderate; >25 = moderate to severe). If the patient indicates a problem with item 4 (oozing, liquid stool), the possibility of impaction should be considered (McMillan & Williams, 1989).

Accuracy: The CAS is commonly used to evaluate severity of constipation in patients with cancer and for patients receiving neurotoxic chemotherapeutic agents, narcotic analgesics, antidepressants, tranquilizers, and muscle relaxants; the CAS has been shown to be valid and reliable with sensitivity to differentiate between moderate and severe symptoms of constipation (Curtiss, 1996; McMillan & Williams, 1989; McMillan, 1999; McMillan, 2002; McMillan & Moody, 2003).

Administration Time: <3 minutes by self-administration.

References

Broussard BS: The Constipation Assessment Scale for pregnancy, *JOGNN* 27:297-301, 1998.

Curtiss CP: Constipation. In Groenwald SL, editor. *Cancer symptom management.* Boston, 1996, Jones & Bartlett.

McMillan SC: Assessing and managing narcotic-induced constipation in adults with cancer, *JMCC* 6:198-204, 1999.

McMillan SC: Presence and severity of constipation in hospice patients with advanced cancer, *Am J Hosp Palliat Care* 19:426-430, 2002.

McMillan SC, Moody LE: Hospice patient and caregiver congruence in reporting patients' symptom intensity, *Cancer Nurs* 26:113-118, 2003.

McMillan SC, Williams FA: Validity and reliability of the Constipation Assessment Scale, *Cancer Nurs* 12:183-188, 1989.

McSahen RE, McLane AM: Constipation. Consensual and empirical validation, *Nurs Clin North Am* 20:801-808, 1985.

UROLOGY AND SEXUAL FUNCTION

Androgen Deficiency in Aging Males (ADAM) Questionnaire

Authors: Morley JE, Perry HM, 1999.

Source: The Androgen Deficiency in Aging Males (ADAM) Questionnaire is reprinted here and can also be found online by using any search engine.

Targeted Population: Older adult males.

Description: The ADAM Questionnaire was developed at St. Louis University Medical School to detect the symptom complex related to decreased testosterone levels in older men. The questionnaire contains 10 questions with yes/no responses.

Scores: A patient who gives a "yes" answer to question 1 or 7 or any three other questions has a high likelihood of having a low testosterone level.

Accuracy: The questionnaire was demonstrated to have high sensitivity and adequate specificity for detecting decreased testosterone levels (Morley et al, 2000). The authors suggest that testosterone treatment in older men with hypogonadism results in the reversal of most of the symptoms reported on the ADAM Questionnaire.

Administration Time: <2 minutes by self-administration.

References

Morley JE, Charlton E, Patrick P, et al: Validation of a screening questionnaire for androgen deficiency in aging males, *Metabolism* 49:1239-1242, 2000.

Morley JE, Perry HM: Androgen deficiency in aging men, *Med Clin North Am* 83:1279-1289, 1999.

Brief Male Sexual Function Inventory for Urology

Authors: O'Leary MP et al, 1995.

Targeted Population: Adult males.

Description: The Brief Male Sexual Function Inventory for Urology consists of 11 validated questions developed to measure sexual function and satisfaction. This instrument includes subscales for sexual drive (two items), erections (three items), ejaculation (two items), problem assessment (three items), and overall satisfaction (one item). A 5-point Likert-type scale is used, and patients choose a response for each of the 11 items. This tool is a brief questionnaire that is ideal for the office setting (Chun & Carson, 2001).

Scores: Item scores range from 0 (least satisfactory) to 4 (most satisfactory). All items may be summed for a total score; however, the authors do not recommend this approach because sexual function is multidimensional (O'Leary et al, 1995). Subscale scores may be calculated or individual questions may be examined as the preferred methods to characterize sexual function and satisfaction. **Accuracy:** Test-retest reliabilities, internal consistencies, and construct validities were examined with satisfactory findings; self-assessments of ejaculate volume were problematic (O'Leary et al, 1995). Rosen (1996), in a comment on this tool, criticized the omission of questions on orgasm in the absence of ejaculation, the occurrence of premature ejaculation, and the patient's ability to sustain erection after penetration.

Administration Time: <5 minutes by self-administration.

References

Chun J, Carson CC: Physician-patient dialogue and clinical evaluation of erectile dysfunction, *Urol Clin North Am* 28:249-258, viii. 2001.

O'Leary MP, Fowler FJ, Lenderking WR, et al: A brief male sexual function inventory for urology, *Urology* 46:697-706, 1995.

Rosen RC: Brief Male Sexual Function Inventory for urology, *Urology* 47:782-783, 1996.

American Urological Association (AUA) Symptom Index   i

Authors: Barry MJ et al, 1992a.

Source: The American Urological Association (AUA) Symptom Index is widely available online for downloading and can be found at http://www.prostate-cancer.org/tools/forms/aua_symptom_form.html.

Targeted Population: Adult males.

Description: The AUA Symptom Index was developed to categorize benign prostatic hyperplasia (BPH) symptoms. This questionnaire has been adopted worldwide and is also known as the *International Prostate Symptom Score* (*IPSS*). It is sometimes seen with a quality-of-life scale at the end of the questionnaire. The AUA Symptom Index contains seven items covering incomplete emptying, frequency, intermittency, urgency, weak urinary stream, straining, and nocturia. Items are rated on a 6-point Likert-type scale for frequency of symptoms occurring in the past month.

Scores: Items are scored as follows: 0 points = not at all; 1 point = less than 1 in 5 times (<20%); 2 points = less than half the time (<50%); 3 points = about half the time (50%); 4 points = more than half the time (>50%); 5 points = almost always (>80%). Scores for the seven items are summed for a total score. Suggested interpretation for total scores is as follows: <7 = mild BPH symptoms; 8 to 19 = moderate BPH symptoms; >20 = severe BPH symptoms.

Accuracy: The AUA Symptom Index has been validated by a multidisciplinary measurement committee of the AUA (Barry et al, 1992a). Results showed internal consistency, excellent test-retest reliability, high correlation to subjects' global ratings of the magnitude of their urinary problems, and good discrimination between patients with BPH and control subjects. When used as an outcome measure, the AUA Symptom Index demonstrated good

sensitivity to change after prostatectomy (Barry et al, 1992a) and was a good indicator for the presence of re-stenosis after urethroplasty (Aydos et al, 2001). The AUA Symptom Index correlates well with other measures (Barry et al, 1992b) and was found to be more sensitive to differences in symptoms than the general quality-of-life measures (Fowler & Barry, 1993).

Administration Time: <2 minutes by self-administration

References

Aydos MM, Memis A, Yakupoglu YK, et al: The use and efficacy of the American Urological Association Symptom Index in assessing the outcome of urethroplasty for post-traumatic complete posterior urethral strictures, *BJU Int* 88:382-384, 2001.

Barry MJ, Fowler FJ Jr, O'Leary MP, et al: The American Urological Association symptom index for benign prostatic hyperplasia. The Measurement Committee of the American Urological Association, *J Urol* 148:1549-1557, 1992a.

Barry MJ, Fowler FJ Jr, O'Leary MP, et al: Correlation of the American Urological Association symptom index with self-administered versions of the Madsen-Iversen, Boyarsky and Maine Medical Assessment Program symptom indexes. Measurement Committee of the American Urological Association, *J Urol* 148:1558-1563, 1992b.

Fowler FJ Jr, Barry MJ: Quality of life assessment for evaluating benign prostatic hyperplasia treatments. An example of using a condition-specific index, *Eur Urol* 24(suppl 1):24-27, 1993.

Incontinence Impact Questionnaire (IIQ-7) and Urogenital Distress Inventory (UDI-6)

Authors: Shumaker SA et al, 1994.

Source: The Incontinence Impact Questionnaire (IIQ-7) and Urogenital Distress Inventory (UDI-6) are reprinted here and are also available online at many locations including http://www.uab.edu/obesitysurgery/beta/IncontinenceImpactQuest.pdf, http://www.urologychannel.com/drjuma/incontinence.pdf, and http://www.urologychannel.com/drjuma/urogenital.pdf. Long forms of the IIQ and UDI are available at http://www.medal.org/ch1.html (IIQ) and http://www.medal.org/ch14.html (UDI).

Targeted Population: Adult females.

Description: The IIQ and UDI were designed to assess the impact of urinary incontinence on activities and emotions in women and the degree to which symptoms associated with incontinence are troubling (Shumaker et al, 1994; Uebersax et al, 1995). Each tool has a long form and a short form. The IIQ contains 30 questions covering four domains: physical activity, social relationships, travel, and emotional health. The short form of the IIQ (IIQ-7) contains seven questions from the IIQ. The UDI contains 19 questions in three domains: symptoms related to stress urinary incontinence, detrusor overactivity, and bladder outlet obstruction. The short form of the UDI (UDI-6) contains six questions from the UDI. Responses to the short and long forms of both tools are on a 4-point Likert-type scale rating the extent to which urinary incontinence affects daily functioning (IIQ) and the degree to which symptoms are problematic (UDI).

The IIQ and UDI are used worldwide as standard measures of incontinence impact on quality of life and are frequently used in outcomes studies.

Scores: Points are assigned to responses as follows: 0 = not at all, 1 = slightly, 2 = moderately, and 3 = greatly. Points are summed for a total score and may be calculated for domain scores on the long forms. The minimum score for all forms is 0; maximum scores are as follows: 90 for the IIQ, 57 for the UDI, 21 for the IIQ-7, and 18 for the UDI-6. The average score for each form may be calculated and correlated to the response for that number to determine the overall degree of impact on activities (IIQ) and the level of distress (UDI).

Accuracy: Shumaker et al (1994) assessed the validity, reproducibility, and sensitivity to change of the IIQ and UDI in women with demonstrated urodynamic diagnoses, finding a low but significant correlation with incontinence severity on the 1-hour pad test. More recently, van der Vaart et al (2003) tested the IIQ and UDI in clinical and control groups, finding the subscales to be reliable, valid, and of clinical use. They identified a fifth subscale for the IIQ (embarrassment) and five subscales for the UDI (discomfort/pain, urinary incontinence, overactive bladder, genital prolapse, and obstructive micturition). Hagen et al (2002) also found that the UDI and IIQ had good psychometric properties, including test-retest reliability. In examination of the short forms, FitzGerald et al (2001) found that UDI-6 and IIQ-7 scores changed after reconstructive pelvic surgery; patients who were subjectively continent had lower postoperative scores on both scales.

The scales have not always been found to be useful in predicting urodynamic diagnoses, nor have scores necessarily correlated with the severity of objectively measured urinary incontinence (FitzGerald & Brubaker, 2002;

Harvey et al, 2001). However, as a quality-of-life instrument, these measures are intended to evaluate the patient's subjective perception of symptoms, which may also be influenced by coexisting conditions (Melville et al, 2002), cultural background, and other biases.

Administration Time: <5 minutes by self-administration for IIQ-7 and UDI-6 taken together.

References

FitzGerald MP, Kenton K, Shott S, et al: Responsiveness of quality of life measurements to change after reconstructive pelvic surgery, *Am J Obstet Gynecol* 185:20-24, 2001.

FitzGerald MP, Brubaker L: Urinary incontinence symptom scores and urodynamic diagnoses, *Neurourol Urodyn* 21:30-35, 2002.

Hagen S, Hanley J, Capewell A: Test-retest reliability, validity, and sensitivity to change of the urogenital distress inventory and the incontinence impact questionnaire, *Neurourol Urodyn* 21:534-539, 2002.

Harvey MA, Kristjansson B, Griffith D, et al: The Incontinence Impact Questionnaire and the Urogenital Distress Inventory: a revisit of their validity in women without a urodynamic diagnosis, *Am J Obstet Gynecol* 185:25-31, 2001.

Melville JL, Walker E, Katon W, et al: Prevalence of comorbid psychiatric illness and its impact on symptom perception, quality of life, and functional status in women with urinary incontinence, *Am J Obstet Gynecol* 187:80-87, 2002.

Shumaker SA, Wyman JF, Uebersax JS, et al: Health-related quality-of-life measures for women with urinary incontinence—the incontinence impact questionnaire and the urogenital distress inventory, *Qual Life Res* 3:291-306, 1994.

Uebersax JS, Wyman JF, Shumaker SA, et al: Continence Program for Women Research Group. Short forms to assess life quality and symptom distress for urinary incontinence in women: the incontinence impact questionnaire and the urogenital distress inventory, *Neurourol Urodyn* 14:131-139, 1995.

van der Vaart CH, de Leeuw JR, Roovers JP, et al: Measuring health-related quality of life in women with urogenital dysfunction: the Urogenital Distress Inventory and Incontinence Impact Questionnaire revisited, *Neurourol Urodyn* 22:97-104, 2003.

ROSENBAUM POCKET VISION SCREENER

	Point	Jaeger	distance equivalent
95			$\frac{20}{800}$
874			$\frac{20}{400}$
2843	26	16	$\frac{20}{200}$
6 3 8 E Ш Ǝ X O O	14	10	$\frac{20}{100}$
8 7 4 5 Ǝ m Ш O X O	10	7	$\frac{20}{70}$
6 3 9 2 5 m E Ǝ X O X	8	5	$\frac{20}{50}$
4 2 8 3 6 5 Ш E m O X O	6	3	$\frac{20}{40}$
3 7 4 2 5 8 Ǝ Ш Ǝ X X O	5	2	$\frac{20}{30}$
9 3 7 8 2 6 Ш m E X O O	4	1	$\frac{20}{25}$
4 2 8 7 3 9 E Ш m O O X	3	1+	$\frac{20}{20}$

Card is held in good light 14 inches from eye. Record vision for each eye separately with and without glasses. Presbyopic patients should read thru bifocal segment. Check myopes with glasses only.

DESIGN COURTESY J. G. ROSENBAUM, M.D.

PUPIL GAUGE (mm.)

2   3   4   5   6   7   8   9

Amsler Grid

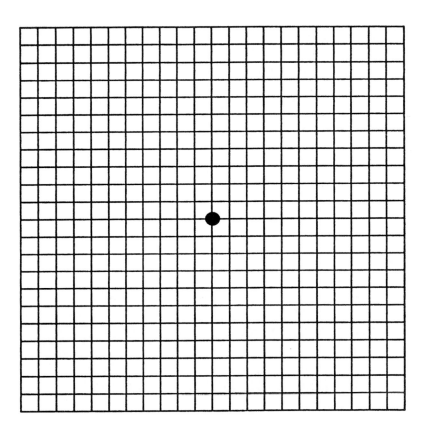

Self-Assessment Hearing Test

Name: _____

Date: _____

The onset of hearing loss is usually very gradual. It may take place over 25-30 years or it may happen more rapidly if you are exposed to loud noises at work or through hobbies. Because it usually does occur slowly, you may not even be aware you have a problem until someone else brings it to your attention. Here is a simple test you can take to determine if you have a hearing problem. Please circle the correct response, yes or no.

1.	Do you have to turn the volume up on the television?	Yes	No
2.	Do you frequently have to ask others to repeat something?	Yes	No
3.	Do you have difficulty understanding when in groups or in noisy situations?	Yes	No
4.	Do you have to sit up front in meetings or in church in order to understand?	Yes	No
5.	Do you have difficulty understanding women or young children?	Yes	No
6.	Do you have trouble knowing where sounds are coming from?	Yes	No
7.	Are you unable to understand when someone talks to you from another room?	Yes	No
8.	Have others told you that you don't seem to hear them?	Yes	No
9.	Do you avoid family meetings or social situations because you "can't understand"?	Yes	No
10.	Do you have ringing or other noises (tinnitus) in your ears?	Yes	No

Scoring:

Answered Yes to less than 3 of the questions: No significant hearing loss present
Answered Yes to between 3 and 5 questions: You may have a slight hearing problem*
Answered Yes to between 5 and 7 questions: You have a moderate hearing problem*
Answered Yes to more than 7 questions: You have a significant hearing problem*

*In order to determine the exact degree of hearing loss present, you should have your hearing evaluated by a licensed hearing professional.

Adapted from hearingloss.org. Self-Help for Hard of Hearing People (CHHH). http://www.shhh.org/html/self-assessment.html.

Epworth Sleepiness Scale (ESS)

Name: _____

Date: _____

Age: _____   *Gender:* Male   Female

Height: _____ *Weight:* _____

Please indicate the likelihood that you would fall asleep in the following situations. This refers to your usual way of life in recent times. Use the following scale to circle the <u>most appropriate</u> number for each situation:

0 = Would ***never*** doze

1 = ***Slight*** chance of dozing

2 = ***Moderate*** chance of dozing

3 = ***High*** chance of dozing

Situation				
Sitting and reading	0	1	2	3
Watching TV	0	1	2	3
Sitting, inactive in a public place (e.g., a theatre or a meeting)	0	1	2	3
As a passenger in a car for an hour without a break	0	1	2	3
Lying down to rest in the afternoon when circumstances permit	0	1	2	3
Sitting and talking to someone	0	1	2	3
Sitting quietly after lunch without alcohol	0	1	2	3
In a car, while stopped for a few minutes in traffic	0	1	2	3

Total Score: _____

THANK YOU FOR YOUR COOPERATION

Adapted from Johns MW: A new method for measuring daytime sleepiness: the Epworth Sleepiness Scale, *Sleep* 14:540-545, 1991.

Headache Diary

Name _____

Week of: _____

Directions: Complete this diary every day, even when you do not have a headache. Women should circle the dates of menstrual flow. Use the lists below to help describe your headache.

Date	Pain Intensity	Location	Symptoms	Hours Lasted	Headache Triggers	Headache Medications	Relief Measures	Other Medications Taken	Hours of Sleep	Mood

Comments: _____

Pain Intensity (choose 1-10)

0—No Headache
1 to 3—Mild
4 to 6—Moderate
7 to 10—Severe

Location

1. Behind/between eyes
2. Front/temples
3. Top of head
4. Back of head
5. Neck
6. One side (specify R or L)

Symptoms

1. Nausea
2. Vomiting
3. Sensitivity to light
4. Sensitivity to sound
5. Mood changes
6. Muscle pain/tenderness

Headache Triggers

1. Alcohol
2. Chocolate
3. Aged cheese
4. Citrus fruits
5. Cured meats
6. MSG
7. NutraSweet®

Headache Triggers (continued)

8. Skipped meals
9. Other foods (specify)
10. Excess caffeine
11. Odors (specify)
12. Fatigue
13. Stress
14. Missed medication
15. Eyestrain/visual triggers
16. Allergies/sinus
17. Weather changes
18. Physical exercise
19. Sexual activity
20. Other (specify)

Relief Measures:

1. Ice pack
2. Bed rest
3. Dark room
4. Medication (name & dosage)
5. Relaxation techniques
6. Massage
7. Other (specify)

Mood

1. Happy
2. Nervous
3. Downhearted
4. Tired
5. Hopeless

Berg Balance Scale

Name: _____

Date: _____

General Instructions

Please demonstrate each task and/or give instructions as written below. When scoring, please record the lowest response category that applies for each item.

In most items, the subject is asked to maintain a given position for a specific time. Progressively more points are deducted if the time or distance requirements are not met, if the subject's performance warrants supervision, or if the subject touches an external support or receives assistance from the examiner. Subjects should understand that they must maintain their balance while attempting the tasks. The choices of which leg to stand on or how far to reach are left to the subject. Poor judgment will adversely influence the performance and the scoring.

Equipment required for testing are a stopwatch or watch with a second hand and a ruler or other indicator of 2, 5, and 10 inches (5, 12.5, and 25 cm). Chairs used during testing should be of reasonable height. Either a step or a stool (of average step height) may be used for item #12.

Item	Description	Score (0-4)
1.	Sitting to standing	_____
2.	Standing unsupported	_____
3.	Sitting unsupported	_____
4.	Standing to sitting	_____
5.	Transfers	_____
6.	Standing with eyes closed	_____
7.	Standing with feet together	_____
8.	Reaching forward with outstretched arm	_____
9.	Retrieving object from floor	_____
10.	Turning to look behind	_____
11.	Turning 360 degrees	_____
12.	Placing alternate foot on stool	_____
13.	Standing with one foot in front	_____
14.	Standing on one foot	_____
	Total	_____

1. Sitting to Standing
INSTRUCTIONS: Please stand up. Try not to use your hands for support.
( ) 4   able to stand without using hands and stabilize independently
( ) 3   able to stand independently using hands
( ) 2   able to stand using hands after several tries
( ) 1   needs minimal aid to stand or to stabilize
( ) 0   needs moderate or maximal assist to stand

2. Standing Unsupported
INSTRUCTIONS: Please stand for two minutes without holding.
( ) 4   able to stand safely 2 minutes
( ) 3   able to stand 2 minutes with supervision
( ) 2   able to stand 30 seconds unsupported
( ) 1   needs several tries to stand 30 seconds unsupported
( ) 0   unable to stand 30 seconds unassisted

If a subject is able to stand 2 minutes unsupported, score full points for sitting unsupported. Proceed to item #4.

Berg Balance Scale - 2

3. Sitting with Back Unsupported But Feet Supported on Floor or on a Stool
INSTRUCTIONS: Please sit with arms folded for 2 minutes.

( ) 4   able to sit safely and securely 2 minutes
( ) 3   able to sit 2 minutes under supervision
( ) 2   able to sit 30 seconds
( ) 1   able to sit 10 seconds
( ) 0   unable to sit without support 10 seconds

4. Standing to Sitting
INSTRUCTIONS: Please sit down.

( ) 4   sits safely with minimal use of hands
( ) 3   controls descent by using hands
( ) 2   uses back of legs against chair to control descent
( ) 1   sits independently but has uncontrolled descent
( ) 0   needs assistance to sit

5. Transfers
INSTRUCTIONS: Arrange chair(s) for a pivot transfer. Ask subject to transfer one way toward a seat with armrests and one way toward a seat without armrests. You may use two chairs (one with and one without armrests) or a bed and a chair.

( ) 4   able to transfer safely with minor use of hands
( ) 3   able to transfer safely; definite need of hands
( ) 2   able to transfer with verbal cueing and/or supervision
( ) 1   needs one person to assist
( ) 0   needs two people to assist or supervise to be safe

6. Standing Unsupported with Eyes Closed
INSTRUCTIONS: Please close your eyes and stand still for 10 seconds.

( ) 4   able to stand 10 seconds safely
( ) 3   able to stand 10 seconds with supervision
( ) 2   able to stand 3 seconds
( ) 1   unable to keep eyes closed 3 seconds but stays steady
( ) 0   needs help to keep from falling

7. Standing Unsupported with Feet Together
INSTRUCTIONS: Place your feet together and stand without holding.

( ) 4   able to place feet together independently and stand for 1 minute safely
( ) 3   able to place feet together independently and stand for 1 minute with supervision
( ) 2   able to place feet together independently and to hold for 30 seconds
( ) 1   needs help to attain position but able to stand for 15 seconds with feet together
( ) 0   needs help to attain position and unable to hold for 15 seconds

8. Reaching Forward with Outstretched Arm While Standing
INSTRUCTIONS: Lift arm to 90 degrees. Stretch out your fingers and reach forward as far as you can. (Examiner places a ruler at end of fingertips when arm is at 90 degrees. Fingers should not touch the ruler while subject is reaching forward. The recorded measure is the distance forward that the fingers reach while the subject is in the most forward leaning position. When possible, ask subject to use both arms when reaching to avoid rotation of the trunk.)

( ) 4   can reach forward confidently >25 cm (10 inches)
( ) 3   can reach forward >12.5 cm safely (5 inches)
( ) 2   can reach forward >5 cm safely (2 inches)
( ) 1   reaches forward but needs supervision
( ) 0   loses balance while trying/requires external support

9. Pick Up Object from the Floor from a Standing Position
INSTRUCTIONS: Pick up the shoe/slipper that is placed in front of your feet.
( ) 4   able to pick up slipper safely and easily
( ) 3   able to pick up slipper but needs supervision

( ) 2   unable to pick up slipper but reaches 2-5 cm (1-2 inches) from slipper and keeps balance independently
( ) 1   unable to pick up slipper and needs supervision while trying
( ) 0   unable to try/needs assist to keep from losing balance or falling

10. Turning to Look Behind Over Left and Right Shoulders While Standing
INSTRUCTIONS: Turn to look **directly** behind you over toward left shoulder. Repeat to the right.
Examiner may pick an object to look at directly behind the subject to encourage a better twist turn.

( ) 4   looks behind from both sides and weight shifts well
( ) 3   looks behind one side only; other side shows less weight shift
( ) 2   turns sideways only but maintains balance
( ) 1   needs supervision when turning
( ) 0   needs assist to keep from losing balance or falling

11. Turn 360 Degrees
INSTRUCTIONS: Turn completely around in a full circle. Pause. Then turn a full circle in the other direction.

( ) 4   able to turn 360 degrees safely in 4 seconds or less
( ) 3   able to turn 360 degrees safely one side only in 4 seconds or less
( ) 2   able to turn 360 degrees safely but slowly
( ) 1   needs close supervision or verbal cueing
( ) 0   needs assistance while turning

12. Placing Alternate Foot on Step or Stool While Standing Unsupported
INSTRUCTIONS: Place each foot alternately on the step/stool. Continue until each foot has touched the step/stool four times.

( ) 4   able to stand independently and safely and complete 8 steps in 20 seconds
( ) 3   able to stand independently and complete 8 steps >20 seconds
( ) 2   able to complete 4 steps without aid with supervision
( ) 1   able to complete >2 steps; needs minimal assist
( ) 0   needs assistance to keep from falling/unable to try

13. Standing Unsupported One Foot in Front
INSTRUCTIONS: (Demonstrate to Subject) Place one foot directly in front of the other. If you feel that you cannot place your foot directly in front, try to step far enough ahead that the heel of your forward foot is ahead of the toes of the other foot. (To score 3 points, the length of the step should exceed the length of the other foot and the width of the stance should approximate the subject's normal stride width)

( ) 4   able to place foot tandem independently and hold 30 seconds
( ) 3   able to place foot ahead of other independently and hold 30 seconds
( ) 2   able to take small step independently and hold 30 seconds
( ) 1   needs help to step but can hold 15 seconds
( ) 0   loses balance while stepping or standing

14. Standing on One Leg
INSTRUCTIONS: Stand on one leg as long as you can without holding.

( ) 4   able to lift leg independently and hold >10 seconds
( ) 3   able to lift leg independently and hold 5-10 seconds
( ) 2   able to lift leg independently and hold = or >3 seconds
( ) 1   tries to lift leg; unable to hold 3 seconds but remains standing independently
( ) 0   unable to try or needs assist to prevent fall

( ) Total Score (Maximum = 56)

From Berg K, Wood-Dauphinee S, Williams JL, et al: Measuring balance in the elderly: preliminary development of an instrument, *Phsyiotherapy Canada* 41:304-331, 1989.

Abnormal Involuntary Movement Scale (AIMS) - Screening for Tardive Dyskinesia

Patient Name: _____   Examiner: _____

Date of Visit: _____

> **Examination Procedure[a]**   Either before or after completing the EXAMINATION PROCEDURE observe the patient unobtrusively, at rest (eg, in the waiting room). The chair to be used in this examination should be a hard, firm one without arms.

1) Ask patient whether there is anything in his/her mouth (eg, gum, candy, etc.) and if there is, to remove it.
2) Ask patient about the <u>current</u> condition of his/her teeth. Ask patient if he/she wears dentures. Do teeth or dentures bother patient now?
3) Ask patient whether he/she notices any movements in mouth, face, hands, or feet. If yes, ask to describe and to what extent they <u>currently</u> bother patient or interfere with his/her activities.
4) Have patient sit in chair with hands on knees, legs slightly apart, and feet flat on floor. (Look at entire body for movements while patient is in this position.)
5) Ask patient to sit with hands hanging unsupported: [for a male patient, hands hanging between his legs, and for a female patient wearing dress, hands hanging over her knees].[b] (Observe hands and other body areas.)
6) Ask patient to open mouth. (Observe tongue at rest within mouth.) Do this twice.
7) Ask patient to protrude tongue. (Observe abnormalities of tongue movement.) Do this twice.
8) Ask patient to tap thumb, with each finger, as rapidly as possible for 10-15 seconds, separately with right hand, then with left hand. (Observe facial and leg movements.)
9) Flex and extend patient's left and right arms (one at a time). (Note any rigidity.)
10) Ask patient to stand up. (Observe in profile. Observe all body areas again, hips included.)
11) Ask patient to extend both arms outstretched in front with palms down. (Observe trunk, legs, and mouth.)
12) Have patient walk a few paces, turn, and walk back to chair. (Observe hands and gait.) Do this twice.

> **Movement Ratings[a,b]**   Complete EXAMINATION PROCEDURE (above) before making ratings for the MOVEMENT RATINGS, rate the highest severity observed.
>
> 0 = none
> 1 = minimal (may be extreme normal)
> 2 = mild
> 3 = moderate
> 4 = severe

FACIAL & ORAL MOVEMENTS:

❶ **Muscles of facial expression** (eg, movements of forehead, eyebrows, periorbital area, cheeks; Include frowning, blinking, smiling, grimacing [of upper face].) — 0 1 2 3 4

❷ **Lips and perioral area** (eg, puckering, pouting, smacking) — 0 1 2 3 4

❸ **Jaw** (eg, biting, clenching, chewing, mouth opening, lateral movement) — 0 1 2 3 4

❹ **Tongue** (Rate only increase in movement both in and out of mouth, NOT inability to sustain a movement.) — 0 1 2 3 4

EXTREMITY MOVEMENTS:

❺ **Upper** *(arms, wrists, hands, fingers)* Include choreic movements, (ie, rapid, objectively purposeless, irregular, spontaneous), athetoid movements (ie, slow, irregular, complex, serpentine). Do NOT include tremor (ie, repetitive, regular rhythmic) — 0 1 2 3 4

❻ **Lower** *(legs, knees, ankles, toes)* eg, lateral knee movement, foot tapping, heel dropping, foot squirming, inversion & eversion of foot) — 0 1 2 3 4

TRUNK MOVEMENTS:

❼ **Neck, shoulders, hips** (eg, rocking, twisting, squirming, pelvic gyrations) Include diaphragmatic movements. — 0 1 2 3 4

GLOBAL JUDGMENTS: [score based on highest single score on items 1-7 above]

❽ Severity of abnormal movement — 0 1 2 3 4

❾ Incapacitation due to abnormal movement — 0 1 2 3 4

❿ Patient's awareness of abnormal movement (Rate only patient's report.) — 0 1 2 3 4
   0 = no awareness;   1 = aware, no distress;   2 = aware, mild distress;
   3 = aware, moderate distress;   4 = aware, severe distress.

Rate item 10 according to reported level of distress

DENTAL STATUS

⓫ Current problems with teeth and/or dentures — No: 0   Yes: 1

⓬ Does patient usually wear dentures? — No: 0   Yes: 1

[a]Munetz & Benjamin (1988) offer a detailed review of the Examination Procedure as well as a detailed proposal for how to score the Movement Ratings. The authors note the recommendation that the AIMS be administered twice per year beginning prior to the start of neuroleptic (antipsychotic) drug therapy. (Baldressarini et al, 1980) They also note that although ratings above 0 may suggest tardive dyskinesia, it is important to determine if the abnormal movement is clinically significant. Also, nonmedication causes should be ruled out. The original AIMS scoring directed that movements (re: Examination Procedure items 8, 11, and 12) be scored 1 point less if they did not occur spontaneously. However, Munetz and Benjamin recommend not following this direction. Schooler and Kane (1982) propose the following criteria for a diagnosis of probable tardive dyskinesia: (a) exposure to neuroleptics for a total of at least 3 months, (b) score of 2 for at least 2 body areas, or score of 3 for at least 1 body area, and (c) rule out other causes for abnormal movement.

[b]AIMS text in brackets was added or rephrased by Munetz and Benjamin (1988).

From Guy W: *ECDEU Assessment Manual for Psychopharmacology*, revised edition. Washington, DC, 1976, US Department of Health, Education, and Welfare. Modified by Munetz MR, Benjamin S: How to examine patients using the Abnormal Involuntary Movement Scale, *Hospital Com Psychiatry* 39(11):1172-1177, 1988.

Rhodes Index of Nausea and Vomiting—Revised (INVR)

Patient Name: _____

Date: _____

Time: _____

Directions: Please mark the box in each row that most clearly corresponds to your experience. Please make *one* mark on each *line.*

1. In the last 12 hours, I threw up ___ times.	7 or more	5-6	3-4	1-2	I did not throw up
2. In the last 12 hours, from retching or dry heaves I have felt ____ distress.	no	mild	moderate	great	severe
3. In the last 12 hours, from vomiting or throwing up, I have felt ____ distress.	severe	great	moderate	mild	no
4. In the last 12 hours, I have felt nauseated or sick at my stomach ____.	not at all	1 hour or less	2-3 hours	4-6 hours	more than 6 hours
5. In the last 12 hours, from nausea/ sickness at my stomach, I have felt ____ distress.	no	mild	moderate	great	severe
6. In the last 12 hours, each time I threw up I produced a ____ amount.	very large (3 cups or more)	large (2-3 cups)	moderate (½-2 cups)	small (up to ½ cup)	I did not throw up
7. In the last 12 hours, I have felt nauseated or sick at my stomach ____ times.	7 or more	5-6	3-4	1-2	no
8. In the last 12 hours, I have had periods of retching or dry heaves without bringing anything up ____ times.	no	1-2	3-4	5-6	7 or more

Note: Copyright 1983 by Verna Rhodes; revised 1996. Reprinted with permission.

DIRECTIONS FOR USE

Complete *one* INVR Scale starting at 7, 8, or 9 pm on (date). Choose the best hour for your schedule. Beginning with your chosen hour, complete *one* INVR Scale every 12 hours at the *same* clock hour for six times. Example: 7 pm-7 am; 8 pm-8 am; 9 pm-9 am

DIRECTIONS FOR SCORING

To score the INVR, reverse items 1, 3, 6, and 7. Assign a numeric value to each response from 0, the least amount of distress, to 4, the most distress. Total symptom experience from nausea and vomiting is calculated by summing the patient's responses to each of the eight items on the Rhodes INV. The potential range of scores is from a low of 0 to a maximum of 32. Subscale scores also can be obtained from the Rhodes INV for the following.

CALCULATION OF SUBSCALE SCORES

Subscales for Symptom Experience	Items on Scale	Potential Range of Scores
Nausea experience	4, 5, 7	0-12
Vomiting experience	1, 3, 6	0-12
Retching experience	2, 8	0-8
Total experience score	All items	0-32

Subscales for Symptom Occurrence	Items on Scale	Potential Range of Scores
Nausea occurrence	4, 7	0-8
Vomiting occurrence	1, 6	0-8
Retching occurrence	8	0-4
Total occurrence score	All items	0-20

Subscales for Symptom Distress	Items on Scale	Potential Range of Scores
Nausea distress	5	0-4
Vomiting distress	3	0-4
Retching distress	2	0-4
Total distress score	All items	0-12

Constipation Assessment Scale (CAS)

Name: _____

Date: _____

Directions: Circle the appropriate number to indicate whether, during the past three days, you have had NO PROBLEM, SOME PROBLEM, or A SEVERE PROBLEM with each of the items listed below.

Item	*No Problem*	*Some Problem*	*Severe Problem*
1. Abdominal distention or bloating	0	1	2
2. Change in amount of gas passed rectally	0	1	2
3. Less frequent bowel movements	0	1	2
4. Oozing liquid stool	0	1	2
5. Rectal fullness or pressure	0	1	2
6. Rectal pain with bowel movement	0	1	2
7. Small stool size	0	1	2
8. Urge but inability to pass stool	0	1	2

Total Score: _____

Rater: _____

From McMillan SC, Williams F: Validity and reliability of the constipation assessment scale, *Cancer Nurs* 12:183-188, 1989.

Androgen Deficiency in Aging Males (ADAM) Questionnaire

Name: _____

Date: _____

Choose the answers below that best describe how you have been feeling. Answers will help your health care provider and you to better manage your medical needs.

1. Do you have a decrease in libido (sex drive)?	Yes	No
2. Do you have a lack of energy?	Yes	No
3. Do you have a decrease in strength and/or endurance?	Yes	No
4. Have you lost height?	Yes	No
5. Have you noticed a decreased "enjoyment of life"?	Yes	No
6. Are you sad and/or grumpy?	Yes	No
7. Are your erections less strong?	Yes	No
8. Have you noticed a recent deterioration in your ability to play sports?	Yes	No
9. Are you falling asleep after dinner?	Yes	No
10. Has there been a recent deterioration in your work performance?	Yes	No

If you answered yes to #1, #7, or any three others, you may have symptoms associated with low testosterone.

Other Comments:

Thank you for your responses.

From Morley JE, Perry HM: Androgen deficiency in aging men, *Med Clin North Am*, 83(5):1279–1289, 1999.

Brief Male Sexual Function Inventory For Urology

Name: _____

Date: _____

SEXUAL DRIVE					
Let's define sexual drive as a feeling that may include wanting to have a sexual experience (masturbation or intercourse), thinking about having sex, or feeling frustrated due to lack of sex.					
1. During the past 30 days, on how many days have you felt sexual drive?	No days 0	Only a few days 1	Some days 2	Most days 3	Almost every day 4
2. During the past 30 days, how would you rate your level of sexual drive?	None at all 0	Low 1	Medium 2	Medium High 3	High 4
ERECTIONS					
3. Over the past 30 days, how often have you had partial or full sexual erections when you were sexually stimulated in any way?	Not at all 0	A few times 1	Fairly often 2	Usually 3	Always 4
4. Over the past 30 days, when you had erections, how often were they firm enough to have sexual intercourse?	0	1	2	3	4
5. How much difficulty did you have getting an erection during the past 30 days?	Did not get erections at all 0	A lot of difficulty 1	Some difficulty 2	Little difficulty 3	No difficulty 4
EJACULATION					
6. In the past 30 days, how much difficulty have you had ejaculating when you have been sexually stimulated?	Have had no sexual stimulation in past month 0	A lot of difficulty 1	Some difficulty 2	Little difficulty 3	No difficulty 4
7. In the past 30 days, how much did you consider the amount of semen you ejaculate to be a problem for you?	Did not climax 0	Big problem 1	Medium problem 2	Small problem 3	No problem 4
PROBLEM ASSESSMENT					
8. In the past 30 days, to what extent have you considered a lack of sex drive to be a problem?	Big problem 0	Medium problem 1	Small problem 2	Very small problem 3	No problem 4
9. In the past 30 days, to what extent have you considered your ability to get and keep erections to be a problem?	0	1	2	3	4
10. In the past 30 days, to what extent have you considered your ejaculation to be a problem?	0	1	2	3	4
OVERALL SATISFACTION					
11. Overall, during the past 30 days, how satisfied have you been with your sex life?	Very dissatisfied 0	Mostly dissatisfied 1	Neutral or mixed (about equally satisfied and dissatisfied) 2	Mostly satisfied 3	Very satisfied 4

From O'Leary MP, Fowler FJ, Lenderking WR, et al: A brief male sexual function inventory for urology, *Urology* 46:697-706, 1995.

440

Incontinence Impact Questionnaire (IIQ-7)

Name: _____

Date: _____

Has urine leakage affected your:

("X one for each question)

	Not at all	Slightly	Moderately	Greatly
1. Ability to do household chores (cooking, housecleaning, laundry)?	☐	☐	☐	☐
2. Physical recreation such as walking, swimming, or other exercise?	☐	☐	☐	☐
3. Entertainment activities (movies, concerts, etc.)?	☐	☐	☐	☐
4. Ability to travel by car or bus more than 30 minutes from home?	☐	☐	☐	☐
5. Participation in social activities outside your house?	☐	☐	☐	☐
6. Emotional health (nervousness, depression, etc.)?	☐	☐	☐	☐
7. Feeling frustrated?	☐	☐	☐	☐

Urogenital Distress Inventory (UDI-6)

Do you experience, and if so,
How much are you bothered by:

("X" one for each question)

	Not at all	Slightly	Moderately	Greatly
1. Frequent urination?	☐	☐	☐	☐
2. Urine leakage related to the feeling of urgency?	☐	☐	☐	☐
3. Urine leakage related to physical activity, coughing, or sneezing?	☐	☐	☐	☐
4. Small amounts of urine leakage drops?	☐	☐	☐	☐
5. Difficulty emptying your bladder?	☐	☐	☐	☐
6. Pain or discomfort in the lower abdominal or genital area?	☐	☐	☐	☐

From Shumaker SA, Wyman JF, Uebersax JS, et al: Health-related quality-of-life measures for women with urinary incontinence, *Qual Life Res* 3(5):291-306, 1994.

CHAPTER 16

Social and Spiritual Assessment Tools

Chapter Contents

ICON KEY: 📄 Tool Printed ✏ Tool on CD-ROM ∞ Customizable Tool **i** Information and Resources Provided for Further Acquisition

Introduction to Social Support and Spiritual Measures

Social health has been described as a dimension of individual well-being distinct from physical and mental health, defined in terms of interpersonal interactions, and portrayed as the degree to which a person functions as a member of the community (Bowling, 1997). Social integration, the level of social support that one experiences, and personal concepts of spirituality all contribute to the overall wellness of an individual. Measurement of the level of social support has increased because of growing evidence of the effect that support has on an individual's response to disease, use of primary care services, and self-care behaviors (Broadhead et al, 1988). As the emphasis in medicine has moved away from treating just a disease toward treating the whole person (body, mind, and spirit) and helping people lead independent, productive lives, tools have been developed to assist researchers and clinicians in evaluating the quality of and need for social support.

A great number of instruments that measure various aspects of social functioning are available. Examination of social roles, satisfaction with relationships, adjustment to life situations, and presence of emotional support are all qualitative aspects of social functioning that these tools attempt to assess. A difficulty in attempting to measure social support is in the subjective nature of a person's perception of such support. Perception may be influenced by underlying depression and other psychologic or physical influences. Objective questions about social networks, such as number and frequency of social encounters, may be inadequate for assessing a person's response to availability of such support. Clinicians using social measurement tools need to validate—through dialogue, interview, or confirmation of information with another person—the results of a social functioning measure.

Measures of spirituality have also been developed, particularly in support of care for the terminally ill. Spirituality may be defined as "that which gives meaning to one's life and draws one to transcend oneself" (Puchalski, 1998). Expressions of spirituality may include religion, meditation, prayer, interactions with others or nature, and a personal relationship with God or a higher power. Assessment of the degree of spirituality influencing a person's well-being has become important; the clinician can use the results of an assessment to assist or guide the patient in personal development and integration of life's experiences. Because the meanings of spirituality and religiousness are subjective, these types of measures are diverse and may be focused on a particular philosophy or religious ideation.

References

Bowling A: *Measuring health: a review of quality of life measurement scales,* Philadelphia, 1997, Open University Press.

Broadhead WE, Gehlbach SH, de Gruy FV, et al: The Duke-UNC Functional Social Support Questionnaire. Measurement of social support in family medicine patients, *Med Care* 26(7):709-723, 1988.

Puchalski C: *Spirituality,* Washington, DC, 1998, Washington University: Center to Improve Care of the Dying. Available at http://www.gwu.edu/~cicd/toolkit/spiritual.htm.

Chapter Contents

This chapter contains widely used measures of social support and spiritual well-being. Most of these instruments measure subjective perceptions of satisfaction, support, and well-being; several tools contain objective questions on the quantity of interactions or social encounters. Tools in this chapter focus on family functioning, caregiver stress, social support and social networks, loneliness, spiritual well-being, and pain attitudes. Because of the subjective understanding of the questions by the patient and the analysis of the responses by the clinician, a broad range of interpretation is possible with these tools. Therefore scores are not absolute indicators of social or spiritual functioning but should be considered together with the overall clinical impression and dialogue with the patient in order to offer effective therapeutic interventions.

The Family APGAR

Author: Smilkstein G, 1978, 1982.

Targeted Population: Adults and children ages 10 and older.

Description: The Family APGAR was developed to measure satisfaction in five dimensions of family function: adaptation, partnership, growth, affection, and resolve. The Family APGAR was initially introduced by

Smilkstein in 1978, and a "friends" component was added in 1982 to more fully explore social support and provide a better understanding of its impact on the individual. The same five question items used in the family segment were directed to the respondent's friends. A third component, the companion questionnaire, was also added to provide information on the respondent's relationships with family, friends, and a significant other. Smilkstein et al (1982) report offering the Family APGAR to all newly registered patients as part of a self-administered general medical and family history questionnaire in the clinical setting.

Scores: Three possible responses to each of the five items in the "family" and "friends" sections of the questionnaire are scored as follows: 2 (almost always), 1 (some of the time), and 0 (hardly ever). Scores for each item are summed and range from 0 (low satisfaction) to 10 (high satisfaction) for each component of the Family APGAR.

Accuracy: The Family APGAR was initially reported to be reliable and valid based on a variety of population group responses (Smilkstein et al, 1982). However, the construct validity of the Family APGAR has been questioned in subsequent studies. Mengel (1987) found that knowledge of the APGAR score did not increase the frequency with which physicians evaluated family function or diagnosed family dysfunction. Gwyther et al (1993) also found that the Family APGAR failed to detect family dysfunction revealed by psychologic interviewing. Smucker et al (1995) reported that child psychosocial problems were more than twice as likely to be present when the Family APGAR score was low (<5). However, there was poor correlation between the Family APGAR scores and physicians' detection of child psychosocial problems, suggesting that family functioning is related to child psychosocial problems but that the Family APGAR may not improve screening for child psychosocial problems. In 1998, Murphy et al reported that a lack of family social support is associated with child psychosocial dysfunction as assessed by two different measures. However, the Family APGAR was not a sensitive measure of child psychosocial problems, suggesting that it supplements, but does not replace, information concerning the child's overall psychosocial functioning. In another large study that included more than 22,000 pediatric office visits, Family APGAR scores were negative for 73% of clinician-identified dysfunctional families, and clinicians did not identify dysfunction for 83% of Family APGAR–identified dysfunctions (Gardner et al, 2001). This study also revealed that scores on the initial visit often differed from scores at follow-up visits, leading the authors to conclude that data did not support the use of the Family APGAR as a measure of family dysfunction in the primary care setting. The Family APGAR did identify significant family functioning issues in a small group of patients with advanced cancer (Powazki et al, 2002).

The Family APGAR is included here because of its popularity and the desire by many primary care providers to have a brief family functioning screening tool. However, the previously mentioned studies highlight the fact that caution is recommended in interpreting the results of any screen measuring family dysfunction until more sophisticated test construction is presented. Sound clinical judgment always supercedes screening test results.

Administration Time: 5 to 10 minutes by self-administration.

References

Gardner W, Nutting PA, Kelleher KJ, et al: Does the family APGAR effectively measure family functioning? *J Fam Pract* 50:19-25, 2001.

Gwyther RE, Bentz EJ, Drossman DA, et al: Validity of the Family APGAR in patients with irritable bowel syndrome, *Fam Med* 25: 21-25, 1993.

Mengel M: The use of the family APGAR in screening for family dysfunction in a family practice center, *J Fam Pract* 24:394-398, 1987.

Murphy JM, Kelleher K, Pagano ME, et al: The family APGAR and psychosocial problems in children: a report from ASPN and PROS, *J Fam Pract* 46:54-64, 1998.

Powazki RD, Walsh D: Family distress in palliative medicine: a pilot study of the family APGAR scale, *Am J Hosp Palliat Care* 19:392-396, 2002.

Smilkstein G: The Family APGAR: a proposal for a family function test and its use by physicians, *J Fam Pract* 6:1231-1239, 1978.

Smilkstein G, Ashworth C, Montano D: Validity and reliability of the Family APGAR as a test of family function, *J Fam Pract* 15:303-311, 1982.

Smucker WD, Wildman BG, Lynch TR, et al: Relationship between the family APGAR and behavioral problems in children, *Arch Fam Med* 4:535-539, 1995.

Zarit Burden Interview (ZBI)

Author: Zarit S, 1980; revised 1985.

Source: For more information about caregiver stress and the Zarit Burden Interview (ZBI), please see http://www.caregiving-solutions.com/carstres.html. This site provides a link to an article by Parks and Novielli (2000) in which they discuss a systematic approach for assessing the degree of caregiver burden.

Targeted Population: Adult caregivers of the elderly.

Description: The ZBI has become a widely used caregiver burden measure in gerontological research and clinical practice. Designed to assess the stress experienced by caregivers of patients with dementia, the ZBI consists of 22 questions that examine the impact of the patient's disabilities on the caregiver's well-being. For each item, the caregivers choose one of five responses (never, rarely, sometimes, quite frequently, nearly always) that best represents how often they experience the problem described in the question.

Scores: Twenty-two items are scored from 0 (never) to 4 (nearly always). The total score ranges from 0 to 88, with higher scores indicating a greater level of burden.

Accuracy: The ZBI was developed by examination of caregiver experiences, an in-depth community study of caregivers and care recipients, and analysis of prior research on caregiver stress (Zarit et al, 1980). The ZBI has demonstrated excellent internal consistency (Majerovitz, 1995; Zarit et al, 1987). Hébert et al (2000)

found that the ZBI score was more strongly correlated to the depressive mood of the caregivers and the behavior problems of the care recipients than to the recipients' cognitive and functional status.

A short version (12-item; questions 2, 3, 5, 6, 9, 10, 11, 12, 17, 19, 20, and 21) and a screening version (4-item; questions 2, 3, 9, and 19) of the ZBI have been developed with excellent correlation to the full version (Bédard et al, 2001). Reducing the number of items did not affect the properties of the ZBI, and the authors propose that clinicians and researchers use the short version. They identify a score of 17 on the short version and a score of 8 on the screening version as indicative of significant burden.

Administration Time: 10 to 20 minutes by self-administration or interview.

References

Bédard M, Molloy DW, Squire L, et al: The Zarit Burden Interview: a new short version and screening version, *Gerontologist* 41:652-657, 2001.

Hébert R, Bravo G, Preville M: Reliability, validity and reference values of the Zarit Burden Interview for assessing informal caregivers of community-dwelling older persons with dementia, *Can J Aging* 19:494-507, 2000.

Majerovitz SD: Role of family adaptability in the psychological adjustment of spouse caregivers to patients with dementia, *Psychol Aging* 10:447-457, 1995.

Parks SM, Novielli KD: A practical guide to caring for caregivers, *Am Fam Physician* 62: 2613-2622, 2000.

Zarit SH, Anthony C, Boutselis M: Interventions with care givers of dementia patients: comparison of two approaches, *Psychol Aging* 2:225-232, 1987.

Zarit SH, Orr NK, Zarit JM: *The hidden victims of Alzheimer's disease: families under stress.* New York, 1985, New York University Press.

Zarit SH, Reever KE, Bach-Peterson J: Relatives of the impaired elderly: correlates of feelings of burden, *Gerontologist* 20:649-655, 1980.

Support for Caregivers Questionnaire

Authors: George LK, Gwyther LP, 1983, 1986.

Targeted Population: Caregivers of the elderly.

Description: This simple questionnaire is designed to assist the caregiver with determining the need for caregiver support. Thirteen questions are presented with a 5-point answer scale ranging from "never" to "regularly." The questions pertain to tasks for which the caregiver is responsible and serve to identify the level of assistance the caregiver has with the tasks. The primary helper to the caregiver is identified for each task. Because this is a qualitative questionnaire, no formal scoring is involved; the answers assist the clinician in guiding the caregiver to family, community, and professional resources.

Administration Time: 2 to 5 minutes by self-administration or interview.

References

George LK, Gwyther LP: Caregiver well-being: a multidimensional examination of family caregivers of demented adults, *Gerontologist* 26:253-259, 1986.

George LK, Gwyther LP: *Duke University Caregiver Well-Being Survey*: Durham, NC, 1983, Duke University Center for the Study of the Aging and Human Development.

Duke UNC (University of North Carolina) Functional Social Support (DUFSS) Questionnaire

Authors: Broadhead WE et al, 1988.

Source: The Duke-UNC (University of North Carolina) Functional Social Support (DUFSS) Questionnaire is reprinted in this text and may also be viewed at http://www.medal.org/ch1.html.

Targeted Population: Adults at risk of isolation.

Description: The DUFSS Questionnaire assesses quality of social support by measuring a person's satisfaction with the support. Originally constructed as a 14-item measure, psychometric testing by the authors refined the DUFSS Questionnaire to an eight-item functional social support instrument intended for primary care practice. Social support is measured on two scales: affective support (items 1, 2, and 8) and confidant support (remaining five items).

Please note that this questionnaire is not to be confused with the lengthier Duke Social Support Index or the Duke Social Support and Stress Scale.

Scores: Each of the eight items is answered on a 5-point scale, which ranges from "as much as I would like" (5 points) to "much less than I would like" (1 point). A total score may be obtained from adding the item scores. As with other qualitative tools, the item scores may offer more insight into perceived satisfaction than a summary score.

Accuracy: Reliability, as tested by the authors, was adequate. Validity, particularly correlation with other social support instruments, was low. The population from which the scale was derived was primarily female, white, and younger than 45 years. McDowell and Newell (1996) suggest further testing on agreement with other social support measures. Testing on more diverse populations would also strengthen the applicability of this tool.

Administration Time: 1 to 2 minutes by self-administration.

References

Broadhead WE, Gehlbach SH, de Gruy FV, et al: The Duke-UNC Functional Social Support Questionnaire. Measurement of social support in family medicine patients, *Med Care* 26:709-723, 1988.

McDowell I, Newell C: *Measuring health: a guide to rating scales and questionnaires*. ed 2. New York, 1996, Oxford University Press, pp. 140-142.

Lubben Social Network Scale (LSNS)

Author: Lubben JE, 1988.

Source: The Lubben Social Network Scale (LSNS) is reprinted in this text and may also be viewed at http://www.medal.org/ch1.html.

Targeted Population: Elderly adults.

Description: The LSNS consists of 10 items that measure levels of social interaction with relatives and friends. Three of the items deal with family relationships, three items deal with relationships with friends, and four items concern interdependent relationships (confidant relationships, helping others, living arrangements). Answers are arranged on a 6-point (0 to 5) scale, which grades frequency of interactions and numbers of confidants.

Scores: The total LSNS score is a sum of the 10-item scores. The total score ranges from 0 to 50. A score below 20 suggests an extreme risk for limited social networks. Rubinstein et al (1994) grouped total scores into four types: isolated (<20), high risk (21-25), moderate risk (26-30), and low risk (31+).

Accuracy: Lubben (1988) examined the relationship of the LSNS and three health indicators (past hospitalizations, a mental health measure, and a health practices checklist) in a diverse sample of elderly persons. The LSNS demonstrated internal consistency and correlated strongly with all three health measures. Rubinstein et al (1994) compared LSNS scores with social worker evaluations, with a resulting strong consensus.

Administration Time: 5 to 10 minutes by self-administration or interview.

References

Lubben JE: Assessing social networks among elderly populations, *Fam Commun Health* 11:42-52, 1988.

Rubinstein RL, Lubben JE, Mintzer JE: Social isolation and social support: an applied perspective, *J Appl Gerontol* 13:58-72, 1994.

UCLA Loneliness Scale (Version 3)

Author: Russell DW, 1996.

Source: The UCLA Loneliness Scale (Version 3) is reprinted in this text. A summary description of the measure, with contact information for the author is available at http://www.psychology.iastate.edu/faculty/ccutrona/uclalone.htm.

Targeted Population: Adults.

Description: The UCLA Loneliness Scale is the most well-known measure of loneliness (Bowling, 1997). Version 3 of the UCLA Loneliness Scale evolved from two prior versions; understandability was improved and social desirability and population biases were reduced in the course of its development (Russell, 1996). Version 3 consists of 11 negatively worded (or "lonely") items and 9 positively worded (or "non-lonely") items. This version has also been reworded to facilitate personal or telephone interviews.

Scores: Each item is answered by writing a number from 1 to 4, indicating "never" (1), "rarely" (2), "sometimes" (3), or "always" (4). The 10 positively worded items (1, 5, 6, 9, 10, 15, 16, 19, and 20) are reverse-scored (i.e., 1 = 4, 2 = 3, 3 = 2, 4 = 1), and the scores for each item are summed. Higher scores indicate greater degrees of loneliness.

Accuracy: The author reports Version 3 to be highly reliable across varied populations, including internal consistency and test-retest reliability (Russell, 1996). Convergent and construct validity for the scale was demonstrated by significant correlations with other measures of loneliness and significant relations with measures of the adequacy of the individual's interpersonal relationships.

Administration Time: 2 to 5 minutes by self-administration or interview.

References

Russell DW: UCLA Loneliness Scale (Version 3): reliability, validity, and factor structure, *J Pers Assess* 66:20-40, 1996.

Bowling A: *Measuring health: a review of quality of life measurement scales*, Philadelphia, 1997, Open University Press, pp. 108-110.

JAREL Spiritual Well-Being Scale

Authors: Hungelmann J et al, 1996.

Targeted Population: Older adults.

Description: The JAREL Spiritual Well-Being Scale was developed by nurse researchers as an assessment tool for spiritual well-being. A 21-item scale resulted from grounded theory-based research; items were grouped into three domains as follows: Factor I, faith/belief dimension; Factor II, life/self-responsibility; and Factor III, life satisfaction/self-actualization. A 6-point Likert-type scale is used to rate responses from "strongly agree" to "strongly disagree." As an interesting aside, the name of this tool was taken from the first letters of the primary authors' first names.

Scores: Responses for Factors I and III are scored from 6 (strongly agree) to 1 (strongly disagree). Factor II is reverse-scored. A total score by factor group may be summed; however, the authors note that the total score is not as important as the identification of individual strengths and needs or concerns. The clinician is encouraged to use the individual item scores to guide interventions with the client. A high score on a particular item may guide the clinician to encourage the client to realize his or her potential for enhanced spiritual well-being. A lower score on an item may lead the clinician to further explore the client's perception of spirituality or spiritual distress. The authors describe four nursing interventions for spiritual diagnoses: affirmation, therapeutic communication, reminiscence, and referral.

Accuracy: Little psychometric testing of this scale has been published. Foley et al (1998) reported good to excellent reliability, including internal consistency and test-retest reliability. Correlation with another spiritual assessment scale was also good.

Administration Time: 5 to 10 minutes by self-administration or interview.

References

Foley L, Wagner J, Waskel SA: Spirituality in the lives of older women, *J Women Aging* 10:85-91, 1998.

Hungelmann J, Kenkel-Rossi E, Klassen L, et al: Focus on spiritual well-being: harmonious interconnectedness of mind-body-spirit, Use of the JAREL spiritual well-being scale. *Geriatr Nurs* 17:262-266, 1996.

Survey of Pain Attitudes (SOPA-35)

Authors: Jensen MP et al, 1987; revised 2000.

Targeted Population: Adults with chronic pain.

Description: Pain specialists stress the importance of tracking patient pain beliefs, because beliefs may affect treatment response. Changes in pain beliefs during treatment may also affect outcomes (Jensen et al, 2000). This pain beliefs assessment tool has been extensively studied and is widely used for both research and clinical applications. Originally published in 1987 (Jensen et al), the Survey of Pain Attitudes (SOPA) has undergone three major and two abbreviated revisions. Seven pain-related belief areas (scales) are assessed: Pain control, Disability, Medical Cures, Solicitude, Medication, Emotion, and Harm. The goal for creation of the brief version was that it reflect the original SOPA scales as closely as possible. The version reprinted in this text has 35 items related to patient beliefs about pain. Responses are indicated on a 5-point Likert-type scale, ranging from 1 (this is very untrue for me) to 5 (this is very true for me).

Scores: Responses to the 35 items are scored on a scale of 1 to 5, with 12 items reverse-scored. All ratings for each scale are summed after reverse scoring; the sum is then divided by the number of items responded to within each scale. The resulting number indicates the level of belief regarding the scale dimension.

Accuracy: Since its inception, the SOPA has shown strong psychometric properties and good relationship to treatment outcomes. Jensen et al (2000) state that the SOPA-35 conforms closely to the original 57-item SOPA. With the exception of the SOPA-35 Harm scale, this brief version has excellent internal consistency. The SOPA-35 has demonstrated validity and shows greater similarity to the 57-item SOPA than other versions (Jensen et al, 2000). Although it is not interchangeable with the long version because of scale score differences, the SOPA-35 is a brief measure suitable for assessment of general belief dimensions.

Administration Time: 2 to 5 minutes by self-administration or interview.

References

Jensen MP, Karoly P, Huger R: The development and preliminary validation of an instrument to assess patients' attitudes toward pain, *J Psychosom Res* 31:393-400, 1987.

Jensen MP, Turner JA, Romano JM: Pain belief assessment: a comparison of the short and long versions of the surgery of pain attitudes, *J Pain* 1:138-150, 2000.

McDowell I, Newell C: *Measuring health: a guide to rating scales and questionnaires*. ed 2. New York, 1996, Oxford University Press, pp. 323-324.

Other Measures:

Medical Outcomes Study Social Support Survey (MOS-SSS) i

Author: Sherbourne CD, Stewart AL, 1991.

Source: The Medical Outcomes Study Social Support Survey (MOS-SSS) and scoring instructions are available at http://www.rand.org/health/surveys/mos.descrip.html. The surveys that appear on the RAND Health site are public documents, available without charge to all researchers. The authors request appropriate citation when the surveys found on the site are used.

Targeted Population: Adults.

Description: This brief, self-administered social support survey was developed for patients in the Medical Outcomes Study, a 2-year study of patients with chronic conditions. The survey consists of 19 items within four separate social support subscales: emotional/informational support (8 items), tangible support (4 items), affectionate support (3 items), and positive social interaction (3 items) plus a separate last item (Sherbourne & Stewart, 1991; Sherbourne et al, 1992).

Scores: Responses are recorded on a 5-point Likert-type scale indicating how often each kind of support is available if needed. Answers range from "none of the time" (1 point) to "all of the time" (5 points). The average of the scores for each item in the subscale is calculated. For the purpose of obtaining an overall support index, the average of (1) the scores for all 18 items included in the four subscales and (2) the score for the last item in the survey is calculated. Scale scores may also be transformed to a scale of 0 to 100 with a formula available on the website. A higher score for an individual scale or for the overall support index indicates more support.

Accuracy: In demonstrating that patients with higher levels of support, as measured by the MOS-SSS, had better levels of physical functioning and emotional well-being than those with low levels of support, Sherbourne and Stewart (1991) provide support for construct validity. Reliability is also good, including item-scale correlations. Bowling (1997) notes that the scale is based on subjective perceptions; therefore another measure needs to be used for objective study of the support structure. Despite this limitation, the scale merits wider use.

Administration Time: 2 to 5 minutes by self-administration.

References

Bowling A: *Measuring health: a review of quality of life measurement scales,* Philadelphia, 1997, Open University Press, pp. 55-56.

Sherbourne CD, Meredith LS, Rogers W, et al: Social support and stressful life events: age differences in their effects on health related quality of life among the chronically ill, *Qual Life Res* 1:235-246, 1992.

Sherbourne CD, Stewart AL: The MOS Social Support Survey, *Soc Sci Med* 32:705-714, 1991.

Spiritual Involvement and Beliefs Scale (SIBS)   i

Author: Hatch RL et al, 1998.

Source: The Spiritual Involvement and Beliefs Scale (SIBS) is available online at http://www.mywhatever.com/cifwriter/content/41/pe1182.html. The tool may be printed and copied for personal use from this site.

Targeted Population: Adults.

Description: The SIBS was designed to be widely applicable across religious traditions; the instrument assesses actions, as well as beliefs. This questionnaire contains 34 statements regarding spiritual and religious beliefs, with a 7-point Likert-type response scale. Five additional items assess actions related to spirituality, with the same response scale.

Scores: Patients indicate their agreement with statements on a scale ranging from "strongly agree" (7 points) to "strongly disagree" (1 point). Points are summed and range from 39 to 273, with higher scores indicating a higher level of spiritual orientation.

Accuracy: Reliability and validity appear good, including internal consistency, test-retest reliability, and high correlation with another established measure of spirituality, the Spiritual Well-Being Scale. More testing is recommended.

Administration Time: 5 to 10 minutes by self-administration.

Reference

Hatch RL, Burg MA, Naberhaus DS, et al: The Spiritual Involvement and Beliefs Scale: development and testing of a new instrument, *J Fam Pract* 46:476-486, 1998.

Spiritual Well-Being Scale (SWBS)   i

Authors: Paloutzian RF, Ellison CW, 1982.

Source: The Spiritual Well-Being Scale (SWBS) can be ordered directly through Life Advance, Inc., at http://www.lifeadvance.com/swbs.htm. Information provided in this section may also be found at this site.

Targeted Population: Adults.

Description: The SWBS is a 20-item scale with two dimensions: religious and existential. Designed as a general indicator of well-being, it provides an overall measure of the perception of spiritual quality of life. Two subscales are included: the Religious Well-Being subscale (RWB), which consists of 10 religious items containing a reference to God, and the Existential Well-Being subscale (EWB), which consists of 10 items with no reference to God. Half the items from each subscale are worded in positive and negative directions. The clinician may use the RWB or EWB scores alone. The SWBS is useful for evaluation of the well-being of clinical patients and counseling clients in both individual and group settings.

Scores: Patients indicate their agreement with statements on a 6-point scale, ranging from "strongly agree" to strongly disagree." Half of the items from each subscale are reverse-scored. A total SWBS score and scores for the RWB and EWB subscales may be summed. Subscale scores are useful, because the sense of religious well-being and the sense of existential well-being may be expressed differently. Higher scores indicate spiritual well-being.

Accuracy: Reliability is reported to be good, including internal consistency and test-retest reliability. Validity is also good because SWB scores correlate in predicted ways with several other scales.

Administration Time: 10 to 15 minutes by self-administration.

Reference

Paloutzian RF, Ellison CW: Loneliness, spiritual well-being and quality of life. In Peplau LA, Perlman D, editors. *Loneliness: a sourcebook of current theory, research, and therapy.* New York, 1982, John Wiley & Sons.

Index of Core Spiritual Experiences (INSPIRIT)

i

Author: Kass J et al, 1991.

Source: The Index of Core Spiritual Experiences (INSPIRIT) is available at http://www.spirituality-health.com/newsh/items/selftest/item_234.html. The resource includes the instrument, a scale of well-being, and analysis of responses to the online screening.

Targeted Population: Adults.

Description: The INSPIRIT is an 18-item interview scale used for spiritual assessment in general populations and populations of hospital patients. The items assess the degree to which one has beliefs and experiences of a higher power and one's relationship to that power. The first six items measure the beliefs regarding spirituality, religion, and God; the next 12 items assess spiritual experiences. The author notes that these measurements can provide helpful guideposts for those in search of a closer connection to their spiritual core.

Scores: A 4-point Likert scale format records responses for each question. The total INSPIRIT score ranges from 7 to 28.

Accuracy: No specific reliability or validity psychometric studies are available. INSPIRIT scores have been statistically related to increases in life purpose and satisfaction and to decreases in the average frequency of medical symptoms (Kass, 1996). McBride et al (1998) found significant correlation between patient health and spirituality, as measured by the INSPIRIT. Kass et al (1991) recommends that this tool be used in conjunction with a general well-being and stress assessment for a more complete understanding of the effect of spirituality on overall health.

Administration Time: 2 to 5 minutes.

References

Kass J: Spirituality and well-being, *Spirituality and Health Online*, 1996. Available at http://www.spiritualityhealth.com/newsh/items/selftest/more_234.html.

Kass J, Friedman R, Leserman J, et al: Health outcomes and a new measure of spiritual experience, *J Sci Study Rel* 30:203-211, 1991.

McBride JL, Arthur G, Brooks R, et al: The relationship between a patient's spirituality and health experiences, *Fam Med* 30:122-126, 1998.

Online Resources

Center to Improve Care of the Dying–Spirituality: This site provides reviews of 30 instruments. They are divided into four groups of scales that measure quality of life, attitudes, religiousness, and spirituality. Available at http://www.gwu.edu/~cicd/toolkit/spiritual.htm.

Toolkit of Instruments to Measure End-of-Life Care: Caregiver Well-Being: This resource cites and reviews 35 general instruments and 19 disease-specific instruments pertaining to caregiver well-being. Disease-specific instruments are for caregivers of people with Alzheimer's disease, dementia, stroke survivors, and patients with acquired immunodeficiency syndrome. Available at http://www.chcr.brown.edu/PCOC/familyburden.htm.

RAND Health–Quality Improvement Tools: This site provides access or reference to many practical tools and surveys for improving quality of care. Included in this group are tools for assessing quality of life and health status, assessment tools for quality of care for vulnerable older adults, health plan questionnaires, and many other care assessment instruments. Instruments include or refer to many of the Medical Outcomes Study (MOS) measures, patient satisfaction questionnaires, and disease-specific surveys. Available at http://www.rand.org/health/tools/; Surveys: http://www.rand.org/health/surveys.html.

The Family APGAR

Name: _____

Date: _____

Date of Birth: _____ *Gender:* Male Female

The following questions have been designed to help us better understand you and your friends. Friends are non-relatives from your school or community with whom you have a sharing relationship.

Comment space should be used if you wish to give additional information or if you wish to discuss the way the question applies to your friends. Please try to answer all questions.

The following questions have been designed to help us better understand you and your family. You should feel free to ask questions about any item in the questionnaire.

Comment space should be used if you wish to give additional information or if you wish to discuss the way the question applies to your family. Please try to answer all questions.

"Family" is the individual(s) with whom you usually live. If you live alone, consider family as those with whom you now have the strongest emotional ties.

For each question, check only one box

	Almost always	Some of the time	Hardly ever
I am satisfied that I can turn to my friends for help when something is troubling me. Comments:	☐	☐	☐
I am satisfied with the way my friends talk over things with me and share problems with me. Comments:	☐	☐	☐
I am satisfied that my friends accept and support my wishes to take on new activities or directions. Comments:	☐	☐	☐
I am satisfied with the way my friends express affection, and respond to my emotions, such as anger, sorrow, or love. Comments:	☐	☐	☐
I am satisfied with the way my friends and I share time together. Comments:	☐	☐	☐

	Almost always	Some of the time	Hardly ever
I am satisfied that I can turn to my family for help when something is troubling me. Comments:	☐	☐	☐
I am satisfied with the way my family talks over things with me and shares problems with me. Comments:	☐	☐	☐
I am satisfied that my family accepts and supports my wishes to take on new activities or directions. Comments:	☐	☐	☐
I am satisfied with the way my family expresses affection, and responds to my emotions, such as anger, sorrow, or love. Comments:	☐	☐	☐
I am satisfied with the way my family and I share time together. Comments:	☐	☐	☐

The Family APGAR - 2

Who lives in your home?* List by relationship (e.g., spouse, significant other,† child, or friend).

Please check below the column that best describes how you now get along with each member of the family listed.

Relationship	Age	Sex	Well	Fairly	Poorly
_____	_____	_____	☐	☐	☐
_____	_____	_____	☐	☐	☐
_____	_____	_____	☐	☐	☐

If you don't live with your own family, please list below the individuals to whom you turn for help most frequently. List by relationship, (e.g., family member, friend, associate at work, or neighbor).

Please check below the column that best describes how you now get along with each person listed.

Relationship	Age	Sex	Well	Fairly	Poorly
_____	_____	_____	☐	☐	☐
_____	_____	_____	☐	☐	☐
_____	_____	_____	☐	☐	☐

*If you have established your own family, consider home to be the place where you live with your spouse, children, or significant other; otherwise, consider home as your place of origin, e.g., the place where your parents or those who raised you live.

†"Significant other" is the partner you live with in a physically and emotionally nurturing relationship, but to whom you are not married.

Zarit Burden Interview (ZBI)

Name: _____

Date: _____

Date of Birth: _____   *Gender:* Male   Female

Circle the response that best describes how you feel.	Never	Rarely	Sometimes	Quite frequently	Nearly always
1. Do you feel that your relative asks for more help than he/she needs?	0	1	2	3	4
2. Do you feel that because of the time you spend with your relative that you don't have enough time for yourself?	0	1	2	3	4
3. Do you feel stressed between caring for your relative and trying to meet other responsibilities for your family or work?	0	1	2	3	4
4. Do you feel embarrassed over your relative's behavior?	0	1	2	3	4
5. Do you feel angry when you are around your relative?	0	1	2	3	4
6. Do you feel that your relative currently affects your relationships with other family members or friends in a negative way?	0	1	2	3	4
7. Are you afraid what the future holds for your relative?	0	1	2	3	4
8. Do you feel your relative is dependent on you?	0	1	2	3	4
9. Do you feel strained when you are around your relative?	0	1	2	3	4
10. Do you feel your health has suffered because of your involvement with your relative?	0	1	2	3	4
11. Do you feel that you don't have as much privacy as you would like because of your relative?	0	1	2	3	4

Zarit Burden Interview (ZBI) - 2

Circle the response that best describes how you feel.	Never	Rarely	Sometimes	Quite frequently	Nearly always
12. Do you feel that your social life has suffered because you are caring for your relative?	0	1	2	3	4
13. Do you feel uncomfortable about having friends over because of your relative?	0	1	2	3	4
14. Do you feel that your relative seems to expect you to take care of him/her as if you were the only one he/she could depend on?	0	1	2	3	4
15. Do you feel that you don't have enough money to take care of your relative in addition to the rest of your expenses?	0	1	2	3	4
16. Do you feel that you will be unable to take care of your relative much longer?	0	1	2	3	4
17. Do you feel you have lost control of your life since your relative's illness?	0	1	2	3	4
18. Do you wish you could leave the care of your relative to someone else?	0	1	2	3	4
19. Do you feel uncertain about what to do about your relative?	0	1	2	3	4
20. Do you feel you should be doing more for your relative?	0	1	2	3	4
21. Do you feel you could do a better job in caring for your relative?	0	1	2	3	4
22. Overall, how burdened do you feel in caring for your relative?	0	1	2	3	4

Instructions for caregiver: The questions above reflect how persons sometimes feel when they are taking care of another person. After each statement, circle the word that best describes how often you feel that way. There are no right or wrong answers.

Scoring instructions: Add the scores for the 22 questions. The total score ranges from 0 to 88. A high score correlates with higher level of burden.

Support for Caregivers Questionnaire

Name: _____

Date: _____

Date of Birth: _____ Gender: Male Female

"Now I'd like to ask you about some of the ways your family and friends may help you out—either how they help you personally or the way they help you to care for your confused relative. For each question below, please check one column to indicate how often your family or friends give you that kind of help. Then please tell us the relationship of the person who gives you the most help of that type (for example, sister, friend, daughter-in-law)."

Type of help Do your family or friends:	How often do you receive this help?					
	Never	Rarely	Only if I ask	Now and then	Regularly	Relationship of helper
1. Help you out when you are sick?						
2. Shop or run errands for you?						
3. Help you out with money or bills?						
4. Fix things around your house?						
5. Keep house for you or do household chores?						
6. Give you advice on business or finances?						
7. Provide companionship for you?						
8. Give you advice on dealing with problems?						
9. Provide transportation for you or your confused relative?						
10. Prepare or provide meals?						
11. Stay with your confused relative while you are away?						
12. Provide personal grooming services for your confused relative?						
13. Do you wish that your family and friends would give you more help with these kinds of things? 1. No 2. Yes						

From George LK, Gwyther LP: Duke University Caregiver Well-Being Survey, Durham, NC, 1983, Duke University Center for the Study of Aging and Human Development; Caregiver well-being: a multidimensional examination of family caregivers of demented adults, *Gerontologist* 26:253, 1986.

Duke-UNC Functional Social Support (DUFSS) Questionnaire

Name: _____

Date: _____

Date of Birth: _____   *Gender:* Male Female

HERE IS A LIST OF SOME THINGS THAT OTHER PEOPLE DO FOR US OR GIVE US THAT MAY BE HELPFUL OR SUPPORTIVE. PLEASE READ EACH STATEMENT CAREFULLY AND PLACE A CHECK (✔) IN THE BLANK THAT IS <u>CLOSEST</u> TO YOUR SITUATION.

HERE IS AN EXAMPLE:

	As much as I would like				Much less than I would like
I get enough vacation time		✔			

If you put a check where we have, it means that you get <u>almost</u> as much vacation time as you would like, but not quite as much as you would like.

ANSWER EACH ITEM AS BEST YOU CAN. THERE ARE <u>NO</u> RIGHT OR WRONG ANSWERS.

I get: . . .	As much as I would like				Much less than I would like
1. people who care what happens to me					
2. love and affection					
3. chances to talk to someone about problems at work or with my housework					
4. chances to talk to someone I trust about my personal and family problems					
5. chances to talk about money matters					
6. invitations to go out and do things with other people					
7. useful advice about important things in life . . .					
8. help when I'm sick in bed					

From George LK, Gwyther LP: Duke University Caregiver Well-Being Survey, Durham, NC, 1983, Duke University Center for the Study of Aging and Human Development; George LK, Gwyther LP: Caregiver well-being: a multidimensional examination of family caregivers of demented adults, *Gerontologist* 26:253-259, 1986.

Lubben Social Network Scale (LSNS)

Name: _____

Date: _____

Date of Birth: _____   *Gender:* Male   Female

Family Networks

Q1. How many relatives do you see or hear from at least once a month? (NOTE: Include in-laws with relatives.)

0 = zero	3 = three or four
1 = one	4 = five to eight
2 = two	5 = nine or more

Q1 _____

Q2. Tell me about the relative with whom you have the most contact. How often do you see or hear from that person?

0 = <monthly	3 = weekly
1 = monthly	4 = a few times a week
2 = a few times a month	5 = daily

Q2 _____

Q3. How many relatives do you feel close to? That is, how many of them do you feel at ease with, can talk to about private matters, or can call on for help?

0 = zero	3 = three or four
1 = one	4 = five to eight
2 = two	5 = nine or more

Q3 _____

Friends Networks

Q4. Do you have any close friends? That is, do you have any friends with whom you feel at ease, can talk to about private matters, or can call on for help? If so, how many?

0 = zero	3 = three or four
1 = one	4 = five to eight
2 = two	5 = nine or more

Q4 _____

Q5. How many of these friends do you see or hear from at least once a month?

0 = zero	3 = three or four
1 = one	4 = five to eight
2 = two	5 = nine or more

Q5 _____

Q6. Tell me about the friend with whom you have the most contact. How often do you see or hear from that person?

0 = <monthly	3 = weekly
1 = monthly	4 = a few times a week
2 = a few times a month	5 = daily

Q6 _____

Lubben Social Network Scale (LSNS) -2

Confidant Relationships

Q7. When you have an important decision to make, do you have someone you can talk to about it?

Q7 _____

Always	Very often	Often	Sometimes	Seldom	Never
5	4	3	2	1	0

Q8. When other people you know have an important decision to make, do they talk to you about it?

Q8 _____

Always	Very often	Often	Sometimes	Seldom	Never
5	4	3	2	1	0

Helping Others

Q9a. Does anybody rely on you to do something for them each day?
For example: shopping, cooking dinner, doing repairs, cleaning house, providing child care, etc.

NO—if no, go on to Q9b.
YES—if yes, Q9 is scored "5" and skip to Q10

Q9b. Do you help anybody with things like shopping, filling out forms, doing repairs, providing child care, and so on?

Q9 _____

Always	Very often	Often	Sometimes	Seldom	Never
5	4	3	2	1	0

Living Arrangements

Q10. Do you live alone or with other people? (NOTE: Include in-laws with relatives.)

Q10 _____

5 Live with spouse
4 Live with other relatives or friends
1 Live with other unrelated individuals (e.g., paid help)
0 Live alone

TOTAL LSNS SCORE: _____

Scoring:

The total LSNS score is obtained by adding up scores from each of the 10 individual items. Thus total LSNS scores can range from 0 to 50. Scores on each item were anchored between 0 and 5 to permit equal weighting of the 10 items. It is suggested that a score below 20 indicates an extreme risk for limited social networks.

From Lubben JE: Assessing social networks among elderly populations, *Fam Comm Health* 11:1988.

UCLA Loneliness Scale

Name: _____

Date: _____

Date of Birth: _____ *Gender:* Male Female

Instructions: The following statements describe how people sometimes feel. For each statement, please indicate how often you feel the way described by placing a check in the space provided. Here is an example:

How often do you feel happy?

If you never felt happy, you would check "never"; if you always feel happy, you would check "always."

	NEVER 1	RARELY 2	SOMETIMES 3	ALWAYS 4
*1. How often do you feel that you are "in tune" with the people around you?				
2. How often do you feel that you lack companionship?				
3. How often do you feel that there is no one you can turn to?				
4. How often do you feel alone?				
*5. How often do you feel part of a group of friends?				
*6. How often do you feel that you have a lot in common with the people around you?				
7. How often do you feel that you are no longer close to anyone?				
8. How often do you feel that your interests and ideas are not shared by those around you?				
*9. How often do you feel outgoing and friendly?				
*10. How often do you feel close to people?				
11. How often do you feel left out?				
12. How often do you feel that your relationships with others are not meaningful?				
13. How often do you feel that no one really knows you well?				
14. How often do you feel isolated from others?				
*15. How often do you feel you can find companionship when you want it?				
*16. How often do you feel that there are people who really understand you?				
17. How often do you feel shy?				
18. How often do you feel that people are around you but not with you?				
*19. How often do you feel that there are people you can talk to?				
*20. How often do you feel that there are people you can turn to?				

Scoring:
Items that are asterisked should be reversed (i.e., 1 = 4, 2 = 3, 3 = 2, 4 = 1), and the scores for each item then summed together. Higher scores indicate greater degrees of loneliness.

From Russell DW: UCLA Loneliness Scale (Version 3): reliability, validity, and factor structure, *J Pers Assess* 66:20-40, 1996.

JAREL Spiritual Well-Being Scale

Name: _____

Date: _____

Date of Birth: _____ Gender: Male Female

DIRECTIONS: Please circle the choice that best describes how much you agree with each statement. Circle only <u>one</u> answer for each statement. There is no right or wrong answer.

	Strongly Agree	Moderately Agree	Agree	Disagree	Moderately Disagree	Strongly Disagree
1. Prayer is an important part of my life.	SA	MA	A	D	MD	SD
2. I believe I have spiritual well-being.	SA	MA	A	D	MD	SD
3. As I grow older, I find myself more tolerant of others' beliefs.	SA	MA	A	D	MD	SD
4. I find meaning and purpose in my life.	SA	MA	A	D	MD	SD
5. I feel there is a close relationship between my spiritual beliefs and what I do.	SA	MA	A	D	MD	SD
6. I believe in an afterlife.	SA	MA	A	D	MD	SD
7. When I am sick I have less spiritual well-being.	SA	MA	A	D	MD	SD
8. I believe in a supreme power.	SA	MA	A	D	MD	SD
9. I am able to receive and give love to others.	SA	MA	A	D	MD	SD
10. I am satisfied with my life.	SA	MA	A	D	MD	SD
11. I set goals for myself.	SA	MA	A	D	MD	SD
12. God has little meaning in my life.	SA	MA	A	D	MD	SD
13. I am satisfied with the way I am using my abilities.	SA	MA	A	D	MD	SD
14. Prayer does not help me in making decisions.	SA	MA	A	D	MD	SD
15. I am able to appreciate differences in others.	SA	MA	A	D	MD	SD
16. I am pretty well put together.	SA	MA	A	D	MD	SD
17. I prefer that others make decisions for me.	SA	MA	A	D	MD	SD
18. I find it hard to forgive others.	SA	MA	A	D	MD	SD
19. I accept my life situations.	SA	MA	A	D	MD	SD
20. Belief in a supreme being has no part in my life.	SA	MA	A	D	MD	SD
21. I cannot accept change in my life.	SA	MA	A	D	MD	SD

Factor I
Faith/Belief Dimension
(Scoring: SA = 6   SD = 1)
Item 1 _____
Item 2 _____
Item 3 _____
Item 4 _____
Item 5 _____
Item 6 _____
Item 8 _____   Subscore _____

Factor II
Life/Self-Responsibility
(Reverse Scoring: SA 1   SD6)
Item 7 _____
Item 12 _____
Item 14 _____
Item 17 _____
Item 18 _____
Item 20 _____
Item 21 _____   Subscore _____

Factor III
Life Satisfaction/Self-Actualization
(Scoring SA 6   SD 1)
Item 9 _____
Item 10 _____
Item 11 _____
Item 13 _____
Item 15 _____
Item 16 _____
Item 19 _____   Subscore _____

Total score _____

From Hungelmann J, Kenkel-Rossi E, Klassen L, et al, 1987. Copyright Marquette University College of Nursing, Milwaukee, Wisconsin.

Survey of Pain Attitudes (SOPA-35)

Name: _____

Date: _____

Date of Birth: _____   Gender: Male   Female

Please indicate how much you agree with each of the following statements about your pain problem by using the response key below.

Response key	Very untrue	Somewhat untrue	Neither true nor untrue (or does not apply)	Somewhat true	Very true
1. The pain I feel is a sign that damage is being done.					
2. I will probably always have to take pain medications.					
3. When I hurt, I want my family to treat me better.					
4. If my pain continues at its present level, I will be unable to work.					
5. The amount of pain I feel is out of my control.					
6. I do not expect a medical cure for my pain.					
7. Pain does not have to mean that my body is being harmed.					
8. I have had the most relief from pain with the use of medications.					
9. Anxiety increases the pain I feel.					
10. There is little that I can do to ease my pain.					
11. When I am hurting, I deserve to be treated with care and concern.					
12. I pay doctors so they will cure me of my pain.					
13. My pain problem does not need to interfere with my activity level.					
14. It is the responsibility of my family to help me when I feel pain.					
15. Stress in my life increases the pain I feel.					
16. Exercise and movement are good for my pain problem.					
17. Medicine is one of the best treatments for chronic pain.					
18. My family needs to learn how to take better care of me when I am in pain.					
19. Depression increases the pain I feel.					
20. If I exercise, I could make my pain problem much worse.					

Survey of Pain Attitudes (SOPA-35) - 2

Response key	Very untrue	Somewhat untrue	Neither true nor untrue (or does not apply)	Somewhat true	Very true
21. I can control my pain by changing my thoughts.					
22. I need more tender loving care than I am now getting when I am in pain.					
23. I consider myself to be disabled.					
24. I have learned to control my pain.					
25. I trust that doctors can cure my pain.					
26. My pain does not stop me from leading a physically active life.					
27. My physical pain will never be cured.					
28. There is a strong connection between my emotions and my pain level.					
29. I am not in control of my pain.					
30. No matter how I feel emotionally, my pain stays the same.					
31. When I find the right doctor, he or she will know how to reduce my pain.					
32. If my doctor prescribed pain medications for me, I would throw them away.					
33. I will never take pain medications again.					
34. Exercise can decrease the amount of pain I experience.					
35. My pain would stop anyone from leading an active life.					

SOPA-35 scoring key:

Control: 5*, 10*, 21, 24, 29*
Disability: 4, 13*, 23, 26*, 35
Harm: 1, 7*, 16*, 20, 34*
Emotion: 9, 15, 19, 28, 30
*Reverse-scored items.

Medication: 2, 8, 17, 32*, 33*
Solicitude: 3, 11, 14, 18, 22
Medical Cure: 6*, 12, 25, 27*, 31

Sum all ratings provided for each scale (transform reverse-scored items [ie, 4 minus rating given], before summing with other ratings) and divide by the number of items responded to within each scale.

From Jensen MP, Turner JA, Romano JM: Pain belief assessment: a comparison of the short and long versions of the surgery of pain attitudes, *J Pain* 1(2):138-150, 2000. Copyright American Pain Society.

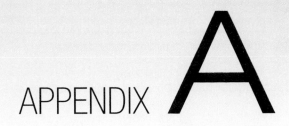

Abbreviations

Abbreviation	Definition
6CIT	6-Item Cognitive Impairment Test
A	abortion
A&P	auscultation and percussion
A/Ab	abnormal
AAA	abdominal aortic aneurism
AAP	American Academy of Pediatrics
ABG	arterial blood gas
ACC	American College of Cardiology
ADA	American Dietetic Association
ADAM	Androgen Deficiency in Aging Males Questionnaire
ADHD	attention-deficit/hyperactivity disorder
ADL	activities of daily living
AF	anterior fontanelle
AHA	American Heart Association
AHCPR	Agency for Health Care Policy and Research
AHRQ	Agency for Healthcare Research and Quality
AIMS	Abnormal Involuntary Movement Scale
AIMS	Arthritis Impact Measurement Scales
AMA	American Medical Association
AMD	age-related macular degeneration
ASA	American Society of Anesthesiologists
ASQ	Ages and Stages Questionnaire
AUA	American Urological Association
AUDIT	Alcohol Use Disorders Identification Test
AV	anteverted
BAI	Beck Anxiety Inventory
BARS	Brief Agitation Rating Scale
BASE	Brief Abuse Screen for the Elderly
BCIS	Bureau of Citizenship and Immigration Services
BCRS	Brief Cognitive Rating Scale
BDI	Batelle Developmental Inventory
BDI	Beck Depression Inventory
BDST	Burke Dysphagia Screening Test
BF	breastfeeding
BHS	Beck Hopelessness Scale
BINS	Bayley Infant Neurodevelopmental Screener
BM	bowel movement
BMI	body mass index
BP	blood pressure

Abbreviation	Definition
BPH	benign prostatic hyperplasia
BPI	Brief Pain Inventory
BRBPR	bright red blood per rectum
BS	bowel sounds
BSS	Beck Scale for Suicidal Ideation
BT	bleeding time
BUN	blood urea nitrogen
BUS	Bartholin, urethral, and Skene glands
BV	bacterial vaginosis
CA	cancer
CABG	coronary artery bypass graft
CAD	coronary artery disease
CAPE	Clifton Assessment Procedures for the Elderly
CAS	Colored Analog Scale
CAS	Constipation Assessment Scale
CASE	Caregiver Abuse Screen
CBC	complete blood count
CC	chief complaint
CDC	Centers for Disease Control and Prevention
CDI	Child Development Inventories
CDL	commercial driver's license
CDR	Clinical Dementia Rating
CDT	Clock Drawing Test
CES-D	Center for Epidemiologic Studies–Depression Scale
CES-DC	Center for Epidemiologic Studies-Depression Scale for Children
CFT	capillary filling time
CHAT	Checklist for Autism in Toddlers
CHEOPS	Children's Hospital of Eastern Ontario Pain Scale
CHF	congestive heart failure
CHO	carbohydrate
CMT	cervical motion tenderness
CN	cranial nerve
COPD	chronic obstructive pulmonary disease
CRS-R	Conners' Rating Scales–Revised
CSDD	Cornell Scale for Depression in Dementia
CT	computed tomography
CTS	Conflict Tactics Scale
CV	cardiovascular
CVA	cerebrovascular accident

Abbreviation	Definition
CVD	cardiovascular disease
CX	cervix
CXR	chest x-ray
CY-BOCS	Children's Yale-Brown Obsessive Compulsive Scale
D/C	discharge
DAST	Drug Abuse Screening Test
DAST	Dyslexia Adult Screening Test
DEST	Dyslexia Early Screening Test
DM	diabetes mellitus
DNR	do not resuscitate
DOB	date of birth
DOE	dyspnea on exertion
DSM	*Diagnostic and Statistical Manual of Mental Disorders*
DST	Dyslexia Screening Test
DT	diphtheria, tetanus
DTaP	diphtheria, tetanus, acellular pertussis
DTP	diphtheria, tetanus, pertussis
DTR	deep tendon reflex
DUFSS	Duke University of North Carolina Functional Social Support
DUI	driving under the influence
DVT	deep vein thrombosis
EAT-26	Eating Attitudes Test
EBM	expressed breast milk
ECG	electrocardiogram
ED	erectile dysfunction
EDC	estimated date of confinement
EDI-2	Eating Disorders Inventory–Second Edition
EG	external genitalia
EGA	estimated gestational age
EKG	electrocardiogram
EOM	extraocular movements
EPDS	Edinburgh Postnatal Depression Scale
ERT	estrogen replacement therapy
ESI-R	Early Screening Inventory–Revised
ESP	Eating Disorder Screen for Primary Care
ESS	Epworth Sleepiness Scale
ETOH	alcohol
F to N	finger to nose
FBG	fasting blood glucose
FBS	fasting blood sugar
FH	family history
FIM	Functional Independence Measure
FMCSA	Federal Motor Carrier Safety Administration
FOBT	fecal occult blood test
FOCI	Florida Obsessive-Compulsive Inventory
FSI	Functional Status Index
G	gravida
GAF	Global Assessment of Functioning Scale
GAPS	Guidelines for Adolescent Preventive Services
GAS	Global Assessment Scale
GBD	gall bladder disease
GC	gonococcal
GDS	Geriatric Depression Scale
GERD	gastroesophageal reflux disease
GI	gastrointestinal
GU	genitourinary
H&P	history and physical

Abbreviation	Definition
HA	headache
HAM-D	Hamilton Rating Scale for Depression
HAQ	Health Assessment Questionnaire
HARS	Hamilton Anxiety Rating Scale
Hb	hemoglobin
HbA$_{1c}$	hemoglobin A$_{1c}$ level
HC	head circumference
HCG	human chorionic gonadotropin
Hct	hematocrit
HDL	high-density lipoprotein
HEDIS	Health Plan Employer Data and Information
HEENT	head, ears, eyes, nose, and throat
HHIE-S	Hearing Handicap Inventory for the Elderly–Screening Version
HHS	Department of Health and Human Services
Hib	*Haemophilus influenzae* type B
HIS	Hachinski Ischemic Score
HIV	human immunodeficiency virus
HPI	history of present illness
HRSD	Hamilton Rating Scale for Depression
HRT	hormone replacement therapy
HSV	herpes simplex virus
HTN	hypertension
I&O	ins and outs
IADL	instrumental activities of daily living
IBW	ideal body weight
ICD-10-CM	*International Classification of Diseases,* 10th Revision
ICP	intracranial pressure
IIQ-7	Incontinence Impact Questionnaire
IMC	Information-Memory-Concentration Test
INR	international normalized ratio (prothrombin)
INSPIRIT	Index of Core Spiritual Experiences
INVR	Rhodes Index of Nausea and Vomiting–Revised
IPV	inactivated polio vaccine
ISA	Index of Spouse Abuse
IUGR	intrauterine growth retardation
IV	intravenous
IVR	interactive voice response
JCAHO	Joint Commission on Accreditation for Healthcare Organizations
L	living
L&D	labor and delivery
LDL	low-density lipoprotein
LE	lower extremity
LFT	liver function test
LMP	last menstrual period
LOC	level of consciousness
LSAS	Liebowitz Social Anxiety Scale
LSNS	Lubben Social Network Scale
MAC	mid-arm circumference
MADRS	Montgomery-Åsberg Depression Rating Scale
MAMC	mid-arm muscle circumference
MAST	Michigan Alcoholism Screening Test
M-CHAT	Modified Checklist for Autism in Toddlers
MCL	mid-clavicular line
MET	metabolic equivalent levels
MGF	maternal grandfather

Abbreviation	Definition
MGM	maternal grandmother
MI	myocardial infarction
MIDAS	Migraine Disability Assessment
MMR	measles, mumps, rubella
MMSE	Mini-Mental State Examination
MNA	Mini Nutritional Assessment
MOS-12	Medical Outcomes Study Short Form 12
MOS-36	Medical Outcomes Study Short Form 36
MOS-SSS	Medical Outcomes Study Social Support Survey
MPQ	McGill Pain Questionnaire
MRI	magnetic resonance imaging
MRSA	methicillin-resistant *Staphylococcus aureus*
MS/MSK	musculoskeletal
N	normal
NCQA	National Committee for Quality Assurance
NGC	National Guideline Clearinghouse
NHP	Nottingham Health Profile
NICHQ	National Initiative for Children's Healthcare Quality
NIPS	Neonatal Infant Pain Scale
NKDA	no known drug allergies
NL	normal
NPUAP	National Pressure Ulcer Advisory Panel
NRS	Numeric Rating Scale
NSVD	normal spontaneous vaginal delivery
NYHA	New York Heart Association
OARS	Older American Resources and Services
OAS-M	Overt Aggression Scale–Modified
OCD	obsessive compulsive disorder
OFC	occipital-frontal circumference
ORIF	open reduction, internal fixation
OTC	over-the-counter
P	para
P	premature
PCM	protein-calorie malnutrition
PCP	primary care provider
PCV	pneumococcal vaccine
PDI	Pain Disability Index
PE	premature ejaculation
PE	pulmonary embolism
PEDS	Parents' Evaluation of Developmental Status
PERRL	pupils equally round and reactive to light
PF	posterior fontanelle
PFM	peak flow meter
PGF	paternal grandfather
PGM	paternal grandmother
PHQ-9	Patient Health Questionnaire 9-Item Depression Module
PHS	Public Health Service
PID	pelvic inflammatory disease
PIH	pregnancy-induced hypertension
PMH	past medical history
PMI	point of maximal impulse
PMS	premenstrual syndrome
PND	paroxysmal nocturnal dyspnea
POSIT	Problem Oriented Screening Instrument for Teenagers
PPD	packs per day

Abbreviation	Definition
PPD	purified protein derivative (tuberculin)
PPE	preparticipation physical evaluation
PPIP	Put Prevention Into Practice
PRIME-MD	Primary Care Evaluation of Mental Disorders
PSA	prostate-specific antigen
PSC	Pediatric Symptom Checklist
PSH	past surgical history
PT	pain thermometer
PT	prothrombin time
PTCA	percutaneous transluminal coronary angioplasty
PTT	partial thromboplastin time
PUD	peptic ulcer disease
PUSH	Pressure Ulcer Scale for Healing
PVD	peripheral vascular disease
Q-EDD	Questionnaire for Eating Disorder Diagnoses
QL	quality of life
QOLID	Quality of Life Instruments Database
RADS-2	Reynolds Adolescent Depression Scale–2nd Edition
RAGE	Rating Scale for Aggressive Behavior in the Elderly
RAM	rapid alternating movements
RAT	Risk Assessment Tool for Falls
RBG	random blood glucose
RBS	random blood sugar
RCDS	Reynolds Child Depression Scale
RDA	Recommended Dietary Allowance
RISK	Reassessment is Safe "Kare" Tool
RLCQ	Recent Life Changes Questionnaire
ROM	range of motion
ROS	review of systems
RPR	rapid plasma reagin (syphilis screening test)
RSQ-4	4-Item Risk of Suicide Questionnaire
RSV	respiratory syncytial virus
RV	retroverted
Rx	prescriptive
S/P	status post
SAILS	Structured Assessment of Independent Living Skills
SAS	Zung Self-Rating Anxiety Scale
SBE	self-breast examination
SCA	sickle cell anemia
SDS	Zung Self-Rating Depression Scale
SH	social history
SI	suicidal ideation
SIBS	Spiritual Involvement and Beliefs Scale
SIP	Sickness Impact Profile
SIQ	Suicidal Ideation Questionnaire
SMAC 7	blood chemistry panel
SOB	shortness of breath
SOI	Special Olympics International
SOPA	Survey of Pain Attitudes
SPE	Skill Performance Evaluation
SPS	Suicide Probability Scale
STD	sexually transmitted disease
SWBS	Spiritual Well-Being Scale
SWILS	Safety Word Inventory and Literacy Screener

Abbreviation	Definition
T	term
T&A	tonsillectomy & adenoidectomy
TB	tuberculosis
Td	tetanus, diphtheria
TG	triglycerides
TIA	transient ischemic attack
TIPP	The Injury Prevention Program
TM	tympanic membrane
TMJ	temporal mandibular joint
TNR	tonic neck reflex
TP	thin prep
TSE	testicular self-examination
TSF	triceps skinfold
TSH	thyroid-stimulating hormone
UA	urinalysis
UC	urine culture
UDI-6	Urogenital Distress Inventory

Abbreviation	Definition
UDS	Uniform Data System for Medical Rehabilitation
UE	upper extremity
URI	upper respiratory tract infection
US	ultrasound
USCIS	United States Citizenship and Immigration Services
USDA	U.S. Department of Agriculture
USPSTF	U.S. Preventive Services Task Force
UTI	urinary tract infection
VAS	Visual Analogue Scale
VBS	Verbal Descriptor Scale
VF	visual fields
VRE	vancomycin-resistant *Enterococci*
Y-BOCS	Yale-Brown Obsessive Compulsive Scale
ZBI	Zarit Burden Interview

Permissions for Use and Copyright Information

Reprinted in this text are many rating scales, questionnaires, and forms that are copyright protected, with ownership held by the author or distributor of the tool. The information listed in this appendix notes whether a tool is copyright protected or lies within public domain. If the tool is copyright protected, contact the source (as listed) and request permission to use the tool.

A work in the public domain may be freely reproduced, distributed, transmitted, used, modified, or otherwise exploited by anyone for any purpose, commercial or noncommercial. For more information on public domain definitions, please see http://www.unc.edu/~unclng/public-d.htm.

The reader is advised to use discretion as to when, where, and how the material will be used, and should there be any uncertainties, to contact the copyright holder for further use authorization or questions concerning use of the material.

Chapter 1

Printed and customizable forms:
  Comprehensive Adult History and Physical Form
  Adult History and Physical Form–Female
  Adult History and Physical Form–Male
  Adult History and Physical–Female Short Form
  Adult History and Physical–Male Short Form
  Well-Woman History and Physical Form
  Comprehensive Older Adult History and Physical Form
  Office Visit Form
  Medication History
The printed forms listed above are copyrighted by Elsevier. They are available for personal practice and individual educational use only and may not be distributed, reproduced for commercial purposes, sold, or altered without permission from Elsevier.

All customizable versions of the foregoing forms on CD-ROM are permitted to be altered and used by the reader for personal practice and individual educational use. The templates for the customizable forms are copyright protected and may not be distributed, reproduced for commercial purposes, or sold without permission from the publisher.

Chapter 2

Printed and customizable forms:
  Adult Health Profile
  Adult Health Care Maintenance Record
  Medication Log
  Medication Refill Log
  Injection Record
  Adult Vaccine and PPD Administration Record
  Pediatric Vaccine and PPD Administration Record
  Laboratory Results Log
  X-Ray and Special Procedure Results Log
  Coagulation Monitoring Log
  Blood Pressure Log
  Vital Signs Flow Sheet
  Diabetes Monitoring Log
  Asthma Monitoring Log
The printed forms listed above are copyrighted by Elsevier. They are available for personal practice and individual educational use only and may not be distributed, reproduced for commercial purposes, sold, or altered without permission from Elsevier.

All customizable versions of the foregoing forms on CD-ROM are permitted to be altered and used by the reader for personal practice and individual educational use. The templates for the customizable forms are copyright protected and may not be distributed, reproduced for commercial purposes, or sold without permission from the publisher.

Telephone Triage Call Record. From Wheeler S: Telephone triage: SAVED by the form, *Nursing 2000* 30:54-55, 2000.

Chapter 3

Printed and customizable forms:
  Pediatric Initial Health Questionnaire
  Pediatric History and Physical Forms: Ages 0-1
    month to 18-20 year well-visit forms
  With permission, adapted from:17 Child & Teen
    Checkups (C&TC) Provider Documentation Forms;
    with acknowledgements to Allina Health Systems/
    Medica Health Plans, Blue Cross and Blue Shield/
    Blue Plus of Minnesota, Children's Physician
    Network, HealthPartners, Hennepin County
    Community Health, Hennepin County Medical
    Center, Metropolitan Health Plan, Minnesota
    Department of Health, Minnesota Department of
    Human Services, UCare, University Affiliated
    Family Physicians, University of Minnesota, and
    many other individuals who contributed valuable
    feedback throughout the development process.
  Pediatric Well-Care Summaries: Newborn to 18 Years
  Periodic Blood Lead Screening Risk Questionnaire
  Tuberculosis Risk Questionnaire
  Adolescent Risk Monitoring Log

The printed forms listed above are copyrighted by Elsevier. They are available for personal practice and individual educational use only and may not be distributed, reproduced for commercial purposes, sold, or altered without permission from Elsevier.

All customizable form versions of the foregoing forms on CD-ROM are permitted to be altered and used by the reader for personal practice and individual educational use. The templates for the customizable forms are copyright protected and may not be distributed, reproduced for commercial purposes, or sold without permission from the publisher.

Screening Form for Early Follow-Up of Breastfed Infants. Copyright © Marianne Neifert, MD. Handout may be purchased from HealthONE Alliance Lactation Program, Denver, Colo; phone: 303-320-7081.

Breastfeeding Infant Triage Form. Copyright © Christine M. Betzold, NP, IBCLC, MSN. http://www.theBFclinic.com. This form may be used by the reader for clinical purposes, and not be sold or distributed without permission of the copyright holder.

Adolescent Questionnaire. Adapted, with permission, from Guidelines for Adolescent Preventive Services (GAPS). Younger Adolescent Questionnaire and Middle/Older Adolescent Questionnaire. Adapted from http://www.ama-assn.org/ama/pub/category/2280.html. Additional comprehensive forms designed by the American Medical Association (AMA) to support the implementation of the Guidelines for Adolescent Preventive Services (GAPS) are available at the previously mentioned URL and include younger adolescent, middle/older adolescent, and parent/guardian questionnaires in English and Spanish.

HEADSSS. From Goldenring JM, Cohen R: Getting into adolescents heads, *Contemp Pediatr* 5:75-90, 1988. Copyright © Thomson Medical Economics.
SAFETEENS. From Gilchrist VJ: Preventive health care for the adolescent, *Am Fam Physician* 43:869-78, 1991.

Chapter 4

Preparticipation Physical Evaluation
Preparticipation Physical Evaluation Clearance Form: Copyright © 1997 American Academy of Family Physicians, American Academy of Pediatrics, American Medical Society for Sports Medicine, American Orthopaedic Society for Sports Medicine, and American Osteopathic Academy of Sports Medicine. Release of the third edition of this monograph containing all revised preparticipation evaluation forms is scheduled for the later half of 2004.
Patient-Runner History Form. Adapted, with permission, from Kirby KAS, Valmassy RL: The runner-patient history: what to ask and why, *Journal of the American Podiatry Association* 73:39-43, 1983.
Sample Special Olympics Athlete Application for Participation Form. This form, courtesy of Massachusetts Special Olympics, is reprinted for informational purposes only. There is no national Special Olympics Athlete Application form for medical examination. Special Olympics authorizes individual state programs to implement athlete participation forms at their discretion. State contact information can be accessed online at http://www.specialolympics.org/ by clicking on "Find a Location."

Chapter 5

Mental Health Assessment Form. Adapted from Varcarolis EM: *Foundations of psychiatric mental health nursing,* ed 3, Philadelphia, 1998, WB Saunders.
Child Psychiatry Emergency Consultation Mental Status Examination Checklist. Modified from an unpublished working draft. Reprinted with permission from Brad Peterson, MD, Melvin Lewis, MD, and Robert King, MD. In Lewis M, editor: *Child and adolescent psychiatry: a comprehensive textbook,* ed 2, Baltimore, MD, 1996, Williams & Wilkins, pp. 440-457.
Substance Use History and Physical Examination. From Nordsey D, Smith N: *Protocol for medical assessment,* Hanover, NH, 1989, Project Cork Weekend Program. Available from http://www.projectcork.org.
Abuse Assessment Screen. From Soeken KL, McFarlane J, Parker B, et al: The abuse assessment screen: a clinical instrument to measure frequency, severity and perpetrator of abuse against women. In Campbell JC, editor: *Empowering survivors of abuse: health care for battered women and their children,* Thousand Oaks, Calif, 1998, Sage.

Spouse Abuse—Assessing Level of Violence in the Home Questionnaire. From Jezierski M: Abuse of women by male partners: basic knowledge for emergency nurses, *J Emerg Nurs* 20:361-368, 1994. The Emergency Nurses Association.

Use Your "RADAR"—Recognizing and Treating Partner Violence Screening Tool. Copyright © 1992, 1996, 1999 Massachusetts Medical Society.

BATHE Technique. From Lieberman JA III: BATHE: an approach to the interview process in the primary care setting, *J Clin Psychiatry* 58(suppl 3):3-6, 1997.

HOPE Questionnaire. From Anandarajah G, Hight E: Spirituality and medical practice: using the HOPE question as a practical tool for spiritual assessment, *Am Fam Physician* 63:81-89, 2001.

SPIRIT: A framework for spiritual assessment. From Maugans TA: The SPIRITual history, *Arch Fam Med* 5:11-16, 1996.

ETHNIC: A framework for culturally competent clinical practice. Developed by Steven Levin, MD, Robert Like, MD, MS, Jan Gottlieb, MPH. Department of Family Medicine, University of Medicine and Dentistry of New Jersey, Robert Wood Johnson Medical School, 1997.

Chapter 6

General Nutritional Assessment Forms:
- Level I Screen
- Level II Screen
- Determine Your Nutritional Health
- Medications Use Checklist

The Nutrition Screening Initiative, a project of the American Academy of Family Physicians, The American Dietetic Association, and the National Council on the Aging, Inc., and funded in part by a grant from Ross Products Division, Abbott Laboratories. No permission is needed; these forms are available for public use.

Food Intake Record. Copyright © 1998 American Dietetic Association. From American Dietetic Association: *Medical nutrition therapy across the continuum of care,* ed 2, Chicago, 1998, American Dietetic Association.

Nutrition History Form. From Hark L, Deen D: Taking a nutrition history: a practical approach for family physicians, *Am Fam Physician* 59:1521-1528, 1531-1532, 1999.

Initial Nutrition Assessment Form. Copyright © 1998 American Dietetic Association. From American Dietetic Association: *Medical nutrition therapy across the continuum of care,* ed 2, Chicago, 1998, American Dietetic Association.

General Food Frequency Questionnaire. From Mahan LK, Escott-Stump S: *Krause's food, nutrition, & diet therapy,* ed 11, Philadelphia, 2004, WB Saunders.

Food Diaries:
Food Diary
One-Day (24 Hour) Record of Food Intake

The foregoing food diaries may be used for personal and clinical practice.

Perinatal Nutrition Screening/Assessment Form. Northside Hospital, Atlanta, GA.

Eating Disorder Nutritional Assessment Form. From Mahan LK, Escott-Stump S: *Krause's food, nutrition, & diet therapy,* ed 11, Philadelphia, 2004, WB Saunders.

Herbal, Botanical and Dietary Supplement Intake Form. Copyright © 2000 American Dietetic Association. From *American Dietetic Association: Sports nutrition: a guide for the professional working with active people,* 2000, Chicago, IL:American Dietetic Association, 2000; and The American Dietetic Association. Special report from the Joint Working Group on Dietary Supplements, 2000.

Chapter 7

Printed and customizable forms:
    Pre-Operative Clearance Evaluation Form–Adult
    Pre-Operative Clearance Evaluation Form–Pediatric

The printed forms listed above are copyrighted by Elsevier. They are available for personal practice and individual educational use only and may not be distributed, reproduced for commercial purposes, sold, or altered without permission from Elsevier.

All customizable form versions of the foregoing forms on CD-ROM are permitted to be altered and used by the reader for personal practice and individual educational use. The templates for the customizable forms are copyright protected and may not be distributed, reproduced for commercial purposes, or sold without permission from the publisher.

Stepwise Approach to Preoperative Cardiac Assessment. From ACC/AHA Guidelines for the Perioperative Cardiovascular Evaluation for Noncardiac Surgery, *J Am Coll Cardiol* 27:910-948, 1996. Copyright © 2002 American College of Cardiology and the American Heart Association, Inc.

American Society of Anesthesiologists (ASA) Physical Status Classification System. From American Society of Anesthesiologists, 2003. American Society of Anesthesiologists, 520 North Northwest Highway, Park Ridge, IL 60068-2573.

Forms listed below for Chapter 7 are within the public domain.

Commercial Driver Fitness Evaluation–US Department of Transportation (DOT):
- Medical Examination Report for Commercial Driver Fitness Determination (649-F (6045))
- Medical Examiner's Certificate

Evaluation for Adjustment of Immigrant Status–US Department of Homeland Security (DHS): US Citizenship and Immigration Services (USCIS):
- Medical Examination of Aliens Seeking Adjustment of Status (I-693)

Chapter 8

Maturational Assessment of Gestational Age (New Ballard Score). From Ballard JL, Khoury JC, Wedig K, et al: New Ballard Score expanded to include extremely premature infant, *J Pediatr* 119:417, 1991.

Centers for Disease Control and Prevention 2000 Growth Charts for the United States. No permission is needed; these are in the public domain.

Growth Charts for Children with Down Syndrome. No permission needed; these are in the public domain.

Apgar Scoring System. Modified from Apgar V: A proposal for a new method of evaluation of the newborn infant, *Res Anesth Analg* 32:260-267, 1953.

Baby Check Scoring System. From London: The Foundation for the Study of Infants. Deaths. Reprinted with permission from Child Growth Foundation.
Morley CJ, Thornton AJ, Cole TJ, et al: Baby Check: a scoring system to grade the severity of acute systemic illness in babies under 6 months old, *Arch Dis Child* 66:100-105, 1991.

Injury Behavior Checklist. From Speltz ML, Gonzales N. Sulzbacher S, et al: Assessment of injury risk in children: a preliminary study of the Injury Behavior Checklist, *J Pediatr Psychol* 15:373-383, 1990. Oxford University Press.

Checklist for Autism in Toddlers (CHAT). From Baron-Cohen S, Allen J, Gillberg C: Can autism be detected at 18 months? The needle, the haystack, and the CHAT, *Brit J Psychiat* 161:839-843, 1992; and Baron-Cohen S, Cox A, Baird G, et al: Psychological markers of autism at 18 months of age in a large population, *Brit J Psychiat* 168:158-163, 1996.

Chapter 9

Global Assessment of Functioning Scale (GAF)/Global Assessment Scale (GAS). From the *Diagnostic and statistical manual of mental disorders,* ed 4, text revision, Washington, DC, 2000, American Psychiatric Association. Copyright © 2000 American Psychiatric Association. Permission to copy or reprint the GAF Scale should be obtained from the American Psychiatric Publishing, Inc., 1000 Wilson Blvd, Suite 1825, Arlington, VA 22209-3901; phone: 703-907-7322 or 800-368-5777.

POSIT: Problem Oriented Screening Instrument for Teenagers. From Rahdert E, editor: *The adolescent assessment/referral system manual,* Rockville, MD, 1991, National Institute on Drug Abuse. DHHS Pub. No (ADM) 91-1735. This form is available for public use.

Center for Epidemiologic Studies–Depression Scale (CES-D). From Radloff LS: The CES-D Scale: a self-report depression scale for research in the general population, *Appl Psychol Measure* 1:385-401, 1977.

Hamilton Rating Scale for Depression. From Hamilton M: A rating scale for depression, *J Neurol Neurosurg Psychiatry* 25:56-62, 1960.

Montgomery Åsberg Depression Rating Scale. From Montgomery S, Åsberg M: A new depression scale designed to be sensitive to change, *Br J Psychiatry* 134:382-389, 1979.

Primary Care Evaluation of Mental Disorders: Patient Health Questionnaire 9-Item Depression Module (PRIME-MD PHQ-9). Developed by Drs. Robert L. Spitzer, Janet B. W. Williams, and Kurt Kroenke with an educational grant from Pfizer, Inc. For research information, contact Dr. Spitzer at rls8@columbia.edu. The names PRIME-MD® and PRIME-MD TODAY® are trademarks of Pfizer, Inc.

Zung's Self-Rating Depression Scale. From Zung WK: A self-rating depression scale, *Arch Gen Psychiatry* 12:63-70, 1965. Copyright © 1965 American Medical Association.

Edinburgh Postnatal Depression Scale. From Cox JL, Holden JM, Sagovsky R: Detection of postnatal depression: development of the 10-item Edinburgh Postnatal Depression Scale, *Br J Psychiatry* 150: 782-786, 1987. Copyright © 1987 Royal College of Psychiatrists.

Geriatric Depression Scale. From Yesavage JA, Brink TL, Rose TL, et al: Development and validation of a geriatric depression screening scale: a preliminary paper, *J Psychiatr Res* 17:37-49, 1983. Copyright © 1983 Elsevier Science. The original scale is in the public domain, being partly the result of Federal support.

Cornell Scale for Depression in Dementia. From Alexopoulos GS, Agrams RC, Young RC, et al: Cornell Scale for Depression Dementia, *Biol Psychiatry* 23:271-284, 1988. Copyright © 1988 Society of Biological Psychiatry.

Hamilton Anxiety Rating Scale. From Hamilton M: The assessment of anxiety states by rating, *Br J Med Psychol* 32:50-55, 1959. Copyright © 1959 British Psychological Society.

Zung Anxiety Scale. From Zung WWK: A rating instrument for anxiety disorders, *Psychosomatics* 12:371-379, 1971. Copyright © 1971 American Psychiatric Association.

Yale-Brown Obsessive Compulsive Scale (Y-BOCS). From Goodman WK, Price LH, Rasmussen SA, et al: The Yale-Brown Obsessive Compulsive Scale. I. Development, use, and reliability, *Arch Gen Psychiatry* 46:1006-1011, 1989. Copyright © 1989 American Medical Association.

Florida Obsessive Compulsive Inventory. Copyright © Wayne K. Goodman, MD, 1994. Permission is required to use this screening tool in clinical practice and may be obtained by contacting Wayne K. Goodman, MD, care of Beverly Hollingsworth, University of Florida, College of Medicine, Department of Psychiatry, PO Box 100256,

Gainesville, FL 32610-0256; phone: 352-392-3681; fax: 352-392-9887.

Liebowitz Social Anxiety Scale. From Liebowitz MR: Social phobia, *Mod Probl Pharmacopsychiatry* 22: 141-173, 1987. Reprinted with permission from S Karger A.G.

Recent Life Changes Questionnaire. From Miller RA, Rahe RH: Life changes scaling for the 1990's, *J Psychosom Res* 43:279-292, 1997. Richard H. Rahe, MD, President, Health Assessment Programs Inc., 5209 Boulevard Extension Rd, SE, Olympia, WA 98501; Web site: http://www.DrRichardRahe.com. Reprinted by permission from the author, Richard H. Rahe, M.D.

Life-Changing Event Questionnaire. Adapted from Rahe R: Psychosocial stressors and adjustment disorder: Van Gogh's life chart illustrates stress and disease, *J Clin Psychiatry* 51(suppl 1):15, 1990. Physicians Postgraduate Press.

Overt Aggression Scale–Modified. Copyright © 1991 Emil Coccaro, MD.

Rating Scale for Aggressive Behavior in the Elderly (RAGE). From Patel V, Hope RA: A rating scale for aggressive behavior in the elderly—the RAGE, *Psychol Med* 22:211-221, 1992. Cambridge University Press.

HITS Screening Tool. From Sherin KM, Sinacore JM, Li XQ, et al: HITS: a short domestic violence screening tool for use in a family practice setting, *Fam Med* 30:508-512, 1998. The Society of Teachers of Family Medicine; Web site: http://www.stfm.org

Modified SAD Persons Scale. From Hockberger RS, Rothstein RJ: Assessment of suicide potential by nonpsychiatrists using the SAD PERSONS Score, *J Emerg Med* 6:99-107, 1988.

4-Item Risk of Suicide Questionnaire (RSQ-4). From Horowitz LM, Wang PS, Koocher GP, et al: Detecting suicide risk in a pediatric emergency department: development of a brief screening tool, *Pediatrics* 107:1133-1137, 2001.

CAGE Questionnaire. From Ewing JA: Detecting alcoholism: the CAGE questionnaire, *JAMA* 252:1905-1907, 1984. Copyright © 1984 American Medical Association. Researchers and clinicians who are publishing studies using the CAGE Questionnaire should cite the above reference. No other permission is necessary unless used in a profit-making endeavor.

T-ACE Questionnaire. From Sokol RJ, Martier SS, Ager JW: The T-ACE questions: practical prenatal detection of risk drinking, *Am J Obstet Gynecol* 160:863-868, 1989.

Michigan Alcoholism Screening Test (MAST). From Selzer ML: The Michigan Alcoholism Screening Test: the quest for a new diagnostic instrument, *Am J Psychiatry* 127:1653-1658, 1971. No permission is needed; this is in the public domain.

Alcohol Use Disorders Identification Test (AUDIT). From Babor TF, de la Fuente JR, Saunders J, et al:

AUDIT—The Alcohol Use Identification Test: guidelines for use in primary health care, Geneva, 1992, World Health Organization. The AUDIT questionnaire is copyrighted but may be reproduced without permission.

Drug Abuse Screening Test (DAST). From Skinner HA: *Drug Abuse Screening Test (DAST), Addict Behav* 7:363-371, 1982, Elsevier Science. Copyright © 1982 Elsevier Science.

CRAFFT Questionnaire. From Knight JR, Shrier LA, Bravender TD, et al: A new brief screening for adolescent substance abuse, *Arch Pediatr Adolesc Med* 153:591-596, 1999. Copyright © 1999 American Medical Association. The CRAFFT may be used clinically without permission.

SCOFF Questionnaire. From Morgan JF, Reid F, Lacey H: The SCOFF Questionnaire: assessment of a new screening tool for eating disorders, *BMJ* 319:1467-1468, 1999.

Eating Disorder Screen for Primary Care. From Cotton M, Ball C, Robinson P: Four simple questions can help screen for eating disorders, *J Gen Intern Med* 18:53-56, 2003.

Eating Attitudes Test (EAT-26). From Garner DM, Olmsted MP, Bohr Y, et al: The eating attitudes test: psychometric features and clinical correlates, *Psychol Med* 12:871-878, 1982. Cambridge University Press.

Chapter 10

Instrumental Activities of Daily Living Scale. From Lawton MP, Brody E: Assessment of older people: self-maintaining and instrumental activities of daily living, *Gerontologist* 9:179-186, 1969.

Structured Assessment of Independent Living Skills (SAILS). From Mahurin RK, DeBettignies BH, Pirozzolo FJ: Structured assessment of independent living skills: preliminary report of a performance measure of functional abilities in dementia, *J Gerontol* 46:58-66, 1991.

Five Instrumental Activities of Daily Living Items. Adapted from the Older American Resources and Services (OARS) multidimensional functional assessment questionnaire. From Fillenbaum GG: Screening the elderly: a brief instrumental activities of daily living measure, *J Am Geriatr Soc* 33:698-706, 1985. Blackwell Publishing, Ltd.

Hearing Handicap Inventory for the Elderly—Screening Version (HHIE-S). From Ventry IM, Weinstein BE: Identification of elderly people with hearing problems, *ASHA* 25:37-42, 1983. Copyright © American-Speech-Language-Hearing Association. Reprinted with permission of copyright holder; author permission waived.

Tinetti Balance and Gait Assessment Tool. From Tinetti ME: Performance-oriented assessment of mobility problems in elderly patients, *J Am Geriatr Soc* 34: 119-126, 1986. Blackwell Publishing, Ltd.

"Get Up and Go" Test. From Mathias S, Nayok U, Isaacs B: Balance in elderly patients: the "Get Up and Go" test, *Arch Phys Med Rehabil* 67:387-389, 1986.

Timed "Up and Go" Test. From Podsiadlo D, Richardson S: The timed "Up and Go": a test of basic functional mobility for frail, elderly persons, *J Am Geriatr Soc* 39:142-148, 1991. Blackwell Publishing, Ltd.

Risk Assessment Tool (RAT) for Falls. From Brians LK, Alexand K, Grota P, et al: The development of the RISK tool for fall prevention, *Rehabil Nurs* 16:67-69, 1991. Reprinted from *Rehabilitation Nursing*, with permission of the Association of Rehabilitation Nurses, 4700 West Lake Avenue, Glenview, IL, 60025-1485. Copyright © 1997.

Reassessment is Safe "KARE" (RISK) Tool. From Brians LK, Alexand K, Grota P, et al: The development of the RISK tool for fall prevention, *Rehabil Nurs* 16:67-69, 1991. Reprinted from *Rehabilitation Nursing*, with permission of the Association of Rehabilitation Nurses, 4700 West Lake Avenue, Glenview, IL 60024-1485. Copyright © 1997.

Guidelines for Home Safety Assessment. From Stanhope M, Knollmueler RN: *Handbook of community-based and home health nursing practice: tools for assessment, intervention, and education,* ed 3, St Louis, 2000, Mosby. Modified from Yoshikawa TT, Cobbs EL, Brummel-Smith K: *Practical ambulatory geriatrics,* St Louis, 1998, Mosby.

Environmental Assessment for the Elderly. From Kane R, Ouslander J, Abrass I: *Essentials of clinical geriatrics,* ed 3, New York, 1994, McGraw-Hill.

Driving Skills Quiz. From Mayo Foundation for Medical Education and Research: Driving: How safe are you behind the wheel? *Mayo Clin Health Lett* 14(4):7, 1996. Based in part on materials developed by the American Association of Retired Persons (AARP); visit http://www.aarp.org/drive for more information.

Brief Abuse Screen for the Elderly (BASE). From Reis M, Nahmiash D: *When seniors are abused: a guide to intervention,* Concord, Ontario, Canada, 1995, Captus Press. Reprinted with permission of Captus Press, Inc., Units 14 and 15, 1600 Steeles Ave, West, Concord, Ontario, Canada L4K 4M4; E-mail: info@captus.com; Web site: http://www.captus.com

Caregiver Abuse Screen (CASE). From Reis M, Nahmiash D: *When seniors are abused: a guide to intervention,* Concord, Ontario, Canada, 1995, Captus Press, Inc., Units 14 and 15, 1600 Steeles Ave, Concord, Ontario, Canada L4K 4M5; E-mail: info@captus.com; Web site: http://www.captus.com

Blessed Dementia Rating Scale. From Blessed G, Tomlinson BF, Roth M: The association between quantitative measures of dementia and senile change in the cerebral gray matter of elderly subjects, *Br J Psychiatry* 114:797-811, 1968.

FROMAJE Mental Status Guide. From Libow LS: A rapidly administered, easily remembered mental status evaluation: FROMAJE. In Libow LS, Sherman FT, editors: *The core of geriatric medicine,* St Louis, 1980, Mosby.

SET Test. From Isaacs B, Kennie AT: The Set Test: an aid to the detection of dementia in old people, *Br J Psychiatry* 123:467-470, 1973.

Clock Drawing Task and Interpretation Scale. From Sunderland T, Hill JL, Mellow AM, et al: Clock drawing in Alzheimer's disease: a novel measure of dementia severity, *J Am Geriatr Soc* 37:725-729, 1989. Blackwell Publications, Ltd.

Six-Item Cognitive Impairment Test. From Brooke P, Bullock R: Validation of the 6-item cognitive impairment test with a view to primary care, *Int J Geriatr Psychiatry* 14:936-940, 1999. Copyright © 1999 John Wiley and Sons Limited. Copyright for the revised 6-Item Cognitive Impairment Test (6CIT) is held by Kingshill (Version 2000©). For information on this tool and access to this version, please visit http://www.kingshill-research.org/kresearch/6cit.ASP.

Hachinski Ischemic Score for Multi-Infarct Dementia. From Hachinski VC, Iliff LD, Silhka E, et al: Cerebral blood flow in dementia, *Arch Neurol* 32:632-637, 1975.

Chapter 11

Spitzer Quality of Life. From Spitzer WO, Dobson AJ, Hall J, et al: Measuring the quality of life of cancer patients: a concise QL-index for use by physicians, *J Chronic Dis* 34:585-597, 1981.

COOP Functional Assessment Charts. Copyright © Trustees of Dartmouth College/COOP Project 2003, Dartmouth Medical School, Butler Building, HB 7265, Hanover, NH 03755; phone: 603-650-1220; fax: 603-650-1331. The charts are available and permissible for personal use at http://www.dartmouth.edu/~coopproj/figure1.html.

Duke Health Profile. From Parkerson GR, Broadhead WE, Tse C-KJ: The Duke Health Profile: a 17-item measure of health and dysfunction, *Med Care* 28:1056-1072, 1990. The developers of the Duke Health Profile encourage its use by others. The measure is copyrighted; however, permission to use it for clinical and research purposes is granted upon request, usually without charge. For further information, contact the Department of Community and Family Medicine, Duke University Medical Center, Durham, NC 27710; phone: 919-681-3043; E-mail: parke001@mc.duke.edu.

Arthritis Impact Measurement Scales 2 (AIMS2). From Meenan RF, Mason JH, Anderson JJ, et al: AIMS2: the content and properties of a revised and expanded Arthritis Impact Measurement Scales health status questionnaire, *Arthritis Rheum* 35:1-10, 1992. See http://www.qolid.org/public/aims/cadre/guide.pdf and uplink for copyright and usage information.

Arthritis Impact Measurement Scales 2–Short Form (AIMS2-SF). From Guillemin F, Coste J, Pouchot J, et al: The AIMS2-SF: a short form of the Arthritis Impact Measurement Scales 2, French Quality of Life in Rheumatology Group, *Arthritis Rheum* 40:1267-1274, 1997. See http://www.qolid.org/public/aims/cadre/guide.pdf and uplink for copyright and usage information.

Barthel Index. From Mahoney R, Barthel D: Functional evaluation: The Barthel Index. *Maryland State Medical Journal* 14:61-5, 1965. Copyright © Maryland State Medical Society. The Barthel Index may be used freely for noncommercial purposes with citation by Mahoney and Barthel (1965). Permission is required to modify the Barthel Index or use it for commercial purposes.

Katz Index of Daily Living Activities. From Katz S, Downs TD, Cash HR, et al: Progress in the development of the Index of ADL, *Gerontologist* 10:20-30, 1970.

Katz Index of Independence in Activities of Daily Living: Scoring and Definitions. From Katz S, Downs TD, Cash HR, et al: Progress in development of the Index of ADL, *Gerontologist* 10:20-30, 1970.

Functional Status Index. From Jette AM.: Functional capacity evaluation: an empirical approach. *Arch Phys Med Rehabil* 61(2):85-89, 1980. No permission is needed; this is in the public domain.

FIM™ Instrument. Copyright © 1997 Uniform Data System for Medical Rehabilitations (UDSMR), a division of UB Foundation Activities, Inc. (UBFA). Reprinted with permission of UDSMR. All marks associated with FIM and UDSMR are owned by UBFA. For further information on the FIM(™), please contact Uniform Data System for Medical Rehabilitation, 232 Parker Hall, University at Buffalo, 3435 Main St, Buffalo, NY 14214-3007; phone: 716-829-2076; fax: 716-829-2080; E-mail: fimnet@ubvms.cc.buffalo.edu or info@udsmr.org; Web site: http://www.udsmr.org.

Pain Disability Index. From Pollard CA: Preliminary validity of the Pain Disability Index, *Percept Mot Skills* 59:974, 1984. Copyright © Perceptual and Motor Skills.

Chapter 12

Wong/Baker Faces Rating Scale. From Wong DL, Hockenberry-Eaton M, Wilson D, et al: *Wong's essentials of pediatric nursing*, ed 6, St Louis, 2001, Mosby. Copyright © Mosby, Inc. Permissions for use form may be found online at http://www3.us.elsevierhealth.com/WOW/facesPermission.html.

Oucher Scale (African-American). The African-American version of the Oucher Scale was developed and copyrighted in 1990 by Mary J. Denyes, PhD, RN, Wayne State University, and Antonio M. Villarruel, PhD, RN, University of Michigan. Cornelia P. Porter, PhD, RN, and Charlotta Marshall, MSN, RN, contributed to the development of this scale.

Oucher Scale (Caucasian). The Caucasian version of the Oucher Scale was developed and copyrighted in 1983 by Judith E. Beyer, PhD, RN, currently at the University of Missouri–Kansas City School of Nursing.

Oucher Scale (Hispanic). The Hispanic version of the Oucher Scale was developed and copyrighted in 1990 by Antonio M. Villarruel, PhD, RN, University of Michigan, and Mary J. Denyes, PhD, RN, Wayne State University.

The Faces Pain Scale—Revised. From Hicks CL, von Baeyer CL, Spafford van Korlaar I, et al: The Faces Pain Scale—Revised: toward a common metric in pediatric pain measurement, *Pain* 93:173-183, 2001. Scale adapted from Bieri D, Reeve R, Champion GD, et al: The Faces Pain Scale for the self-assessment of the severity of pain experienced by children: development, initial validation and preliminary investigation for ration scale properties, *Pain* 41:139-150, 1990. The International Association for the Study of Pain.

McGill Pain Questionnaire–Long Form. From Melzack R: The McGill Pain Questionnaire: major properties and scoring methods, *Pain* 1:277-299, 1975.

McGill Pain Questionnaire–Short Form. From Melzack R: The short form McGill Pain Questionnaire, *Pain* 30:191-197, 1987.

Brief Pain Inventory. Copyright © 1991 Charles S. Cleeland, PhD, Pain Research Group. Used by permission. Permission to use the short and long versions of this tool must be obtained from the author with agreement to not alter its format; permission is granted free of charge at http://www.mdanderson.org/departments/prg/ by clicking on "Symptom Assessment Tools," following links to "The Brief Pain Inventory (BPI)," then on "Permission Form."

CHEOPS. From McGrath PJ, Johnson G, Goodman JT, et al: The CHEOPS: a behavioral scale to measure postoperative pain in children. Chapman J, Fields HL, Dubner R, et al, editors: *Advances in pain research and therapy*, vol. 9, New York, 1985, Raven Press.

NIPS. From Lawrence J, Alcock D, McGrath P, et al: The development of a tool to assess neonatal pain, *Neonatal Netw* 12:59-65, 1993.

Body Outline Tool. Copyright © 2004 Elsevier. No permission is needed for personal use.

Geriatric Pain Assessment Form. From Stein WM, Ferrell BA: Pain in the nursing home, *Clin Geriatr Med* 12:601-613, 1996.

Chapter 13

National Pressure Ulcer Advisory Panel (NPUAP) Staging System for Pressure Ulcerations. From Agency for Health Care Policy and Research. Panel for the Prediction and Prevention of Pressure Ulcers in

Adults: *Pressure ulcers in adults: prediction and prevention*, Rockville, Md, 1992, AHCP Research, Public Health Service, U.S. Department of Health and Human Services. Clinical practice guideline, Number 3. AHCPR Publication No. 92-0047. No permission is needed; this is in the public domain.

Wagner Wound Classification. From Wagner FW Jr: A dysvascular foot: a system for diagnosis and treatment, *Foot Ankle* 2:64-122, 1981.

University of Texas Health Science Center, San Antonio, Diabetic Wound Classification System. From Lavery LA, Armstrong DG, Harkless LB, Copyright 1996 by the American College of Foot and Ankle Surgeons, originally published in the *Journal of Foot and Ankle Surgery*, November/December, 1996, Volume 35, Number 6, pages 528-531, and reproduced here with permission.

Norton Pressure Ulcer Prediction Scale. From Norton D, McLaren R, Exton-Smith AN: *An investigation of geriatric nursing problems in hospital*, London, England, 1962, National Corporation for the Care of Old People. Copyright © National Corporation for the Care of Old People (now Centre for Policy on Ageing), London, England.

Braden Scale for Predicting Pressure Sore Risk. Copyright © 1988 Barbara Braden and Nancy Bergstrom. Permission for use may be granted at no charge to professionals who agree not to resell it or to profit from its use. Permission is readily given to those using the tool in research, scholarly publications, or programs of prevention in clinical agencies. For more information and permission for use, see http://www.bradenscale.com.

Chapter 14

Tools listed below for Chapter 14 are within the public domain and are available for use without permission.

Body-Mass Index
USDA Food Guide Pyramid
Food Guide Pyramid for Young Children

Height and Weight Assessment. Copyright © 1996, 1999 Metropolitan Life Insurance Company. All rights reserved.

Mini Nutritional Assessment MNA®. Copyright © Nestle, 1994, Revision 1998, Societe des Produits Nestle S.A.

Willett's Healthy Eating Pyramid. From Willett WC: *Eat, drink, and be healthy*, New York, 2001, Simon & Schuster Adult Publishing Group. Copyright © 2001 President and Fellows of Harvard College.

Food Guide Pyramid for Vegetarian Meal Planning. From Position of the American Dietetic Association: Messina VK, Burke KI: Position of the American Dietetic Association: vegetarian diets, *J Am Diet Assoc* 97:1317-21, 1997. Copyright © 1997 American Dietetic Association.

Chapter 15

Tools listed below for Chapter 15 are within the public domain and are available for use without permission.

New York Heart Association (NYHA) Classification for Congestive Heart Failure (CHF)
Rosenbaum Chart
Amsler Grid
Self-Assessment Hearing Test
Constipation Assessment Scale

American College of Cardiology (ACC/AHA) 2001 Guidelines: Stages of Heart Failure. Copyright © 2002 American College of Cardiology and American Heart Association, Inc.

FACES Screening Tool for Heart Failure. Adapted from the Heart Failure Society of America. http://www.abouthf.org/hf_awareness_materials.htm.

Revised Cardiac Risk Index. Adapted from Lee TH, Marcantonio ER, Mangione CM, Thomas EJ, et al: Derivation and prospective validation of a simple index for prediction of cardiac risk of major noncardiac surgery, *Circulation* 100:1043-1049, 1999.

Burke Dysphagia Screening Test. From DePippo KL, Holas MA, Reding MJ: The Burke dysphagia screening test: validation of its use in patient with stroke, *Arch Phys Med Rehabil* 75:1284-1286, 1994. The American Congress of Rehabilitation Medicine and the American Academy of Physical Medicine and Rehabilitation.

Epworth Sleepiness Scale. Adapted from Johns MW: A new method for measuring daytime sleepiness: The Epworth Sleepiness Scale, *Sleep* 14:540-545, 1991.

Glascow Coma Scale. From Teasdale G, Jennett B: Assessment of coma and impaired consciousness. A practical scale. *Lancet* 2(7872):81-84, 1974.

Modified Glascow Coma Scale. From Reilly PL, Simpson DA, Sprod R, et al: Assessing the conscious level in infants and young children: a paediatric version of the Glascow Coma Scale, *Childs Nerv Syst* 4:30-33, 1988.

Headache Diary. Copyright © 2004 Elsevier. No permission is needed for personal use.

Berg Balance Scale. From Berg K, Wood-Dauphinee S, Williams JL, et al: Measuring balance in the elderly: preliminary development of an instrument, *Physiotherapy Canada* 41:304-331, 1989.

Abnormal Involuntary Movement Scale. From Guy W: *ECDEU assessment manual for psychopharmacology*, rev. ed., Washington, DC, 1976, U.S. Department of Health, Education, and Welfare. Modified by Munetz MR, Benjamin S: How to examine patients using the Abnormal Involuntary Movement Scale, *Hosp Commun Psychiatry* 39:1172-1177, 1988.

Rhodes Index of Nausea, Vomiting, and Retching. Copyright © 1996. Curators of Missouri, Verna A. Rhodes, RN, EdS, FAAN.

Androgen Deficiency in Aging Males (ADAM) Questionnaire. From Morley JE, Perry HM: Androgen deficiency in aging men, *Med Clin North Am* 83:1279-1289, 1999.

Brief Male Sexual Function Inventory for Urology. From O'Leary MP, Fowler FJ, Lenderking WR, et al: A brief male sexual function inventory for urology, *Urology* 46:697-706, 1995.

Incontinence Impact Questionnaire (IIQ-7) and Urogenital Distress Syndrome (UDI-6). From Shumaker SA, Wyman JF, Uebersax JS, et al: Health-related quality-of-life measures for women with urinary incontinence, *Qual Life Res* 3:291-306, 1994.

Chapter 16

Family APGAR. From Smilkstein G: The Family APGAR: a proposal for a family function test and its use by physicians, *J Fam Pract* 6:1231-1239, 1978. Dowden Health Media.

Zarit Burden Interview. From Zarit SH, Reever KE, Bach-Peterson J. Relatives of the impaired elderly: correlates of feelings of burden. *Gerontologist* 20:649-655, 1980. Copyright © Steven Zarit.

Support for Caregiver Questionnaire. From George LK, Gwyther LP: Duke University Caregiver Well-Being Survey, Durham, NC, 1983, Duke University Center for the Study of Aging and Human Development; George LK, Gwyther LP. Caregiver well-being: a multidimensional examination of family caregivers of demented adults, *Gerontologist* 26:253-259, 1986.

Duke-UNC Functional Social Support Questionnaire. From Broadhead WE, Gehlbach SH, deGruv FV, et al: The Duke-UNC functional support questionnaire: measurement of social support in family medicine patients, *Med Care* 26:722-723, 1988.

Lubben Social Network Scale. From Lubben JE: Assessing social networks among elderly populations, *Fam Comm Health* 11:42-45, 1988.

UCLA Loneliness Scale. From Russell DW: UCLA Loneliness Scale (Version 3): reliability, validity, and factor structure, *J Pers Assess* 66:20-40, 1996.

JAREL Spiritual Well-Being Scale. From Hungelmann J, Kenkel-Rossi E, Klassen L, et al: Focus on spiritual well-being: harmonious interconnectedness of mind-body-spirit, Use of the JAREL spiritual well-being scale, *Geriatr Nurs* 17:262-266, 1996. Copyright © Marquette University College of Nursing, Milwaukee, Wisconsin.

Survey of Pain Attitudes (SOPA-35). From Jensen MP, Turner JA, Romano JM: Pain belief assessment: a comparison of the short and long versions of the survey of pain attitudes, *J Pain* 1:138-150, 2000. Copyright © American Pain Society.

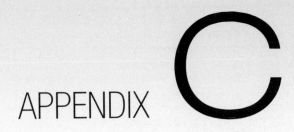

CD-ROM Table of Contents

Italicized forms also have a customizable version.

Substance Use History and Physical Examination Form
Abuse Assessment Screen
Partner Violence Screen
Spouse Abuse: Assessing Level of Violence in the Home
SAFE Technique
RADAR Screening Tool
SIG E CAPS
SALSA
BATHE
HOPE
SPIRIT
ETHNIC

6 Nutrition Forms

Level I Screen
Level II Screen
Determine Your Nutritional Health
Medications Use Checklist
Nutrition History
General Food Frequency Questionnaire
Food Intake Record
Nutrition History Form (ADA)
Initial Nutrition Assessment
Food Diary
A One-Day (24 Hour) Record of Food Intake
Perinatal Nutrition Screening/Assessment Form
Eating Disorder Nutritional Assessment Form
Herbal, Botanical, and Dietary Supplement Intake Form

7 Specialized Forms

Stepwise Approach to Preoperative Cardiac Assessments
American Society of Anesthesiologists Physical Status Classification System
Preoperative Clearance Evaluation Form: Adult
Preoperative Clearance Evaluation Form: Pediatric
Medical Examination Report for Commercial Driver Fitness Determination (649-F [6045])
Physical Qualifications for Drivers (49 CFR 391.41)
Instructions to the Medical Examiner: Federal Motor Carrier Safety Regulations-Advisory Criteria
Medical Examiner's Certificate (650-FS-L2 [6046])
Medical Examination of Aliens Seeking Adjustment of Status (I-693)
Medical Clearance Requirements for Aliens Seeking Adjustment of Status

8 Developmental and Pediatric Tools

Maturational Assessment of Gestational Age (New Ballard Score)
Centers for Disease Control and Prevention 2000 Growth Charts for the United States
    Boys 0-36 Months: Length for Age/Weight for Age
    Boys 0-36 Months: Head Circumference for Age/Weight for Length

Girls 0-36 Months: Length for Age/Weight for Age
    Girls 0-36 Months: Head Circumference for Age/Weight for Length
    Boys 2-20 Years: Stature for Age/Weight for Age
    Boys 2-20 Years: Body Mass Index for Age
    Boys 2-20 Years: Weight for Stature
    Girls 2-20 Years: Stature for Age/Weight for Age
    Girls 2-20 Years: Body Mass Index for Age
    Girls 2-20 Years: Weight for Stature
Growth Charts for Children with Down Syndrome
    Weight: Birth-3 Years, Girls
    Weight: 2-18 Years, Girls
    Weight: Birth-3 Years, Boys
    Weight: 2-18 Years, Boys
    Length: Birth-3 Years, Girls
    Height: 2-18 Years, Girls
    Length: Birth-3 Years, Boys
    Height: 2-18 Years, Boys
    Head Circumference: Birth-3 Years, Girls
    Head Circumference: Birth-3 Years, Boys
Tanner Stages of Development
Apgar Newborn Scoring System
Baby Check Scoring System
The Injury Behavior Checklist
CHAT (Checklist for Autism in Toddlers)

9 Behavioral and Psychiatric Instruments

Problem Oriented Screening Instrument for Teenagers (POSIT)
Hamilton Rating Scale for Depression (HRSD)
Montgomery Åsberg Depression Rating Scale (MADRS)
Primary Care Evaluation of Mental Disorders: Patient Health Questionnaire 9-Item Depression Module (PRIME-MD PHQ-9)
Geriatric Depression Scale (GDS)
Cornell Scale for Depression in Dementia (CSDD)
Hamilton Anxiety Rating Scale (HARS)
Zung Self-Rating Anxiety Scale (SAS)
Yale-Brown Obsessive Compulsive Scale (Y-BOCS)
Y-BOCS Symptom Checklist
Florida Obsessive-Compulsive Inventory (FOCI)
Liebowitz Social Anxiety Scale (LSAS)
Recent Life Changes Questionnaire (RLCQ)
Rating Scale for Aggressive Behavior in the Elderly (RAGE)
HITS-Safety Questionnaire
Modified SAD PERSONS Scale
4-Item Risk of Suicide Questionnaire (RSQ-4)
T-ACE Questionaire
Michigan Alcoholism Screening Test (MAST)
Alcohol Use Disorders Identification Test (AUDIT)
Drug Abuse Screening Test (DAST)
SCOFF Questionnaire
Eating Disorder Screen for Primary Care (ESP)
Eating Attitudes Test (EAT-26)

Index